Medical Terminology
An Illustrated Guide

body Fluoride mito

pulmonic

ation

ous body dend

jaundice

oma ossicle

limbic system

RON-ik endos

hypoba

rtex

Medical
Terminology
An Illustrated Guide

Fourth Edition

Barbara Janson Cohen, MEd

Associate Professor

Delaware County Community College

Media, Pennsylvania

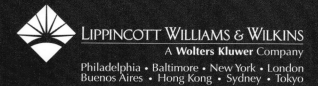

LIPPINCOTT WILLIAMS & WILKINS

A **Wolters Kluwer** Company

Philadelphia • Baltimore • New York • London
Buenos Aires • Hong Kong • Sydney • Tokyo

Senior Acquisitions Editor: John Goucher
Development Editor: Rose G. Foltz
Managing Editor: Karen Gulliver
Senior Project Editor: Karen Ruppert
Senior Marketing Manager: Aimee Sirmon
Designer: Doug Smock
Compositor: Circle Graphics
Printer: Donnelley

Library of Congress Cataloging-in-Publication Data

Cohen, Barbara J.
    Medical terminology : an illustrated guide / Barbara Janson Cohen.—4th ed.
        p. cm.
    Includes index.
    ISBN 0-7817-3688-9
    1. Medicine—Terminology. I. Title

    R123.C56 2004
    610'.1'4—dc21

                                                                    2003044697

05 06 07 08
3 4 5 6 7 8 9 10

Preface

Every career in health care begins with learning the vast and challenging language of medical terminology. Without adequate learning and teaching resources, it can be an overwhelming challenge for students and faculty. This new edition of *Medical Terminology: An Illustrated Guide* meets that challenge with a clear organizational scheme, full-color illustrations with a strong clinical focus, a wide array of effective pedagogical features, a variety of activities, and useful ancillaries to make teaching and learning more effective. Because the content is so accessible and logically organized, the text can be used as part of classroom instruction, for independent study, or for distance learning.

Organization and Approach

Medical Terminology: An Illustrated Guide takes a stepwise approach to learning the language of medical terminology. Part 1 describes how medical terms are built, and Part 2 introduces body structure, disease, and treatment. These chapters should be studied before proceeding to Part 3, which describes each of the body systems. Individual chapters also build on knowledge in stages, with Key Terms sections listing those terms most commonly used and specialized terms included in a later section entitled Supplementary Terms. The latter terms may be studied according to time available and student needs.

Each chapter opens with a chapter outline and a list of student objectives—goals to be accomplished by the completion of the chapter. In Part 3, the chapters begin with an overview of the normal structure and function of the system under study, followed by a list of key terms with definitions (the roots used in the accompanying chapter exercises are included in these definitions). Word parts related to each topic are then presented and illustrated, along with exercises on the new material. Next, there is an overview of clinical information pertaining to the system, also followed by a list of key terms with definitions. Many chapters contain displays that unify and simplify material on specific topics.

New to this edition is information on complementary and alternative medicine and special interest boxes with information on word derivations and usage.

Learning Resources

Features of *Medical Terminology: An Illustrated Guide* were designed to bring the content alive and to aid in student understanding and retention (also see the User's Guide).

- **Illustrations**—Detailed, full-color anatomical drawings and photographs illuminate the text. Approximately 100 new drawings were added to this edition.
- **Case Studies**—Case studies that present terminology in the context of a medical report are included in all chapters, followed by related questions (answers at the ends of the chapters). Professionals in a variety of health professions figure in these scenarios to represent the diverse work settings students may encounter. Because they may include information learned in a previous chapter, the case studies also serve as an excellent mode of review.
- **Pronunciations**—The text places great emphasis on pronunciation, and phonetic pronunciations are included with all new terms. It is important to practice saying these words and to be able to recognize them when they are heard.
- **Exercises**—Exercises accompany the introduction of all material, and review exercises conclude each chapter. Many of the illustrations have corresponding labeling exercises that include alphabetical word lists to aid in the labeling. Students are actively involved in the learning process, answering questions on new material, checking answers with nearby answer keys, correcting mistakes, and keeping track of progress with review exercises.
- **Glossaries of Word Parts**—In working through the exercises, students can refer to complementary lists at the end of the text. Appendix 3 lists word parts and their meanings, and Appendix 4 lists meanings with corresponding word parts.
- **Crossword Puzzles**—To exercise the student's newfound knowledge, each chapter on the body systems includes a crossword puzzle. Answers to these puzzles are found at the end of the chapter.
- **Flashcards**—Because flashcards offer an excellent way to learn this new vocabulary, a flashcard section is included at the back of the text. Flashcard content is presented in chapter order so that the cards can be removed in sequence as one progresses through the book. Although additional flashcards have been included with this edition, these cards represent only a portion of the necessary vocabulary, and students should add to the collection with personalized cards (some blank cards are included for this purpose).
- **Interactive CD-ROM**—A CD-ROM is included with the text, containing practice tests, word-building exercises, labeling exercises, crossword puzzles, additional case studies, and audio pronunciations.

Students are also encouraged to create their own learning aids, such as devising a practice test by covering lists of words and testing themselves on the definitions, or by covering definitions and testing themselves on the words. The same can be done with the charts on word parts and their definitions. It is also helpful to keep a personal list of words that the student finds difficult to spell or pronounce.

Teaching Resources

A strong package of ancillary materials is available to instructors with this edition. These resources include:

- **Instructor's Manual**—This valuable teaching resource contains Comments to supplement the text; Supplementary Activities; Spelling and Pronunciation Lists; Word Groups for Writing Case Studies; Word Search Puzzles; and Multiple-Choice Test Files.
- **Test Generator**—A computerized test generator containing more than 1,200 questions is packaged in the back of the Instructor Manual.
- **Connection Site**—A customized web site (http://connection.lww.com/go/cohen4e) has been developed with access to an image bank containing many of the beautiful text illustrations, Instructor's Manual content, and conversion guides from the text that you may be using in your course.
- **Transparencies**—Fifty full-color transparencies for overhead projection are available on request.
- **WebCT and Blackboard Online Course**—Customized course content has been developed for use with your learning management system.

An understanding of medical terminology provides an essential foundation for any career in health care. *Medical Terminology: An Illustrated Guide,* 4th Edition, both the textbook and its ancillaries, makes learning and teaching medical terminology a rewarding and exciting process.

User's Guide

This User's Guide shows you how to put the features of *Medical Terminology: An Illustrated Guide*, 4th Edition to work for you.

TERMINOLOGY

Terminology is presented in a consistent and logical manner. Phonetic pronunciations are included with all new terms.

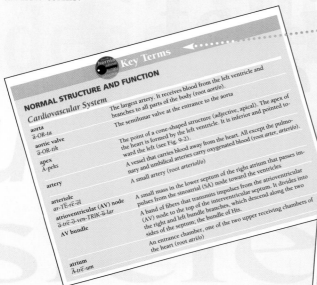

Key Terms include the most commonly used words.

Supplementary Terms list more specialized words.

Abbreviations for common terms.

Key Clinical Terms list medical terms pertinent to the body system under discussion.

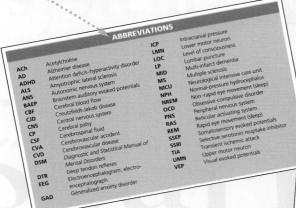

SPECIAL INTEREST BOXES

Special interest boxes appear throughout the book and contain information on word derivations and usage.

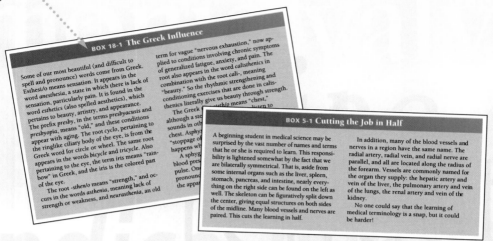

BOX 18-1 The Greek Influence

Some of our most beautiful (and difficult to spell and pronounce) words come from Greek. Esthesi/o means sensation. It appears in the word *anesthesia*, a state in which there is lack of sensation, particularly pain. It is found in the word *esthetics* (also spelled aesthetics), which pertains to beauty, artistry, and appearance. The prefix *presby*, in the terms presbyacusis and presbyopia, means "old," and these conditions appear with aging. The root *cyclo*, pertaining to the ringlike ciliary body of the eye, is from the Greek word for circle or wheel. The same root appears in the words bicycle and tricycle. Also pertaining to the eye, the term iris means "rainbow" in Greek, and the iris is the colored part of the eye.

The root *-sthen/o* means "strength," and occurs in the words asthenia, meaning lack of strength or weakness, and *neurasthenia*, an old term for vague "nervous exhaustion," now applied to conditions involving chronic symptoms of generalized fatigue, anxiety, and pain. This root also appears in the word *calisthenics* in combination with the root *cali-*, meaning "beauty." So the rhythmic strengthening and conditioning exercises that are done in calisthenics literally give us beauty through strength.

The Greek *...eth/o* means "chest," although a ste... sounds in oth... chest. Asphy... "stoppage o... happens wh...

A sphygm... blood pres... pulse. On... pronounc... the appa...

BOX 5-1 Cutting the Job in Half

A beginning student in medical science may be surprised by the vast number of names and terms that he or she is required to learn. This responsibility is lightened somewhat by the fact that we are bilaterally symmetrical. That is, aside from some internal organs such as the liver, spleen, stomach, pancreas, and intestine, nearly everything on the right side can be found on the left as well. The skeleton can be figuratively split down the center, giving equal structures on both sides of the midline. Many blood vessels and nerves are paired. This cuts the learning in half.

In addition, many of the blood vessels and nerves in a region have the same name. The radial artery, radial vein, and radial nerve are parallel, and all are located along the radius of the forearm. Vessels are commonly named for the organ they supply: the hepatic artery and vein of the liver, the pulmonary artery and vein of the lungs, the renal artery and vein of the kidney.

No one could say that the learning of medical terminology is a snap, but it could be harder!

DISPLAYS

Displays organize information on specific topics and serve as references and reviews.

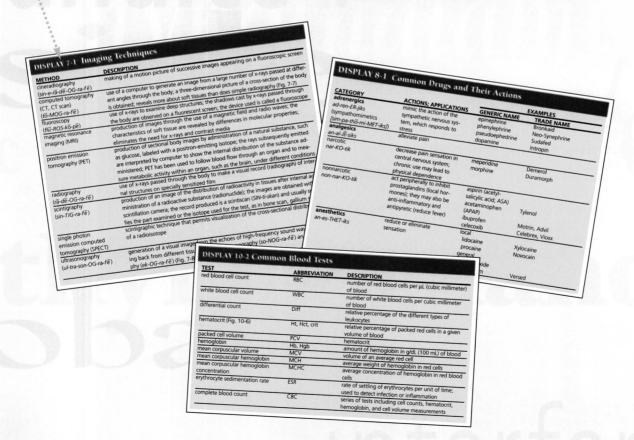

DISPLAY 7-1 Imaging Techniques

METHOD	DESCRIPTION
cineradiography (sin-e-rā-dē-OG-ra-fē)	making of a motion picture of successive images appearing on a fluoroscopic screen
computed tomography (CT, CT scan) (tō-MOG-ra-fē)	use of a computer to generate an image from a large number of x-rays passed at different angles through the body, a three-dimensional picture of a cross-section of the body is obtained; reveals more about soft tissues than does simple radiography (Fig. 7-7)
fluoroscopy (flū-ROS-kō-pē)	use of x-rays to examine deep structures; the shadows cast by x-rays passed through the body are observed on a fluorescent screen; the device used is called a fluoroscope
magnetic resonance imaging (MRI)	production of images through the use of a magnetic field and radio waves; the characteristics of soft tissue are revealed by differences in molecular properties; eliminates the need for x-rays and contrast media
positron emission tomography (PET)	production of sectional body images by administration of a natural substance, such as glucose, labeled with a positron-emitting isotope; the rays subsequently emitted are interpreted by computer to show the internal distribution of the substance administered; PET has been used to follow blood flow through an organ and to measure metabolic activity within an organ, such as the brain, under different conditions
radiography (rā-dē-OG-ra-fē)	use of x-rays passed through the body to make a visual record (radiograph) of internal structures on specially sensitized film
scintigraphy (sin-TIG-ra-fē)	production of an image of the distribution of radioactivity in tissues after internal administration of a radioactive substance (radionuclide); the images are obtained with a scintillation camera; the record produced is a scintiscan (SIN-ti-skan) and usually specifies the part examined or the isotope used for the test, as in bone scan, gallium scan
single photon emission computed tomography (SPECT)	scintigraphic technique that permits visualization of the cross-sectional distribution of a radioisotope
ultrasonography (ul-tra-son-OG-ra-fē)	generation of a visual image from the echoes of high-frequency sound waves traveling back from different tissues ...nography (so-NOG-ra-fē) an...phy (ek-OG-ra-fē) (Fig. 7-8...

DISPLAY 8-1 Common Drugs and Their Actions

CATEGORY	ACTIONS; APPLICATIONS	GENERIC NAME	EXAMPLES TRADE NAME
adrenergics ad-ren-ER-jiks (sympathomimetics (sim-pa-thō-mi-MET-iks))	mimic the action of the sympathetic nervous system, which responds to stress	epinephrine phenylephrine pseudoephedrine dopamine	Bronkaid Neo-Synephrine Sudafed Intropin
analgesics an-al-JĒ-siks	alleviate pain		
narcotic nar-KO-tik	decrease pain sensation in central nervous system; chronic use may lead to physical dependence	meperidine morphine	Demerol Duramorph
nonnarcotic non-nar-KO-tik	act peripherally to inhibit prostaglandins (local hormones); they may also be anti-inflammatory and antipyretic (reduce fever)	aspirin (acetyl-salicylic acid; ASA) acetaminophen (APAP) ibuprofen celecoxib	Tylenol Motrin, Advil Celebrex, Vioxx
anesthetics an-es-THET-iks	reduce or eliminate sensation	local lidocaine procaine general ...xide ...m	Xylocaine Novocain Versed

DISPLAY 10-2 Common Blood Tests

TEST	ABBREVIATION	DESCRIPTION
red blood cell count	RBC	number of red blood cells per μL (cubic millimeter) of blood
white blood cell count	WBC	number of white blood cells per cubic millimeter of blood
differential count	Diff	relative percentage of the different types of leukocytes
hematocrit (Fig. 10-6)	Ht, Hct, crit	relative percentage of packed red cells in a given volume of blood
packed cell volume	PCV	hematocrit
hemoglobin	Hb, Hgb	amount of hemoglobin in g/dL (100 mL) of blood
mean corpuscular volume	MCV	volume of an average red cell
mean corpuscular hemoglobin	MCH	average weight of hemoglobin in red cells
mean corpuscular hemoglobin concentration	MCHC	average concentration of hemoglobin in red blood cells
erythrocyte sedimentation rate	ESR	rate of settling of erythrocytes per unit of time; used to detect infection or inflammation
complete blood count	CBC	series of tests including cell counts, hematocrit, hemoglobin, and cell volume measurements

FULL-COLOR ARTWORK AND PHOTOS

Beautiful **full-color art** throughout the book brings the content to life and illustrates the most important information.

Illustrations bring complex information to life.

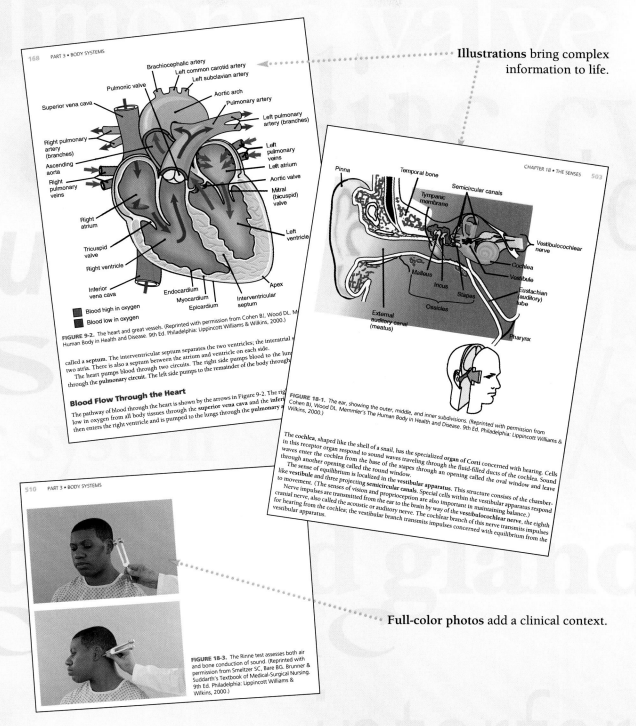

168   PART 3 • BODY SYSTEMS

FIGURE 9-2. The heart and great vessels. (Reprinted with permission from Cohen BJ, Wood DL. Memmler's Human Body in Health and Disease. 9th Ed. Philadelphia: Lippincott Williams & Wilkins, 2000.)

called a **septum**. The interventricular septum separates the two ventricles; the interatrial septum separates the two atria. There is also a septum between the atrium and ventricle on each side.

The heart pumps blood through two circuits. The right side pumps blood to the lungs through the **pulmonary circuit**. The left side pumps to the remainder of the body through the

Blood Flow Through the Heart

The pathway of blood through the heart is shown by the arrows in Figure 9-2. The right side pumps blood low in oxygen from all body tissues through the **superior vena cava** and the **inferior vena cava**. Blood then enters the right ventricle and is pumped to the lungs through the **pulmonary artery**.

CHAPTER 18 • THE SENSES   503

FIGURE 18-1. The ear, showing the outer, middle, and inner subdivisions. (Reprinted with permission from Cohen BJ, Wood DL. Memmler's The Human Body in Health and Disease. 9th Ed. Philadelphia: Lippincott Williams & Wilkins, 2000.)

The **cochlea**, shaped like the shell of a snail, has the specialized **organ of Corti** concerned with hearing. Cells in this receptor organ respond to sound waves traveling through the fluid-filled ducts of the cochlea. Sound waves enter the cochlea from the base of the stapes through an opening called the oval window and leave through another opening called the round window.

The sense of equilibrium is localized in the **vestibular apparatus**. This structure consists of the chamber-like **vestibule** and three projecting **semicircular canals**. Special cells within the vestibular apparatus respond to movement. (The senses of vision and proprioception are also important in maintaining balance.)

Nerve impulses are transmitted from the ear to the brain by way of the **vestibulocochlear nerve**, the eighth cranial nerve, also called the acoustic or auditory nerve. The cochlear branch of this nerve transmits impulses for hearing from the cochlea; the vestibular branch transmits impulses concerned with equilibrium from the vestibular apparatus.

510   PART 3 • BODY SYSTEMS

FIGURE 18-3. The Rinne test assesses both air and bone conduction of sound. (Reprinted with permission from Smeltzer SC, Bare BG. Brunner & Suddarth's Textbook of Medical-Surgical Nursing. 9th Ed. Philadelphia: Lippincott Williams & Wilkins, 2000.)

Full-color photos add a clinical context.

CASE STUDIES

Case studies illustrate terminology in the context of a medical report.
These are followed by questions about terms used in the cases.

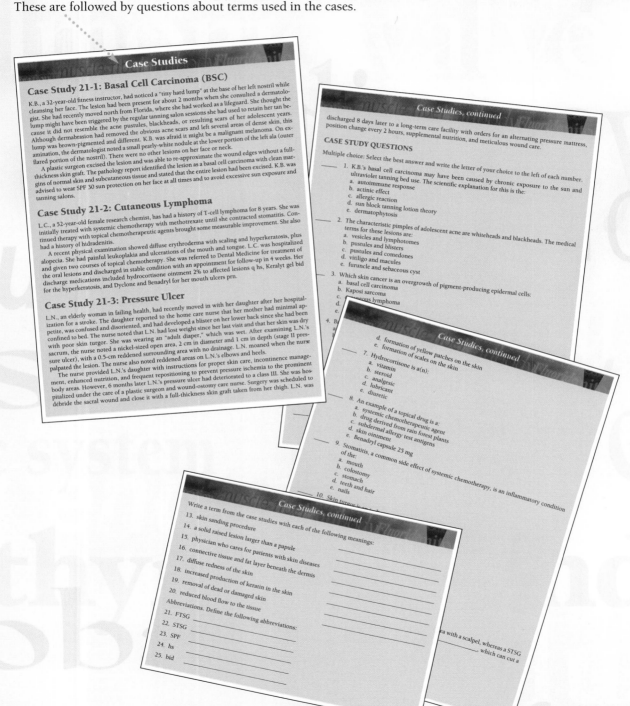

Case Studies

Case Study 21-1: Basal Cell Carcinoma (BSC)

K.B., a 32-year-old fitness instructor, had noticed a "tiny hard lump" at the base of her left nostril while cleansing her face. The lesion had been present for about 2 months when she consulted a dermatologist. She had recently moved north from Florida, where she had worked as a lifeguard. She thought the lump might have been triggered by the regular tanning salon sessions she had used to retain her tan because it did not resemble the acne pustules, blackheads, or resulting scars of her adolescent years. Although dermabrasion had removed the obvious acne scars and left several areas of dense skin, this lump was brown-pigmented and different. K.B. was afraid it might be a malignant melanoma. On examination, the dermatologist noted a small pearly-white nodule at the lower portion of the left ala (outer flared portion of the nostril). There were no other lesions on her face or neck.

A plastic surgeon excised the lesion and was able to re-approximate the wound edges without a full-thickness skin graft. The pathology report identified the lesion as a basal cell carcinoma with clean margins of normal skin and subcutaneous tissue and stated that the entire lesion had been excised. K.B. was advised to wear SPF 30 sun protection on her face at all times and to avoid excessive sun exposure and tanning salons.

Case Study 21-2: Cutaneous Lymphoma

L.C., a 52-year-old female research chemist, has had a history of T-cell lymphoma for 8 years. She was initially treated with systemic chemotherapy with methotrexate until she contracted stomatitis. Continued therapy with topical chemotherapeutic agents brought some measurable improvement. She also had a history of hidradenitis.

A recent physical examination showed diffuse erythroderma with scaling and hyperkeratosis, plus alopecia. She had painful leukoplakia and ulcerations of the mouth and tongue. L.C. was hospitalized and given two courses of topical chemotherapy. She was referred to Dental Medicine for treatment of the oral lesions and discharged in stable condition with an appointment for follow-up in 4 weeks. Her discharge medications included hydrocortisone ointment 2% to affected lesions q hs, Keralyt gel bid for the hyperkeratosis, and Dyclone and Benadryl for her mouth ulcers prn.

Case Study 21-3: Pressure Ulcer

L.N., an elderly woman in failing health, had recently moved in with her daughter after her hospitalization for a stroke. The daughter reported to the home care nurse that her mother had minimal appetite, was confused and disoriented, and had developed a blister on her lower back since she had been confined to bed. The nurse noted that L.N. had lost weight since her last visit and that her skin was dry with poor skin turgor. She was wearing an "adult diaper," which was wet. After examining L.N.'s sacrum, the nurse noted a nickel-sized open area, 2 cm in diameter and 1 cm in depth (stage II pressure ulcer), with a 0.5-cm reddened surrounding area with no drainage. L.N. moaned when the nurse palpated the lesion. The nurse also noted reddened areas on L.N.'s elbows and heels.

The nurse provided L.N.'s daughter with instructions for proper skin care, incontinence management, enhanced nutrition, and frequent repositioning to prevent pressure ischemia to the prominent body areas. However, 6 months later L.N.'s pressure ulcer had deteriorated to a class III. She was hospitalized under the care of a plastic surgeon and wound-ostomy care nurse. Surgery was scheduled to debride the sacral wound and close it with a full-thickness skin graft taken from her thigh. L.N. was

---

Case Studies, continued

discharged 8 days later to a long-term care facility with orders for an alternating pressure mattress, position change every 2 hours, supplemental nutrition, and meticulous wound care.

CASE STUDY QUESTIONS

Multiple choice: Select the best answer and write the letter of your choice to the left of each number.

_____ 1. K.B.'s basal cell carcinoma may have been caused by chronic exposure to the sun and ultraviolet tanning bed use. The scientific explanation for this is the:
   a. autoimmune response
   b. actinic effect
   c. allergic reaction
   d. sun block tanning lotion theory
   e. dermatophytosis

_____ 2. The characteristic pimples of adolescent acne are whiteheads and blackheads. The medical terms for these lesions are:
   a. vesicles and lymphotomes
   b. pustules and blisters
   c. pustules and comedones
   d. vitiligo and macules
   e. furuncle and sebaceous cyst

_____ 3. Which skin cancer is an overgrowth of pigment-producing epidermal cells:
   a. basal cell carcinoma
   b. Kaposi sarcoma
   c. cutaneous lymphoma
   d.
   e.

Case Studies, continued

   d. formation of yellow patches on the skin
   e. formation of scales on the skin

_____ 7. Hydrocortisone is a(n):
   a. vitamin
   b. steroid
   c. analgesic
   d. lubricant
   e. diuretic

_____ 8. An example of a topical drug is a:
   a. systemic chemotherapeutic agent
   b. drug derived from rain forest plants
   c. subdermal allergy test antigens
   d. skin ointment
   e. Benadryl capsule 25 mg

_____ 9. Stomatitis, a common side effect of systemic chemotherapy, is an inflammatory condition of the:
   a. mouth
   b. colostomy
   c. stomach
   d. teeth and hair
   e. nails

_____ 10. Skin turgor

Case Studies, continued

Write a term from the case studies with each of the following meanings:

13. skin sanding procedure _____

14. a solid raised lesion larger than a papule _____

15. physician who cares for patients with skin diseases _____

16. connective tissue and fat layer beneath the dermis _____

17. diffuse redness of the skin _____

18. increased production of keratin in the skin _____

19. removal of dead or damaged skin _____

20. reduced blood flow to the tissue _____

Abbreviations. Define the following abbreviations:

21. FTSG _____

22. STSG _____

23. SPF _____

24. hs _____

25. bid _____

area with a scalpel, whereas a STSG
which can cut a

PRACTICE EXERCISES

Exercises are included throughout the book to help you understand the content, assess your progress, and review and prepare for quizzes and tests.

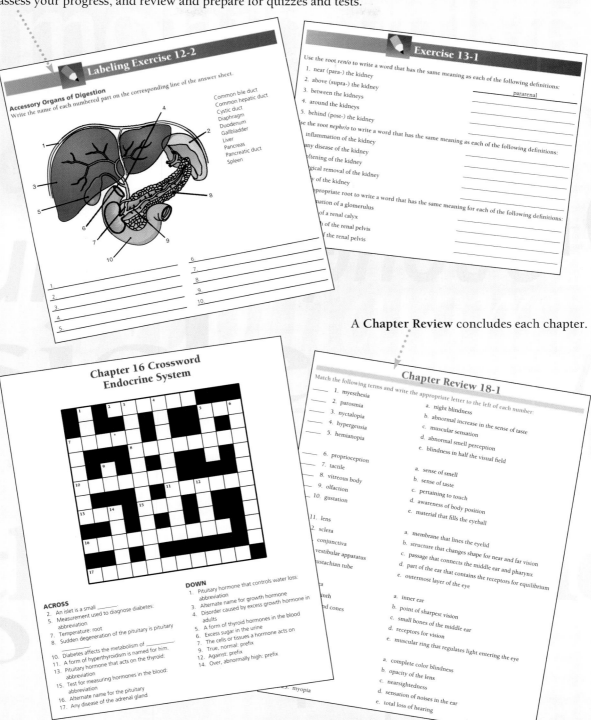

Labeling Exercise 12-2

Accessory Organs of Digestion
Write the name of each numbered part on the corresponding line of the answer sheet.

Common bile duct
Common hepatic duct
Cystic duct
Diaphragm
Duodenum
Gallbladder
Liver
Pancreas
Pancreatic duct
Spleen

1. _____
2. _____
3. _____
4. _____
5. _____
6. _____
7. _____
8. _____
9. _____
10. _____

Exercise 13-1

Use the root *ren/o* to write a word that has the same meaning as each of the following definitions:

1. near (para-) the kidney
2. above (supra-) the kidney
3. between the kidneys   pararenal
4. around the kidneys
5. behind (post-) the kidney

Use the root *nephr/o* to write a word that has the same meaning as each of the following definitions:

inflammation of the kidney
any disease of the kidney
softening of the kidney
gical removal of the kidney
y of the kidney

ppropriate root to write a word that has the same meaning for each of the following definitions:

nation of a glomerulus
of a renal calyx
t of the renal pelvis
f the renal pelvis

A **Chapter Review** concludes each chapter.

Chapter 16 Crossword
Endocrine System

ACROSS
2. An islet is a small _____.
5. Measurement used to diagnose diabetes: abbreviation
7. Temperature: root
8. Sudden degeneration of the pituitary is pituitary _____
10. Diabetes affects the metabolism of _____.
11. A form of hyperthyroidism is named for him.
13. Pituitary hormone that acts on the thyroid: abbreviation
15. Test for measuring hormones in the blood: abbreviation
16. Alternate name for the pituitary
17. Any disease of the adrenal gland

DOWN
1. Pituitary hormone that controls water loss: abbreviation
3. Alternate name for growth hormone
4. Disorder caused by excess growth hormone in adults
5. A form of thyroid hormones in the blood
6. Excess sugar in the urine
7. The cells or tissues a hormone acts on
11. True, normal: prefix
12. Against: prefix
14. Over, abnormally high: prefix

Chapter Review 18-1

Match the following terms and write the appropriate letter to the left of each number:

_____ 1. myesthesia
_____ 2. parosmia
_____ 3. nyctalopia
_____ 4. hypergeusia
_____ 5. hemianopia

a. night blindness
b. abnormal increase in the sense of taste
c. muscular sensation
d. abnormal smell perception
e. blindness in half the visual field

_____ 6. proprioception
_____ 7. tactile
_____ 8. vitreous body
_____ 9. olfaction
_____ 10. gustation

a. sense of smell
b. sense of taste
c. pertaining to touch
d. awareness of body position
e. material that fills the eyeball

_____ 11. lens
_____ 2. sclera
_____ conjunctiva
_____ estibular apparatus
_____ ustachian tube

a. membrane that lines the eyelid
b. structure that changes shape for near and far vision
c. passage that connects the middle ear and pharynx
d. part of the ear that contains the receptors for equilibrium
e. outermost layer of the eye

_____ a
_____ nth
_____ d cones

a. inner ear
b. point of sharpest vision
c. small bones of the middle ear
d. receptors for vision
e. muscular ring that regulates light entering the eye

_____ myopia

a. complete color blindness
b. opacity of the lens
c. nearsightedness
d. sensation of noises in the ear
e. total loss of hearing

FLASHCARDS

A set of **flashcards** is included to help you maximize your study time. Expand your vocabulary by making additional flashcards as you work through the text.

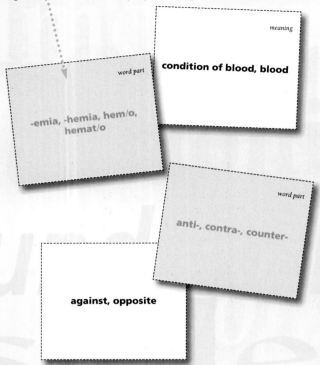

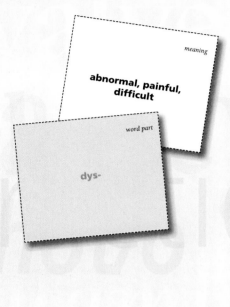

CD-ROM

The free **CD-ROM** includes practice tests, additional exercises to test your knowledge and assess your progress, and a pronunciation glossary. Have fun while you learn!

- The **practice tests** offer an opportunity for you to prepare for assessment.
- **Interactive labeling exercises** help you reinforce your understanding of anatomy.
- The **pronunciation glossary** allows you to hear accurate pronunciations of over 2,500 terms, drawn directly from *Stedman's Medical Dictionary*.

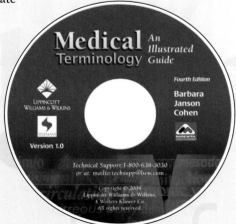

Acknowledgments

I wish to thank the many people who helped in the preparation of this 4th edition of *Medical Terminology: An Illustrated Guide.*

At Lippincott Williams & Wilkins, acquisitions editor John Goucher has worked with me from the early planning stages for the revision and has helped continuously thereafter. Thanks also to editorial assistants Heidi Weinkam and Peter Sabatini. Development editors Nancy Peterson and Jacquelyn Merrell helped oversee the editorial process, while Rose Foltz examined every detail of the text and made many valuable suggestions for illustrations. Karen Gulliver, managing editor, oversaw the art preparation and got the manuscript ready for production, and Karen Ruppert, production editor, oversaw the copyediting and composition.

Special thanks to Craig Durant at Dragonfly Media Group for his wonderful work on the art program, visualizing concepts beautifully and accurately.

I appreciate the assistance of all of the reviewers who gave of their time and expertise in evaluating work in progress and making suggestions for improvement. In addition, Cheryl Meyer and Frederick J. Goldstein helped with the latest information in pharmacology.

Armloads of thanks to Christine Smith for writing the case studies and serving as reviewer and guide on clinical matters. Working with Chris added so much to my enjoyment in preparing this revision. Thanks, Chris, for many late-night E-conferences and for understanding that laughter is the best medicine.

Reviewers

Pam Besser, PhD
Professor
Business Division
Jefferson Community College
Louisville, KY

Dr. Joyce B. Harvey, RHIA, PhD
Associate Professor
Department of Allied Health
Norfolk State University
Norfolk, VA

Les Chatelain
University of Utah
Department of Health Promotion and Education
Salt Lake City, UT

Mary Allbright, RN
Medical Instructor
Department of Business Technology and Paramedic
    Program
Arkansas Valley Technical College
Van Buren, AR

Kimberly Shannon, RN
Surgical Technology Program Coordinator
Moore Norman Technology Center
Norman, OK

Juanita R. Bryant, CMA-A/C
BE, Masters Equivalent
Professor of Medical Terminology
Cabrillo College/Sierra College
Aptos/Rocklin, CA

Margaret Bellak, MN
Professor of Nursing
Nursing and Allied Health Department
Indiana University of Pennsylvania
Indiana, PA

Sharon A. Kerber
Instructor
Department of Education
Missouri College
St. Louis, MO

Cynthia Booth Lord, MHS, PA-C
Assistant Professor and Physician Assistant
    Program Director
Department of Biomedical Science
Quinnipiac University
Hamden, CT

Pamela Van Bevern, PA-C, MPAS
Assistant Professor
Physician Assistant Program
Saint Louis University
St. Louis, MO

Jill E. Winland-Brown, EdD, MSN, ARNP
Professor and Assistant Dean of Undergraduate
    Studies
Christine E. Lynn College of Nursing
Florida Atlantic University
Boca Raton, FL

Contents

Expanded Contents

Medical Terminology
An Illustrated Guide

body *Fluoride* mitoc

ation pulmonic

ous body denot

jaundice

oma ossicle

limbic system

RON-ik

hypobari

ortex

Introduction to Medical Terminology

Chapters 1 through 5, Part 1, present the basics of medical terminology and body structure. Chapters 6 through 8, Part 2, deal with disease and treatment. These beginning chapters form the basis for the chapters on the individual body systems, Part 3.

Concepts of Medical Terminology

Chapter Contents

Objectives

After study of this chapter you should be able to:

1. Explain the purpose of medical terminology.
2. Define the terms *root, suffix*, and *prefix.*
3. Explain what combining forms are and why they are used.
4. Name the languages from which most medical word parts are derived.
5. Pronounce words according to the pronunciation guide used in this text.
6. Analyze a case study with regard to some concepts of medical terminology.

Medical terminology is a special vocabulary used by health care professionals for effective and accurate communication. Because it is based mainly on Greek and Latin words, medical terminology is consistent and uniform throughout the world. It is also efficient; although some of the terms are long, they often reduce an entire phrase to a single word. The one word *gastroduodenostomy*, for example, stands for "a communication between the stomach and the first part of the small intestine" (Fig. 1-1).

The medical vocabulary is vast, and learning it may seem like learning the entire vocabulary of a foreign language. Moreover, like the jargon that arises in all changing fields, it is always expanding. Think of the terms that have been added to our vocabulary with the development of computers, such as software, megabyte, search engine, e-mail, chat room. The task seems overwhelming, but there are methods that can aid in learning and remembering words and can even help in making informed guesses regarding the meanings of unfamiliar words. Most medical terms can be divided into component parts—roots, prefixes, and suffixes—that maintain the same meaning whenever they appear. By learning these meanings, you can analyze and remember many words.

Word Parts

The fundamental unit of each medical word is the **root**. This establishes the basic meaning of the word and is the part to which modifying prefixes and suffixes are added.

A **suffix** is a short word part or series of parts added at the end of a root to modify its meaning. In this book suffixes are indicated by a dash before the suffix, such as *-itis*.

A **prefix** is a short word part added before a root to modify its meaning. In this book prefixes are indicated by a dash after the prefix, such as *pre-*. Shown diagrammatically:

Prefix	—	Root	—	Suffix

Prefix	Root	Suffix

Words are formed from roots, prefixes, and suffixes.   Word

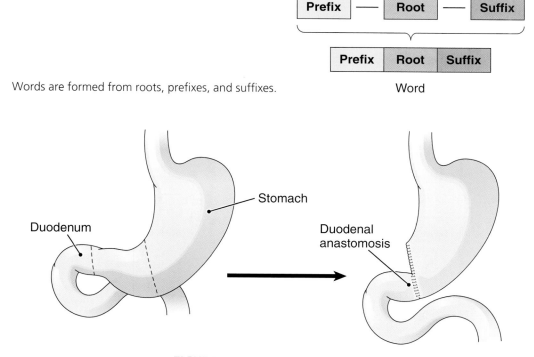

FIGURE 1-1. Gastroduodenostomy

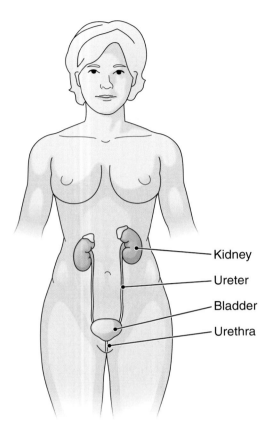

Kidney

Ureter

Bladder

Urethra

FIGURE 1-2. The Greek root *nephr* and the Latin root *ren* are used to refer to the kidney, an organ of the urinary system.

The simple word *learn* can be used as a root to illustrate. If we add the suffix *-er* to form *learner*, we have "one who learns." If we add the prefix *re-* to form *relearn*, we have "to learn again."

Not all roots are complete words. In fact, most medical roots are derived from other languages and are meant to be used in combinations. The Greek word *kardia*, for example, meaning "heart," gives us the root *cardi*. The Latin word *pulmo*, meaning "lung," gives us the root *pulm*. In a few instances, both the Greek and Latin roots are used. We find both the Greek root *nephr* and the Latin root *ren* used in words pertaining to the kidney (Fig. 1-2).

Note that the same root may have different meanings in different fields of study. The root *myel* means "marrow" and may apply to either the bone marrow or the spinal cord. The root *scler* means "hard" but may also apply to the white of the eye. *Cyst* means "a filled sac or pouch" but also refers specifically to the urinary bladder. You will sometimes have to consider the context of a word before assigning its meaning.

Compound words contain more than one root. The words *eyeball*, *bedpan*, *frostbite*, and *wheelchair* are examples. Some compound medical words are *cardiovascular* (pertaining to the heart and blood vessels), *urogenital* (pertaining to the urinary and reproductive systems), and *lymphocyte* (a white blood cell found in the lymphatic system).

Combining Forms

When a suffix beginning with a consonant is added to a root, a vowel (usually an o) is inserted between the root and the suffix to aid in pronunciation.

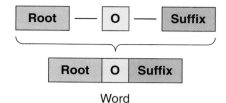

A combining vowel may be added between a root and a suffix.   Word

Thus, when the suffix *-logy*, meaning "study of," is added to the root *neur*, meaning "nerve or nervous system," a combining vowel is added:

neur + o + logy = neurology (study of the nervous system)

Roots shown with a combining vowel are called **combining forms**.

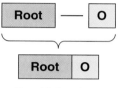

A root with a combining vowel is often called a combining form.   Combining form

In this text, roots are given with their most common combining vowels added after a slash and are referred to simply as roots, as in neur/o. A combining vowel usually is not used if the ending begins with a vowel. The root *neur* is combined with the suffix *-itis*, meaning "inflammation of," in this way:

neur + itis = neuritis (inflammation of a nerve)

There are some exceptions to this rule, particularly when pronunciation or meaning is affected, but you will observe these as you work.

Word Derivations

As mentioned, most medical word parts come from Greek (G) and Latin (L). The original words and their meanings are included in this text only occasionally. They are interesting, however, and may aid in learning. For example, *muscle* comes from a Latin word that means "mouse" because the movement of a muscle under the skin was thought to resemble the scampering of a mouse.

The coccyx, the tail end of the spine, is named for the cuckoo because it was thought to resemble the cuckoo's bill (Fig. 1-3). For those interested in the derivations of medical words, a good medical dictionary will provide this information. Several such books are listed in the bibliography at the end of this text.

Pronunciation

Phonetic pronunciations are provided in the text at every opportunity, even in the answer keys. Take advantage of these aids. Repeat the word aloud as you learn to recognize it in print. Be aware that word parts may change in pronunciation when they are combined in different ways. The following pronunciation guidelines apply throughout the text.

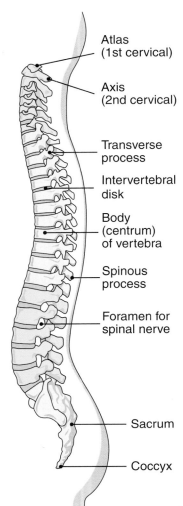

Atlas
(1st cervical)

Axis
(2nd cervical)

Transverse
process

Intervertebral
disk

Body
(centrum)
of vertebra

Spinous
process

Foramen for
spinal nerve

Sacrum

Coccyx

FIGURE 1-3. The coccyx of the spine looks like the bill of a cuckoo. (Reprinted with permission from Cohen BJ, Wood DL. Memmler's The Human Body in Health and Disease. 9th Ed. Philadelphia: Lippincott Williams & Wilkins, 2000.)

A vowel (a, e, i, o, u) gets a short pronunciation if it has no pronunciation mark over it, such as:

a as in hat
e as in met
i as in bin
o as in some
u as in run

A short line over the vowel gives it a long pronunciation:

$\bar{a}$ as in say
$\bar{e}$ as in tea
$\bar{i}$ as in lie
$\bar{o}$ as in hose
$\bar{u}$ as in sue

The accented syllable in each word is shown with capital letters.

Note that pronunciations may vary from place to place. Only one pronunciation for each word is given here, but be prepared for differences.

Soft and Hard *c* and *g*

A soft *c*, as in *racer*, will be written as *s* (RĀ-ser). A hard *c*, as in *candy*, will be written as *k* (KAN-dē). A soft *g*, as in *page*, will be written as *j* (pāj). A hard *g*, as in *grow*, will be written as *g* (grō).

Silent Letters and Unusual Pronunciations

A silent letter or unusual pronunciation can be a problem, especially if it appears at the start of a word that you are trying to look up in the dictionary. See Table 1-1 for some examples.

The combinations in Table 1-1 may be pronounced differently when they appear within a word, as in **ap**nea (*AP-nē-a*), meaning cessation of breathing; nephro**pt**osis (*nef-rop-TŌ-sis*), meaning dropping of the kidney; pro**gn**osis (*prog-NŌ-sis*), meaning prediction of the outcome of disease.

Symbols

Symbols are commonly used in case histories as a form of shorthand. Some examples are Ⓛ and Ⓡ for left and right; ↑ and ↓ for increase and decrease. A list of common symbols appears in Chapter 7 and in Appendix 1.

Abbreviations

Like symbols, abbreviations can save time, but they can also cause confusion if they are not universally understood. Usage varies in different institutions, and the same abbreviation may have different meanings in different fields. An **acronym** is an abbreviation formed from the first letter of each word in a phrase. Some

TABLE 1-1 Silent Letters and Unusual Pronunciations

LETTER(S)	PRONUNCIATION	EXAMPLE	DEFINITION OF EXAMPLE
ch	k	chemical *KEM-i-kl*	pertaining to chemistry
dys	dis	dystrophy *DIS-trō-f ē*	poor nourishment of tissue
eu	u	euphoria *ū-FOR-ē-a*	exaggerated feeling of well-being
gn	n	gnathic *NATH-ik*	pertaining to the jaw
ph	f	pharmacy *FAR-ma-sē*	a drug dispensary
pn	n	pneumonia *nū-MŌ-nē-a*	inflammation of the lungs
ps	s	pseudo- *SŪ-dō*	false
pt	t	ptosis *TŌ-sis*	dropping
rh	r	rheumatic *rū-MAT-ik*	pertaining to rheumatism, a disorder of muscles and joints
x	z	xiphoid *ZIF-oyd*	pertaining to cartilage attached to the sternum

everyday acronyms are ASAP (as soon as possible) and ATM (automated teller machine). In computerese, RAM stands for "random access memory." Acronyms have become popular for saving time and space in naming objects, organizations, and procedures. Only the most commonly used abbreviations are given. These are listed at the end of each chapter, but a complete alphabetical list appears in Appendix 2. An abbreviation dictionary also is helpful.

Words Ending In *x*

When a word ending in *x* has a suffix added, the *x* is changed to a *g* or a *c*. For example, *pharynx* (throat) becomes *pharyngeal* (*fa-RIN-jē-al*), to mean "pertaining to the throat"; *coccyx* (terminal portion of the vertebral column) becomes *coccygeal* (*kok-SIJ-ē-al*), to mean "pertaining to the coccyx"; *thorax* (chest) becomes *thoracotomy* (*thor-a-KOT-ō-mē*) to mean "an incision into the chest."

Suffixes Beginning With *rh*

When a suffix beginning with *rh* is added to a root, the *r* is doubled:

    hem/o (blood) + -rhage (bursting forth) = hemorrhage (a bursting forth of blood)
    men/o (menses) + -rhea (flow, discharge) = menorrhea (menstrual flow)

Key Terms

acronym *AK-rō-nim*	An abbreviation formed from the first letter of each word in a phrase
combining form	A word root in combination with a vowel used to link the root with a suffix. Combining forms are shown with a slash between the root and the vowel, as in *neur/o*.
prefix *PRE-fix*	A word part added before a root to modify its meaning
root	The fundamental unit of a word
suffix *SU-fix*	A word part added to the end of a root to modify its meaning

Chapter Review 1-1

Fill in the blanks:

1. A root with a vowel added to aid in pronunciation is called a(n) _____.

2. A word part that comes before a root is a(n) _____.

3. Combine the word parts *dia-*, meaning "through," and *-rhea*, meaning "flow," to form a word meaning "passage of fluid stool." _____

4. Combine the root *psych*, meaning "mind," with the suffix *-logy*, meaning "study of," to form a word meaning "study of the mind." _____

Multiple choice: Select the best answer and write the letter of your choice to the left of each number.

_____ 5. Which of the following is a compound word?
 a. urinary
 b. skeletal
 c. gastrointestinal
 d. coronary
 e. artery

_____ 6. The adjective for *thorax* is
 a. thoraxic
 b. thoracic
 c. thoral
 d. thorial
 e. thoraxial

_____ 7. An acronym is formed from
 a. a proper name
 b. Latin or Greek
 c. a compound word
 d. the first letter of each word in a phrase
 e. two or more roots

Pronounce the following words:

8. dysfunction

9. rheumatoid

10. chronologic

11. pharynx

Pronounce the following phonetic forms:

12. *nar-KOT-ik*

13. *NĪ-trō-jen*

14. *SUR-fas*

15. *VAS-kū-lar*

16. *thō-RAS-ik*

Case Study

Case Study 1-1: Multiple Health Problems Secondary to Injury

D.S., a 28-year-old woman, was treated for injuries sustained in a train derailment accident. During the course of her treatment, she was seen by several specialists. For pain in her knee and hip joints, she was referred to an orthopedist. For migraine headaches and blurry vision, she consulted a neurologist. For pain on urination and occasional bloody urine, she saw a urologist. Later, for a persistent dry cough and problems resulting from a fractured nose, she was referred to an otorhinolaryngologist. During her initial course of treatment, she had a CT scan of her abdomen and brain and an MRI of her hip and knee. Both imaging studies required her to lie motionless on her back for 45 minutes.

Several months after the accident, D.S. was still experiencing some discomfort, and she decided to investigate alternative therapies. She made an appointment with a naturist practitioner who specialized in homeopathy and herbal medicine. Before her appointment, she browsed in the Nutra-Medica Shop, which carried nutritional supplements, vitamin and mineral products, homeopathic remedies, and herbal formulas. She planned to ask the therapist about some of the products that she saw there, which included remedies with the trade names Pneumogen, Arthogesia-Plus, Renovite, Nephrostat, and Hematone.

CASE STUDY QUESTIONS

Multiple choice: Select the best answer and write the letter of your choice to the left of each number.

_____ 1. The *-ist* in the word neurologist is a:
   a. prefix
   b. root
   c. suffix
   d. combining form
   e. conjunction

Case Study, continued

_____ 2. *Endo-* in endoscopic is a:
   a. root
   b. suffix
   c. combining form
   d. prefix
   e. derivation

_____ 3. MRI stands for magnetic resonance imaging. This term represents a(n):
   a. combining form
   b. acronym
   c. prefix
   d. suffix
   e. abbreviation

_____ 4. D.S. needed plastic surgery on her nose to repair the postfracture deformity. This procedure is called a(n):
   a. septoscope
   b. rhinoplasty
   c. neurectomy
   d. cardioplasty
   e. rhinitis

_____ 5. Several of the radiological imaging studies required D.S. to lie on her back for 45 minutes. This position is referred to as:
   a. supine
   b. prone
   c. lateral recumbent
   d. lithotomy
   e. Trendelenburg

_____ 6. The products Renovite and Nephrostat are named for their action on the:
   a. lung
   b. nerves
   c. liver
   d. heart
   e. kidney

_____ 7. The *pn* in Pneumogen is pronounced as:
   a. p
   b. pa
   c. n
   d. up
   e. f

Fill in the blanks.

8. Use Appendix 4 to find roots that mean *blood*. _____

9. Use the index to find the chapter that contains information on imaging techniques.

_____

Case Study, continued

10. Use the flash cards at the back of this book to find the meaning of the word part *endo-*.
    _____

11. Another word part with the same meaning as *endo-* is _____.

12. Use Appendix 3 to look up the meaning of the roots in *otorhinolaryngology*.
    ot/o _____
    rhino _____
    laryng/o _____

13. Use Appendix 3 to find the meaning of the word part *homeo-*
    _____.

14. When the word *larynx* has a suffix added, the *x* is changed to a
    _____.

15. Appendix 2 tells you that the abbreviation *CT* in CT scan means
    _____.

CHAPTER 1 **Answer Section**

Answers to Chapter Exercises
1. combining form
2. prefix
3. diarrhea
4. psychology
5. c
6. b
7. d
8. *dis-FUNK-shun*
9. *RŪ-ma-toyd*
10. *kron-ō-LOJ-ik*
11. *FAR-inks*
12. narcotic
13. nitrogen
14. surface
15. vascular
16. thoracic

Answers to Case Study Questions
1. c
2. d
3. b
4. b
5. a
6. e
7. c
8. hem/o, hemat/o
9. chapter 7
10. in; within
11. intra-
12. ear; nose; larynx
13. same, unchanging
14. g
15. computed tomography

Suffixes

Chapter Contents

Objectives

After study of this chapter you should be able to:

1. Define a suffix.
2. Give examples of how suffixes are used.
3. Recognize and use some general noun, adjective, and plural suffixes used in medical terminology.
4. Analyze the suffixes used in a case study.

A suffix is a word ending that modifies a root. A suffix may indicate that the word is a noun or an adjective and often determines how the definition of the word will begin. For example, using the root *myel/o*, meaning "bone marrow," the adjective ending *-oid* forms the word *myeloid*, which means "like or pertaining to bone marrow." The ending *-oma* produces *myeloma*, which is a tumor of the bone marrow. Adding another root, *gen*, which represents genesis or origin, and the adjective ending *-ous* forms the word *myelogenous*, meaning "originating in bone marrow."

The suffixes given in this chapter are general ones that are used throughout medical terminology. Additional suffixes will be presented in later chapters, as they pertain to disease states, medical treatment, or specific body systems.

Noun Suffixes

TABLE 2-1 Suffixes That Mean "Condition Of"

SUFFIX	EXAMPLE	DEFINITION OF EXAMPLE
-ia	phobia *FŌ-bē-a*	persistent and exaggerated fear
-ism	alcoholism *AL-kō-hol-izm*	impaired control of alcohol use
-sis*	acidosis *as-i-DŌ-sis*	acid condition of body fluids
-y	tetany *TET-a-nē*	sustained muscle contraction

*The ending *-sis* may appear with a combining vowel, as -osis, -iasis, -esis, or -asis. The first two of these denote an abnormal condition.

Exercise 2-1

Write the suffix that means "condition of" in each of the following words:

1. egotism (exaggerated self-importance)   -ism
   Ē-gō-tizm

2. dysentery (intestinal disorder)   _____
   DIS-en-ter-ē

3. insomnia (inability to sleep)   _____
   in-SOM-nē-a

4. parasitism (infection with parasites or behaving as a parasite)   _____
   PAR-a-sit-izm

5. thrombosis (having a blood clot in a vessel) (Fig. 2-1)   _____
   throm-BŌ-sis

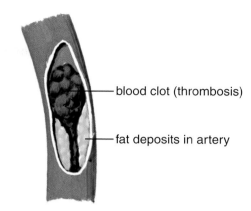

blood clot (thrombosis)

fat deposits in artery

FIGURE 2-1. Thrombosis (formation of a blood clot). (Reprinted with permission from Hosley JB, Jones SA, Molle-Matthews EA. Lippincott's Textbook for Medical Assistants. Philadelphia: Lippincott-Raven Publishers, 1997.)

6. psoriasis (skin disease)
   sō-RĪ-a-sis

7. analgesia (absence of pain)
   an-al-JĒ-zē-a

8. sclerosis (hardening)
   skle-RŌ-sis

9. atony (lack of muscle tone)
   AT-ō-nē

TABLE 2-2 Suffixes for Medical Specialties

SUFFIX	MEANING	EXAMPLE	DEFINITION OF EXAMPLE
-ian	specialist in a field of study	physician *fi-ZISH-un*	practitioner of medicine (from root *physi/o,* meaning "nature")
-iatrics	medical specialty	geriatrics *jer-ē-AT-riks*	study and treatment of the aged (from root *ger/i,* meaning "old age")
-iatry	medical specialty	podiatry *pō-DĪ-a-trē*	study and treatment of the foot (from root *pod/o,* meaning "foot")
-ics	medical specialty	orthopedics *or-thō-PĒ-diks*	study and treatment of the skeleton and joints (from root *ped/o,* meaning "child," and prefix *ortho,* meaning "straight")
-ist	specialist in a field of study	cardiologist *kar-dē-OL-ō-jist*	specialist in the study and treatment of the heart (from root *cardi/o,* meaning "heart")
-logy	study of	physiology *fiz-ē-OL-ō-jē*	Study of function in a living organism (from root *physi/o,* meaning "nature")

Exercise 2-2

Write the suffix in each of the following words that means "study of," "medical specialty," or "specialist in a field of study":

1. dentist (one who treats the teeth and mouth)
    DEN-tist   _____ -ist _____

2. neurology (the study of the nervous system)
    nū-ROL-ō-jē   _____

3. pediatrics (treatment of children) (Fig. 2-2)
    pē-dē-AT-riks   _____

4. technologist (specialist in a technical field)
    tek-NOL-ō-jist   _____

5. psychiatry (study and treatment of mental disorders)
    sī-KĪ-a-trē   _____

Write a word for a specialist in each of the following fields:

6. anatomy (study of body structure)
    a-NAT-ō-mē   _____

7. pediatrics (care and treatment of children)
    pē-dē-AT-riks   _____

8. radiology (use of radiation in diagnosis and treatment)
    rā-dē-OL-ō-jē   _____

9. orthodontics (correction of the teeth)
    or-thō-DON-tiks   _____

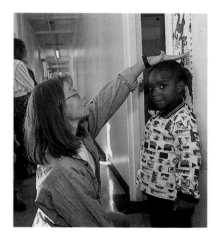

FIGURE 2-2. A practitioner of pediatrics. (Reprinted with permission from Taylor C, Lillis C, LeMone P. Fundamentals of Nursing: The Art and Science of Nursing Care. 4th Ed. Philadelphia: Lippincott, Williams & Wilkins, 2001.)

BOX 2-1 Suffixes With a Meaning All Their Own

Suffixes sometimes take on a color of their own as they are added to different words. The suffix *-thon* is taken from the name of the Greek town Marathon, from which news of a battle victory was carried by a long-distance runner. It has been attached to various words to mean a contest of great endurance. We have bike-athons, dance-athons, telethons, even major charity fund-raisers called thon-a-thons.

The adjective ending *-ish*, as in Scottish, can be added to imply that something is not right on target, as in largish, softish, oldish.

In science and medicine, the ending *-tech* is used to imply high technology, and *-pure* may be added to inspire confidence, as in the company name Genentech and the Multi-Pure water filter. The ending *-mate* suggests a helping device, as in HeartMate, a pump used to assist a damaged heart

Adjective Suffixes

The suffixes below are all adjective endings that mean "pertaining to" or "resembling" (Table 2-3). There are no rules for which ending to use for a given noun. Familiarity comes with practice. When necessary, tips on proper usage are given in the text.

TABLE 2-3 Suffixes That Mean "Pertaining to" or "Resembling"

SUFFIX	EXAMPLE	DEFINITION OF EXAMPLE
-ac	cardiac CAR-dē-ak	pertaining to the heart
-al	skeletal SKEL-e-tal	pertaining to the skeleton
-ar	muscular MUS-kū-lar	pertaining to muscles
-ary	dietary dī-e-tar-ē	pertaining to the diet
-form	muciform MŪ-si-form	like or resembling mucus
-ic*	metric ME-trik	pertaining to a meter (unit of measurement) (Fig. 2-3)
-ical (ic + al)	anatomical an-a-TOM-i-kl	pertaining to anatomy
-ile	febrile FEB-rīl	pertaining to fever
-oid	toxoid TOK-soyd	resembling toxin (poison)
-ory	respiratory RES-pi-ra-tor-ē	pertaining to respiration
-ous	venous VĒ-nus	pertaining to a vein

*For words ending with the suffix *-sis*, the first *s* in the ending is changed to *t* before adding *-ic* to form the adjective, as in psychotic, pertaining to psychosis (a mental disorder), or diuretic, pertaining to diuresis (increased urination).

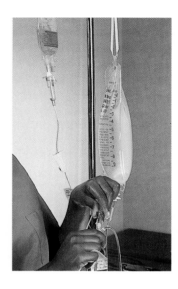

FIGURE 2-3. The metric system is used for all scientific and clinical measurements. (Reprinted with permission from Taylor C, Lillis C, LeMone P. Fundamentals of Nursing: The Art and Science of Nursing Care. 4th Ed. Philadelphia: Lippincott, Williams & Wilkins, 2001.)

 Exercise 2-3

Identify the suffix meaning "pertaining to" or "resembling" in each of the following words:

1. salivary (pertaining to saliva)
   SAL-i-var-ē
   _____ -ary _____

2. pelvic (pertaining to the pelvis)
   PEL-vik
   _____

3. neurotic (pertaining to neurosis)
   nū-ROT-ik
   _____

4. fibrous (pertaining to fibers)
   FĪ-brus
   _____

5. epileptiform (resembling epilepsy)
   ep-i-LEP-ti-form
   _____

6. ovoid (resembling an egg)
   OV-oyd
   _____

7. topical (pertaining to a surface)
   TOP-i-kal
   _____

8. virile (masculine)
   VIR-il
   _____

9. vocal (pertaining to the voice)
   VŌ-kal
   _____

10. surgical (pertaining to surgery)
    SUR-ji-kal
    _____

11. nuclear (pertaining to a nucleus)
    NŪ-klē-ar
    _____

12. urinary (pertaining to urine)
    Ū-ri-nar-ē

    _____

13. circulatory (pertaining to circulation)
    SIR-kū-la-tor-ē

    _____

Forming Plurals

Many medical words have special plural forms based on the ending of the word. Table 2-4 gives some general rules for the formation of plurals along with examples. The plural endings listed in column 2 are substituted for the word endings in column 1.

Some Exceptions to the Rules

There are exceptions to the rules above for forming plurals, some of which will appear in later chapters. For example, the plural of *virus* is *viruses*, and *serums* is sometimes used instead of *sera*. An *-es* ending may be added to words ending in *-ex* or *-ix* to form a plural, as in *appendixes*, *apexes*, and *indexes*.

Some people, in error, use *phalange* as the singular of *phalanges*. Words ending in *-oma*, meaning "tumor," should be changed to *-omata*, but most people just add an s to form the plural. For example, the plural of *carcinoma* (a type of cancer) should be *carcinomata*, but *carcinomas* is commonly used.

TABLE 2-4 Plural Endings

WORD ENDING	PLURAL ENDING	SINGULAR EXAMPLE	PLURAL EXAMPLE
a	ae	gingiva (gum) *JIN-ji-va*	gingivae *JIN-ji-vē*
en	ina	foramen (opening) *fō-RĀ-men*	foramina *fō-RAM-i-na*
ex, ix, yx	ices	appendix (something added) *a-PEN-dix*	appendices *a-PEN-di-sēz*
is	es	diagnosis (identification of disease) *dī-ag-NŌ-sis*	diagnoses *dī-ag-NŌ-sēz*
ma	mata	stigma (mark or scar) *STIG-ma*	stigmata *stig-MAT-a*
nx (anx, inx, ynx)	nges	phalanx (bone of finger or toe) *fa-LANKS*	phalanges *fa-LAN-jēz*
on	a	spermatozoon (male reproductive cell) *sper-ma-tō-ZŌ-on*	spermatozoa *sper-ma-tō-ZŌ-a*
um	a	ovum (egg) *Ō-vum*	ova *Ō-va*
us	ii	embolus *EM-bō-lus*	emboli *EM-bō-lī*

Exercise 2-4

Write the plural form of each of the following words. The word ending is underlined in each.

1. vertebr<u>a</u> (bone of the spine) (Fig. 2-4)   _____vertebrae_____
   VER-te-bra

2. gangli<u>on</u> (mass of nerve tissue)   _____
   GANG-lē-on

3. oment<u>um</u> (abdominal membrane)   _____
   ō-MEN-tum

4. test<u>is</u> (male gonad)   _____
   TES-tis

5. lum<u>en</u> (central opening)   _____
   LU-min

6. matr<u>ix</u> (background substance; mold)   _____
   MĀ-triks

7. ser<u>um</u> (liquid)   _____
   SĒ-rum

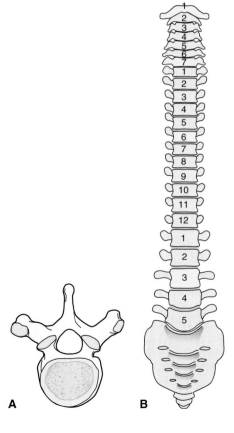

FIGURE 2-4. Each bone of the spine is a vertebra **(A).** The spinal column is made of 26 vertebrae **(B).** (Reprinted with permission from Cohen BJ, Wood DL. Memmler's The Human Body in Health and Disease. 9th Ed. Philadelphia: Lippincott Williams & Wilkins, 2000.)

8. meni<u>nx</u> (membrane around the brain and spinal cord) _____
   ME-ninks

9. foc<u>us</u> (center) _____
   FŌ-kus

10. pelv<u>is</u> (bony hip girdle) _____
    PEL-vis

11. adeno<u>ma</u> (tumor of a gland) _____
    ad-e-NŌ-ma

Chapter Review 2-1

Identify the suffix that means "condition of" in each of the following words:

1. egotism (*E-gō-tizm*) _____

2. anemia (*a-NĒ-mē-a*) _____

3. stenosis (*ste-NŌ-sis*) _____

4. dystrophy (*DIS-trō-fē*) _____

5. acidosis (*as-i-DŌ-sis*) _____

6. anesthesia (*an-es-THĒ-zē-a*) _____

Give the suffix in the following words that means "specialty" or "specialist":

7. psychiatry (*sī-KĪ-a-trē*) _____

8. orthopedist (*or-thō-PĒ-dist*) _____

9. obstetrics (ob-STET-riks) _____

10. urology (*ū-ROL-ō-jē*) _____

Give the name of the specialist in each of the following fields:

11. pediatrics (*pē-dē-A-triks*) _____

12. dermatology (*der-ma-TOL-ō-jē*) _____

13. pharmacy (*FAR-ma-sē*) _____

14. gynecology (*gī-ne-KOL-ō-jē*) _____

Identify the adjective suffix in each of the following words that means "pertaining to" or "resembling":

15. physiologic (*fiz-ē-ō-LOJ-ik*) _____

16. local (*LŌ-kal*) _____

17. cutaneous (*kū-TĀ-nē-us*) _____

18. lymphoid (*LIM-foyd*) _____

19. cellular (*SEL-ū-lar*) _____

20. basic (*BĀ-sik*) _____

21. salivary (*SAL-i-var-ē*) _____

22. oral (*OR-al*) _____

23. rheumatoid (*RŪ-ma-toyd*) _____

24. virile (*VIR-il*) _____

25. anatomical (*an-a-TOM-i-kal*) _____

26. circular (*SIR-ku-lar*) _____

27. exploratory (*ek-SPLOR-a-tor-ē*) _____

Write the plural for each of the following words. The word ending is underlined:

28. patell<u>a</u> (kneecap) _____
    pa-TEL-a

29. prognos<u>is</u> (prediction of disease outcome) _____
    prog-NŌ-sis

30. bacter<u>ium</u> (type of microorganism) _____
    bak-TĒ-rē-um

31. fung<u>us</u> (simple, nongreen plant) _____
    FUN-gus

32. protozo<u>on</u> (single-celled animal) _____
    prō-tō-ZŌ-an

33. phary<u>nx</u> (throat) _____
    FAR-inks

34. ap<u>ex</u> (high point; tip) _____
    Ā-peks

Write the singular form for each of the following words. The word ending is underlined:

35. foram<u>ina</u> (openings) _____
    fō-RAM-i-na

36. nucl<u>ei</u> (center; core) _____
    NU-klē-ī

37. gangl<u>ia</u> (small masses of nerve tissue) _____
    GANG-lē-a

38. vertebr<u>ae</u> (spinal bones) _____
    VER-te-brē

39. ind<u>ices</u> (directories; lists) _____
    IN-di-sēz

40. carcinom<u>ata</u> (cancers) _____
    kar-si-NŌ-ma-ta

Case Study

Case Study 2-1: Health Problems on Return From the Rain Forest

E.G., a 39-year-old archaeologist and university professor, returned from a 6-month expedition in the rain forest of South America suffering from a combination of physical symptoms and conditions that would not subside on their own. He was fatigued, yet unable to sleep through the night. He also had a mild fever, night sweats, occasional dizziness, double vision, and mild crampy abdominal pain accompanied by intermittent diarrhea. In addition, he had a nonhealing wound on his ankle from an insect bite. He made an appointment with his family doctor, an internist.

On examination, E.G. was febrile (feverish) with a temperature of 101°F. His heart and lungs were normal, with a slightly elevated heart rate. His abdomen was tender to palpation (touch), and his bowel sounds were active and gurgling to auscultation (listening with a stethoscope). His skin was dry and warm. He had symmetrical areas of edema (swelling) around both knees and tenderness over both patellae (kneecaps). The ulceration on his left lateral ankle had a ring of necrosis (tissue death) surrounding an area of granulation tissue. There was a small amount of purulent (pus-containing) drainage.

E.G.'s doctor ordered a series of hematology lab studies and stool cultures for ova and parasites. The doctor suspected a viral disease, possibly carried by mosquitoes, indigenous to tropical rain forests. He also suspected a form of dysentery typically caused by protozoa. E.G. was also possibly anemic, dehydrated, and septic (infected). The doctor was confident that after definitive diagnosis and treatment, E.G. would gain relief from his insomnia, diplopia (double vision), and dizziness.

CASE STUDY QUESTIONS

Multiple choice: Select the best answer and write the letter of your choice to the left of each number.

_____ 1. Diplopia, the condition of having double vision, has the suffix:
   a. lopia
   b. opia
   c. ia
   d. pia
   e. plopia

_____ 2. The adjective *septic* is formed from the noun:
   a. sepsis
   b. septosis
   c. septemia
   d. septery
   e. anemia

_____ 3. E.G. was suspected of having anemia (diminished hemoglobin). The adjective form of the noun *anemia* is _____, and the field of health science devoted to the study of blood is called _____.
   a. anemic; hematology
   b. hematosis; hematism
   c. dehemia; hematomegaly
   d. anemic; parasitology
   e. microhematic; hemacology

Case Study, continued

Write the suffix that means "condition of" in each of the following words:

4. necrosis _____

5. dysentery _____

6. insomnia _____

Write the adjective ending of each of the following words:

7. febrile _____

8. symmetrical _____

9. anemic _____

Write the singular form of each of the following words:

10. patellae _____

11. ova _____

12. protozoa _____

Write a word from the case study that means each of the following:

13. The word *virus* used as an adjective _____

14. The noun form of the adjective *necrotic* _____

15. Expert in the field of archeology _____

16. Expert in the field of internal medicine _____

17. The noun *abdomen* used as an adjective _____

CHAPTER 2 Answer Section

Answers to Chapter Exercises

EXERCISE 2-1

1. -ism
2. -y
3. -ia
4. -ism
5. -sis, -osis
6. -sis, -asis
7. -ia
8. -sis, -osis
9. -y

EXERCISE 2-2

1. -ist
2. -logy
3. -iatrics
4. -ist
5. -iatry
6. anatomist

7. pediatrician
8. radiologist
9. orthodontist

EXERCISE 2-3

1. -ary
2. -ic
3. -ic
4. -ous
5. -form
6. -oid
7. -ical
8. –ile
9. -al
10. -ical
11. -ar
12. -ary
13. -ory

EXERCISE 2-4

1. vertebrae (*VER-te-brē*)
2. ganglia (*GANG-lē-a*)
3. omenta (*ō-MEN-ta*)
4. testes (*TES-tēz*)
5. lumina (*LŪ-min-a*)
6. matrices (*MĀ-tri-sēz*)
7. sera (*SĒ-ra*)
8. meninges (*me-NIN-jēz*)
9. foci (*FŌ-si*)
10. pelves (*PEL-vēz*)
11. adenomata (*ad-e-NŌ-ma-ta*)

Answers to Chapter Review 2-1

1. -ism
2. -ia
3. -sis
4. -y
5. -sis
6. -ia
7. -iatry
8. -ist
9. -ics
10. -logy
11. pediatrician
12. dermatologist
13. pharmacist

14. gynecologist
15. -ic
16. -al
17. -ous
18. -oid
19. -ar
20. -ic
21. -ary
22. -al
23. -oid
24. -ile
25. -ical
26. -ar
27. -ory
28. patellae
29. prognoses
30. bacteria
31. fungi
32. protozoa
33. pharynges
34. apices
35. foramen
36. nucleus
37. ganglion
38. vertebra
39. index
40. carcinoma

Answers to Case Study Questions

1. c
2. a
3. a
4. -sis
5. -y
6. -ia
7. -ile
8. -ical
9. -ic
10. patella
11. ovum
12. protozoon
13. viral
14. necrosis
15. archeologist
16. internist
17. abdominal

CHAPTER **3**

Prefixes

Chapter Contents

Objectives

After study of this chapter you should be able to:

1. Define a prefix and explain how prefixes are used.
2. Identify and define some of the prefixes used in medical terminology.
3. Use prefixes to form words used in medical terminology.

A prefix is a short word part added before a word or word root to modify its meaning. For example, the word lateral means "side." Adding the prefix uni-, meaning "one," forms unilateral, which means "affecting or involving one side." Adding the prefix contra-, meaning "against or opposite," forms contralateral, which refers to an opposite side. The term equilateral means "having equal sides." Prefixes in this book will be followed by a hyphen to show that other parts will be added to the prefix to form a word.

This chapter introduces most of the prefixes used in medical terminology. Although the list is long, almost all of the prefixes you will need to work through this book are presented here. There is just one short additional chart of prefixes related to position in Chapter 5 on body structure. The meanings of many of these prefixes will be familiar to you from words that are already in your vocabulary. The words in the charts are given as examples of usage. Almost all of them will reappear in later chapters. If you forget a prefix as you work, you may refer to this chapter or to the alphabetical lists of word parts and meanings in the glossary.

Common Prefixes

TABLE 3-1 Prefixes for Numbers*

PREFIX	MEANING	EXAMPLE	DEFINITION OF EXAMPLE
prim/i-	first	primitive PRIM-i-tiv	occurring first in time
mon/o	one	monocular mon-OK-ū-lar	pertaining to one eye
uni-	one	unicellular ū-ni-SEL-ū-lar	composed of one cell (Fig. 3-1)
hemi-	half; one side	hemisphere HEM-i-sfēr	one half of a rounded structure
semi-	half; partial	semisolid sem-ē-SOL-id	partially solid
bi-	two, twice	bicuspid bī-KUS-pid	a tooth with two points (cusps)
di-	two, twice	dimorphous dī-MOR-fus	having two forms (morph/o)
dipl/o	double	diploid DIP-loyd	having two sets of chromosomes
tri-	three	triplet TRIP-let	one of three offspring produced in a single birth
quadr/i-	four	quadrant KWOD-rant	one-fourth of an area
tetra-	four	tetrahedron tet-ra-HĒ-dron	a figure with four surfaces
multi-	many	multiple MUL-ti-pl	consisting of many parts
poly-	many, much	polysaccharide pol-ē-SAK-a-rīd	substance composed of many sugars

*Prefixes pertaining to the metric system are in the appendix.

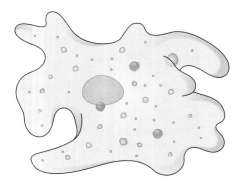

FIGURE 3-1. An amoeba, a unicellular organism.

Exercise 3-1

Fill in the blanks:

1. Monoclonal (*mon-ō-KLŌN-al*) refers to a colony (clone) derived from
   _____ cell(s).

2. The quadriceps (*KWAD-ri-seps*) muscle has _____ part(s).

3. To unify (*Ū-ni-fī*) means to make two or more parts into _____ part(s).

4. The term semilunar (*sem-ē-LŪ-nar*) means _____ moon(s).

5. A dichotomy (*dī-KOT-ō-mē*) has _____ part(s).

6. A multicellular organism has _____ cell(s).

7. A tetralogy (*te-TRAL-ō-jē*) is composed of _____ elements or factors.

8. A triangle (*TRĪ-an-gl*) has _____ angle(s).

9. Bipolar (*bī-PŌ-lar*) means having _____ pole(s).

Give a prefix that is similar in meaning to each of the following:

10. bi- _____

11. poly- _____

12. semi- _____

13. mon/o _____

TABLE 3-2 Prefixes for Colors

PREFIX	MEANING	EXAMPLE	DEFINITION OF EXAMPLE
cyan/o-	blue	cyanosis *sī-a-ON-sis*	bluish discoloration of the skin due to lack of oxygen
erythr/o-	red	erythrocyte *e-RITH-rō-sīt*	a red blood cell

TABLE 3-2 Prefixes for Colors, *continued*

PREFIX	MEANING	EXAMPLE	DEFINITION OF EXAMPLE
leuk/o-	white, colorless	leukoplakia *lū-kō-PLĀ-kē-a*	white patches in the mouth
melan/o-	black, dark	melanin *MEL-a-nin*	the dark pigment that colors the hair and skin
xanth/o-	yellow	xanthoderma *zan-thō-DER-ma*	yellow coloration of the skin

 # Exercise 3-2

Match the following terms and write the appropriate letter to the left of each number:

_____ 1. melanocyte (*MEL-a-nō-sīt*)

_____ 2. xanthoma (*zan-THŌ-ma*)

_____ 3. cyanotic (*sī-a-NOT-ik*)

_____ 4. erythroderma (*e-rith-rō-DER-ma*)

_____ 5. leukemia (*lū-KĒ-mē-a*)

a. pertaining to bluish discoloration

b. redness of the skin

c. yellow raised area on the skin

d. cell that produces dark pigment

e. overgrowth of white blood cells

TABLE 3-3 Negative Prefixes

PREFIX	MEANING	EXAMPLE	DEFINITION OF EXAMPLE
a-, an-	not; without	aseptic *ā-SEP-tik*	free of infectious organisms
anti-	against	antidote *AN-ti-dōt*	means for counteracting a poison
contra-	against, opposite	contraception *kon-tra-SEP-shun*	prevention of conception
de-	down, without	depilatory *dē-PIL-a-tor-ē*	agent used to remove hair (pil/o)
dis-	absence, removal, separation	dissect *di-SEKT*	to separate tissues for anatomical study
in-*; im- (used before b, m, p)	not	insignificant *in-sig-NIF-i-cant*	not important
non-	not	noninfectious *non-in-FEK-shus*	not able to spread disease
un-	not	unconscious *un-KON-shus*	not responsive

*May also mean "in" or "into" as in inject, inhale.

Exercise 3-3

Identify and define the prefix in each of the following words:

	Prefix	Meaning of Prefix
1. amorphous (without form) (root morph/o)	a-	not, without, lack of, absence (a-MOR-fus)
2. antibody	_____	_____
3. amnesia	_____	_____
4. disintegrate	_____	_____
5. contralateral	_____	_____
6. incontinent	_____	_____
7. dehumidify	_____	_____
8. noncontributory	_____	_____

Add a prefix to form the negative of each of the following words:

9. coordinated	uncoordinated
10. adequate	_____
11. infect	_____
12. permeable (capable of being penetrated)	_____
13. congestant	_____
14. compatible	_____

BOX 3-1 Prefix Shorthand

Many prefixes catch on rapidly as a form of shorthand. In everyday life, the prefix e- for electronic has spread to words such as e-mail, e-commerce, e-Bay, and many more. X- for extreme appears in X-games and other X-sports.

The prefix endo- in the names of many surgical instruments signifies new endoscopic instruments that are longer and thinner and have smaller working tips to be used in areas where there is minimal access. Some examples are endoscissors, endosuture, endocautery, endograsper, and endosnare.

Health care products designed for specific age groups are also encoded by prefixes. Geri-, pertaining to old age, as in geriatrics, appears in geri-chair, geri-pads, geri-jacket, and the patent medicine Geritol, among others. Pedi- or pedia-, meaning "child," is found in the names pedi-cath, pedi-dose, pedi-set (instruments), and Pedialyte, a product used for children to replace fluid and electrolytes.

TABLE 3-4 Prefixes for Direction

PREFIX	MEANING	EXAMPLE	DEFINITION OF EXAMPLE
ab-	away from	abduct *ab-DUKT*	to move away from the midline
ad-	toward; near	adhere *ad-HĒR*	to attach or stick together
dia-	through	dialysis *dī-AL-i-sis*	separation (-lysis) by passage through a membrane (Fig. 3-2)
per-	through	percutaneous *per-kū-TĀ-nē-us*	through the skin
trans-	through	transfusion *trans-FŪ-zhun*	introduction of blood or blood components into the bloodstream

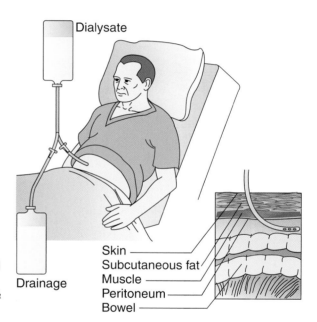

FIGURE 3-2. Peritoneal dialysis, in which the dialysate is infused into the peritoneal cavity by gravity. (Reprinted with permission from Rosdahl, Kowalski. Textbook of Basic Nursing. 8th Ed. Philadelphia: Lippincott Williams & Wilkins, 2003:1208.)

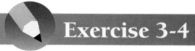

Exercise 3-4

Identify and define the prefix in each of the following words:

	Prefix	Meaning of Prefix
1. perforate	_____	_____
2. adjacent	_____	_____
3. abnormal	_____	_____
4. diarrhea	_____	_____
5. transfer	_____	_____

TABLE 3-5 Prefixes for Degree

PREFIX	MEANING	EXAMPLE	DEFINITION OF EXAMPLE
hyper-	over, excess, abnormally high, increased	hyperventilation *hī-per-ven-ti-LĀ-shun*	excess breathing
hypo-*	under, below, abnormally low, decreased	hypoxia *hī-POK-sē-a*	decreased oxygen in the tissues
olig/o-	few, scanty	oligomenorrhea *ol-i-gō-men-ō-RE-a*	a scanty menstrual flow (men/o)
pan-	all	panacea *pan-a-SĒ-a*	remedy that cures all ills; a cure-all
super-*	above, excess	supernumerary *su-per-NŪ-mer-ar-ē*	in excess number

*May also show position, as in hypodermic, superficial.

Exercise 3-5

Match the following terms and write the appropriate letter to the left of each number:

_____ 1. pandemic (*pan-DEM-ik*)

_____ 2. hyposecretion (*hi-pō-sē-KRĒ-shun*)

_____ 3. hypertension (*hī-per-TEN-shun*)

_____ 4. oligodontia (*ol-i-gō-DON-shē-a*)

_____ 5. superficial (*sū-per-FISH-al*)

a. located at the surface (above other structures)

b. less than the normal number of teeth

c. underproduction of a substance

d. disease affecting an entire population

e. high blood pressure

TABLE 3-6 Prefixes for Size and Comparison

PREFIX	MEANING	EXAMPLE	DEFINITION OF EXAMPLE
equi-	equal, same	equilateral *e-kwi-LAT-er-al*	having equal sides
eu-	true, good, easy, normal	euthanasia *ū-tha-NĀ-zē-a*	easy or painless death (root thanat/o)
hetero-	other, different, unequal	heterosexual *het-er-ō-SEX-ū-al*	pertaining to the opposite sex
homo-, homeo-	same, unchanging	homothermic *hō-mō-THER-mik*	maintaining a constant body temperature (root therm/o); warm blooded
iso-	equal, same	isograft *I-sō-graft*	graft between two genetically identical individuals
macro-	large, abnormally large	macrocyte *MAK-rō-sīt*	extremely large red blood cell

TABLE 3-6 Prefixes for Size and Comparison, *continued*

PREFIX	MEANING	EXAMPLE	DEFINITION OF EXAMPLE
mega-,* megalo-	large; abnormally large	megabladder *meg-a-BLAD-er*	enlargement of the bladder
micro-†	small	microscopic *mī-krō-SKOP-ik*	extremely small; visible only through a microscope
neo-	new	neonate *NĒ-ō-nāt*	a newborn infant (Fig. 3-3)
normo-	normal	normovolemia *nor-mō-vol-Ē-mē-a*	normal blood volume
ortho-	straight, correct, upright	orthotic *or-THOT-ik*	correcting or preventing deformities
poikilo-	varied; irregular	poikiloderma *poy-ki-lō-DER-ma*	mottled condition of the skin
pseudo-	false	pseudoplegia *sū-dō-PLĒ-jē-a*	false paralysis (suffix -plegia)
re-	again; back	regurgitation *rē-gur-ji-TĀ-shun*	backward or return flow, as of blood or stomach contents

*Mega- also means "one million" as in megahertz.
†Micro- also means "one millionth" as in microsecond.

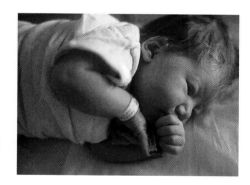

FIGURE 3-3. A neonate (newborn). (Reprinted with permission from Taylor C, Lillis C, LeMone P. Fundamentals of Nursing: The Art and Science of Nursing Care. 4th ed. Philadelphia: Lippincott Williams & Wilkins, 2001.)

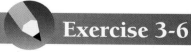 Exercise 3-6

Match the following terms and write the appropriate letter to the left of each number:

_____ 1. reflux (*RĒ-flux*)

_____ 2. orthodontic (*or-thō-DON-tik*)

_____ 3. pseudoreaction (*sū-dō-rē-AK-shun*)

_____ 4. poikilocyte (*POY-kil-ō-sīt*)

_____ 5. normothermic (*nor-mō-THER-mik*)

a. an irregularly shaped cell

b. pertaining to normal body temperature

c. backward flow

d. false response

e. pertaining to straight teeth

Identify and define the prefix in each of the following words:

	Prefix	Meaning of Prefix
6. equidistant	_____	_____
7. orthopedics	_____	_____
8. recuperate	_____	_____
9. euthyroidism	_____	_____
10. neocortex	_____	_____
11. megacolon	_____	_____
12. isometric	_____	_____

Write the opposite of each of the following words:

13. heterogeneous (composed of different materials) _____

14. macroscopic (visible with the naked eye) _____

TABLE 3-7 Prefixes for Time and/or Position

PREFIX	MEANING	EXAMPLE	DEFINITION OF EXAMPLE
ante-	before	antenatal *an-tē-NĀ-tal*	before birth
pre-	before, in front of	predisposing *prē-dis-PŌZ-ing*	leading toward a condition, such as disease
pro-	before, in front of	prodrome *prō-drōm*	symptom that precedes a disease
post-	after, behind	postmenopausal *pōst-men-ō-PAW-sal*	after menopause

 ## Exercise 3-7

Match the following terms and write the appropriate letter to the left of each number:

1. postnasal (*pōst-NĀ-zal*)   a. throwing or extending forward

2. antecedent (*an-tē-SĒ-dent*)   b. occurring before the proper time

3. projection (*prō-JEK-shun*)   c. behind the nose

4. premature (*prē-ma-CHŪR*)   d. before birth

5. prenatal (*prē-NĀ-tal*)   e. occurring before another event

Identify and define the prefix in each of the following words:

	Prefix	Meaning of Prefix
6. premenstrual (prē-MEN-strū-al)	_____	_____
7. post-traumatic (pōst-traw-MAT-ik)	_____	_____
8. progenitor (prō-JEN-i-tor)	_____	_____
9. antedate (an-ti-DĀT)	_____	_____

TABLE 3-8 Prefixes for Position

PREFIX	MEANING	EXAMPLE	DEFINITION OF EXAMPLE
dextr/o-	right	dextrocardia *deks-trō-KAR-dē-a*	location of the heart (cardi/o) in the right side of the chest
sinistr/o-	left	sinistrad *sin-IS-trad*	toward the left
ec-, ecto-	out; outside	ectoderm *EK-tō-derm*	outermost layer of the developing embryo
ex/o-	away from; outside	excise *ek-SĪZ*	to cut out
end/o-	in; within	endoscope *EN-dō-skōp*	device for viewing the inside of a cavity or organ
mes/o-	middle	mesencephalon *mes-en-SEF-a-lon*	midbrain
syn-, sym- (used before b, m, p,)	together	synapse *SIN-aps*	a junction between two nerve cells (Fig. 3-4)
tel/e-, tel/o-	end	telangion *tel-AN-jē-on*	a terminal vessel (root angi/o)

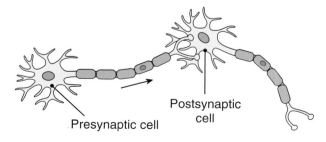

FIGURE 3-4. A synapse. (Reprinted with permission from Cohen BJ, Wood DL. Memmler's The Human Body in Health and Disease. 9th Ed. Philadelphia: Lippincott Williams & Wilkins, 2000.)

Presynaptic cell

Postsynaptic cell

Exercise 3-8

Match the following terms and write the appropriate letter to the left of each number:

_____ 1. endonasal (*en-dō-NĀ-zal*)

_____ 2. syndrome (*SIN-drōm*)

_____ 3. mesoderm (*MES-ō-derm*)

_____ 4. ectocardia (*ek-tō-KAR-dē-a*)

_____ 5. Telophase (*TEL-e-fāz*)

a. placement of the heart outside its normal position

b. middle layer of the developing embryo

c. the last stage of cell division

d. within the nose

e. group of symptoms occurring together

Identify and define the prefix in each of the following words:

	Prefix	Meaning of Prefix
6. synthesis	_____	_____
7. extract	_____	_____
8. ectopic (*ek-TOP-ik*)	_____	_____
9. symbiosis (*sim-bī-Ō-sis*)	_____	_____
10. endoplasm (*en-dō-PLAZM*)	_____	_____

Write the opposite of each of the following words:

11. exogenous (outside the organism) _____
    eks-OJ-e-nus

12. sinistromanual (left handed) _____
    sin-is-trō-MAN-ū-al

13. endoderm (outermost layer of the embryo) _____
    EN-dō-derm

Chapter Review 3-1

Match the following terms and write the appropriate letter to the left of each number:

_____ 1. primary

_____ 2. trisect

_____ 3. unilateral

_____ 4. polymorphous

_____ 5. hemithorax

a. one half or one side of the chest

b. having many forms

c. to cut into three parts

d. pertaining to one side

e. first

_____ 6. neonate

_____ 7. melanoma

a. cell with yellow color

b. through the skin

_____ 8. xanthocyte

_____ 9. percutaneous

_____ 10. leukoderma

c. dark tumor

d. a newborn

e. loss of color in the skin

_____ 11. heterothermic

_____ 12. mesencephalon

_____ 13. panplegia

_____ 14. telencephalon

_____ 15. orthopedic

a. endbrain

b. having varying body temperature

c. total paralysis

d. correcting or preventing deformities

e. midbrain

Match each of the following prefixes with its meaning:

_____ 16. oligo-

_____ 17. pseudo-

_____ 18. eu-

_____ 19. iso-

_____ 20. dextro-

a. equal, same

b. right

c. few, scanty

d. good, true, easy

e. false

Fill in the blanks:

21. A monocular microscope has _____ eyepiece(s).

22. To bisect is to cut into _____ parts.

23. A quadruped animal has _____ feet.

24. Sinistrad means toward the _____.

25. A triad has _____ part(s).

26. A unicellular organism is composed of _____ cell(s).

27. A diatomic molecule has _____ atom(s).

28. A tetralogy is composed of _____ part(s).

Identify and define the prefix in each of the following words:

	Prefix	Meaning of Prefix
29. nonexistent	_____	_____
30. transmit	_____	_____
31. equivalent	_____	_____
32. react	_____	_____
33. exhale	_____	_____
34. absent	_____	_____
35. contraindication	_____	_____
36. detoxify	_____	_____

37. predict   _____   _____

38. perforate   _____   _____

39. adduct   _____   _____

40. dialyze (*DĪ-a-līz*)   _____   _____

41. antiserum   _____   _____

42. microsurgery   _____   _____

43. disease   _____   _____

44. ectoparasite   _____   _____

45. symbiotic (*sim-bī-OT-ik*)   _____   _____

46. prognosis (*prog-NŌ-sis*)   _____   _____

47. inadequate   _____   _____

Opposites. Write a word that means the opposite of each of the following:

48. responsive _____

49. mature _____

50. active _____

51. sufficient _____

52. exotoxin _____

53. macroscopic _____

54. homograft _____

55. hypoactive _____

56. preoperative _____

Synonyms. Write a word that means the same as each of the following:

57. supersensitivity _____

58. megalocyte (extremely large red blood cell) _____

59. antenatal _____

60. equilateral (having equal sides) _____

Case Studies

Case Study 3-1: Displaced Fracture of the Femoral Neck

While walking home from the train station, M.A., a 72-year-old woman with osteoporosis, tripped over a broken curb and fell. In the emergency department, she was assessed for severe pain, swelling, and bruising of her left thigh. A radiograph showed a displaced left femoral neck fracture. M.A. was pre-

Case Studies, continued

pared for surgery and given a preoperative injection of an analgesic to relieve her pain. Intraoperatively, she was given spinal anesthesia and positioned on an operating room table, with her left hip elevated on a small pillow. Intravenous antibiotics were given before the incision. Her left hip was repaired with a bipolar hemiarthroplasty. Postoperative care included maintaining the left hip in abduction, blood and fluid replacement, physical therapy, and vigilance for development of avascular necrosis and possible dislocation.

Case Study 3-2: Intertrochanteric Fracture

A.R., age 88, slipped on the wet grass and fell while gardening in his back yard. His neighbor was unable to help him to a standing position and called for an ambulance. A.R. had excruciating pain in his right leg, which was externally rotated, slightly shorter than his left leg, and adducted. Preoperative radiographs showed a non-displaced right intertrochanteric fracture. Intraoperatively, Mr. R. was given spinal anesthesia and positioned on an orthopedic table with his right hip abducted and secured in traction. He had an open reduction and internal fixation with a compression screw and side plate with screws. His postoperative recovery was unremarkable, although he was at risk for deep vein thrombosis, that is, blood clots in his legs. He was discharged to a rehabilitation facility for several weeks of physical therapy and assistance with activities of daily living, such as personal hygiene, dressing, eating, ambulating, and toileting.

CASE STUDY QUESTIONS

Write a word from the case histories that means the same as each of the following:

1. replacement of half of the joint component _____

2. substances that act against microorganisms _____

3. in a position away from the midline of the body _____

4. position toward the midline of the body _____

Identify and define the prefixes in the following words:

	Prefix	Meaning of Prefix
5. displace and dislocate	_____	_____
6. replacement, recovery, and rehabilitation	_____	_____
7. avascular	_____	_____
8. anesthesia and analgesic	_____	_____
9. orthopedic	_____	_____
10. externally	_____	_____
11. bipolar	_____	_____
12. unremarkable	_____	_____

Case Studies, continued

Fill in the blanks:

13. The adjective for the operative time span from decision for surgery to placement on the operating room table is _____ .

14. The adjective for the operative time span from placement on the operating room table until transfer to postanesthesia recovery unit or intensive care unit is _____ .

15. The adjective for the operative time span from admission to postanesthesia is _____ .

CHAPTER 3 Answer Section

Answers to Chapter Exercises

EXERCISE 3-1

1. one
2. four
3. one
4. half
5. two
6. many
7. four
8. three
9. two
10. di-
11. multi-
12. hemi-
13. uni

EXERCISE 3-2

1. d
2. c
3. a
4. b
5. e

EXERCISE 3-3

1. a-; not, without, lack of, absence
2. anti-; against, opposite
3. a-; not, without (root mnem/o means "memory")
4. dis-; absence, removal, separation
5. contra-; against
6. in-; not
7. de-; down, without, removal, loss
8. non-; not
9. uncoordinated
10. inadequate
11. disinfect
12. impermeable
13. decongestant
14. incompatible

EXERCISE 3-4

1. per-; through
2. ad-; toward, near
3. ab-; away from
4. dia-; through
5. trans-; through

EXERCISE 3-5

1. d
2. c
3. e
4. b
5. a

EXERCISE 3-6

1. c
2. e
3. d
4. a
5. b
6. equi-; equal, same
7. ortho-; straight, correct, upright
8. re-; again, back
9. eu-; true, good, easy, normal

10. neo-; new
11. mega-; large, abnormally large
12. iso-; equal, same
13. homogeneous (hō-mō-JĒ-nē-us)
14. microscopic

EXERCISE 3-7

1. c
2. e
3. a
4. b
5. d
6. pre-; before, in front of
7. post-; after, behind
8. pro-; before, in front of
9. ante-; before

EXERCISE 3-8

1. d
2. e
3. b
4. a
5. c
6. syn-; together
7. ex-; away from, outside
8. ecto-; out, outside
9. sym-; together
10. endo-; in, within
11. endogenous
12. dextromanual
13. ectoderm

Answers to Chapter Review 3-1

1. e
2. c
3. d
4. b
5. a
6. d
7. c
8. a
9. b
10. e
11. b
12. e
13. c
14. a
15. d
16. c
17. e
18. d
19. a
20. b
21. one
22. two

23. four
24. left
25. three
26. one
27. two
28. four
29. non-; not
30. trans-; through, across, beyond
31. equi-; equal, same
32. re-; again, back
33. ex-; away from, outside
34. ab-; away from
35. contra-; against, opposite
36. de-; down, without
37. pre-; before, in front of
38. per-; through
39. ad-; toward, near
40. dia-; through
41. anti-; against
42. micro-; small
43. dis-; absence, removal, separation
44. ecto-; out, outside
45. sym-; together
46. pro-; before, in front of
47. in-; not
48. unresponsive
49. immature
50. inactive
51. insufficient
52. endotoxin
53. microscopic
54. heterograft
55. hyperactive
56. postoperative
57. hypersensitivity
58. macrocyte
59. prenatal
60. isolateral

Answers to Case Study Questions

1. hemiarthroplasty
2. antibiotics
3. abduction
4. adducted
5. dis-; absence, removal, separation
6. re-; again, back
7. a-; not, without
8. an-; not, without
9. ortho-; straight, correct, upright
10. ex-; away from, outside
11. bi-; two, twice
12. un-; not
13. preoperative
14. intraoperative
15. postoperative

Cells, Tissues, and Organs

Objectives

After study of this chapter you should be able to:

1. Describe the main parts of a cell.
2. Label a diagram of a typical cell.
3. Name and give the functions of the four basic types of tissues in the body.
4. Define basic terms pertaining to the structure and function of body tissues.
5. Recognize and use roots and suffixes pertaining to cells, tissues, and organs.
6. Analyze two case studies pertaining to cells and tissues.

The Cell

The body can be studied from its simplest to its most complex level, beginning with the **cell**, the basic unit of living organisms (Fig. 4-1). Cells carry out **metabolism**, the sum of all of the physical and chemical activities that occur in the body. Providing the energy for metabolic reactions is the chemical **ATP** (adenosine triphosphate), commonly described as the energy compound of the cell. The main categories of organic compounds in the body are:

- **Proteins,** which include the enzymes, some hormones, and structural materials.
- **Carbohydrates,** which include sugars and starches. The main carbohydrate is the sugar glucose, which circulates in the blood to provide energy for the cells.
- **Lipids,** which include fats. Some hormones are derived from lipids, and adipose (fat) tissue is designed to store lipids.

Within the **cytoplasm** that fills the cell are subunits called organelles, each with a specific function. The main cell structures are named and described in Display 4-1.

All body functions derive from the activities of billions of specialized cells. The **nucleus** is the control region of the cell. It contains the **chromosomes,** which carry genetic information (Fig. 4-2). Each human

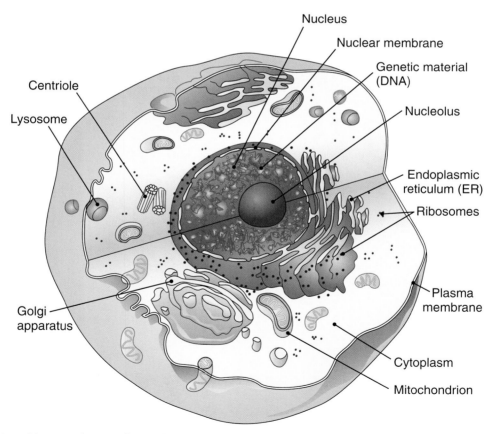

FIGURE 4-1. Diagram of a typical animal cell showing the main organelles. (Reprinted with permission from Cohen BJ, Wood DL. Memmler's The Human Body in Health and Disease. 9th Ed. Philadelphia: Lippincott Williams & Wilkins, 2000.)

DISPLAY 4-1 Cell Structures

NAME	DESCRIPTION	FUNCTION
plasma membrane	outer layer of the cell; composed mainly of lipids and proteins	limits the cell; regulates what enters and leaves the cell
cytoplasm	colloidal suspension that fills cell	holds cell contents
nucleus	large, dark-staining body near the center of the cell; composed of DNA and proteins	contains the chromosomes with the genes (the hereditary material that directs all cell activities)
nucleolus	small body in the nucleus; composed of RNA, DNA, and protein	needed for protein manufacture
endoplasmic reticulum (ER)	network of membranes in the cytoplasm	used for storage and transport; holds ribosomes
ribosomes	small bodies attached to the ER; composed of RNA and protein	manufacture proteins
mitochondria	large organelles with folded membranes inside	convert energy from nutrients into ATP
Golgi apparatus	layers of membranes	put together special substances such as mucus
lysosomes	small sacs of digestive enzymes	digest substances within the cell
centrioles	rod-shaped bodies (usually two) near the nucleus	help separate the chromosomes in cell division
cilia	short, hairlike projections from the cell	create movement around the cell
flagellum	long, whiplike extension from the cell	moves the cell

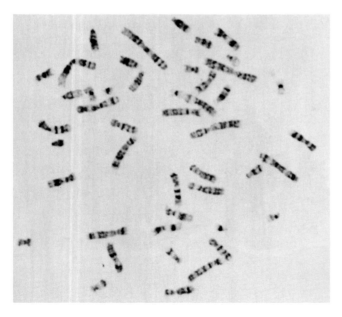

FIGURE 4-2. Human chromosomes. (Reprinted with permission from Cohen BJ, Wood DL. Memmler's The Human Body in Health and Disease. 9th Ed. Philadelphia: Lippincott Williams & Wilkins, 2000.)

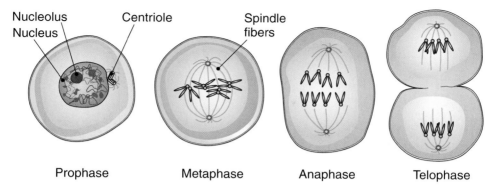

FIGURE 4-3. The stages in cell division (mitosis). (Reprinted with permission from Cohen BJ, Wood DL. Memmler's The Human Body in Health and Disease. 9th Ed. Philadelphia: Lippincott Williams & Wilkins, 2000.)

cell, except for the sex cells, contains 46 chromosomes. The chromosomes are composed of a complex organic substance, **DNA (deoxyribonucleic acid)**, which is organized into separate units called **genes**. Genes control the formation of **enzymes**, the catalysts needed for metabolic reactions. To help manufacture enzymes, the cells use a compound called **RNA (ribonucleic acid)**, which is chemically related to DNA.

When a body cell divides, by the process of **mitosis**, the chromosomes are doubled and then equally distributed to the two daughter cells (Fig. 4-3). Sex cells (egg and sperm) divide by another process (meiosis) that halves the chromosomes in preparation for fertilization.

Tissues

Cells are organized into four basic types of **tissues** that perform specific functions (Fig. 4-4)
- Epithelial (*ep-i-THĒ-lē-al*) tissue covers and protects body structures and lines organs, vessels, and cavities.
- Connective tissue supports and binds body structures. It contains fibers and other nonliving material between the cells. Included are adipose (fat) tissue, cartilage, bone (Chapter 19), and blood (Chapter 10).
- Muscle tissue (root *my/o*) contracts to produce movement. There are three types of muscle tissue:
  - Skeletal or voluntary muscle moves the skeleton. Skeletal muscle is discussed in greater detail in Chapter 20.
  - Cardiac muscle forms the heart. It functions without conscious control and is described as involuntary.
  - Smooth, or visceral, muscle forms the walls of the abdominal organs; it is also involuntary.
- Nervous tissue (root *neur/o*) makes up the brain, spinal cord, and nerves. It coordinates and controls body responses by the transmission of electrical impulses. The nervous system and senses are discussed in Chapters 17 and 18.

The simplest tissues are membranes. Mucous membranes secrete **mucus**, a thick fluid that lubricates surfaces and protects underlying tissue. Serous membranes, which secrete a thin, watery fluid, line body cavities and cover organs.

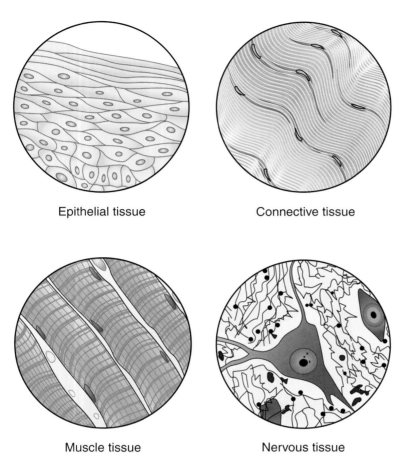

FIGURE 4-4. The four basic types of tissues. (Reprinted with permission from Cohen BJ, Wood DL. Memmler's The Human Body in Health and Disease. 9th Ed. Philadelphia: Lippincott Williams & Wilkins, 2000.)

Organs and Organ Systems

Tissues are arranged into organs, which serve specific functions (Fig. 4-5). The organs, in turn, are grouped into systems. Each of the body systems is discussed in Part 3. Bear in mind, however, that the body functions as a whole—no system is independent of the others. They work together to maintain the body's state of internal stability, termed **homeostasis**.

Key Terms

ATP	The energy compound of the cell; stores energy needed for cell activities. ATP stands for adenosine triphosphate (*a-DEN-ō-sēn trī-FOS-fāt*).
carbohydrate *kar-bō-HĪ-drāt*	The category of organic compounds that includes sugars and starches

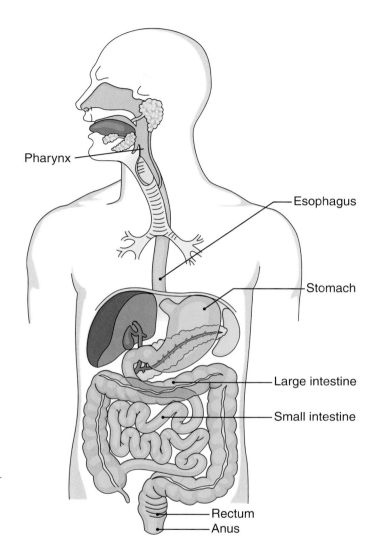

FIGURE 4-5. Organs of the digestive tract. (Reprinted with permission from Cohen BJ, Wood DL. Memmler's The Human Body in Health and Disease. 9th Ed. Philadelphia: Lippincott Williams & Wilkins, 2000.)

cell *sel*	The basic structural and functional unit of the living organism; a microscopic unit that combines with other cells to form tissues (root *cyt/o*)
chromosome *KRŌ-mō-sōm*	A threadlike body in the nucleus of a cell that contains genetic information
cytoplasm *SĪ-tō-plazm*	The fluid that fills a cell and holds the organelles
DNA	The genetic compound of the cell; makes up the genes. DNA stands for deoxyribonucleic (*dē-ok-sē-rī-bō-nū-KLĒ-ik*) acid.
enzyme *EN-zīm*	An organic substance that speeds the rate of metabolic reactions

gene *jēn*	A hereditary unit composed of DNA and combined with other genes to form the chromosomes
glucose *GLŪ-kōs*	A simple sugar that circulates in the blood; the main energy source for metabolism (roots *gluc/o, glyc/o*)
homeostasis *hō-mē-ō-STĀ-sis*	A steady state; a condition of internal stability and constancy
lipid *LIP-id*	A category of organic compounds that includes fats (root *lip/o*)
metabolism *me-TA-bō-lizm*	The sum of all the physical and chemical reactions that occur within an organism
mitosis *mī-TŌ-sis*	Cell division
mucus *MŪ-kus*	A thick fluid secreted by cells in membranes and glands that lubricates and protects tissues (roots *muc/o, myx/o*); the adjective is *mucous*
nucleus *NŪ-klē-us*	The control center of the cell; directs all cell activities based on the information contained in its chromosomes (roots *nucle/o, kary/o*)
protein *PRŌ-tēn*	A category of organic compounds that includes structural materials, enzymes, and some hormones
RNA	An organic compound involved in the manufacture of proteins within cells. RNA stands for ribonucleic (*rī-bō-nū-KLĒ-ik*) acid.
tissue *TISH-ū*	A group of cells that acts together for a specific purpose (root *hist/o, histi/o*)

Word Parts Pertaining to Cells, Tissues, and Organs

TABLE 4-1 Roots for Cells and Tissues

ROOT	MEANING	EXAMPLE	DEFINITION OF EXAMPLE
morph/o	form	polymorphic *pol-ē-MOR-fik*	having many forms
cyt/o, -cyte	cell	cytogenesis *sī-tō-JEN-e-sis*	the formation (-genesis) of cells
nucle/o	nucleus	nuclear *NŪ-klē-ar*	pertaining to a nucleus
kary/o	nucleus	karyotype (Fig. 4-6) *KAR-ē-ō-tīp*	picture of the chromosomes of a cell organized according to size
hist/o, histi/o	tissue	histologist *his-TOL-ō-jist*	specialist in the study of tissue
fibr/o	fiber	fibrosis *fī-BRŌ-sis*	abnormal formation of fibrous tissue

TABLE 4-1 Roots for Cells and Tissues, *continued*

ROOT	MEANING	EXAMPLE	DEFINITION OF EXAMPLE
reticul/o	network	reticulum *re-TIK-ū-lum*	a network
aden/o	gland	adenoma *ad-e-NO-ma*	tumor (-oma) of a gland
papill/o	nipple	papilliform *pa-PIL-i-form*	resembling a nipple
myx/o	mucus	myxadenitis *miks-ad-e-NĪ-tis*	inflammation of a gland that secretes mucus
muc/o	mucus, mucous membrane	mucorrhea *mū-kō-RĒ-a*	increased flow (-rhea) of mucus
somat/o, -some	body	*sō-MAT-ik*	pertaining to the body (as compared with the germ cells or the mind)

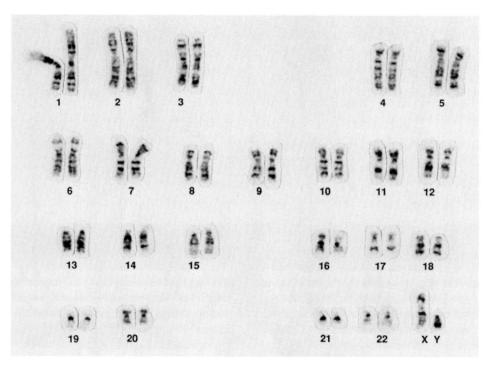

FIGURE 4-6. A karyotype of human chromosomes. (Reprinted with permission from Cohen BJ, Wood DL. Memmler's The Human Body in Health and Disease. 9th Ed. Philadelphia: Lippincott Williams & Wilkins, 2000.)

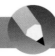 **Exercise 4-1**

Fill in the blanks:

1. Karyomegaly is enlargement (-megaly) of the _____.

2. Adenitis (ad-*e*-NĪ-*tis*) is inflammation (-itis) of a _____.

3. A papilla (*pa*-PIL-*a*) is a projection that resembles a(n) _____.

4. A fibril (FĪ-*bril*) is a small _____.

5. Histogenesis is the formation (-genesis) of _____.

6. A myxoma (*mik*-SŌ-*ma*) is a tumor of tissue that secretes _____.

7. The term reticular (*re*-TIK-*ū*-*lar*) means resembling or pertaining to a(n)
   _____.

8. A dimorphic organism has two _____.

9. The term mucosa (*mu*-KŌ-*sa*) is used to describe a membrane that secretes
   _____.

10. Nucleoplasm (NŪ-*klē*-*ō*-*plazm*) is the material that fills the _____.

11. Somatotropin (*sō*-*ma*-*tō*-TRŌ-*pin*), also called growth hormone, has a general stimulating effect on the
    _____.

Use the suffix -*logy* to build a word with each of the following meanings:

12. The study of cells _____

13. The study of tissues _____

14. The study of form _____

BOX 4-1 Laboratory Study of Tissues

Biopsy is the removal and examination of living tissue to determine a diagnosis. The term is also applied to the specimen itself. Biopsy comes from the Greek word *bios*, meaning "life," plus *opsis*, meaning "vision." Together they mean the visualization of living tissue.

Some other terms that apply to cells and tissues come from Latin. *In vivo* means "in the living body," as contrasted with *in vitro*, which literally means "in glass" and refers to procedures and experiments done in the laboratory, as compared with studies done in living organisms. *In situ* means "in its original place," and is used to refer to tumors that have not spread.

In toto means "whole" or "completely," as in referring to a structure or organ removed totally from the body. *Postmortem* literally means "after death," as in referring to an autopsy performed to determine the cause of death.

TABLE 4-2 Roots for Cell Activity

ROOT	MEANING	EXAMPLE	DEFINITION OF EXAMPLE
blast/o, -blast	immature cell, productive cell, embryonic cell	leukoblast *LŪ-kō-blast*	an immature white blood cell
gen	origin, formation	genetics *je-NET-iks*	the science of genes and heredity
phag/o	eat, ingest	phagocyte *FAG-ō-sīt*	cell that ingests waste and foreign matter
phil	attract, absorb	acidophilic *a-sid-ō-FIL-ik*	attracting acid stain
plas	formation, molding, development	hyperplasia *hī-per-PLĀ-jē-a*	overdevelopment of an organ or tissue
trop	act on, affect	chronotropic *kron-o-TROP-ik*	affecting rate or timing
troph/o	feeding, growth, nourishment	atrophy *AT-rō-fē*	wasting away (lack of nourishment)

The roots in Table 4-2 are often combined with a simple noun suffix (*-in*, *-y*, or *-ia*) or an adjective suffix (*-ic*) and used as word endings. Such combined forms that routinely appear as word endings will simply be described and used as suffixes in this book. Examples from the above list are *-trophy*, *-plasia*, *-tropin*, *-philic*, *-genic*.

Exercise 4-2

Match the following terms and write the appropriate letter to the left of each number:

_____ 1. erythroblast (*e-RITH rō-blast*)   a. organism capable of manufacturing its own food

_____ 2. hypertrophy (*hī-PER-trō-fē*)   b. formation of a nucleus

_____ 3. phagocytosis (*fag-ō-sī-TO-sis*)   c. increased growth of tissue

_____ 4. karyogenesis (*kar-ē-ō-JEN-e-sis*)   d. ingestion of waste by a cell

_____ 5. autotroph (*AW-tō-trof*)   e. immature red blood cell

_____ 6. somatotropic (*sō-mat-ō-TROP-ik*)   a. attracting color

_____ 7. chromophilic (*krō-mō-FIL-ik*)   b. acting on the body

_____ 8. neoplasia (*nē-ō-PLĀ-jē-a*)   c. substance that acts on the sex glands

_____ 9. aplasia (*a-PLĀ-jē-a*)   d. new formation of tissue

_____ 10. gonadotropin (*gon-a-dō-TRŌ-pin*)   e. lack of development

Identify and define the root in each of the following words:

	Root	Meaning of Root
11. esophagus (*e-SOF-a-gus*)	_____	_____
12. normoblast (*NOR-mō-blast*)	_____	_____
13. dystrophy (*DIS-trō-f ē*)	_____	_____
14. aplastic (*a-PLAS-tik*)	_____	_____
15. regenerate (*rē-JEN-e-rāt*)	_____	_____

TABLE 4-3 Suffixes and Roots for Body Chemistry

WORD PART	MEANING	EXAMPLE	DEFINITION OF EXAMPLE
SUFFIXES			
-ase	enzyme	lipase *LĪ-pās*	enzyme that digests fat (lipid)
-ose	sugar	lactose *LAK-tōs*	milk sugar
ROOTS			
hydr/o	water, fluid	hydrophilic *hī-drō-FIL-ik*	attracting water
gluc/o	glucose	glucosuria *glu-kō-SŪ-rē-a*	presence of glucose in the urine (-ur/o)
glyc/o	sugar, glucose	hyperglycemia *hī-per-glī-SĒ-mē-a*	high blood sugar
sacchar/o	sugar	polysaccharide *pol-ē-SAK-a-rīd*	compound containing many sugars
amyl/o	starch	amyloid *AM-i-loyd*	resembling starch
lip/o	lipid, fat	lipogenesis *lip-ō-JEN-e-sis*	formation of fat
adip/o	fat	adipocyte *AD-i-pō-sīt*	cell that stores fat
steat/o	fatty	steatorrhea *stē-a-tō-Rē-a*	discharge (-rhea) of fatty stools
prote/o	protein	protease *PRŌ-tē-ās*	enzyme that digests protein

Exercise 4-3

Fill in the blanks:

1. Amylase (*AM-i-lās*) is an enzyme that digests _____.

2. The ending *-ose* indicates that maltose is a(n) _____.

3. Glucogenesis (*glū-kō-JEN-e-sis*) is the formation of _____.

4. Hydrotherapy is treatment using _____.

5. Liposuction is the surgical removal of _____.

6. Adipose tissue stores _____.

Identify and define the root in each of the following words:

	Root	Meaning of Root
7. glucolytic (*glū-kō-LIT-ik*)	_____	_____
8. asteatosis (*as-tē-a-TŌ-sis*)	_____	_____
9. normoglycemia (*nor-mō-gli-SĒ-mē-a*)	_____	_____
10. lipoma (*lī-PŌ-ma*)	_____	_____

Supplementary Terms

amino acids *a-mē-nō*	The nitrogen-containing compounds that make up proteins
anabolism *a-NAB-ō-lizm*	The type of metabolism in which body substances are made; the building phase of metabolism
catabolism *ka-TAB-ō-lizm*	The type of metabolism in which substances are broken down for energy and simple compounds
collagen *KOL-a-jen*	A fibrous protein found in connective tissue
cortex *KOR-tex*	The outer region of an organ
glycogen *GLĪ-kō-jen*	A complex sugar compound stored in liver and muscles; broken down into glucose when needed for energy
interstitial *in-ter•STISH-al*	Between parts, such as the spaces between cells in a tissue
medulla *me-DUL-la*	The inner region of an organ; marrow (root *medull/o*)
parenchyma *par-EN-ki-ma*	The functional tissue of an organ
parietal *pa-RĪ-e-tal*	Pertaining to a wall; describes a membrane that lines a body cavity
soma *SŌ-ma*	The body. Used as the suffix -some to mean a small body, as in ribosome, lysosome, chromosome
stem cell	An immature cell that has the capacity to develop into any of a variety of different cell types. A precursor cell.
visceral *VIS-er-al*	Pertaining to the internal organs; describes a membrane on the surface of an organ

Labeling Exercise 4-1

Diagram of a Typical Animal Cell

Write the name of each numbered part on the corresponding line of the answer sheet.

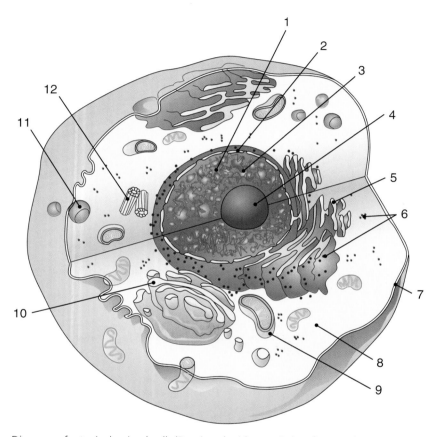

Centriole
Cytoplasm
Endoplasmic reticulum (ER)
Genetic material (DNA)
Golgi apparatus
Lysosome
Mitochondrion
Nuclear membrane
Nucleolus
Nucleus
Plasma membrane
Ribosomes

Diagram of a typical animal cell. (Reprinted with permission from Cohen BJ, Wood DL. Memmler's The Human Body in Health and Disease. 9th Ed. Philadelphia: Lippincott Williams & Wilkins, 2000.)

1. _____   7. _____

2. _____   8. _____

3. _____   9. _____

4. _____   10. _____

5. _____   11. _____

6. _____   12. _____

Chapter Review 4-1

Match the following terms and write the appropriate letter to the left of each number:

_____	1. ribosomes	a. genetic material
_____	2. ATP	b. state of internal stability
_____	3. homeostasis	c. organelles that contain RNA
_____	4. DNA	d. a type of connective tissue
_____	5. cartilage	e. energy compound of the cells

_____	6. cytoplasm	a. organelles that produce ATP
_____	7. metabolism	b. immature red blood cell
_____	8. mitochondria	c. material that fills the cell
_____	9. erythroblast	d. cell division
_____	10. mitosis	e. all the activities of the cell

_____	11. megakaryocyte	a. resembling a gland
_____	12. reticulocyte	b. fibrous tumor
_____	13. chromosome	c. cell with a very large nucleus
_____	14. adenoid	d. cell that contains a network
_____	15. fibroma	e. structure that contains genes

_____	16. fibroplasia	a. without form
_____	17. amorphous	b. wasting of tissue
_____	18. papillary	c. attracting basic stain
_____	19. atrophy	d. formation of fibrous tissue
_____	20. basophilic	e. like or resembling a nipple

_____	21. hyperplasia	a. resembling mucus
_____	22. hypoglycemia	b. low blood sugar
_____	23. amylase	c. enzyme that digests fat
_____	24. mucoid	d. overdevelopment of an organ or tissue
_____	25. lipase	e. enzyme that digests starch

_____ 26. proteolytic   a. pertaining to the body and the mind

_____ 27. nucleosome   b. destroying or dissolving protein

_____ 28. somatotropic   c. cell that contains fat

_____ 29. adipocyte   d. small body in the nucleus

_____ 30. somatopsychic   e. acting on the body

SUPPLEMENTARY TERMS

_____ 31. catabolism   a. building phase of metabolism

_____ 32. collagen   b. outer region of an organ

_____ 33. amino acid   c. building block of protein

_____ 34. anabolism   d. fibrous protein in connective tissue

_____ 35. cortex   e. breakdown phase of metabolism

Fill in the blanks:

36. The four basic tissue types are _____.

37. The simple sugar that is the main energy source for metabolism is _____.

38. The control center of the cell is the _____.

39. The number of chromosomes in each human cell aside from the sex cells is _____.

40. An organic compound that speeds the rate of metabolic reactions is a(n) _____.

41. Karyomegaly (kar-$\bar{e}$-$\bar{o}$-MEG-a-$l\bar{e}$) is enlargement (-megaly) of the _____.

42. A cytotoxic substance is damaging or poisonous to _____.

43. The term *hydration* refers to the relative amount of _____.

44. Adiposuria (ad-i-$p\bar{o}$-$S\bar{U}$-$r\bar{e}$-a) is the presence in the urine of _____.

45. A myxocyte is found in tissue that secretes _____.

Word building. Write a word for each of the following definitions:

46. The study of form and structure _____.

47. The study of tissues _____.

48. The formation of cells (use -*genesis* as an ending)_____.

49. An enzyme that digests proteins_____.

Case Studies

Case Study 4-1: Hematology Laboratory Studies

J.E. had a blood test as required for preoperative anesthesia assessment in preparation for scheduled plastic surgery on her breasts. The report read as follows:

Complete blood count (CBC) and differential
Red blood cell count (RBC)—4.5 million/μL
Hemoglobin (Hgb)—12.6 g/dL
Hematocrit (Hct)—38%
White blood cell count (WBC)—8,500/μL
Neutrophils—58%
Lymphocytes—34%
Monocytes—6%
Eosinophils—2%
Basophils—0.5%
Platelet count—200,000/μL
Prothrombin time (PT)—11.5 seconds
Partial thromboplastin time (PTT)—65 seconds
Blood glucose—84 mg/dL

The surgeon reviewed these results and concluded that they were within normal limits (WNL).

Case Study 4-2: Pathology Laboratory Tests

R.C., the manager of the clinical and pathology laboratory, received several surgical specimens taken from a 26-year-old female patient with a 4-week history of nonspecific pelvic pain. The specimens included several small containers of pink-tinged cloudy fluid labeled *pelvic lavage* (washing) *for cytology*, which R.C. took to the cytology laboratory to be made into slides and checked microscopically for abnormal cells. R.C. also received a tissue specimen labeled *uterine myoma*, a wedge biopsy of right ovarian neoplasm, and four jars each labeled *pelvic lymph nodes*. She took all of the tissue specimens to the pathology laboratory for gross and microscopic evaluation. A test tube half-filled with a cloudy gel and a cotton-tipped applicator labeled *swab of pelvic fluid for culture and sensitivity and Gram stain* was taken to the microbiology laboratory to be streaked on a culture plate and incubated to look for growth. Any organisms that grew out would be Gram-stained and tested for sensitivity to antibiotics that might be used in treatment.

The laboratory form was accompanied by a surgeon's note stating that the patient's preoperative diagnosis was cervical dysplasia with atypical cells and a positive urine leukocyte esterase, indicating a urinary tract infection. R.C. placed a copy of the laboratory forms and surgeon's note on the desk of the pathologist who was involved in carcinogenesis (cancer) research.

CASE STUDY QUESTIONS

Multiple choice: Select the best answer and write the letter of your choice to the left of each number.

_____ 1. J.E.'s blood test results were within normal limits. She could be described as being in a state of:
   a. normosmosis
   b. dysplasia

Case Studies, continued

     c. homeostasis

     d. hematophilia

     e. myogenesis

_____ 2. The suffix in *glucose* indicates that this compound is a:

     a. cervix

     b. enzyme

     c. protein

     d. sugar

     e. fat

_____ 3. The suffix in *esterase* indicates that this compound is a:

     a. sugar

     b. carbohydrate

     c. cell

     d. enzyme

     e. lipid

_____ 4. The root *gen* in carcinogenesis refers to a cancer's:

     a. origin

     b. treatment

     c. location

     d. laboratory results

     e. severity

Identify and give the meaning of the prefixes in each of the following words:

	Prefix	Meaning of Prefix
5. monocytes	_____	_____
6. prothrombin	_____	_____
7. neoplasm	_____	_____
8. atypical	_____	_____
9. leukocyte	_____	_____

Find words in the case studies for the following:

10. Three words that contain a root that means *attract, absorb*:

_____ _____

_____

11. Three words with a root that means *formation, molding, development*:

_____ _____

_____

12. Four words with a root that means *cell*: _____

_____

_____

_____

CHAPTER 4 Answer Section

Answers to Chapter Exercises

EXERCISE 4-1

1. nucleus
2. gland
3. nipple
4. fiber
5. tissue
6. mucus
7. network
8. forms
9. mucus
10. nucleus
11. body
12. cytology ($s\bar{i}$-TOL-$\bar{o}$-$j\bar{e}$)
13. histology (his-TOL-$\bar{o}$-$j\bar{e}$)
14. morphology (mor-FOL-$\bar{o}$-$j\bar{e}$)

EXERCISE 4-2

1. e
2. c
3. d
4. b
5. a
6. b
7. a
8. d
9. e
10. c
11. phag/o; eat, ingest
12. blast; immature cell, productive cell
13. troph; feeding, growth, nourishment
14. plas; formation, molding, development
15. gen; origin, formation

EXERCISE 4-3

1. starch
2. sugar
3. glucose
4. water
5. fat
6. fat
7. gluc/o; glucose
8. steat/o; fatty
9. glyc/o; sugar, glucose
10. lip/o; lipid, fat

LABELING EXERCISE 4-1 DIAGRAM OF A TYPICAL ANIMAL CELL

1. nucleus
2. nuclear membrane
3. genetic material (DNA)
4. nucleolus
5. endoplasmic reticulum (ER)
6. ribosomes
7. plasma membrane
8. cytoplasm
9. mitochondrion
10. Golgi apparatus
11. lysosome
12. centriole

Answers to Chapter Review 4-1

1. c
2. e
3. b
4. a
5. d
6. c
7. e
8. a
9. b
10. d
11. c
12. d
13. e
14. a
15. b
16. d
17. a
18. e
19. b
20. c
21. d
22. b
23. e
24. a
25. c
26. b
27. d
28. e
29. b
30. a
31. e
32. d

33. c
34. a
35. b
36. epithelial, connective, muscle, nervous
37. glucose
38. nucleus
39. 46
40. enzyme
41. nucleus
42. cells
43. water
44. fat
45. mucus
46. morphology
47. histology
48. cytogenesis
49. protease

Answers to Case Study Questions

1. c
2. d
3. d
4. a
5. mono-; one
6. pro-; before, in front of
7. neo-; new
8. a-; not, without
9. leuko-; white, colorless
10. neutrophils, eosinophils, basophils
11. thromboplastin, neoplasm, dysplasia
12. lymphocytes, monocytes, cytology, leukocyte

Body Structure

Chapter Contents

Objectives

After study of this chapter you should be able to:

1. Define the main directional terms used in anatomy.
2. Describe division of the body along three different planes.
3. Locate the dorsal and ventral body cavities.
4. Locate the nine divisions of the abdomen.
5. Locate the four quadrants of the abdomen.
6. Describe the main body positions used in medical practice.
7. Define basic terms describing body structure.
8. Recognize and use roots pertaining to body regions.
9. Recognize and use prefixes pertaining to position and direction.
10. Analyze terms pertaining to body structure in case studies.

Directional Terms

In describing the location or direction of a given point in the body, it is always assumed that the subject is in the **anatomical position**, that is, upright, with face front, arms at the sides with palms forward, and feet parallel, as shown in the small diagram in Figure 5-1. In this stance, the terms illustrated in Figure 5-1 and listed in Display 5-1 are used to designate relative position. Figure 5-2 illustrates planes of section, that is, direc-

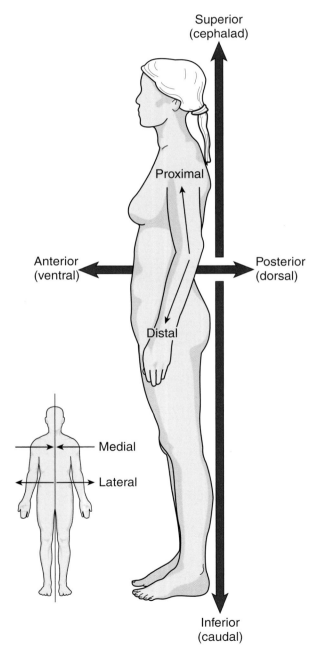

FIGURE 5-1. Directional terms. (Reprinted with permission from Cohen BJ, Wood DL. Memmler's The Human Body in Health and Disease. 9th Ed. Philadelphia: Lippincott Williams & Wilkins, 2000.)

DISPLAY 5-1 Anatomical Directions

TERM	DEFINITION
anterior (ventral)	toward the front (belly) of the body
posterior (dorsal)	toward the back of the body
medial	toward the midline of the body
lateral	toward the side of the body
proximal	nearer to the point of attachment or to a given reference point
distal	farther from the point of attachment or from a given reference point
superior	above
inferior	below
cephalad (cranial)	toward the head
caudal	toward the lower end of the spine (Latin *cauda* means "tail")
superficial (external)	close to the surface of the body
deep (internal)	close to the center of the body

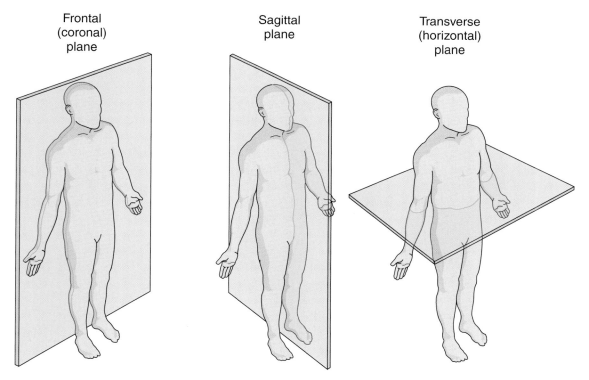

Frontal (coronal) plane

Sagittal plane

Transverse (horizontal) plane

FIGURE 5-2. Planes of division. (Reprinted with permission from Cohen BJ, Wood DL. Memmler's The Human Body in Health and Disease. 9th Ed. Philadelphia: Lippincott Williams & Wilkins, 2000.)

tions in which the body can be cut. A **frontal plane**, also called a coronal plane, is made at right angles to the midline and divides the body into anterior and posterior parts. A **sagittal** (*SAJ-i-tal*) **plane** passes from front to back and divides the body into right and left portions. If the plane passes through the midline, it is a mid-sagittal or medial plane. A **transverse plane** passes horizontally, dividing the body into superior and inferior parts.

Body Cavities

Internal organs are located within dorsal and ventral cavities (Fig. 5-3). The dorsal cavity contains the brain in the **cranial cavity** and the spinal cord in the **spinal cavity (canal)**. The uppermost ventral space, the **thoracic cavity**, is separated from the **abdominal cavity** by the **diaphragm**. There is no anatomical separation between the abdominal cavity and the **pelvic cavity**, which together make up the **abdominopelvic cavity**. The large membrane that lines the abdominopelvic cavity and covers the organs within it is the **peritoneum** (*per-i-tō-NĒ-um*).

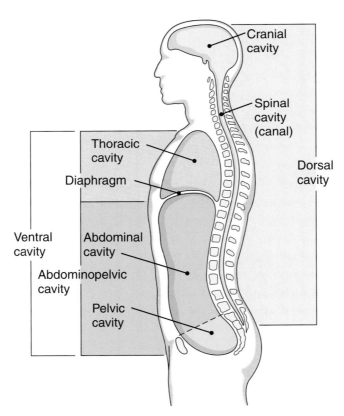

FIGURE 5-3. Side view of the body cavities. (Reprinted with permission from Cohen BJ, Wood DL. Memmler's The Human Body in Health and Disease. 9th Ed. Philadelphia: Lippincott Williams & Wilkins, 2000.)

Body Regions

For orientation, the abdomen can be divided by imaginary lines into nine regions, which are shown in Figure 5-4. The sections down the midline are the:
- epigastric (*ep-i-GAS-trik*) region, located above the stomach
- umbilical (*um-BIL-i-kal*) region, named for the umbilicus, or navel
- hypogastric (*hī-pō-GAS-trik*) region, located below the stomach

The lateral regions are the:
- right and left hypochondriac (*hī-po-KON-drē-ak*) regions, named for their position near the ribs, specifically near the cartilages (root *chondr/o*) of the ribs,
- right and left lumbar (*LUM-bar*) regions, which are located near the small of the back (lumbar region of the spine)
- right and left iliac (*IL-ē-ak*) regions, named for the upper bone of the hip, the ilium. These regions are also called the inguinal (*ING-gwi-nal*) regions, with reference to the groin.

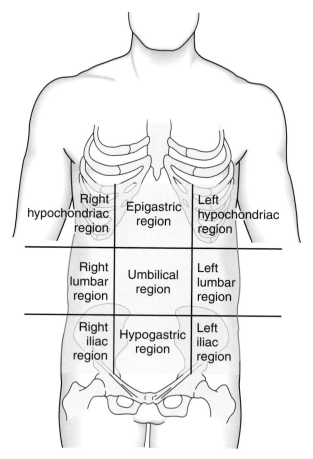

FIGURE 5-4. The nine regions of the abdomen. (Reprinted with permission from Cohen BJ, Wood DL. Memmler's The Human Body in Health and Disease. 9th Ed. Philadelphia: Lippincott Williams & Wilkins, 2000.)

More simply, but less precisely, the abdomen can be divided by a single vertical line and a single horizontal line into four sections (Fig. 5-5), designated the right upper quadrant (RUQ), left upper quadrant (LUQ), right lower quadrant (RLQ), and left lower quadrant (LLQ).

Additional terms for body regions are shown in Figures 5-6 and 5-7. You may need to refer to these illustrations as you work through the book.

Positions

In addition to the anatomical position, there are other standard positions in which the body is placed for examination or medical procedures. The most common of these are described in Display 5-2.

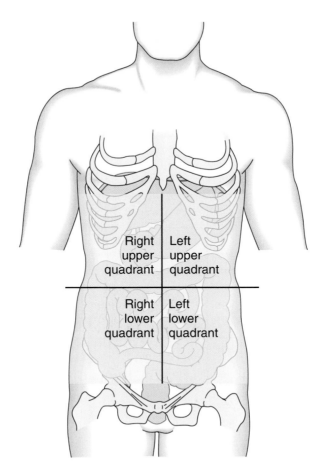

FIGURE 5-5. Quadrants of the abdomen, showing the organs within each quadrant. (Reprinted with permission from Cohen BJ, Wood DL. Memmler's The Human Body in Health and Disease. 9th Ed. Philadelphia: Lippincott Williams & Wilkins, 2000.)

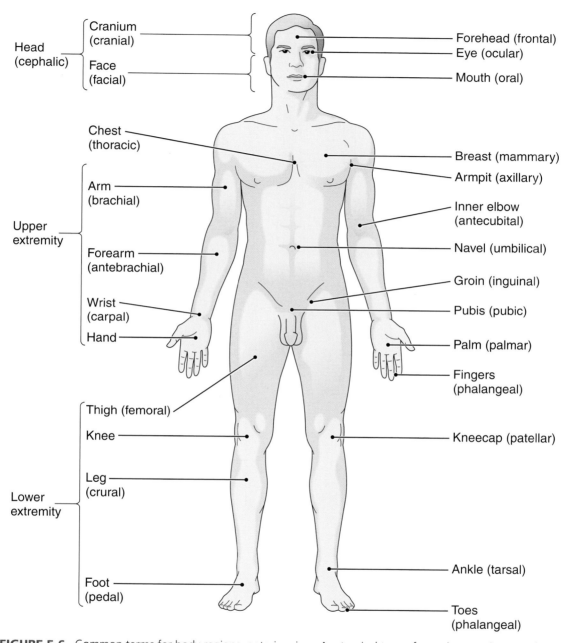

FIGURE 5-6. Common terms for body regions, anterior view. Anatomical terms for regions are in parentheses.

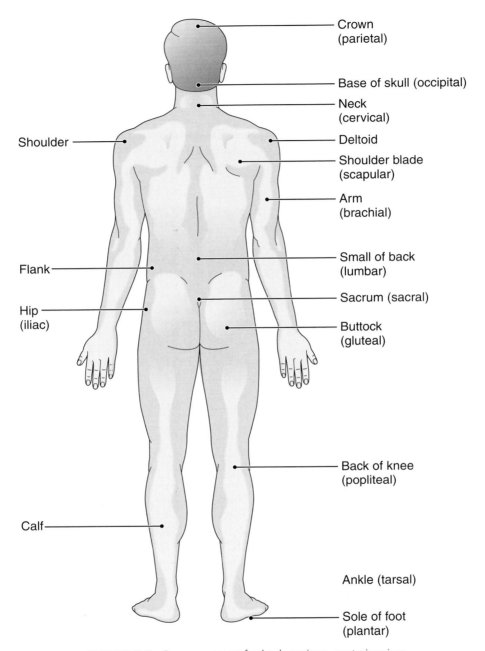

FIGURE 5-7. Common terms for body regions, posterior view.

DISPLAY 5-2 Body Positions

POSITION	DESCRIPTION
anatomical position	standing erect, facing forward, arms at sides, palms forward, legs parallel, toes pointed forward
decubitus position *dē-KŪ-bi-tus*	lying down, specifically according to the part of the body resting on a flat surface, as in left or right lateral decubitus, or dorsal or ventral decubitus
dorsal recumbent position	on back, with legs bent and separated, feet flat
Fowler position	on back, head of bed raised about 18 inches, knees elevated
Kraske (Jackknife) position *KRAS-kē*	prone with the buttocks raised
knee-chest position	on knees, head and upper chest on table, arms crossed above head
lateral recumbent position	on the side with one leg flexed; arm position may vary
lithotomy position *li-THOT-ō-mē*	on back, legs flexed on abdomen, thighs apart
prone	lying face down
Sims position	on left side, right leg drawn up high and forward, left arm along back, chest forward resting on bed
supine* *SŪ-pī-n*	lying face up
Trendelenburg position *tren-DEL-en-berg*	on back with head lowered by tilting bed back at 45° angle

*To remember the difference between prone and supine, look for the word *up* in supine.

Key Terms

abdominal cavity *ab-DOM-i-nal*	The large ventral cavity below the diaphragm and above the pelvic cavity
abdominopelvic cavity *ab-dom-i-nō-PEL-vik*	The large ventral cavity between the diaphragm and pelvis that includes the abdominal and pelvic cavities
anatomic position *an-a-TOM-ik*	Standard position for anatomical studies, in which the body is erect and facing forward, the arms are at the sides with palms forward, and the feet are parallel
cranial cavity *KRĀ-nē-al*	The dorsal cavity that contains the brain
diaphragm *DĪ-a-fram*	The muscle that separates the thoracic from the abdominal cavity
frontal (coronal) plane *ko-RŌN-al*	Plane of section that separates the body into anterior (front) and posterior (back) portions
pelvic cavity *PEL-vik*	The ventral cavity that is below the abdominal cavity

peritoneum *per-i-tō-NĒ-um*	The large serous membrane that lines the abdominopelvic cavity and covers the organs within it
sagittal plane *SAJ-i-tal*	Plane that divides the body into right and left portions
spinal cavity (canal) *SPĪ-nal*	Dorsal cavity that contains the spinal cord
thoracic cavity *thō-RAS-ik*	The ventral cavity above the diaphragm; the chest cavity
transverse (horizontal) plane *trans-VERS*	Plane that divides the body into superior (upper) and inferior (lower) portions

Word Parts Pertaining to Body Structure

TABLE 5-1 Roots for Regions of the Head and Trunk

ROOT	MEANING	EXAMPLE	DEFINITION OF EXAMPLE
cephal/o	head	microcephaly *mī-krō-SEF-a-lē*	abnormal smallness of the head
cervic/o	neck	cervicofacial *ser-vi-kō-FĀ-shal*	pertaining to the neck and face
thorac/o	chest, thorax	extrathoracic *eks-tra-thō-RAS-ik*	outside the thorax
abdomin/o	abdomen	intra-abdominal *in-tra-ab-DOM-i-nal*	within the abdomen
celi/o	abdomen	celiac *SĒ-lē-ak*	pertaining to the abdomen
lapar/o	abdominal wall	laparoscope *LAP-a-rō-skōp*	instrument for viewing the peritoneal cavity through the abdominal wall
lumb/o	lumbar region, lower back	thoracolumbar *thō-rak-ō-LUM-bar*	pertaining to the chest and lumbar region
periton, peritone/o	peritoneum	peritoneal *per-i-tō-NĒ-al*	pertaining to the peritoneum

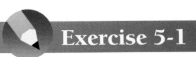

Exercise 5-1

Write the adjective that fits each of the following definitions. The correct suffix is given in parentheses.

1. Pertaining to (-ic) the head _____cephalic_____

2. Pertaining to (-ic) the chest _____

3. Pertaining to (-al) the neck _____

4. Pertaining to (-ar) the lower back _____

5. Pertaining to (-al) the abdomen _____

Fill in the blanks:

6. Peritonitis (*per-i-tō-NĪ-tis*) is inflammation (-itis) of the _____.

7. Celiocentesis (*sē-lē-ō-sen-TĒ-sis*) is surgical puncture (centesis) of the

_____.

BOX 5-1 Cutting the Job in Half

A beginning student in medical science may be surprised by the vast number of names and terms that he or she is required to learn. This responsibility is lightened somewhat by the fact that we are bilaterally symmetrical. That is, aside from some internal organs such as the liver, spleen, stomach, pancreas, and intestine, nearly everything on the right side can be found on the left as well. The skeleton can be figuratively split down the center, giving equal structures on both sides of the midline. Many blood vessels and nerves are paired. This cuts the learning in half.

In addition, many of the blood vessels and nerves in a region have the same name. The radial artery, radial vein, and radial nerve are parallel, and all are located along the radius of the forearm. Vessels are commonly named for the organ they supply: the hepatic artery and vein of the liver, the pulmonary artery and vein of the lungs, the renal artery and vein of the kidney.

No one could say that the learning of medical terminology is a snap, but it could be harder!

TABLE 5-2 Roots for the Extremities

ROOT	MEANING	EXAMPLE	DEFINITION OF EXAMPLE
acro	extremity, end	acrodermatitis *ak-rō-der-ma-TĪ-tis*	inflammation of the skin of the extremities
brachi/o	arm	antebrachium *an-tē-BRĀ-kē-um*	forearm
dactyl/o	finger, toe	polydactyly *pol-ē-DAK-til-ē*	having more than the normal number of fingers or toes
ped/o	foot	dextropedal *deks-TROP-e-dal*	using the right foot in preference to the left
pod/o	foot	podiatric *pō-dē-AT-rik*	pertaining to study and treatment of the foot

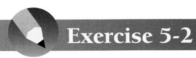

Exercise 5-2

Fill in the blanks:

1. Acrokinesia (*ak-rō-kī-NĒ-sē-a*) is excess motion (-kinesia) of the _____.

2. Animals that brachiate (*BRĀ-kē-āt*), such as monkeys, swing from place to place using their
   _____.

3. A dactylospasm (*DAK-til-o-spazm*) is a cramp (spasm) of the _____.

4. The term brachiocephalic (*brā-kē-ō-se-FAL-ik*) refers to the _____.

5. Podiatry (*pō-DĪ-a-trē*) is a specialty that treats problems of the _____.

6. A bipedal animal has two _____.

TABLE 5-3 Prefixes for Position and Direction

PREFIX	MEANING	EXAMPLE	DEFINITION OF EXAMPLE
circum-	around	circumoral ser-kum-OR-al	around the mouth
peri-	around	perivascular per-ē-VAS-kū-lar	around a vessel (*vascul/o*)
intra-	in, within	intrauterine in-tra-Ū-ter-in	within the uterus
epi-	on, over	epithelium ep-i-THĒ-lē-um	tissue that covers surfaces
extra-	outside	extracellular eks-tra-SEL-ū-lar	outside a cell or cells
infra-*	below	infrapatellar in-fra-pa-TEL-ar	below the kneecap (patella)
sub-*	below, under	sublingual sub-LING-gwal	under the tongue (*lingu/o*)
inter-	between	intercostal in-ter-KOS-tal	between the ribs (*cost/o*)
juxta-	near, beside	juxtaposition juks-ta-pō-ZI-shun	a location near or beside another structure
para-	near, beside behind	parasagittal par-a-SAJ-i-tal	near or beside a sagittal plane
retro-	backward	retroperitoneal re-trō-per-i-tō-NĒ-al	behind the peritoneum
supra-	above	suprascapular su-pra-SKAP-ū-lar	above the scapula (shoulder blade)

*Also indicates degree.

Exercise 5-3

Synonyms. Write a word that has the same meaning as each of the words below:

1. circumoral _____ perioral _____

2. subscapular _____

3. circumocular _____

4. infracostal _____

Opposites. Write a word that means the opposite of each of the following words:

5. infrapatellar _____

6. intracellular _____

Define each of the following terms:

7. paranasal (*par-a-NĀ-zal*) _____

8. retrouterine (*re-trō-Ū-ter-in*) _____

9. suprapelvic (*sū-pra-PEL-vik*) _____

10. intravascular (*in-tra-VAS-kū-lar*) _____

Refer to Figures 5-6 and 5-7 to define the following terms:

11. supracervical (*sū-pra-SER-vi-kal*) _____

_____

12. interphalangeal (*in-ter-fa-LAN-jē-al*) _____

_____

13. epicranial (*ep-i-KRĀ-nē-al*) _____

_____

14. infraumbilical (*in-fra-um-BIL-i-kal*) _____

_____

15. parasacral (*par-a-SĀ-kral*) _____

_____

Supplementary Terms

digit *DIJ-it*	A finger or toe (adjective, digital)
epigastrium *ep-i-GAS-trē-um*	The epigastric region
fundus *FUN-dus*	The base or body of a hollow organ; the area of an organ farthest from its opening
hypochondrium *hī-pō-KON-drē-um*	The hypochondriac region (left or right)
lumen *LŪ-men*	The central opening within a tube or vessel
meatus *mē-Ā-tus*	A passage or opening
orifice *OR-i-fis*	The opening of a cavity
os	Mouth; any body opening
septum *SEP-tum*	A wall dividing two cavities
sinus *SĪ-nus*	A cavity, as within a bone
sphincter *SFINK-ter*	A circular muscle that regulates an opening

ABBREVIATIONS

LLQ	Left lower quadrant	**RLQ**	Right lower quadrant
LUQ	Left upper quadrant	**RUQ**	Right upper quadrant

Labeling Exercise 5-1

Directional Terms

Write the name of each numbered part on the corresponding line of the answer sheet.

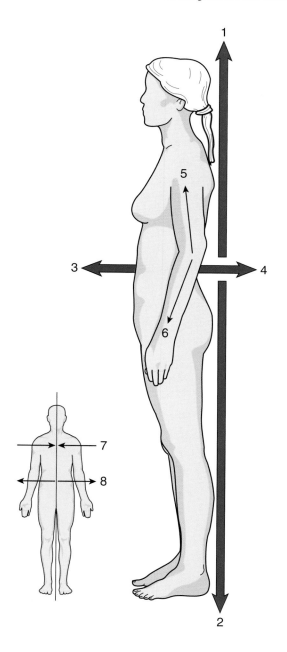

Anterior (ventral)   Medial
Distal   Posterior (dorsal)
Inferior (caudal)   Proximal
Lateral   Superior (cephalad)

1. _____

2. _____

3. _____

4. _____

5. _____

6. _____

7. _____

8. _____

Labeling Exercise 5-2

Planes of Division

Write the name of each numbered part on the corresponding line of the answer sheet.

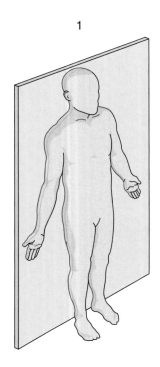

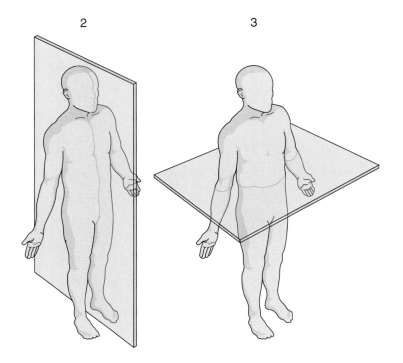

Frontal (coronal) plane
Sagittal plane
Transverse (horizontal) plane

1. _____

2. _____

3. _____

Labeling Exercise 5-3

Side View of the Body Cavities

Write the name of each numbered part on the corresponding line of the answer sheet.

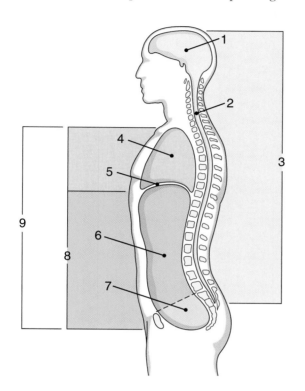

Abdominal cavity
Abdominal pelvic cavity
Cranial cavity
Dorsal cavity
Diaphragm
Pelvic cavity
Spinal cavity (canal)
Thoracic cavity
Ventral cavity

1. _____
2. _____
3. _____
4. _____
5. _____

6. _____
7. _____
8. _____
9. _____

Labeling Exercise 5-4

The Nine Regions of the Abdomen
Write the name of each numbered part on the corresponding line of the answer sheet.

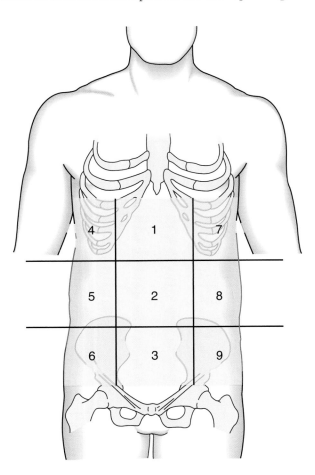

Epigastric region
Hypogastric region
Left hypochondriac region
Left iliac region
Left lumbar region
Right hypochondriac region
Right iliac region
Right lumbar region
Umbilical region

1. _____

2. _____

3. _____

4. _____

5. _____

6. _____

7. _____

8. _____

9. _____

Chapter Review 5-1

Match the following terms and write the appropriate letter to the left of each number:

_____ 1. abrachia   a. incision into the chest

_____ 2. acrocyanosis   b. absence of an arm

_____ 3. laparotomy   c. absence of a finger or toe

_____ 4. adactyly   d. bluish discoloration of the extremities

_____ 5. thoracotomy   e. incision through the abdominal wall

_____ 6. antebrachium   a. fusion of the fingers or toes

_____ 7. celiocentesis   b. excessive size of the feet

_____ 8. macropodia   c. outer layer of the skin

_____ 9. epidermis   d. forearm

_____ 10. syndactyly   e. surgical puncture of the abdomen

SUPPLEMENTARY TERMS

_____ 11. fundus   a. cavity, as in a bone

_____ 12. lumen   b. circular muscle that regulates an opening

_____ 13. sphincter   c. central opening of a tube

_____ 14. septum   d. dividing wall

_____ 15. sinus   e. base of a hollow organ

True-False. Examine each of the following statements. If the statement is true, write T in the first blank. If the statement is false, write F in the first blank and correct the statement by replacing the underlined word in the second blank.

16. The cranial and spinal cavities are the ventral body cavities.   __F__   ____dorsal____

17. The elbow is distal to the wrist.   _____   _____

18. A midsagittal plane divides the body into equal right and left parts. _____   _____

19. A frontal plane divides the body into anterior and posterior parts.   _____   _____

20. The thoracic cavity is inferior to the abdominal cavity.   _____   _____

21. The epigastric region is above the stomach.   _____   _____

22. The right hypochondriac region is in the RUQ.   _____   _____

23. In the supine position, the patient is lying face-down.   _____   _____

Adjectives. Name the part of the body referred to in each of the following adjectives:

24. cervical _____

25. cephalic _____

26. brachial _____

27. celiac _____

28. thoracic _____

29. peritoneal _____

30. pedal _____

Define the following words:

31. intra-abdominal _____

32. retroperitoneal _____

33. sublingual _____

34. intergluteal _____

35. abdominopelvic _____

Synonyms. Write a word that has the same meaning as each of the following words:

36. periocular _____

37. submammary _____

38. posterior _____

39. ventral _____

Opposites. Write a word that has the opposite meaning of each of the following words:

40. macrocephaly _____

41. extracellular _____

42. proximal _____

43. superior _____

44. infrapubic _____

45. superficial _____

Case Study

Case Study 5-1: Emergency Care

During a triathlon, paramedics responded to a scene with multiple patients involved in a serious bicycle accident. B.R., a 20-year-old woman, lost control of her bike while descending a hill at approximately 40 mph. As she fell, two other cyclists collided with her, sending all three crashing to the ground.

Case Study, continued

At the scene, B.R. complained of pain in her head, back, chest, and leg. She also had numbness and tingling in her legs and feet. Other injuries included a cut on her face and on her right arm and an obvious deformity to both her shoulder and knee. She had slight difficulty breathing.

The paramedic did a rapid cephalocaudal assessment and immobilized B.R.'s neck in a cervical collar. She was secured on a backboard and given oxygen. After her bleeding was controlled and her injured extremities were immobilized, she was transported to the nearest emergency department.

During transport, the paramedic in charge radioed ahead to provide a prehospital report to the charge nurse. His report included the following information: occipital and frontal head pain; laceration to right temple, superior and anterior to right ear; lumbar pain; bilateral thoracic pain on inspiration at midclavicular line on right and midaxillary line on the left; dull aching pain of the posterior proximal right thigh; bilateral paresthesia (numbness and tingling) of distal lower legs circumferentially; varus (knock-knee) adduction deformity of left knee; and posterior displacement deformity of left shoulder.

At the hospital, the emergency department physician ordered radiographs for B.R. Before the procedure, the radiology technologist positioned a lead gonadal shield centered on the midsagittal line above B.R.'s symphysis pubis to protect her ovaries from unnecessary irradiation by the primary beam. The technologist knew that gonadal shielding is important for female patients undergoing imaging of the lumbar spine, sacroiliac joints, acetabula, pelvis, and kidneys. Shields should not be used for any examination in which an acute abdominal condition is suspected.

CASE STUDY QUESTIONS

Multiple choice: Select the best answer and write the letter of your choice to the left of each number.

_____ 1. The term for the time span between injury and admission to the emergency department is:
    a. preoperative
    b. prehospital
    c. pre-emergency
    d. pretrauma
    e. intrainjury

_____ 2. A cephalocaudal assessment goes from _____ to _____.
    a. stem to stern
    b. front to back
    c. head to toe
    d. side to side
    e. skin to bone

_____ 3. The victim's injured extremities were immobilized before transport. Immobilized means:
    a. abducted as far as they will go
    b. internally rotated and flexed
    c. adducted so that the limbs are crossed
    d. rotated externally
    e. held in body alignment to keep them from moving

Case Study, continued

_____ 4. A cervical collar was placed on the victim to stabilize and immobilize the _____.
   a. uterus
   b. shoulders
   c. chin
   d. neck
   e. pelvis

_____ 5. The singular form of acetabula is:
   a. acetyl
   b. acetabulum
   c. acetabia
   d. acetab
   e. acetabulae

Draw or shade the appropriate areas on one or both diagrams for each question.

6. Draw a dot over the area of the victim's occipital and frontal pain.

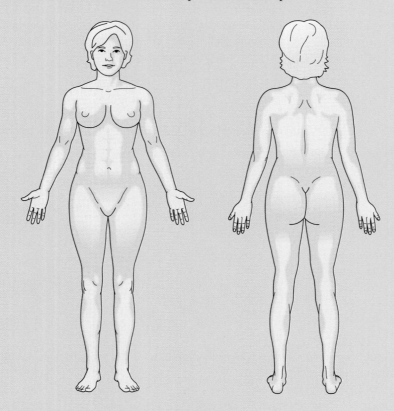

7. Draw a dash (---) over the area of the right temporal laceration—superior and anterior to the right ear.

8. Shade the area of lumbar pain.

Case Study, continued

9. Shade the anterior area of thoracic pain at the midaxillary line on the left.

10. Draw a star at the area of the pain on the right proximal posterior thigh.

11. Shade the area of the bilateral paresthesia of the distal lower legs, circumferentially.

12. Draw an arrow to show the direction of the varus adduction of the left knee.

13. Draw an arrow to show the direction of the posterior displacement of the left shoulder.

14. Draw a fig leaf to show the gonadal shield on the midsagittal line above the symphysis pubis.

15. Draw a circle around the area of the sacroiliac joints.

CHAPTER 5 Answer Section

Answers to Chapter Exercises

EXERCISE 5-1

1. cephalic (se-FAL-ik)
2. thoracic (thō-RAS-ik)
3. cervical (SER-vi-kal)
4. lumbar (LUM-bar)
5. abdominal (ab-DOM-i-nal)
6. peritoneum
7. abdomen

EXERCISE 5-2

1. extremities (hands and feet)
2. arms
3. fingers or toes
4. arms and head
5. one who studies and treats the foot
6. feet

EXERCISE 5-3

1. perioral
2. infrascapular
3. periocular
4. subcostal
5. suprapatellar
6. extracellular
7. near the nose
8. behind the uterus

9. above the pelvis
10. within a vessel
11. above the neck
12. between the fingers or toes
13. on or over the cranium
14. below the navel
15. near the sacrum

LABELING EXERCISE 5-1 DIRECTIONAL TERMS

1. superior (cephalad)
2. inferior (caudal)
3. anterior (ventral)
4. posterior (dorsal)
5. proximal
6. distal
7. medial
8. lateral

LABELING EXERCISE 5-2 PLANES OF DIVISION

1. frontal plane
2. sagittal plane
3. transverse plane

LABELING EXERCISE 5-3 SIDE VIEW OF THE BODY CAVITIES

1. cranial cavity
2. spinal cavity (canal)
3. dorsal activity

4. thoracic cavity
5. diaphragm
6. abdominal cavity
7. pelvic cavity
8. abdominopelvic cavity
9. ventral cavity

LABELING EXERCISE 5-4 THE NINE REGIONS OF THE ABDOMEN

1. epigastric (*ep-i-GAS-trik*) region
2. umbilical (*um-BIL-i-kal*) region
3. hypogastric (*hī-pō-GAS-trik*) region
4. right hypochondriac (*hī-pō-KON-drē-ak*) region
5. right lumbar (*LUM-bar*) region
6. right iliac (*IL-ē-ak*) region; also inguinal (*ING-gwi-nal*) region
7. left hypochondriac region
8. left lumbar region
9. left iliac region; also inguinal (*ING-gwi-nal*) region

Answers to Chapter Review 5-1

1. b
2. d
3. e
4. c
5. a
6. d
7. e
8. b
9. c
10. a
11. e
12. c
13. b
14. d
15. a
16. F dorsal
17. F proximal
18. T
19. T
20. F superior
21. T
22. T
23. F prone
24. neck
25. head
26. arm
27. abdomen
28. thorax, chest
29. peritoneum
30. foot
31. within the abdomen
32. behind the peritoneum

33. under the tongue
34. between the buttocks
35. pertaining to the abdomen and pelvis
36. circumocular
37. inframammary
38. dorsal
39. anterior
40. microcephaly
41. intracellular
42. distal
43. inferior
44. suprapubic
45. deep

Answers to Case Study Questions

1. b
2. c
3. e
4. d
5. b

6–15. See diagram

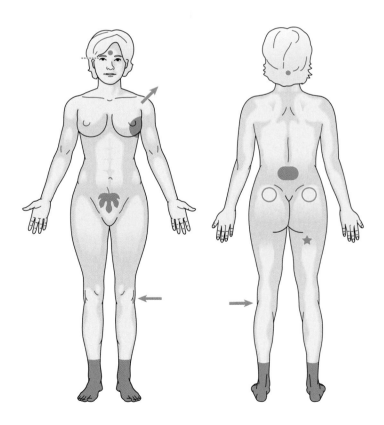

body Fluoride mito

ation pulmo

ous body dendri

jaundice

oma ossicle

limbic

RON-ik

hypoba

ortex

Disease and Treatment

Chapters 6 through 8 in Part 2 cover general terminology related to diseases, diagnosis, and treatment, including information on drugs. More specific information about how diseases affect individual systems and how these diseases are treated will be presented in Part 3.

Disease

Chapter Contents

Objectives

After study of this chapter you should be able to:

1. List the major categories of diseases.
2. Compare the common types of infectious organisms, and list some diseases caused by each.
3. Define and give examples of neoplasia.
4. Identify and use word parts pertaining to diseases.
5. Define the major terms describing types of diseases.
6. List and define the major manifestations of diseases.
7. Analyze the disease terminology in several case studies.

A disease is any alteration from the normal structure or function of any part of the body. Diseases can be grouped into a number of different but often overlapping categories. These include:

- Infectious diseases—caused by microorganisms and other **parasites** that live at the expense of another organism. Any disease-causing organism is described as a **pathogen**.
- Degenerative diseases—resulting from wear and tear, aging, or **trauma** (injury) that can result in a **lesion** (wound) and perhaps **necrosis** (death) of tissue. Common examples include arthritis, cardiovascular problems, and certain respiratory disorders such as emphysema. Structural malformations such as congenital malformations, **prolapse** (dropping), or **hernia** (rupture) may also result in degenerative changes.
- Neoplasia—abnormal and uncontrolled growth of tissue.
- Immune disorders—failures of the immune system, allergies, and autoimmune diseases, in which the body makes antibodies to its own tissues, fall into this category. (Immune disorders are discussed in more detail in Chapter 10.)
- Metabolic disorders—resulting from lack of enzymes or other factors needed for cellular functions. Many hereditary disorders fall into this category. Malnutrition caused by inadequate intake of nutrients or inability of the body to absorb and use nutrients also upsets metabolism. (Metabolic disorders are discussed in more detail in Chapter 12, and hereditary disorders are discussed in Chapter 15.)
- Hormonal disorders—caused by underproduction or overproduction of hormones or by inability of the hormones to function properly. One example is diabetes mellitus. (Hormonal disorders are discussed in more detail in Chapter 16.)
- Mental and emotional disorders—disorders that affect the mind and adaptation of an individual to his or her environment. (Behavioral disorders are discussed in more detail in Chapter 17.)

The cause of a disease is its **etiology** ($\overline{e}$-$t\overline{e}$-OL-$\overline{o}$-$j\overline{e}$), although many diseases have multiple interacting causes. An **acute** disease is sudden and severe and of short duration. A **chronic** disease is of long duration and progresses slowly.

BOX 6-1 Name That Disease

Diseases get their names in a variety of ways. Some are named for the places where they were first found, such as Lyme disease for Lyme, Connecticut; West Nile disease and Rift Valley fever for places in Africa; and hantavirus fever for a river in Korea. Others are named for people who first described them, such as Cooley anemia; Crohn disease, an inflammatory bowel disease; and Hodgkin disease of the lymphatic system.

Many diseases are named on the basis of the symptoms they cause. Tuberculosis causes small lesions known as tubercles in the lungs and other tissues. Skin anthrax produces lesions that turn black, and its name comes from the same root as anthracite coal. In sickle cell anemia, red blood cells become distorted into a crescent shape when they give up oxygen. Having lost their smooth, round form, the cells jumble together, blocking small blood vessels and depriving tissues of oxygen.

Bubonic plague causes painful and enlarged lymph nodes called buboes. Lupus erythematosus, a systemic autoimmune disorder, is named for the Latin term for wolf because the red rash that may form on the face of people with this disease gives them a wolf-like appearance. Yellow fever, scarlet fever, and rubella (German measles) are named for colors associated with the pathology of these diseases.

Infectious Diseases

Infectious diseases are caused by viruses, bacteria, fungi (yeasts and molds), protozoa (single-celled animals), and worms (Display 6-1). In shape, bacteria may be round (cocci, Fig. 6-1), rod-shaped (bacilli, Fig. 6-2), or curved (vibrios and spirochetes, see Fig. 6-2). They may be named according to their shape and by the arrangements they form (see Fig. 6-1). They also are described according to the dyes they take up when stained in the laboratory. The most common laboratory bacterial stain is the **Gram stain**, with which gram-positive organisms stain purple and gram-negative organisms stain red (see Fig. 6-1).

Microorganisms often produce disease by means of the **toxins** (poisons) they release. The presence of harmful microorganisms or their toxins in the body is termed **sepsis**.

DISPLAY 6-1 Common Infectious Organisms

TYPE OF ORGANISM	DESCRIPTION	EXAMPLES OF DISEASES CAUSED
Bacteria *bak-TĒ-rē-a*	simple microscopic organisms that are widespread throughout the world, some of which can produce disease; singular, bacterium (*bak-TĒ-rē-um*)	
cocci *KOK-sī*	round bacteria; may be in clusters (staphylococci), chains (streptococci), and other formations; singular, coccus (*KOK-us*)	pneumonia, rheumatic fever, food poisoning, septicemia, urinary tract infections, gonorrhea
bacilli *ba-SIL-ī*	rod-shaped bacteria; singular, bacillus (*ba-SIL-us*)	typhoid, dysentery, salmonellosis, tuberculosis, botulism, tetanus
vibrios *VIB-rē-ōz*	curved rods	cholera, gastroenteritis
spirochetes *SPĪ-rō-kētz*	corkscrew-shaped bacteria that move with a twisting motion	Lyme disease, syphilis, Vincent disease
chlamydia *kla-MID-ē-a*	organisms smaller than bacteria that, like viruses, grow in living cells but are susceptible to antibiotics	conjunctivitis, trachoma, pelvic inflammatory disease (PID), and other sexually transmitted diseases (STDs)
rickettsia *ri-KET-sē-a*	similar in growth to chlamydia	typhus, Rocky Mountain spotted fever
Viruses *VĪ-rus-es*	submicroscopic infectious agents that can live and reproduce only within living cells	colds, herpes, hepatitis measles, varicella (chickenpox), influenza, AIDS
Fungi *FUN-jī*	simple, nongreen plants, some of which are parasitic; includes yeasts and molds; singular, fungus (*FUN-gus*)	candidiasis, skin infections (tinea, ringworm, valley fever)
Protozoa *prō-tō-ZŌ-a*	single-celled animals; singular, protozoon (*prō-tō-ZŌ-on*)	dysentery, *Trichomonas* infection, malaria
Helminths *HEL-minths*	worms	trichinosis; infestations with roundworms, pinworms, hookworms

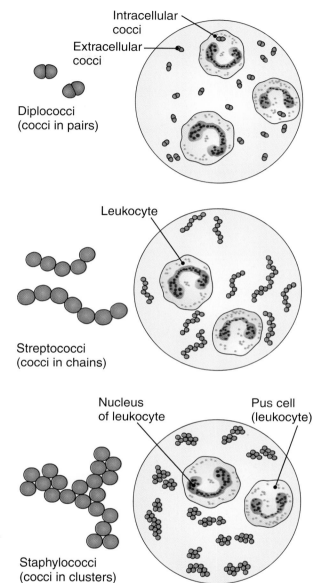

FIGURE 6-1. Round bacteria (cocci), Gram stained. (Reprinted with permission from Cohen BJ, Wood DL. Memmler's The Human Body in Health and Disease. 9th Ed. Philadelphia: Lippincott Williams & Wilkins, 2000.)

Responses to Disease

Inflammation

A common response to infection and to other forms of disease is **inflammation**. When cells are injured, they release chemicals that allow blood cells and fluids to move into the tissues. This inflow of blood results in the four signs of inflammation: heat, pain, redness, and swelling. The suffix -*itis* indicates inflammation, as in appendicitis (inflammation of the appendix) and tonsillitis (inflammation of the tonsils).

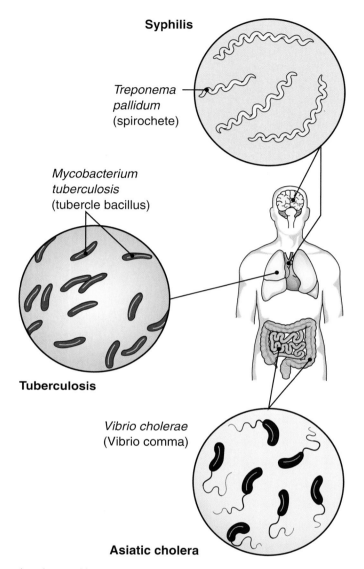

FIGURE 6-2. Rod-shaped and curved bacteria. (Reprinted with permission from Cohen BJ, Wood DL. Memmler's The Human Body in Health and Disease. 9th Ed. Philadelphia: Lippincott Williams & Wilkins, 2000.)

Phagocytosis

The body uses phagocytosis to get rid of invading microorganisms, damaged cells, and other types of harmful debris. Certain white blood cells are capable of engulfing these materials and destroying them internally (Fig. 6-3). Phagocytic cells are found circulating in the blood, in the tissues, and in the lymphatic system (see Chapters 9 and 10). The remains of phagocytosis consist of fluid and white blood cells; this is called **pus.**

Leukocyte   Capillary   Bacteria

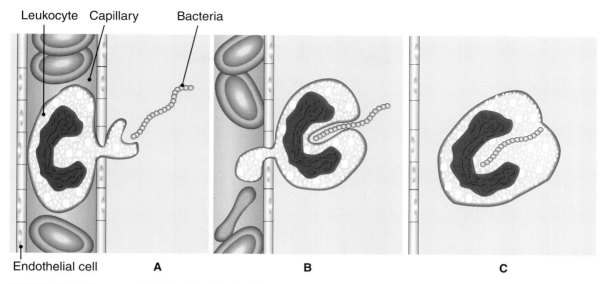

Endothelial cell   A   B   C

FIGURE 6-3. Phagocytosis. **(A)** White blood cell squeezes through a capillary wall in the region of an infection. **(B, C)** White cell engulfs the bacteria. (Reprinted with permission from Cohen BJ, Wood DL. Memmler's The Human Body in Health and Disease. 9th Ed. Philadelphia: Lippincott Williams & Wilkins, 2000.)

Immunity

The immune system mounts our specific responses to disease. Cells of the immune system recognize different foreign invaders, and get rid of them by direct attack and with circulating antibodies that immobilize and help to destroy the cells (see Chapter 10). The immune system also monitors the body continuously for abnormal and malfunctioning cells, such as cancer cells. The system may also overreact to produce allergies, and may react to one's own tissues to cause autoimmune diseases.

Neoplasia

As noted above, a **neoplasm** is an abnormal and uncontrolled growth of tissue—a tumor or growth. A neoplasm that does not spread, that is, **metastasize**, to other tissues is described as **benign**, although it may cause damage at the site where it grows. A neoplasm that metastasizes to other tissues is termed **malignant**, and is commonly called *cancer*. A malignant tumor that involves epithelial tissue is a **carcinoma**. If the tumor arises in glandular epithelium, it is an adenocarcinoma (the root *aden/o* means "gland"); a cancer of pigmented epithelial cells (melanocytes) is a melanoma. A neoplasm that involves connective tissue, muscle, or bone is a **sarcoma**. Cancers of the blood, lymphatic system, and nervous system are classified according to the cell types involved and other clinical features. These are described in Chapters 10 and 17.

Often mistaken for a malignancy is a **cyst**, a sac or pouch filled with fluid or semisolid material that is usually abnormal but not cancerous (Fig. 6-4). Common sites for cyst formation are the breasts, the sebaceous glands of the skin, and the ovaries. Causes of cyst formation include infection or blockage of a duct.

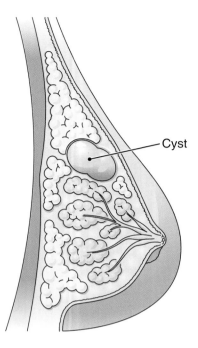

FIGURE 6-4. Cyst in the breast.

Key Terms

acute *a-KŪT*	Sudden, severe; having a short course
benign *bē-NĪN*	Not recurrent or malignant; favorable for recovery; describing tumors that do not spread
carcinoma *kar-si-NŌ-ma*	A malignant neoplasm composed of epithelial cells (from Greek root *carcino,* meaning "crab") (adjective, carcinomatous)
chronic *KRON-ik*	Of long duration; progressing slowly
cyst *sist*	A filled sac or pouch that is usually abnormal (see Fig. 6-4). Used as a root meaning a normal bladder or sac, such as the urinary bladder or gallbladder (root *cyst/o, cyst/i*).
etiology *ē-tē-OL-ō-jē*	The cause of a disease
Gram stain	A laboratory staining procedure that divides bacteria into two groups: gram-positive, which stain blue, and gram-negative, which stain red (see Fig. 6-1)
hernia *HER-nē-a*	Protrusion of an organ through an abnormal opening; a rupture (Fig. 6-5)

inflammation *in-fla-MĀ-shun*	A localized response to tissue injury characterized by heat, pain, redness, and swelling
lesion *LĒ-zhun*	A distinct area of damaged tissue; an injury or wound
malignant *ma-LIG-nant*	Growing worse; harmful; tending to cause death; describing tumors that spread (metastasize)
metastasize *me-TAS-ta-sīz*	To spread from one part of the body to another; characteristic of cancer. The noun is metastasis (*me-TAS-ta-sis*).
necrosis *ne-KRŌ-sis*	Death of tissue
neoplasm *NĒ-ō-plazm*	An abnormal and uncontrolled growth of tissue, namely, a tumor; may be benign or malignant (root *onc/o*, suffix *-oma*)
phagocytosis *fag-ō-sī-TŌ-sis*	The ingestion of organisms, such as invading bacteria or small particles of waste material by a cell; ingested material is then destroyed by the phagocytic cell, or phagocyte (root *phag/o* means "to eat")
parasite *PAR-a-sīt*	An organism that grows on or in another organism (the host), causing damage to it
pathogen *PATH-ō-jen*	An organism capable of causing disease (root *path/o*)
prolapse *PRŌ-laps*	A dropping or downward displacement of an organ or part; ptosis
pus	A product of inflammation consisting of fluid and white blood cells (root *py/o*)
sarcoma *sar-KŌ-ma*	A malignant neoplasm arising from connective tissue (from Greek root *sarco*, meaning "flesh") (adjective, sarcomatous)
sepsis *SEP-sis*	The presence of harmful microorganisms or their toxins in the blood or other tissues (adjective, septic)
toxin *TOKS-in*	A poison (adjective, toxic; roots *tox/o*, *toxic/o*)
trauma *TRAW-ma*	A physical or psychological wound or injury

See also Display 6-1 on infectious diseases.

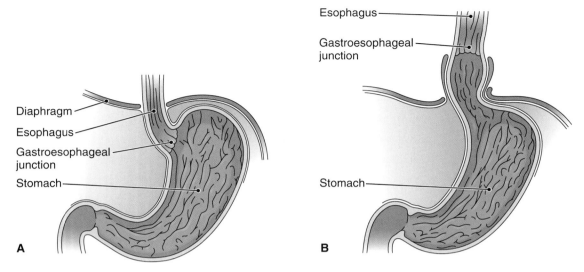

FIGURE 6-5. **(A)** Normal. **(B)** Hiatal hernia. The stomach protrudes through the diaphragm into the thoracic cavity, raising the level of the junction between the esophagus and the stomach. (Reprinted with permission from Cohen BJ, Wood DL. Memmler's The Human Body in Health and Disease. 9th Ed. Philadelphia: Lippincott Williams & Wilkins, 2000.)

Word Parts Pertaining to Disease

TABLE 6-1 Roots for Disease

ROOT	MEANING	EXAMPLE	DEFINITION OF EXAMPLE
alg/o, algi/o, algesi/o	pain	algesia al-JĒ-zē-a	condition of having pain
carcin/o	cancer, carcinoma	carcinogen kar-SIN-ō-jen	substance that produces cancer
cyst/o, cyst/i	filled sac or pouch, cyst, bladder	cystic SIS-tik	pertaining to or having cysts
lith	calculus, stone	lithiasis lith-Ī-a-sis	stone formation
onc/o	tumor	oncogene ON-kō-jēn	gene that causes a tumor
path/o	disease	pathogen PATH-ō-jen	organism that produces disease
py/o	pus	pyocyst PĪ-ō-sist	a sac or cyst containing pus
pyr/o, pyret/o	fever, fire	pyretic pī-RET-ik	pertaining to fever
scler/o	hard	sclerosis skle-RŌ-sis	hardening of tissue
tox/o, toxic/o	poison	exotoxin eks-ō-TOK-sin	toxin secreted by bacterial cells

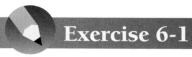

Exercise 6-1

Identify and define the root in each of the following words:

	Root	Meaning of Root

1. pyrexia
   pī-REK-sē-a

2. intoxicate
   in-TOK-si-kāt

3. empyema
   em-pī-Ē-ma

4. pathology
   pa-THOL-ō-jē

Fill in the blanks:

5. Carcinolysis (*kar-sin-OL-i-sis*) is the destruction (-lysis) of a(n) _____.

6. A urolith (*Ū-rō-lith*) is a(n) _____ in the urinary tract (*ur/o*).

7. Oncology (*on-KOL-ō-jē*) is the study and treatment of _____.

8. The term *pathogenic* means producing _____.

9. Pyorrhea (*pī-ō-RĒ-a*) is the discharge (-*rhea*) of _____.

10. Arteriosclerosis (*ar-tē-rē-ō-skle-RŌ-sis*) is a(n) _____ of the arteries.

11. The term toxoid (*TOK-soyd*) means like a(n) _____.

12. An algesimeter (*al-je-SIM-e-ter*) is used to measure sensitivity to _____.

TABLE 6-2 Prefixes for Disease

PREFIX	MEANING	EXAMPLE	DEFINITION OF EXAMPLE
brady-	slow	bradypnea *brad-ip-NĒ-a*	slow breathing (-pnea)
dys-	abnormal, painful, difficult	dysplasia *dis-PLĀ-jē-a*	abnormal development of tissue
mal-	bad, poor	maladaptive *mal-a-DAP-tiv*	poorly suited to a specific use or to the environment
pachy-	thick	pachyemia *pak-ē-Ē-mē-a*	thickness of the blood (-emia)
tachy-	rapid	tachycardia *tak-i-KAR-dē-a*	rapid heart (cardi) rate
xero-	dry	xerosis *zē-RŌ-sis*	dryness of the skin or membranes

Exercise 6-2

Match the following terms and write the appropriate letter to the left of each number:

_____ 1. dystrophy (*DIS-trō-fē*)

_____ 2. tachypnea (*tak-ip-NĒ-a*)

_____ 3. bradycardia (*brad-e-KAR-dē-a*)

_____ 4. xeroderma (*zē-rō-DER-ma*)

_____ 5. dysphagia (*dis-FĀ-jē-a*)

a. dryness of the skin

b. rapid breathing

c. difficulty in swallowing

d. slow heart rate

e. poor nourishment of tissue

Identify and define the prefix in each of the following words:

	Prefix	Meaning of Prefix
6. malnutrition (*mal-nū-TRISH-un*)	_____	_____
7. dysentery (*DIS-en-ter-ē*)	_____	_____
8. pachyderma (*pak-ē-DER-ma*)	_____	_____

TABLE 6-3 Suffixes for Disease

SUFFIX	MEANING	EXAMPLE	DEFINITION OF EXAMPLE
-algia, -algesia	pain	myalgia *mī-AL-jē-a*	pain in a muscle (my/o)
-cele	hernia, localized dilation	hydrocele *HĪ-drō-sēl*	localized dilation containing fluid
-clasis, -clasia	breaking	osteoclasis *os-tē-OK-la-sis*	breaking of a bone (oste/o)
-itis	inflammation	meningitis *men-in-JĪ-tis*	inflammation of the membranes around the brain (meninges)
-megaly	enlargement	hepatomegaly *hep-a-tō-MEG-a-lē*	enlargement of the liver (hepat/o)
-odynia	pain	urodynia *ū-rō-DIN-ē-a*	pain on urination (ur/o)
-oma*	tumor	blastoma *blas-TŌ-ma*	tumor of immature cells
-pathy	any disease of	cardiopathy *kar-dē-OP-a-thē*	any disease of the heart (cardi/o)
-rhage†, -rhagia†	bursting forth, profuse flow, hemorrhage	hemorrhage *HEM-or-ij*	profuse flow of blood
-rhea†	flow, discharge	mucorrhea *mū-kō-rē-a*	discharge of mucus
-rhexis†	rupture	amniorrhexis *am-nē-ō-REK-sis*	rupture of the amniotic sac (bag of waters)
-schisis	fissure, splitting	retinoschisis *ret-i-NOS-ki-sis*	splitting of the retina of the eye

*Plural: -omas, -omata.

†Remember to double the r when adding this suffix to a root.

Exercise 6-3

Match the following terms and write the appropriate letter to the left of each number:

_____ 1. thoracoschisis (*thō-ra-KOS-ki-sis*)   a. breaking of a nucleus

_____ 2. adipocele (*AD-i-pō-sēl*)   b. congenital fissure of the chest

_____ 3. karyoclasis (*kar-ē-OK-la-sis*)   c. tumor of pigmented cells

_____ 4. lipoma (*lip-Ō-ma*)   d. hernia containing fat

_____ 5. melanoma (*mel-a-NŌ-ma*)   e. fatty tumor

_____ 6. hemorrhagic (*hem-or-AJ-ik*)   a. rupture of the liver

_____ 7. hepatorrhexis (*hep-a-tō-REK-sis*)   b. substance that counteracts fever

_____ 8. analgesia (*an-al-JĒ-zē-a*)   c. absence of pain

_____ 9. antipyretic (*an-ti-pī-RET-ik*)   d. pain in a gland

_____ 10. adenodynia (*ad-e-nō-DIN-ē-a*)   e. pertaining to a profuse flow of blood

The root *gastr/o* means "stomach." Define the following terms:

11. gastromegaly (*gas-trō-MEG-a-lē*)   _____ enlargement of the stomach _____

12. gastritis (*gas-TRĪ-tis*)   _____

13. gastropathy (*gas-TROP-a-thē*)   _____

14. gastrocele (*GAS-trō-sēl*)   _____

Some words pertaining to disease are used as suffixes in compound words. As previously noted, the term suffix is used in this book to mean any word part that consistently appears at the end of words. This may be a simple suffix (such as -y, -ia, -ic), a word, or a root–suffix combination (such as -megaly, -rhagia, -pathy).

The words toxic, toxin, and sclerosis are also used as suffixes in compound words. The words carcinoma and sarcoma are used as suffixes to indicate malignant tumors, as in adenocarcinoma and fibrosarcoma.

TABLE 6-4 Words for Disease Used as Suffixes

WORD	MEANING	EXAMPLE	DEFINITION OF EXAMPLE
dilation*, dilatation*	expansion, widening	vasodilation *vas-ō-dī-LĀ-shun*	widening of blood vessels (vas/o)
ectasia, ectasis	dilation	bronchiectasis *brong-kē-EK-ta-sis*	chronic dilation of a bronchus (bronchi/o)
edema	accumulation of fluid, swelling (Fig. 6-6)	lymphedema *lim-fe-DĒ-ma*	swelling of tissues as a result of lymphatic blockage
lysis*	separation, loosening, dissolving, destruction	dialysis *dī-AL-i-sis*	separation of substances by passage through a membrane
malacia	softening	splenomalacia *splē-nō-ma-LĀ-shē-a*	softening of the spleen (splen/o)

TABLE 6-4 Words for Disease Used as Suffixes, *continued*

WORD	MEANING	EXAMPLE	DEFINITION OF EXAMPLE
necrosis	death of tissue	osteonecrosis *os-tē-ō-ne-KRŌ-sis*	death of bone tissue (oste/o)
ptosis	dropping, downward displacement, prolapse	blepharoptosis *blef-e-rop-TŌ-sis*	drooping of the eyelid (blephar/o; Fig. 6-7)
spasm	sudden contraction, cramp	bronchospasm *BRONG-kō-spazm*	spasm of a bronchus (bronch/o)
stasis*	suppression, stoppage	menostasis *men-OS-ta-sis*	suppression of menstrual (men/o) flow
stenosis	narrowing, constriction	arteriostenosis *ar-tēr-ē-ō-ste-NŌ-sis*	narrowing of an artery

*May also refer to treatment.

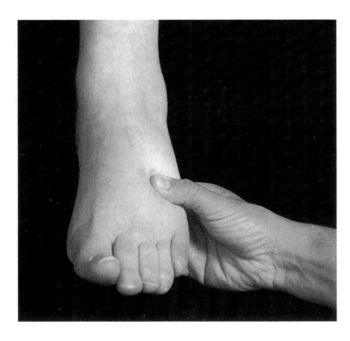

FIGURE 6-6. Edema of the foot. (Reprinted with permission from Bickley LS. Bate's Guide to Physical Examination and History Taking. 8th Ed. Philadelphia: Lippincott Williams & Wilkins, 2003.)

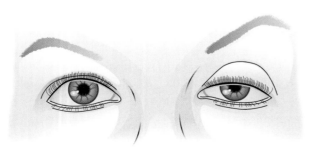

Normal lid   Drooping lid

FIGURE 6-7. Blepharoptosis (drooping of the eyelid).

Exercise 6-4

Match the following terms and write the appropriate letter to the left of each number:

_____ 1. osteonecrosis (os-tē-ō-ne-KRŌ-sis)

_____ 2. craniomalacia (krā-nē-ō-ma-LĀ-shē-a)

_____ 3. hemostasis (hē-mō-STĀ-sis)

_____ 4. gastrectasia (gas-trek-TĀ-sē-a)

_____ 5. hemolysis (hē-MOL-i-sis)

a. destruction of blood cells

b. stoppage of blood flow

c. softening of the skull

d. dilatation of the stomach

e. death of bone tissue

The root *bronch/o* means "bronchus," an air passageway in the lungs. Define the following words:

6. bronchodilation (brong-kō-dī-LĀ-shun)   _____widening of a bronchus_____

7. bronchoedema (brong-kō-e-DĒ-ma)   _____

8. bronchospasm (BRONG-kō-spazm)   _____

9. bronchostenosis (brong-kō-ste-NO-sis)   _____

TABLE 6-5 Prefixes and Roots for Infectious Diseases

WORD PART	MEANING	EXAMPLE	DEFINITION OF EXAMPLE
PREFIXES			
staphyl/o	grapelike cluster	staphylococcus staf-i-lō-KOK-us	a round bacterium that forms clusters
strept/o	twisted chain	streptobacillus strep-tō-ba-SIL-us	a rod-shaped bacterium that forms chains
ROOTS			
bacill/i, bacill/o	bacillus	bacilluria bas-i-LŪ-rē-a	bacilli in the urine (-uria)
bacteri/o	bacterium	bactericide bak-TER-i-sīd	agent that kills (-cide) bacteria
myc/o	fungus, mold	mycosis mī-KŌ-sis	any disease condition caused by a fungus
vir/o	virus	viremia vī-RĒ-mē-a	presence of viruses in the blood (-emia)

Exercise 6-5

Fill in the blanks:

1. The term bacillary (BAS-il-a-rē) means pertaining to _____.

2. The prefix *staphyl/o-* means _____.

3. The prefix *strept/o-* means _____.

Use the suffix -logy to write a word that means the same as each of the following:

4. Study of viruses _____

5. Study of fungi _____

6. Study of bacteria _____

Supplementary Terms

GENERAL TERMS PERTAINING TO DISEASE

acid-fast stain	A laboratory staining procedure used mainly to identify the tuberculosis organism
exacerbation *eks-zas-er-BĀ-shun*	Worsening of disease; increase in severity of a disease or its symptoms
iatrogenic *ī-at-rō-JEN-ik*	Caused by the effects of treatment (from Greek root *iatro-*, meaning "physician")
idiopathic *id-ē-ō-PATH-ik*	Having no known cause
in situ *in SĪ-tū*	Localized, noninvasive (literally "in position"); said of tumors that do not spread, such as carcinoma in situ (CIS)
nosocomial *nos-ō-KŌ-mē-al*	Describing an infection acquired in a hospital (root *nos/o* means "disease," and *comial* refers to a hospital). Such infections can be a serious problem, especially if they are resistant to antibiotics; for example, there are now strains of methicillin-resistant *Staphylococcus aureus* (MRSA) and vancomycin-resistant *S. aureus* (VRSA), which cause troublesome infections in hospital settings.
opportunistic *op-por-tū-NIS-tik*	Describing an infection that occurs because of a poor or altered condition of the host
remission *rē-MISH-un*	A lessening of disease symptoms; the period during which such lessening occurs
septicemia *sep-ti-SĒ-mē-a*	Presence of pathogenic bacteria in the blood; blood poisoning
systemic *sis-TEM-ik*	Pertaining to the whole body

MANIFESTATIONS OF DISEASE

abscess *AB-ses*	A localized collection of pus
adhesion *ad-HĒ-zhun*	A uniting of two surfaces or parts that may normally be separated

Manifestations of Disease, continued

anaplasia *a-na-PLĀ-jē-a*	Lack of normal differentiation, as shown by cancer cells
ascites *a-SĪ-tēz*	Accumulation of fluid in the peritoneal cavity
cellulitis *sel-ū-LĪ-tis*	A spreading inflammation of tissue
effusion *e-FŪ-zhun*	Escape of fluid into a cavity or other body part
exudate *EKS-ū-dāt*	Material that escapes from blood vessels as a result of injury to tissues
fissure *FISH-ur*	A groove or split
fistula *FIS-tū-la*	An abnormal passage between two organs or from an organ to the surface of the body
gangrene *GANG-grēn*	Death of tissue, usually caused by lack of blood supply; may be associated with bacterial infection and decomposition
hyperplasia *hī-per-PLĀ-jē-a*	Excessive growth of normal cells in normal arrangement
hypertrophy *hī-PER-trō-fē*	An increase in size of an organ without increase in the number of cells; may result from an increase in activity, as in muscles
induration *in-dū-RĀ-shun*	Hardening; an abnormally hard spot or place
metaplasia *met-a-PLĀ-jē-a*	Conversion of cells to a form that is not normal for that tissue (prefix *meta-* means "change")
polyp *POL-ip*	A tumor attached by a thin stalk
purulent *PUR-ū-lent*	Forming or containing pus
suppuration *sup-ū-RĀ-shun*	Pus formation

ABBREVIATIONS

CA	Cancer		**staph**	Staphylococcus
CIS	Carcinoma in situ		**strep**	Streptococcus
FUO	Fever of unknown origin		**VRSA**	Vancomycin-resistant
MRSA	Methicillin-resistant *Staphylococcus aureus*			*Staphylococcus aureus*

Chapter Review 6-1

Match the following terms and write the appropriate letter to the left of each number:

_____	1. carcinogenic	a. enlargement of the liver
_____	2. pathogenic	b. causing cancer
_____	3. adenocarcinoma	c. cancer of glandular tissue
_____	4. encephalitis	d. causing disease
_____	5. hepatomegaly	e. inflammation of the brain

_____	6. apyrexia	a. incision to remove a stone
_____	7. detoxification	b. hardened
_____	8. sclerotic	c. absence of a fever
_____	9. oncolysis	d. destruction of a tumor
_____	10. lithotomy	e. removal of poisons

_____	11. xerotic	a. dry
_____	12. dyskinesia	b. thickness of the blood
_____	13. pachyemia	c. swelling of the fingers or toes
_____	14. pyorrhea	d. abnormal movement
_____	15. dactyledema	e. discharge of pus

_____	16. lesion	a. self-destruction
_____	17. nephroptosis	b. local wound or injury
_____	18. hemostasis	c. dilatation
_____	19. ectasia	d. stoppage of blood flow
_____	20. autolysis	e. dropping of the kidney

_____	21. cardiorrhexis	a. any disease of a gland
_____	22. stenosis	b. rupture of the heart
_____	23. cephaledema	c. narrowing
_____	24. adenopathy	d. presence of pathogens in the blood
_____	25. septicemia	e. accumulation of fluid in the head

_____	26. bacilli	a. round bacteria in clusters
_____	27. helminths	b. round bacteria in chains

_____ 28. streptococci   c. fungal infection

_____ 29. mycosis   d. rod-shaped bacteria

_____ 30. staphylococci   e. worms

SUPPLEMENTARY TERMS

_____ 31. purulent   a. having no known cause

_____ 32. idiopathic   b. hospital-acquired

_____ 33. adhesion   c. tumor attached by a thin stalk

_____ 34. nosocomial   d. forming or containing pus

_____ 35. polyp   e. union of two surfaces or parts

Fill in the blanks:

36. Any abnormal and uncontrolled growth of tissue, whether benign or malignant, is called a(n)
_____.

37. Heat, pain, redness, and swelling are the four major signs of _____.

38. A disease of long duration that progresses slowly is described as _____.

39. The spreading of cancer to other parts of the body is called _____.

40. A malignant tumor of connective tissue is called _____.

41. Toxicology is the study of _____.

42. Death of tissue is called _____.

43. A sudden contraction or cramp is called a(n) _____.

44. Protrusion of an organ through an abnormal opening is a(n) _____.

Word building. Use the suffix _-genesis_ to write words with the following meanings:

45. Formation of cancer   _____ carcinogenesis _____

46. Origin of any disease   _____

47. Formation of a tumor   _____

48. Formation of pus   _____

The root _neur/o_ pertains to the nervous system or a nerve. Add a suffix to this root to form words with the following meanings:

49. Any disease of the nervous system   _____

50. Inflammation of a nerve   _____

51. Pain in a nerve   _____

52. Tumor of nervous tissue   _____

Use the root *oste/o*, meaning "bone," to form words with the following meanings:

53. Softening of a bone   _____

54. Tumor of a bone   _____

55. Destruction of bone tissue   _____

56. Breaking of a bone   _____

Case Studies

Case Study 6-1: Esophageal Spasm

B.R., a 53-year-old woman, consulted with her primary physician because of occasional episodes of dysphagia with moderate to severe tight, gripping pain in her midthorax. She reported that the onset was sudden after ingestion of certain foods or beverages, beginning retrosternally and radiating to the cervical and dorsal regions. The pain was not relieved by assuming a supine position or holding her breath. B.R. also stated that she felt like her heart was racing and that she might be having a heart attack. She denied any dyspepsia, vomiting, or dyspnea. Her doctor suspected acute esophageal spasm or possibly a paraesophageal hiatal hernia and referred B.R. to a gastroenterologist for a gastroscopy and esophageal manometry study (pressure measurement). She also underwent a barium swallow study under fluoroscopic imaging.

Case Study 6-2: HIV Infection and Tuberculosis

T.H., a 48-year-old man, was an admitted intravenous (IV) drug user and occasionally abused alcohol. Over 4 weeks, he had experienced fever, night sweats, malaise, a cough, and a 10-lb. weight loss. He was also concerned about several discolored lesions that had erupted weeks before on his arms and legs.

T.H. made an appointment with a physician assistant (PA) at the neighborhood clinic. On examination, the PA noted bilateral anterior cervical and axillary lymphadenopathy and pyrexia. T.H.'s temperature was 39°C. The PA sent T.H. to the hospital for further studies.

T.H.'s chest radiograph (x-ray image) showed paratracheal adenopathy and bilateral interstitial infiltrates, suspicious of tuberculosis (TB). His blood study results were positive for human immunodeficiency virus (HIV) and showed a low lymphocyte count. Sputum and bronchoscopic lavage (washing) fluid were positive for an acid-fast bacillus (AFB), and a PPD (purified protein derivative) skin test result was also positive. Based on these findings, T.H. was diagnosed with HIV, TB, and Kaposi sarcoma related to past IV drug abuse.

Case Study 6-3: Endocarditis

D.A., a 37-year-old alcoholic man, sought treatment after experiencing several days of high fever and generalized weakness on return from his vacation. D.A.'s family doctor suspected cardiac involvement because of D.A.'s history of rheumatic fever. The doctor was concerned because D.A.'s brother had died of acute malignant hyperpyrexia during surgery at the age of 12. D.A. was referred to a cardiologist, who scheduled an electrocardiogram (ECG) and a transesophageal echocardiogram (TEE).

D.A. was admitted to the hospital with subacute bacterial endocarditis (SBE) and placed on high-dose IV antibiotics and bed rest. He had also developed a heart murmur, which was diagnosed as idiopathic hypertrophic subaortic stenosis (IHSS).

Case Studies, continued

CASE STUDY QUESTIONS

Multiple choice: Select the best answer and write the letter of your choice to the left of each number.

_____ 1. The cervical region is the region of the:
    a. heart
    b. uterus
    c. neck
    d. leg
    e. head

_____ 2. A word that has the same meaning as dorsal is:
    a. anterior
    b. posterior
    c. caudal
    d. inferior
    e. superior

_____ 3. In referring to tissues, the term interstitial means:
    a. around cells
    b. under cells
    c. between cells
    d. through cells
    e. within cells

_____ 4. The term axillary refers to the:
    a. bladder
    b. abdomen
    c. wrist
    d. armpit
    e. groin

_____ 5. The term pyrexia refers to a(n):
    a. fever
    b. stone
    c. tumor
    d. spasm
    e. poison

_____ 6. Dyspepsia refers to indigestion. Dysphagia and dyspnea refer to difficulty with _____ and _____.
    a. breathing and coughing
    b. swallowing and urinating
    c. walking and chewing gum
    d. swallowing and breathing
    e. sleeping and breathing

Case Studies, continued

_____ 7. Paraesophageal and paratracheal refer to _____ the esophagus and trachea.
   a. under
   b. superior to
   c. near or beside
   d. in between
   e. within

_____ 8. The endocardium is the lining of the inside of the heart. Endocarditis refers to a(n) _____ of the lining of the heart.
   a. narrowing
   b. inflammation
   c. overgrowth of tissue
   d. cancerous growth
   e. thinning

_____ 9. D.A.'s heart murmur was caused by a stenosis, or _____ of the aortic valve of his heart.
   a. narrowing
   b. inflammation
   c. overgrowth of tissue
   d. cancerous growth
   e. thinning

_____ 10. The term for a condition or disease of unknown etiology is:
   a. stenosis
   b. hypertrophic
   c. chronic
   d. acute
   e. idiopathic

Fill in the blanks:

11. The word in the case studies that means "protrusion of an organ through an abnormal body opening" is a(n) _____.

12. Adenopathy is any disease of a(n) _____.

13. Tuberculosis is caused by a rod-shaped bacterium described as a(n) _____.

14. A malignant neoplasm arising from muscle, connective, or bone tissue is a(n) _____.

15. A disease condition that can be fatal, rapidly spreads to the entire body, and is characterized by a very high fever is called _____.

Case Studies, continued

Give the meaning of the following abbreviations:

16. HIV _____

17. PPD _____

18. ECG _____

19. AFB _____

CHAPTER 6 Answer Section

Answers to Chapter Exercises

EXERCISE 6-1

1. pyr/o; fever
2. toxic/o; poison
3. py/o; pus
4. path/o; disease
5. cancer, carcinoma
6. calculus, stone
7. tumors
8. disease
9. pus
10. hardening
11. poison, toxin
12. pain

EXERCISE 6-2

1. e
2. b
3. d
4. a
5. c
6. mal-; bad, poor
7. dys-; abnormal, painful, difficult
8. pachy-; thick

EXERCISE 6-3

1. b
2. d
3. a
4. e
5. c
6. e
7. a
8. c
9. b
10. d
11. enlargement of the stomach
12. inflammation of the stomach
13. any disease of the stomach
14. hernia of the stomach

EXERCISE 6-4

1. e
2. c
3. b
4. d
5. a
6. widening of a bronchus
7. accumulation of fluid in or swelling of a bronchus
8. sudden contraction (spasm) of a bronchus
9. narrowing of a bronchus

EXERCISE 6-5

1. bacilli or a bacillus
2. grapelike cluster
3. twisted chains
4. virology ($v\bar{i}$-ROL-$\bar{o}$-$j\bar{e}$)

5. mycology ($m\bar{i}$-KOL-$\bar{o}$-$j\bar{e}$)
6. bacteriology (bak-$t\bar{e}r$-$\bar{e}$-OL-$\bar{o}$-$j\bar{e}$)

Answers to Chapter Review 6-1

1. b
2. d
3. c
4. e
5. a
6. c
7. e
8. b
9. d
10. a
11. a
12. d
13. b
14. e
15. c
16. b
17. e
18. d
19. c
20. a
21. b
22. c
23. e
24. a
25. d
26. d
27. e
28. b
29. c
30. a
31. d
32. a
33. e
34. b
35. c
36. neoplasm
37. inflammation
38. chronic
39. metastasis
40. sarcoma
41. toxins; poisons
42. necrosis
43. spasm
44. hernia
45. carcinogenesis
46. pathogenesis
47. oncogenesis
48. pyogenesis
49. neuropathy ($n\bar{u}$-ROP-a-$th\bar{e}$)
50. neuritis ($n\bar{u}$-R$\bar{I}$-tis)
51. neuralgia ($n\bar{u}$-RAL-$j\bar{e}$-a)
52. neuroma ($n\bar{u}$-R$\bar{O}$-ma)
53. osteomalacia (os-$t\bar{e}$-$\bar{o}$-ma-L$\bar{A}$-$sh\bar{e}$-a)
54. osteoma (os-$t\bar{e}$-$\bar{O}$-ma)
55. osteolysis (os-$t\bar{e}$-OL-i-sis)
56. osteoclasis (os-$t\bar{e}$-OK-la-sis)

Answers to Case Study Questions

1. c
2. b
3. c
4. d
5. a
6. d
7. c
8. b
9. a
10. e
11. hernia
12. gland
13. bacillus
14. sarcoma
15. malignant hyperpyrexia (also called hyperthermia or MH)
16. human immunodeficiency virus
17. purified protein derivative
18. electrocardiogram
19. acid-fast bacillus

Diagnosis and Treatment; Surgery

Chapter Contents

Objectives

After study of this chapter you should be able to:

1. List the main components of a patient history.
2. Describe the main methods used in examination of a patient.
3. Name and describe nine imaging techniques.
4. Name possible forms of treatment.
5. Describe theories of alternative and complementary medicine and some healing practices used in these fields.
6. Describe staging and grading as they apply to cancer.
7. Define basic terms pertaining to medical examination, diagnosis, and treatment.
8. Identify and use the roots and suffixes pertaining to diagnosis and surgery.
9. Interpret symbols and abbreviations used in diagnosis and treatment.
10. Interpret a case history containing terms related to diagnosis and treatment.

Diagnosis

Medical **diagnosis**, the determination of the nature and cause of an illness, begins with a patient history. This includes a history of the present illness with a description of symptoms, a past medical history, and a family and a social history.

A physical examination, which includes a review of all systems and observation of any signs of illness, follows the history taking. Practitioners use the following techniques in performing physicals:
- Inspection: visual examination.
- Palpation: touching the surface of the body with the hands or fingers.
- Percussion: tapping the body and listening to the sounds produced (Fig. 7-1).
- Auscultation: listening to body sounds with a stethoscope (Fig. 7-2).

Vital signs (VS) are also recorded for comparison with normal ranges. Vital signs are measurements that reflect basic functions necessary to maintain life and include:
- Temperature (T).
- Pulse rate, measured in beats per minute (bpm) (Fig. 7-3).
- Respiration rate (R), measured in breaths per minute.

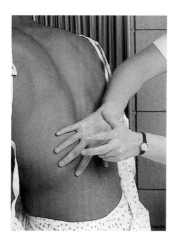

FIGURE 7-1. Percussion. (Reprinted with permission from Taylor C, Lillis C, LeMone P. Fundamentals of Nursing: The Art and Science of Nursing Care. 4th Ed. Philadelphia: Lippincott Williams & Wilkins, 2001.)

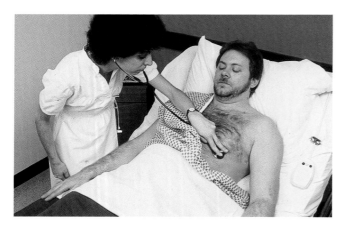

FIGURE 7-2. Auscultation using a stethoscope. (Reprinted with permission from Taylor C, Lillis C, LeMone P. Fundamentals of Nursing: The Art and Science of Nursing Care. 4th Ed. Philadelphia: Lippincott Williams & Wilkins, 2001.)

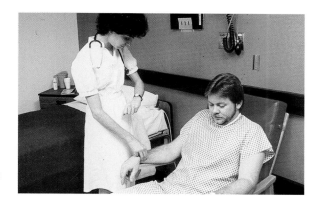

FIGURE 7-3. Measuring the pulse rate. (Reprinted with permission from Taylor C, Lillis C, LeMone P. Fundamentals of Nursing: The Art and Science of Nursing Care. 4th Ed. Philadelphia: Lippincott Williams & Wilkins, 2001.)

- Blood pressure (BP), measured in millimeters mercury (mm Hg) and recorded when the heart is contracting (systolic pressure) and relaxing (diastolic pressure) (Fig. 7-4). There is more information on blood pressure in Chapter 9.

Additional tools used in physical examinations include the **ophthalmoscope** (Fig. 7-5A), for examination of the eyes; the **otoscope** (Fig. 7-5B), for examination of the ears; hammers, for testing reflexes, and the blood pressure cuff or **sphygmomanometer** (*sfig-mō-ma-NOM-e-ter*) (see Fig. 7-4).

The skin, hair, and nails provide easily observable indications of a person's state of health. Such features of the skin as color, texture, thickness, and presence of lesions (local injuries) are noted throughout the course of the physical examination. Chapter 21 contains a discussion of the skin and skin diseases.

Diagnosis is further aided by laboratory test results. These may include tests on blood, urine, and other body fluids, and the identification of infectious organisms. Additional tests may include study of the electrical activity of tissues such as the brain and heart, examination of body cavities by means of an **endoscope** (Fig. 7-6), and imaging techniques. **Biopsy** is the removal of tissue for microscopic examination. Biopsy specimens can be obtained by needle withdrawal (aspiration) of fluid, as from the chest or from a cyst; by a small punch, as of the skin; by endoscopy, as from the respiratory or digestive tract; or by surgical removal, as of a tumor or node.

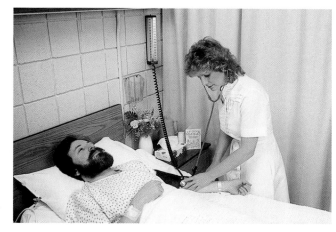

FIGURE 7-4. Measuring blood pressure with a sphygmomanometer. (Reprinted with permission from Taylor C, Lillis C, LeMone P. Fundamentals of Nursing: The Art and Science of Nursing Care. 4th Ed. Philadelphia: Lippincott Williams & Wilkins, 2001.)

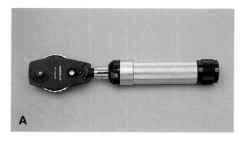 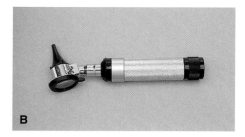

FIGURE 7-5. (A) Ophthalmoscope. **(B)** Otoscope. (Reprinted with permission from Taylor C, Lillis C, LeMone P. Fundamentals of Nursing: The Art and Science of Nursing Care. 4th Ed. Philadelphia: Lippincott Williams & Wilkins, 2001. Photos courtesy of Ken Kasper.)

Imaging Techniques

Imaging techniques are the use of various physical forces to produce visual images of the body. The most fundamental imaging method is **radiography**, which uses x-rays to produce a picture (radiograph) on sensitized film. Radiography is best at showing dense tissues, such as bone, but views of soft tissue can be enhanced by using a contrast medium, such as a barium mixture, to outline the tissue. Other forms of energy used to produce diagnostic images include sound waves, radioactive isotopes, radio waves, and magnetic fields. See Display 7-1 for a description of imaging methods.

Treatment

If diagnosis so indicates, treatment, also termed **therapy**, is begun. This may consist of counseling, drugs, surgery, radiation, physical therapy, occupational therapy, psychiatric treatment, or a combination of these. See Chapter 8 for a discussion of drugs and their actions. During diagnosis and throughout the course of treatment, a patient is evaluated to establish a **prognosis**, that is, a prediction of the outcome of the disease.

Box 7-1 Terminology Evolves With Medical Science

The science of medicine never stands still, nor does its terminology. One can never say that his or her work in learning medical terminology is complete because vocabulary is constantly being added as new diagnoses, treatments, and technologies are discovered or developed.

A generation ago, gene therapy, genetic engineering, in vitro fertilization, cloning, and stem cell research were unknown to the public. PET scans, MRI, DNA fingerprinting, radio immunoassay, bone density scans for identifying osteoporosis, and other diagnostic techniques were not in use. Some of the new categories of drugs, such as statins for reducing cholesterol, antiviral agents, histamine antagonists for treating ulcers, ACE inhibitors for treating hypertension, and breast cancer preventives were undiscovered. The genes associated with certain forms of cancer and with certain hereditary abnormalities had yet to be isolated.

Each of these advances brings new terminology into use. Anyone who wants to keep current with medical terminology has a lifetime of learning ahead.

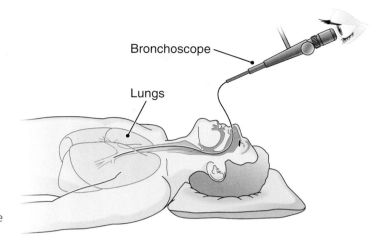

Bronchoscope

Lungs

FIGURE 7-6. Use of a bronchoscope, a type of endoscope.

DISPLAY 7-1 Imaging Techniques

METHOD	DESCRIPTION
cineradiography (sin-e-rā-dē-OG-ra-fē)	making of a motion picture of successive images appearing on a fluoroscopic screen
computed tomography (CT, CT scan) (tō-MOG-ra-fē)	use of a computer to generate an image from a large number of x-rays passed at different angles through the body; a three-dimensional picture of a cross-section of the body is obtained; reveals more about soft tissues than does simple radiography (Fig. 7-7)
fluoroscopy (flū-ROS-kō-pē)	use of x-rays to examine deep structures; the shadows cast by x-rays passed through the body are observed on a fluorescent screen; the device used is called a fluoroscope
magnetic resonance imaging (MRI)	production of images through the use of a magnetic field and radio waves; the characteristics of soft tissue are revealed by differences in molecular properties; eliminates the need for x-rays and contrast media
positron emission tomography (PET)	production of sectional body images by administration of a natural substance, such as glucose, labeled with a positron-emitting isotope; the rays subsequently emitted are interpreted by computer to show the internal distribution of the substance administered; PET has been used to follow blood flow through an organ and to measure metabolic activity within an organ, such as the brain, under different conditions
radiography (rā-dē-OG-ra-fē)	use of x-rays passed through the body to make a visual record (radiograph) of internal structures on specially sensitized film
scintigraphy (sin-TIG-ra-fē)	production of an image of the distribution of radioactivity in tissues after internal administration of a radioactive substance (radionuclide); the images are obtained with a scintillation camera; the record produced is a scintiscan (SIN-ti-skan) and usually specifies the part examined or the isotope used for the test, as in bone scan, gallium scan
single photon emission computed tomography (SPECT)	scintigraphic technique that permits visualization of the cross-sectional distribution of a radioisotope
ultrasonography (ul-tra-son-OG-ra-fē)	generation of a visual image from the echoes of high-frequency sound waves traveling back from different tissues; also called sonography (so-NOG-ra-fē) and echography (ek-OG-ra-fē) (Fig. 7-8)

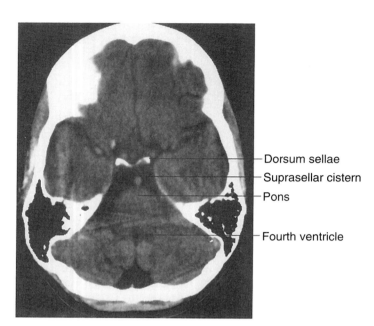

— Dorsum sellae
— Suprasellar cistern
— Pons

— Fourth ventricle

FIGURE 7-7. CT scan of a normal adult human brain. (Reprinted with permission from Erkonen WE, Smith WL. Radiology 101: Basics and Fundamentals of Imaging. Philadelphia: Lippincott Williams & Wilkins, 1998.)

Surgery

Surgery is a method for treating disease or injury by manual operations. Surgery may be done through an existing body opening, but usually it involves cutting or puncturing tissue with a sharp instrument in the process of **incision**. (See Display 7-2 for descriptions of surgical instruments and Figure 7-9 for pictures of surgical instruments.) Some form of **anesthesia** to dull or eliminate pain is usually required. After surgery, incisions must be closed for proper healing. Conventionally, this is done using stitches or **sutures**, but adhesive strips, staples, and skin glue also are used.

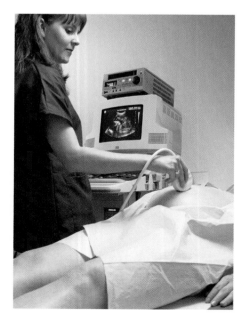

FIGURE 7-8. Use of ultrasound during pregnancy. (Reprinted with permission from Pillitteri A. Maternal and Child Health Nursing: Care of the Childbearing and Childrearing Family. 4th Ed. Philadelphia: Lippincott Williams & Wilkins, 2003).

Many types of operations are now performed using a laser beam. This is an intense beam of light that can be used for surgery and for diagnosis. Some procedures require destruction of tissue by a harmful agent, such as by heat or a chemical, in the process of **cautery** or cauterization.

Some of the purposes of surgery include:

- Treatment: For **excision** (cutting out) of diseased or abnormal tissue, such as a tumor or an inflamed appendix. Surgical methods are also used to repair wounds or injuries, as in skin grafting for burns or realigning broken bones. Surgical methods are used to correct circulatory problems and to return structures to their normal position, as in raising a prolapsed organ, such as the bladder, in a surgical **fixation** procedure.
- Diagnosis: To remove tissue for laboratory study in a biopsy, as described above. Exploratory surgery to investigate the cause of symptoms is performed less frequently now because of advances in non-invasive diagnostic and imaging techniques.
- Restoration: Surgery may compensate for lost function, as when a section of the intestine is redirected in a colostomy, a tube is inserted to allow breathing in a tracheostomy, a feeding tube is inserted, or an organ is transplanted. Plastic or reconstructive surgery may be done to accommodate a prosthesis, to restore proper appearance, or for cosmetic reasons.
- Relief: **Palliative** treatment is any therapy that provides relief but is not intended as a cure. Surgery is done to relieve pain or discomfort, as by cutting the nerve supply to an organ or reducing the size of a tumor to relieve pressure.

Surgery may be done in an emergency or urgent situation under conditions of acute danger, as in traumatic injury or severe blockage. Other procedures, such as cataract removal from the eye, may be planned when convenient. Elective or optional surgery would not cause serious consequences if delayed or not done.

Over time, surgery has extended beyond the classic operating room of a hospital to other hospital areas and to private surgical facilities where people can be treated within 1 day as outpatients. Preoperative care is given before surgery and includes examination, obtaining the patient's informed consent for the procedure, and preadmission testing. Postoperative care includes recovery from anesthesia, follow-up evaluations, and instructions for home care.

Alternative and Complementary Medicine

During the last century, the leading causes of death in industrialized countries gradually shifted from infectious diseases to chronic diseases of the cardiovascular and respiratory systems and cancer. In addition to advancing age, these conditions are greatly influenced by life habits and the environment. As a result, many people have begun to consider healing practices from other philosophies and cultures as alternatives and complements to conventional Western medicine. Some of these philosophies include **osteopathy**, **naturopathy**, **homeopathy**, and **chiropractic**. Techniques of **acupuncture**, **biofeedback**, massage, and meditation may also be used, as well as herbal remedies (see Chapter 8) and nutritional counseling on diet, vitamins, and minerals.

With complementary and alternative therapies, emphasis is placed on maintaining health rather than treating disease and on allowing the body opportunity to heal itself. The U.S. government has established the National Center for Complementary and Alternative Medicine (NCCAM) within the National Institutes of Health (NIH) to study these therapies.

Cancer

Methods used in the diagnosis of cancer include physical examination, biopsy, imaging techniques, and laboratory test results for abnormalities, or "markers," associated with specific types of malignancies. Some cancer markers are byproducts, such as enzymes, hormones, and cellular proteins, that are abnormal or

DISPLAY 7-2 Surgical Instruments

INSTRUMENT	DESCRIPTION
bougie (*BOO-zhē*)	slender, flexible instrument for exploring and dilating tubes
cannula (*KAN-ū-la*)	tube enclosing a trocar (see below) that allows escape of fluid or air after removal of the trocar
clamp	instrument used to compress tissue
curet (curette) (*KŪ-ret*)	spoon-shaped instrument for removing material from the wall of a cavity or other surface (see Fig. 7-9)
elevator (*EL-e-vā-tor*)	instrument for lifting tissue or bone
forceps (*FOR-seps*)	instrument for holding or extracting (see Fig. 7-9)
Gigli saw (*JĒL-yēz*)	flexible wire saw
hemostat (*HĒ-mō-stat*)	small clamp for stopping blood flow from a vessel (see Fig. 7-9)
rasp	surgical file
retractor (*rē-TRAK-tor*)	instrument used to maintain exposure by separating a wound and holding back organs or tissues (see Fig. 7-9)
rongeur (*ron-ZHUR*)	gouge forceps
scalpel (*SKAL-pel*)	surgical knife with a sharp blade (see Fig. 7-9)
scissors (*SIZ-ors*)	a cutting instrument with two opposing blades
sound (*sownd*)	instrument for exploring a cavity or canal (see Fig. 7-9)
trocar (*TRŌ-kar*)	sharp pointed instrument contained in a cannula used to puncture a cavity

are produced in abnormal amounts. Researchers are also linking specific genetic mutations to certain forms of cancer.

Two methods, grading and staging, are used to classify cancers to select and evaluate therapy and estimate the outcome of the disease. **Grading** is based on histologic changes observed in the tumor cells when they are examined microscopically. Grades increase from I to IV with the increasing abnormality of the cells.

Staging is a procedure for establishing the clinical extent of tumor spread, both at the original site and in other parts of the body (metastases). The TNM system is commonly used. These letters stand for primary tumor (T), regional lymph nodes (N), and distant metastases (M). Evaluation in these categories varies for each type of tumor. Based on TNM results, a stage ranging from I–IV in severity is assigned. Cancers of the blood, lymphatic system, and nervous system are evaluated by different standards.

The most widely used methods for treatment of cancer are surgery, radiation therapy, and **chemotherapy** (treatment with chemicals). Newer methods of **immunotherapy** use substances that stimulate the immune system as a whole or vaccines prepared specifically against a tumor. Hormone therapy may also be effective against certain types of tumors. When no active signs of the disease remain, the cancer is said to be in **remission**.

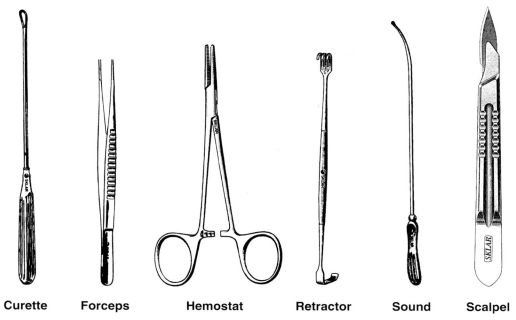

| Curette | Forceps | Hemostat | Retractor | Sound | Scalpel |

FIGURE 7-9. Surgical instruments.

Key Terms

anesthesia *an-es-thē-zē-a*	Loss of the ability to feel pain, as by administration of a drug
auscultation *aws-kul-TĀ-shun*	Listening for sounds within the body, usually within the chest or abdomen (see Fig. 7-2)
biopsy *BĪ-op-sē*	Removal of a small amount of tissue for microscopic examination
cautery *KAW-ter-ē*	Destruction of tissue by a damaging agent, such as a harmful chemical, heat, or electric current (electrocautery); cauterization
chemotherapy *kē-mō-THER-a-pē*	The use of chemicals to treat disease
diagnosis *dī-ag-NŌ-sis*	The process of determining the cause and nature of an illness
endoscope *EN-dō-skōp*	An instrument for examining the inside of an organ or cavity through a body opening or small incision; most endoscopes use fiberoptics for viewing (see Fig. 7-6)
excision *ek-SIZH-un*	Removal by cutting (suffix *-ectomy*)

fixation *fik-SĀ-shun*	Holding or fastening a structure in a fixed position (suffix *-pexy*)
grading *GRĀ-ding*	A method for evaluating a tumor based on microscopic examination of the cells
immunotherapy *im-ū-nō-THER-a-pē*	Treatment that involves stimulation or suppression of the immune system, either specifically or nonspecifically
incision *in-SIZH-un*	A cut, as for surgery; also the act of cutting (suffix *-tomy*)
inspection *in-SPEK-shun*	Visual examination of the body
laser *LĀ-zer*	A device that transforms light into a beam of intense heat and power; used for surgery and diagnosis
ophthalmoscope *of-THAL-mō-skōp*	An instrument for examining the interior of the eye (see Fig. 7-5A)
otoscope *Ō-tō-skōp*	Instrument used to examine the ears (see Fig. 7-5B)
palliative *PAL-ē-a-tiv*	Providing relief but not cure; a treatment that provides such relief
palpation *pal-PĀ-shun*	Examining by placing the hands or fingers on the surface of the body to determine such characteristics as texture, temperature, movement, and consistency
percussion *per-KUSH-un*	Tapping the body lightly but sharply to assess the condition of the underlying part by the sounds obtained (see Fig. 7-1)
prognosis *prog-NŌ-sis*	Prediction of the course and outcome of a disease
radiography *rā-dē-OG-ra-fē*	Use of x-rays passed through the body to make a visual record (radiograph) of internal structures on specially sensitized film
radionuclide *rā-dē-ō-NŪ-klīd*	A substance that gives off radiation; used for diagnosis and treatment; also called radioisotope or radiopharmaceutical
remission *rē-MISH-un*	A lessening of the symptoms of a disease; the period during which this decrease occurs or the period when no sign of a disease exists
sign *sīn*	An objective evidence of disease that can be observed or tested; examples are fever, rash, high blood pressure, and blood or urine abnormalities; an objective symptom
sphygmomanometer *sfig-mō-ma-NOM-e-ter*	The blood pressure apparatus or blood pressure cuff; pressure is read in millimeters of mercury (mm Hg) when the heart is contracting (systolic pressure) and when the heart is relaxing (diastolic pressure) and is reported as systolic/diastolic (see Fig. 7-2)
staging *STĀ-jing*	The process of classifying malignant tumors for diagnosis, treatment, and prognosis

stethoscope *STETH-ō-skōp*	An instrument used for listening to sounds produced within the body (from the Greek root *steth/o*, meaning "chest") (see Fig. 7-2)
surgery *SUR-jer-ē*	A method for treating disease or injury by manual operations
suture *SŪ-chur*	To unite parts by stitching them together; also the thread or other material used in that process or the seam formed by surgical stitching (suffix *-rhaphy*)
symptom *SIM-tum*	Any evidence of disease; sometimes limited to subjective evidence of disease, as experienced by the individual, such as pain, dizziness, weakness
therapy *THER-a-pē*	Treatment; intervention

Alternative and Complementary Medicine

acupuncture *AK-ū-punk-chur*	An ancient Chinese method of inserting thin needles into the body at specific points to relieve pain, induce anesthesia, or promote healing; similar effects can be obtained by using firm finger pressure at the surface of the body in the technique of *acupressure*
biofeedback *bī-ō-FĒD-bak*	A method for learning control of involuntary physiologic responses by using electronic devices to monitor bodily changes and feed this information back to a person
chiropractic *kī-rō-PRAK-tik*	A science that stresses the condition of the nervous system in diagnosis and treatment of disease; often, the spine is manipulated to correct misalignment; most patients consult for musculoskeletal pain and headaches (from Greek *cheir*, meaning "hand")
homeopathy *hō-mē-OP-a-thē*	A philosophy of treating disease by administering drugs in highly diluted form along with promoting healthy life habits and a healthy environment (from *home/o*, meaning "same," and *path*, meaning "disease")
naturopathy *nā-chur-OP-a-thē*	A therapeutic philosophy of helping people to heal themselves by developing healthy lifestyles, naturopaths may use some of the methods of conventional medicine (from *nature* and *path/o*, meaning "disease")
osteopathy *os-tē-OP-a-thē*	A system of therapy based on the theory that the body can overcome disease when it has normal structure, a favorable environment, and proper nutrition; osteopaths use standard medical practices for diagnosis and treatment but stress the identification and correction of faulty body structure (from *oste/o*, meaning "bone," and *path*, meaning "disease")

Word Parts Pertaining to Diagnosis and Treatment

TABLE 7-1 Roots for Physical Forces

ROOT	MEANING	EXAMPLE	DEFINITION OF EXAMPLE
aer/o	air, gas	aerobic er-Ō-bik	requiring air (oxygen)
bar/o	pressure	barotrauma bar-ō-TRAW-ma	injury caused by pressure
chrom/o, chromat/o	color, stain	achromatous a-KRŌ-ma-tus	lacking color
chron/o	time	synchronous SIN-krō-nus	occurring at the same time
cry/o	cold	cryoprobe KRĪ-ō-prōb	instrument used to apply extreme cold
electro/o	electricity	electrolysis ē-lek-TROL-i-sis	destruction (-lysis) by means of electric current
erg/o	work	synergistic sin-er-JIS-tik	working together with increased effect, such as certain drugs in combination
phon/o	sound, voice	phonograph FŌ-nō-graf	instrument used to reproduce sound
phot/o	light	photography fō-TOG-ra-fē	using light to record an image on light-sensitive paper
radi/o	radiation, x-ray	radioactive ra-dē-ō-AK-tiv	giving off radiation
son/o	sound	ultrasonic ul-tra-SON-ik	pertaining to high-frequency sound waves (beyond human hearing)
therm/o	heat, temperature	hypothermia hī-pō-THER-mē-a	abnormally low body temperature

Exercise 7-1

Match the following terms and write the appropriate letter to the left of each number:

_____ 1. asynchronous (*a-SIN-krō-nus*)   a. abnormally high body temperature

_____ 2. hypobaric (*hī-pō-BAR-ik*)   b. study and use of radiation

_____ 3. chromophilic (*krō-mō-FIL-ik*)   c. pertaining to decreased pressure

_____ 4. hyperthermia (*hī-per-THER-mē-a*)   d. not occurring at the same time

_____ 5. radiology (*ra-dē-OL-ō-jē*)   e. attracting color (stain)

Identify and define the root in each of the following words:

	Root	Meaning of Root
6. homeothermic ($h\bar{o}$-$m\bar{e}$-$\bar{o}$-THER-mik)	therm/o	heat
7. anaerobic (an-er-$\bar{O}$-bik)	_____	_____
8. exergonic (ex-er-GON-ik)	_____	_____
9. chronic (KRON-ik)	_____	_____

Fill in the blanks:

10. Cryalgesia ($kr\bar{i}$-al-$J\bar{E}$-$z\bar{e}$-a) is pain caused by _____.

11. Phonetics ($f\bar{o}$-NET-iks) is the study of _____.

12. The term electroconvulsive ($\bar{e}$-lek-$tr\bar{o}$-con-VUL-siv) means causing convulsions by means of

    _____.

13. Ultrasonography (ul-tra-son-OG-ra-$f\bar{e}$) is a method for diagnosis that uses

    _____.

14. A barometer (ba-ROM-e-ter) is an instrument used to measure _____.

15. A photoreaction is a response to _____.

TABLE 7-2 Suffixes for Diagnosis

SUFFIX	MEANING	EXAMPLE	DEFINITION OF EXAMPLE
-graph	instrument for recording data	polygraph POL-$\bar{e}$-graf	instrument used to record many physiologic responses simultaneously; lie detector
-graphy	act of recording data*	radiography $r\bar{a}$-$d\bar{e}$-OG-ra-$f\bar{e}$	obtaining pictures using x-rays
-gram†	a record of data	sonogram SON-$\bar{o}$-gram	record obtained by use of ultrasound (ultrasonography)
-meter	instrument for measuring	audiometer aw-$d\bar{e}$-OM-e-ter	instrument for measuring hearing (audi/o)
metry	measurement of	ergometry er-GOM-e-$tr\bar{e}$	measurement of work done
-scope	instrument for viewing or examining	endoscope EN-$d\bar{o}$-$sk\bar{o}p$	instrument for viewing the inside of an organ or cavity
-scopy	examination of	laparoscopy lap-a-ROS-$k\bar{o}$-$p\bar{e}$	examination of the abdomen through the abdominal wall (lapar/o)

*This ending is often used to mean not only the recording of data but also the evaluation and interpretation of the data.

†A picture taken simply using x-rays is called a radio*graph*. When special techniques are used to image an organ or region with x-rays, the ending -*gram* is used with the root for that area, as in urogram (urinary tract), angiogram (blood vessels), mammogram (breast).

Exercise 7-2

Match the following terms and write the appropriate letter to the left of each number:

_____ 1. audiometry (*aw-dē-OM-e-trē*)

_____ 2. microscope (*MĪ-krō-skōp*)

_____ 3. phonogram (*FŌ-nō-gram*)

_____ 4. echography (*ek-OG-ra-fē*)

_____ 5. thermometer (*ther-MOM-e-ter*)

a. a record of sound

b. instrument for measuring temperature

c. measurement of hearing

d. instrument for examining very small objects

e. producing images by use of ultrasound

_____ 6. calorimeter (*kal-ō-RIM-e-ter*)

_____ 7. electroencephalogram (*e-lek-trō-en-SEF-a-lō-gram*)

_____ 8. bronchoscopy (*brong-KOS-kō-pē*)

_____ 9. celioscope (*SĒ-lē-ō-skōp*)

_____ 10. chronometer (*kron-OM-e-ter*)

a. instrument for examining the abdominal cavity

b. instrument for measuring time

c. instrument for measuring the energy content of food

d. endoscopic examination of breathing passages

e. record of the brain's electrical activity

TABLE 7-3 Suffixes for Surgery

SUFFIX	MEANING	EXAMPLE	DEFINITION OF EXAMPLE
-centesis	puncture, tap	thoracentesis *thor-a-sen-TĒ-sis*	puncture of the chest
-desis	binding, fusion	pleurodesis *plū-ROD-e-sis*	binding of the pleural membranes (around the lungs)
-ectomy	excision, surgical removal	hysterectomy *his-te-REK-tō-mē*	excision of the uterus (*hyster/o*)
-pexy	surgical fixation	cystopexy *SIS-tō-pek-sē*	surgical fixation of the bladder (*cyst/o*)
-plasty	plastic repair, plastic surgery, reconstruction	rhinoplasty *RĪ-nō-plas-tē*	plastic surgery of the nose
-rhaphy	surgical repair, suture	herniorrhaphy *her-nē-OR-a-fē*	surgical repair of a hernia (*herni/o*)
-stomy	surgical creation of an opening	colostomy *kō-LOS-tō-mē*	creation of an opening into the colon
-tome	instrument for incising (cutting)	microtome *MĪ-krō-tōm*	instrument for cutting thin sections of tissue for microscopic study
-tomy	incision, cutting	tracheotomy *trā-kē-OT-ō-mē*	surgical incision of the trachea
-tripsy	crushing	lithotripsy *LITH-ō-trip-sē*	crushing of a stone

Exercise 7-3

Match the following terms and write the appropriate letter to the left of each number:

_____ 1. laparotomy (*lap-a-ROT-ō-mē*)   a. plastic surgery of the breast

_____ 2. neurotripsy (*NŪ-rō-trip-sē*)   b. excision of a gland

_____ 3. mammoplasty (*MAM-ō-plas-tē*)   c. surgical incision of the abdomen

_____ 4. arthrocentesis (*ar-thrō-sen-TĒ-sis*)   d. crushing of a nerve

_____ 5. adenectomy (*ad-e-NEK-tō-mē*)   e. puncture of a joint

The root *arthr/o* means "joint." Use this root to write a word that has the same meaning as each of the following words:

6. Fusion of a joint   arthrodesis
   _____

7. Incision of a joint   _____

8. Plastic repair of a joint   _____

9. Instrument for incising a joint   _____

The root *hepat/o* means "liver." Use this root to write a word that has the same meaning as each of the following words:

10. Surgical repair of the liver   _____

11. Incision into the liver   _____

12. Excision of liver tissue   _____

13. Surgical fixation of the liver   _____

Build a word for each of the following definitions using the roots given:

14. Creation of an opening in the trachea (root *trache/o*)   _____

15. Incision into the stomach (root *gastr/o*)   _____

16. An instrument for cutting skin (root *derm/o*)   _____

Supplementary Terms

SYMPTOMS

clubbing *KLUB-ing*	Enlargement of the ends of the fingers and toes because of growth of the soft tissue around the nails; seen in a variety of diseases, especially lung and heart diseases (Fig. 7-10)
colic *KOL-ik*	Acute abdominal pain associated with smooth muscle spasms

Symptoms, continued

cyanosis *sī-a-NŌ-sis*	Bluish discoloration of the skin due to lack of oxygen
diaphoresis *dī-a-fō-RĒ-sis*	Profuse sweating
malaise *ma-LĀZ*	A feeling of discomfort or uneasiness, often indicative of infection
nocturnal *nok-TUR-nal*	Pertaining to or occurring at night (roots *noct/i* and *nyct/o* mean "night")
pallor *PAL-or*	Paleness; lack of color
prodrome *PRŌ-drōm*	A symptom indicating an approaching disease
sequela *se-KWEL-a*	A lasting effect of a disease (plural, sequelae)
syncope *SIN-kō-pē*	A temporary loss of consciousness because of inadequate blood flow to the brain; fainting

DIAGNOSIS

alpha-fetoprotein (AFP) *al-fa fē-to-prō-tēn*	A fetal protein that appears in the blood of adults with certain types of cancer
bruit *brwē*	A sound, usually abnormal, heard in auscultation
facies *FĀ-shē-ēz*	The expression or appearance of the face
febrile *FEB-ril*	Pertaining to fever
nuclear medicine	The branch of medicine concerned with the use of radioactive substances (radionuclides) for diagnosis, therapy, and research
radiology *rā-dē-OL-ō-jē*	The branch of medicine that uses radiation, such as x-rays, in the diagnosis and treatment of disease; a specialist in this field is a radiologist
speculum *SPEK-ū-lum*	An instrument for examining a canal (Fig. 7-11)
syndrome *SIN-drōm*	A group of signs and symptoms that together characterize a disease condition

TREATMENT

catheter *KATH-e-ter*	A thin tube that can be passed into the body; used to remove fluids from or introduce fluids into a body cavity
clysis *KLĪ-sis*	The introduction of fluid into the body, other than orally, as into the rectum or abdominal cavity; also refers to the solution thus used

Treatment, continued

lavage *la-VAJ*	The washing out of a cavity; irrigation
normal saline solution (NSS) *SĀ-lēn*	A salt (NaCl) solution compatible with living cells; also called physiologic saline solution (PSS)
paracentesis *par-a-sen-TĒ-sis*	Puncture of a cavity for removal of fluid
prophylaxis *prō-fi-LAK-sis*	Prevention of disease

SURGERY

drain	Device for allowing matter to escape from a wound or cavity; common types include Penrose (cigarette), T-tube, Jackson-Pratt (J-P), and Hemovac
ligature *LIG-a-chur*	A tie or bandage; the process of binding or tying (also called ligation)
resection *rē-SEK-shun*	Partial excision of a structure
stapling *STĀ-pling*	In surgery, the joining of tissue by using wire staples that are pushed through the tissue and then bent
surgeon *SUR-jun*	One who specializes in surgery

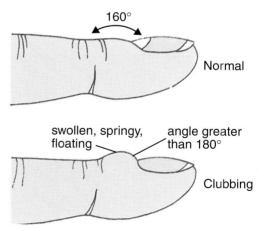

FIGURE 7-10. Clubbing. (Reprinted with permission from Taylor C, Lillis C, LeMone P. Fundamentals of Nursing: The Art and Science of Nursing Care. 4th Ed. Philadelphia: Lippincott Williams & Wilkins, 2001.)

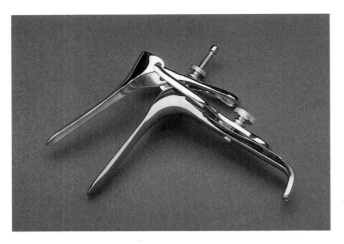

FIGURE 7-11. Vaginal speculum. (Reprinted with permission from Taylor C, Lillis C, LeMone P. Fundamentals of Nursing: The Art and Science of Nursing Care. 4th Ed. Philadelphia: Lippincott Williams & Wilkins, 2001. Photo courtesy of Ken Kasper.)

Symbols

1^{<o>}	primary
2^{<o>}	secondary (to)
Δ	change (Greek, delta)
Ⓛ	left
Ⓡ	right
↑	increase(d)
↓	decrease(d)
♂	male
♀	female
°	degree
>	greater than
<	less than
#	number, pound
×	times

ABBREVIATIONS

History and Physical Examination

ADL	Activities of daily living
BP	Blood pressure
bpm	Beats per minute
C	Celsius (centigrade)
CC	Chief complaint
c/o	Complains of
EOMI	Extraocular muscles intact
ETOH	Alcohol (ethyl alcohol)
F	Fahrenheit
HEENT	Head, eyes, ears, nose, and throat
h/o	History of
H & P	History and physical
HPI	History of present illness
HR	Heart rate
Hx	History
I & O	Intake and output
IPPA	Inspection, palpation, percussion, auscultation
IVDA	Intravenous drug abuse
NAD	No apparent distress
NKDA	No known drug allergies

ABBREVIATIONS

P	Pulse		PET	Positron emission tomography
PE	Physical examination		PICC	Peripherally inserted central catheter
PE(R)RLA	Pupils equal (regular) react to light and accommodation		postop	Postoperative
			preop	Preoperative
PMH	Past medical history		PSS	Physiologic saline solution
pt	Patient		RATx	Radiation therapy
R	Respiration		Rx	Drug, prescription, therapy
R/O	Rule out		SPECT	Single photon emission computed tomography
ROS	Review of systems			
T	Temperature		TNM	(Primary) tumor, (regional lymph) nodes, (distant) metastases
TPR	Temperature, pulse, respiration			
VS	Vital signs		UV	Ultraviolet
WD	Well developed			
WNL	Within normal limits			
w/o	Without			

Views for Radiography

AP	Anteroposterior
LL	Left lateral
PA	Posteroanterior
RL	Right lateral

Diagnosis and Treatment

ABC	Aspiration biopsy cytology
AFP	Alpha-fetoprotein
BS	Bowel sounds
bx	Biopsy
CAM	Complementary and alternative medicine
Ci	Curie (unit of radioactivity)
C & S	Culture and (drug) sensitivity (of bacteria)
CT	Computed tomography
D/C, dc	Discontinue, discharge
Dx	Diagnosis
EBL	Estimated blood loss
ICU	Intensive care unit
I & D	Incision and drainage
MET	Metastasis
MRI	Magnetic resonance imaging
NSS	Normal saline solution
PCA	Patient-controlled analgesia

Orders

AMA	Against medical advice
AMB	Ambulatory
BRP	Bathroom privileges
CBR	Complete bed rest
DNR	Do not resuscitate
KVO	Keep vein open
NPO	Nothing by mouth (Latin, *non per os*)
OOB	Out of bed
QNS	Quantity not sufficient
QS	Quantity sufficient
STAT	Immediately
TKO	To keep open

Drug abbreviations are located in Chapter 8.

Chapter Review 7-1

Match the following terms and write the appropriate letter to the left of each number:

_____ 1. prognosis

_____ 2. suture

_____ 3. staging

a. evidence of disease

b. prediction of the outcome of disease

c. to unite parts by stitching them together

_____ 4. symptom

_____ 5. biopsy

d. removal of tissue for microscopic examination

e. classification of malignant tumors

_____ 6. echogram

_____ 7. scintiscan

_____ 8. excision

_____ 9. radiotherapy

_____ 10. syndrome

a. treatment with radiation

b. a group of symptoms that characterizes a disease

c. sonogram

d. image obtained with a radionuclide

e. removal by cutting

_____ 11. radiograph

_____ 12. baroreceptor

_____ 13. osteotome

_____ 14. lithotripsy

_____ 15. arthroscope

a. instrument for cutting bone

b. image taken using x-rays

c. device for examining the inside of a joint

d. crushing of a stone

e. structure sensitive to pressure

_____ 16. chemocautery

_____ 17. chromatin

_____ 18. gastrorrhaphy

_____ 19. cryotherapy

_____ 20. hepatectomy

a. excision of liver tissue

b. destruction of tissue with chemicals

c. surgical repair of the stomach

d. cellular material that stains easily

e. treatment by use of cold

SUPPLEMENTARY TERMS

_____ 21. catheter

_____ 22. malaise

_____ 23. paracentesis

_____ 24. resection

_____ 25. pallor

a. partial excision

b. paleness

c. feeling of discomfort

d. thin tube

e. puncture of a cavity for removal of fluid

_____ 26. febrile

_____ 27. nocturnal

_____ 28. clubbing

_____ 29. prodrome

_____ 30. speculum

a. occurring at night

b. symptom of an approaching disease

c. instrument for examining a canal

d. enlargement of the ends of the fingers and toes

e. pertaining to fever

_____ 31. bruit

_____ 32. prophylaxis

_____ 33. diaphoresis

_____ 34. colic

_____ 35. lavage

a. profuse sweating

b. washing out of a cavity

c. prevention of disease

d. sound heard on auscultation

e. acute abdominal pain

Identify and define the root in each of the following words:

	Root	Meaning of Root
36. allergy		
37. radiology		
38. chronology		
39. hyperbaric		
40. anaerobic		

Word building. Use the root -cyst/o, meaning "urinary bladder," to write a word with each of the following meanings:

41. Suture of the bladder _____

42. Plastic repair of the bladder _____

43. Incision of the bladder _____

44. Surgical fixation of the bladder _____

45. Surgical creation of an opening in the bladder _____

Eliminations. In each of the sets below, underline the word that does not fit in with the rest and explain the reason for your choice:

46. percussion	auscultation	palpation	inspection	chemotherapy
47. ophthalmoscope	stethoscope	otoscope	syncope	endoscope
48. trocar	scalpel	sequela	hemostat	forceps
49. TMN	CT	MRI	PET	SPECT

Word analysis. Define each of the following words, and give the meaning of the word parts in each. Use a dictionary if necessary.

50. synergy (SIN-er-jē)_____
    a. syn- _____
    b. erg/o _____
    c. -y _____

51. chromogenesis (*krō-mō-JEN-e-sis*)_____
    a. chrom/o _____
    b. gen/e _____
    c. -sis _____

52. phonostethograph (*fō-nō-STETH-ō-graf*)_____
    a. phon/o _____
    b. steth/o _____
    c. -graph _____

Case Studies

Case Study 7-1: Comprehensive History and Physical

C.F., a 46-year-old married Asian woman, works as an office manager for an insurance company. This morning, she had a follow-up visit with her oncologist and was sent to the hospital for immediate admission for possible recurrence or sequelae of her ovarian cancer. She is alert, articulate, and a reliable reporter.

CC: C.F. presents with mild, low, aching pelvic pain and low abdominal fullness. She states, "I feel like I have cramps and am bloated. I've even gained 6 pounds. Sometimes I'm so tired I cannot do my work without a short nap."

HPI: C.F. has been in remission for 14 months from aggressively treated ovarian carcinoma. She presents with mild abdominal distention and tenderness on deep palpation of the lower pelvis. C.F. claims a feeling of fullness in the lower abdomen, loss of appetite, and inability to sleep through the night. She is afraid that her cancer was not cured. Sometimes her heart races and she cannot catch her breath, but with two children in college, she cannot afford to miss work.

MEDS: Therapeutic vitamin × 1/day. Valium 5 mg every 6 hours (q6h) as needed (prn) for anxiety. Benadryl 25 mg at bedtime (hs) prn for insomnia. Echinacea tea 3 cups per day to prevent colds or flu. Ginkgo biloba 3 caps/day for energy.

ALLERGIES: NKDA; no food allergies

PMH: C.F. was diagnosed with ovarian CA 4 years ago and treated with surgery, radiation, and chemotherapy. A total abdominal hysterectomy (removal of the uterus) with bilateral removal of the oviducts and ovaries was performed. At the time of surgery, the pelvic lymph nodes tested negative for disease. Chemotherapy and radiation therapy occurred after surgical recovery. C.F. has been well and capable of full ADL until 4 weeks ago. Childhood history is unremarkable, with normal childhood diseases, including measles, mumps, and chicken pox. C.F. was born and raised in this country. She has no other adult diseases, surgery, or injuries.

CURRENT HEALTH Hx: Denies tobacco, ETOH, or recreational drugs or substances. She exercises 3 to 5 times per week with aerobic exercise class and treadmill. She is a vegetarian and drinks 1 to 5 cups of green tea per day. Immunizations are up to date; unsure of last tetanus booster. Recent negative mammogram and negative TB test (PPD).

FAMILY Hx: Both parents alive and well. Maternal aunt died of "stomach tumor" at age 37.

TPR & BP & PAIN: 37C-96-22 126/72 in no acute distress

HEENT: WNL. Normocephalic, fundi benign, PERRLA, uncorrected 20/20 vision, mouth clear, good dental health, neck supple w/o rigidity, thyromegaly, or cervical lymphadenopathy; trachea midline. No carotid bruits (sounds).

LUNGS: All lobes clear to auscultation and percussion

HEART: Rate 96 bpm, regular; no murmurs, gallops, or rubs

BREASTS: Symmetrical, w/o masses or discharge

ABDOMEN: Skin intact with healed suprapubic midline surgical incision and a symmetrical area of discoloration and dermal thickness from radiation therapy. Bowel sounds active and normal. Suprapubic tenderness on palpation. No hepatosplenomegaly. Absence of inguinal lymph nodes on palpation. Kidneys palpable. Rectal exam WNL. Hemoccult test (stool test for blood) result negative.

GU: Unremarkable. Surgical menopause.

MUSCULOSKELETAL: WNL. No weakness, limitation of mobility, joint pain, stiffness, or edema.

NEUROLOGIC: All reflexes intact. No syncope, paralysis, numbness.

DIAGNOSTIC IMPRESSION: Possible recurrence of ovarian CA, ascites

TREATMENT PLAN: Send blood for CA-125 (genetic marker for ovarian cancer). Schedule abdominal paracentesis and second-look diagnostic laparoscopy with biopsy and tissue staging. D/C all herbal supplements.

Case Study 7-2: Diagnostic Laparoscopy

For a laparoscopy, C.F. was given general anesthesia and her trachea was intubated. She was placed in lithotomy position with arms abducted. Her abdomen was insufflated with carbon dioxide (CO_2) through a thin needle placed below the umbilicus. Three trocar punctures were made to insert the telescope with camera and the cutting and grasping instruments. Biopsies were taken of several pelvic lymph nodes and sent to the pathology laboratory. There were many adhesions from prior surgery, which were lysed to mobilize her organs and enhance visualization. A loop of small bowel, which had adhered to the anterior abdominal wall, had been punctured when the trocar was introduced. The surgeon repaired the defect with an endoscopic stapler and irrigated the abdomen with 3 L of NSS mixed with antibiotic solution.

Case Study 7-3: Postoperative Care

After surgery, C.F. complained of numbness, tingling, and paralysis in her right arm and bilateral subscapular pain when she stood. The retained CO_2 was eventually absorbed, and the subscapular pain diminished. A consult with a neurologist confirmed that she sustained a nerve injury during surgery from hyperabduction of the arm.

Biopsy results were negative, there was no fluid found on paracentesis, and the CA-125 was below 35U/mL, which is negative for recurrence. She was referred to physical therapy to strengthen and maintain range of motion (ROM) in her arm. Occupational therapy was scheduled to help her gain independence with ADL, along with psychological counseling to help her verbalize her fears and gain a sense of control.

Case Studies, continued

CASE STUDY QUESTIONS

Write the word from the case study that completes each of the following statements:

1. Secondary conditions, complications, or lasting effects of C.F.'s cancer would be called
   _____.

2. Examination by touching the surface of the body is _____.

3. The size and shape of C.F.'s head was described as _____.

4. A collection of abdominal fluid (ascites) would be drained by a cavity puncture and drainage
   procedure called a(n) _____.

5. Removal of tissue for microscopic examination is _____.

6. A surgical procedure in which an endoscope is inserted through the abdominal wall to visualize
   the abdominal cavity and determine the cause of a disorder is a(n)
   _____.

7. Extreme or overextension of an arm or leg away from the midline of the body is
   _____.

Multiple choice: Select the best answer and write the letter of your choice to the left of each
number.

_____ 8. C.F.'s cancer was in a state of apparent cure with no active signs of disease. This state is
       called _____.
       a. exacerbation
       b. syndrome
       c. remission
       d. sequelae
       e. tumor staging

_____ 9. C.F. claimed that her heart races and she cannot catch her breath. The terms for these con-
       ditions are _____ and _____.
       a. tachypnea and dyspnea
       b. tachycardia and dyspnea
       c. dyspnea and tachycardia
       d. tachycardia and bradypnea
       e. bradycardia and tachypulmono

_____ 10. Hepatosplenomegaly means:
       a. removal of the liver and spleen
       b. prolapse of the heart and spleen
       c. hemorrhage of the liver and spleen
       d. enlargement of the liver and spleen
       e. surgical repair of the kidney and liver

Case Studies, continued

_____ 11. C.F.'s abdominal cavity and organs were bound with fibrous tissue bands, which had to be lysed during surgery. These bands are called _____.
   a. prodromes
   b. sequelae
   c. adhesions
   d. ascites
   e. fibroids

_____ 12. The incidental (accidental) puncture of the intestines and nerve injury to C.F.'s arm are not expected outcomes of surgery. They are critical incidents and occurred despite attempts to protect her from harm. The term for this type of disorder is _____ (see Chapter 6).
   a. iatrogenic
   b. nosocomial
   c. idiopathic
   d. etiologic
   e. surgical misadventure

Give the meaning of each of the following abbreviations:

13. HPI _____

14. CA _____

15. ADL _____

16. TPR _____

17. bpm _____

18. WNL _____

19. D/C _____

20. NSS _____

CHAPTER 7 **Answer Section**

Answers to Chapter Exercises

EXERCISE 7-1

1. d
2. c
3. e
4. a
5. b
6. therm/o; heat
7. aer/o; air (oxygen)
8. erg/o; work
9. chron/o; time
10. cold
11. sound
12. electricity
13. sound, ultrasound
14. pressure
15. light

EXERCISE 7-2

1. c
2. d
3. a
4. e
5. b
6. c
7. e
8. d
9. a
10. b

EXERCISE 7-3

1. c
2. d
3. a
4. e
5. b
6. arthrodesis (*ar-thrō-DĒ-sis*)
7. arthrotomy (*ar-THROT-ō-mē*)
8. arthroplasty (*AR-thrō-plas-tē*)
9. arthrotome (*AR-thrō-tōm*)
10. hepatorrhaphy (*hep-a-TOR-a-fē*)
11. hepatotomy (*hep-a-TOT-ō-mē*)
12. hepatectomy (*hep-a-TEK-tō-mē*)
13. hepatopexy (*HEP-a-tō-pek-sē*)
14. tracheostomy (*trā-kē-OS-tō-mē*)
15. gastrotomy (*gas-TROT-ō-mē*)
16. dermatome (*DER-ma-tōm*)

CHAPTER REVIEW 7-1

1. b
2. c
3. e
4. a
5. d
6. c
7. d
8. e
9. a
10. b
11. b
12. e
13. a
14. d
15. c
16. b
17. d
18. c
19. e
20. a
21. d
22. c
23. e
24. a
25. b
26. e
27. a
28. d
29. b
30. c
31. d
32. c
33. a
34. e
35. b
36. erg/o; work
37. radi/o; radiation, x-ray
38. chron/o; time
39. bar/o; pressure
40. aer/o; air, oxygen
41. cystorrhaphy (*sis-TOR-a-fē*)
42. cystoplasty (*SIS-tō-plas-tē*)
43. cystotomy (*sis-TOT-ō-mē*)
44. cystopexy (*SIS-tō-pek-sē*)

45. cystostomy (*sis-TOS-tō-mē*)
46. Chemotherapy. The others are examining methods; chemotherapy is treatment with chemicals.
47. Syncope. The others are examining instruments; syncope is fainting.
48. Sequela. The others are surgical instruments; sequela is a lasting effect of disease.
49. TMN. The others are abbreviations for imaging techniques; TMN is an abbreviation for a system of staging cancer.
50. working together of parts or drugs
    a. together
    b. work
    c. condition of
51. Formation of color or pigment
    a. color
    b. origin, formation
    c. condition of
52. instrument for recording chest sounds
    a. sound
    b. chest
    c. instrument for recording data

Answers to Case Study Questions

1. sequelae
2. palpation
3. normocephalic
4. paracentesis
5. biopsy
6. diagnostic laparoscopy
7. hyperabduction
8. c
9. b
10. d
11. c
12. a
13. history of present illness
14. cancer
15. activities of daily living
16. temperature, pulse, respiration
17. beats per minute
18. within normal limits
19. discontinue
20. normal saline solution

Drugs

Chapter Contents

Objectives

After study of this chapter you should be able to:

1. Explain the difference between over-the-counter and prescription drugs.
2. List some potential adverse effects of drugs.
3. Explain ways in which drugs can interact.
4. Explain the difference between the generic name and the trade name of a drug.
5. List several drug references.
6. Describe some of the issues involved in the use of herbal medicines.
7. Identify and use word parts pertaining to drugs.
8. Recognize the major categories of drugs and how they act.
9. List some common herbal medicines and how they act.
10. List common routes for drug administration.
11. List standard forms in which liquid and solid drugs are prepared.
12. Define abbreviations related to drugs and their use.
13. Analyze the terminology related to drugs in several case studies.

A drug is a substance that alters body function. Traditionally, drugs have been derived from natural plant, animal, and mineral sources. Today, most are manufactured synthetically by pharmaceutical companies. A few, such as certain hormones and enzymes, have been produced by genetic engineering. Many drugs, described as over-the-counter (OTC) drugs, are available without **prescription**. Others require a health care provider's prescription for use. Responsibility for the safety and **efficacy** of all drugs sold in the United States lies with the Federal Food and Drug Administration (FDA), which must approve all drugs before they are sold.

Adverse Drug Effects

Most drugs have potential adverse effects or **side effects** that must be evaluated before being prescribed. In addition, there may be **contraindications**, or reasons not to use a particular drug for a specific individual based on that person's medical conditions, current medications, sensitivity, or family history. Also, while a patient is under treatment, it is important to be alert for signs of adverse effects such as digestive upset, changes in the blood, or signs of allergy, such as hives or skin rashes. **Anaphylaxis** is an immediate and severe allergic reaction that may be caused by a drug. It can lead to life-threatening respiratory distress and circulatory collapse.

Because drugs given in combination may interact, the prescriber must know of any drugs the patient is taking before prescribing another. In some cases, a combination may result in **synergy** or **potentiation**, meaning that the drugs together have a greater effect than either of the drugs acting alone. In other cases, one drug may act as an **antagonist** of another, interfering with its action. Drugs may also react adversely with certain foods or substances used socially, such as alcohol and tobacco.

Drugs that act on the central nervous system may lead to a psychological or physical **substance dependence**, in which a person has a chronic or compulsive need for a drug regardless of its bad effects. With repeated use, a person may develop a drug **tolerance**, whereby a constant dose has less effect and the dose must be increased to produce the original response. Cessation of the drug then leads to symptoms of substance **withdrawal**, a state that results from reduction or removal of a drug. Certain symptoms are associated with withdrawal from specific drugs.

Drug Names

Drugs may be cited by either their generic or their trade names. The **generic name** is usually a simple version of the chemical name for the drug and is not capitalized. The **trade name** (brand name, proprietary name) is a registered trademark of the manufacturer and is written with an initial capital letter. The same drug may be marketed by different companies under different trade names.

Drug Information

In the United States, the standard for drug information is the *United States Pharmacopeia* (USP). This reference is published by a national committee of pharmacologists and other scientists. It contains formulas for drugs sold in the United States and standards for testing the strength, quality, and purity of drugs and standards for the preparation and dispensing of drugs. There is also the *Hospital Formulary*, published by the American Society of Health System Pharmacists, and the *Physicians' Desk Reference*, published yearly by Medical Economics Books, with information supplied by the manufacturers. Another excellent source of up-to-date information on drugs is a community or hospital pharmacist.

Box 8-1 Where Do They Get Those Names?

Drug names are derived in a variety of ways. Some are named for their origin. Adrenaline, for example, is named for its source, the adrenal gland. Even its generic name, epinephrine, informs us that it comes from the gland that is above the kidney. Pitocin, a drug used to induce labor, is named for its source, the pituitary gland, combined with the chemical name of the hormone, oxytocin. Botox, currently injected into the skin for cosmetic removal of wrinkles, is the toxin from the organism that causes botulism, a type of food poisoning. Aspirin (an anti-inflammatory agent), Taxol (an antitumor agent), digitalis (used to treat heart failure), and atropine (a smooth muscle relaxant) are all named for the plants they come from. For example, aspirin is named for the blossoms of Spiraea, from which it comes. Taxol is named for the genus *Taxus*, of the yew from which it comes. Digitalis comes from purple foxglove, genus *Digitalis*. Atropine comes from the plant *Atropa belladonna*.

Some names tell about the drug or its actions. The name for Humulin, which is a form of insulin made by genetic engineering, points up the fact that this is human insulin and not a hormone from animal sources. Lomotil reduces intestinal motility and is used to treat diarrhea. The name belladonna is from Italian and means "fair lady," because this drug dilates the pupils of the eyes, making women appear more beautiful.

Herbal Medicines

For hundreds of years, people have used plants to treat diseases, a practice described as herbal medicine or **phytomedicine.** Many people in industrialized countries are now turning to herbal products as alternatives or complements to conventional medicines. Although plants are the source of many conventional drugs, the active ingredients in these drugs usually are purified, measured, and often modified or synthesized rather than being used in their natural state.

Some issues have arisen with the increased use of herbals, including questions about their purity, safety, concentration, and efficacy. Another issue is drug interactions. Health care providers should ask about the use of herbal remedies when taking a patient's drug history, and patients should report any herbal medicines they take when under treatment. The FDA does not test or regulate herbal medicines, and there are no requirements to report adverse effects. There are, however, restrictions on the health claims that can be made by the manufacturers of herbal medicines. The U.S. government has established the Office of Dietary Supplements (ODS) to support and coordinate research in this field.

Displays 8-1 through 8-5 (after the word exercises) summarize information on drugs. Display 8-1 outlines the major categories of drugs, with examples cited by both generic and trade names. Display 8-2 lists some common herbal medicines and their uses. Displays 8-3 through 8-5 have information on routes of administration, drug preparations, and injectable drugs. Refer to these displays as needed as you work through Part 3 of the text.

Key Terms

anaphylaxis *an-a fi-LAK-sis*	An extreme allergic reaction that can lead to respiratory distress, circulatory collapse, and death
antagonist *an-TAG-o-nist*	A substance that interferes with or opposes the action of a drug

contraindication *kon-tra-in-di-KĀ-shun*	A factor that makes the use of a drug undesirable or dangerous
efficacy *EF-i-ka-sē*	The power to produce a specific result; effectiveness
generic name	The nonproprietary name of a drug, that is, a name that is not privately owned or trademarked; usually a simplified version of the chemical name; not capitalized
potentiation *pō-ten-shē-Ā-shun*	Increased potency created by two drugs acting together
prescription (Rx) *prē-SKRIP-shun*	Written and signed order for a drug with directions for its administration
side effect	An undesirable effect of treatment with a drug or other form of therapy
substance dependence	A condition that may result from chronic use of a drug, in which a person has a chronic or compulsive need for a drug regardless of its adverse effects; dependence may be psychological or physical
synergy *SIN-er-jē*	Combined action of two or more drugs working together to produce an effect greater than any of the drugs could produce when acting alone; also called synergism (*SIN-er-jizm*)
tolerance	A condition in which chronic use of a drug results in loss of effectiveness and the dose must be increased to produce the original response
trade name	The brand name of a drug, a registered trademark of the manufacturer; written with a capital letter
withdrawal	A condition that results from cessation or reduction of a drug that has been used regularly

TABLE 8-1 Word Parts Pertaining to Drugs

WORD PART	MEANING	EXAMPLE	DEFINITION OF EXAMPLE
SUFFIXES			
-lytic	dissolving, reducing, loosening	anxiolytic *ang-zī-ō-LIT-ik*	agent that reduces anxiety
-mimetic	mimicking, simulating	sympathomimetic *sim-pa-thō-mi-MET-ik*	mimicking the effects of the sympathetic nervous system
-tropic	acting on	inotropic *in-ō-TROP-ik*	acting on the force of muscle contraction (*in/o* means "fiber")
PREFIXES			
anti-	against	antidote *AN-ti-dōt*	substance that counteracts a poison

TABLE 8-1 Word Parts Pertaining to Drugs, *continued*

WORD PART	MEANING	EXAMPLE	DEFINITION OF EXAMPLE
contra-	against	contraceptive *kon-tra-SEP-tiv*	preventing conception
counter-	opposite, against	countercurrent *kown-ter-KUR-ent*	flowing in an opposite direction
ROOTS			
alg/o, algi/o, algesi/o	pain	algesic *al-JE-sik*	painful
chem/o	chemical	chemotherapy *kē-mō-THER-a-pē*	treatment with drugs
hypn/o	sleep	hypnosis *hip-NŌ-sis*	an altered state with increased responsiveness to suggestion
narc/o	stupor	narcotic *nar-KOT-ik*	drug that induces stupor
pharmac/o	drug	pharmacy *FAR-ma-sē*	the science of preparing and dispensing drugs, or the place where these activities occur
pyr/o, pyret/o	fever	antipyretic *an-ti-pī-RET-ik*	counteracting fever
tox/o, toxic/o	poison, toxin	toxic *TOK-sik*	poisonous
vas/o	vessel	vasomotor *vas-ō-MŌ-tor*	pertaining to change in vessel diameter

Exercise 8-1

Identify and define the suffix in each of the following words:

	Suffix	Meaning of Suffix
1. thrombolytic (*throm-bō-LIT-ik*)	_____	_____
2. parasympathomimetic (*par-a-sim-pa-thō-mi-MET-ik*)	_____	_____
3. chronotropic (*kron-ō-TROP-ik*)	_____	_____

Using the prefixes listed in Table 8-1, write the opposite of each of the following words:

4. pyretic   _____

5. indicated   _____

6. inflammatory   _____

7. balance   _____

8. septic   _____

9. conception   _____

Identify and define the root in each of the following words:

	Root	Meaning of Root
10. hypnotic	_____	_____
11. toxicity	_____	_____
12. chemistry	_____	_____
13. narcosis	_____	_____
14. pharmacist	_____	_____

Define each of the following words:

15. vasoconstriction _____

16. pharmacology _____

17. gonadotropic _____

18. antitoxin _____

ABBREVIATIONS

Drugs and Drug Formulations

APAP	Acetaminophen
ASA	Acetylsalicylic acid (aspirin)
cap	Capsule
elix	Elixir
FDA	Food and Drug Administration
INH	Isoniazid (antitubercular drug)
MED(s)	Medicine(s), medication(s)
NCCAM	National Center for Complementary and Alternative Medicine
NSAID(s)	Nonsteroidal anti-inflammatory drug(s)
ODS	Office of Dietary Supplements
OTC	Over-the-counter
PDR	*Physicians' Desk Reference*
Rx	Prescription
supp	Suppository
susp	Suspension
tab	Tablet
tinct	Tincture
USP	*United States Pharmacopeia*
ung	Ointment

Dosages and Directions

ā	Before (Latin, *ante*)
āā	Of each (Greek, *ana*)

ac	Before meals (Latin, *ante cibum*)
ad lib	As desired (Latin, *ad libitum*)
aq	Water (Latin, *aqua*)
bid	Twice a day (Latin, *bis in die*)
c̄	With (Latin, *cum*)
cc	Cubic centimeter
D/C, dc	Discontinue
ds	Double strength
gt(t)	Drop(s) (Latin, *gutta*)
hs	At bedtime (Latin, *hora somni*)
IM	Intramuscular(ly)
IU	International unit
IV	Intravenous(ly)
mcg	Micrograms
mg	Milligrams
LA	Long-acting
NS	Normal saline
p	After, post
pc	After meals (Latin, *post cibum*)
po	By mouth (Latin, *per os*)
pp	Postprandial (after a meal)
prn	As needed (Latin, *pro re nata*)
qam	Every morning (Latin, *quaque ante meridiem*)
qd	Every day (Latin, *quaque die*)
qh	Every hour (Latin, *quaque hora*)
q ____ h	Every ____ hours

ABBREVIATIONS

qid	Four times a day (Latin, *quater in die*)	**SR**	Sustained release
qod	Every other day (Latin, *quaque* [other] *die*)	**s̄s**	Half (Latin, *semis*)
s̄	Without (Latin, *sine*)	**tid**	Three times per day (Latin, *ter in die*)
SA	Sustained action	**U**	Unit(s)
SC, SQ, subcu	Subcutaneous(ly)	**x**	Times

DISPLAY 8-1 Common Drugs and Their Actions

CATEGORY	ACTIONS; APPLICATIONS	EXAMPLES GENERIC NAME	EXAMPLES TRADE NAME
adrenergics ad-ren-ER-jiks (sympathomimetics [sim-pa-thō-mi-MET-iks])	mimic the action of the sympathetic nervous system, which responds to stress	epinephrine phenylephrine pseudoephedrine dopamine	Bronkaid Neo-Synephrine Sudafed Intropin
analgesics an-al-JĒ-siks	alleviate pain		
narcotic nar-KO-tik	decrease pain sensation in central nervous system; chronic use may lead to physical dependence	meperidine morphine	Demerol Duramorph
nonnarcotic non-nar-KO-tik	act peripherally to inhibit prostaglandins (local hormones); they may also be anti-inflammatory and antipyretic (reduce fever)	aspirin (acetyl-salicylic acid; ASA) acetaminophen (APAP) ibuprofen celecoxib	Tylenol Motrin, Advil Celebrex, Vioxx
anesthetics an-es-THET-iks	reduce or eliminate sensation	local lidocaine procaine general nitrous oxide midazolam	Xylocaine Novocain Versed
anticoagulants an-ti-kō-AG-ū-lants	prevent coagulation and formation of blood clots	heparin warfarin	Coumadin
anticonvulsants an-ti-kon-VUL-sants	suppress or reduce the number and/or intensity of seizures	phenobarbital phenytoin carbamazepine valproic acid	Dilantin Tegretol Depakene
antidiabetics an-ti-dī-a-BET-iks	prevent or alleviate diabetes	insulin chlorpropamide glyburide metformin acarbose	Humulin (injected) Diabinese (oral) Micronase Glucophage Precose

DISPLAY 8-1 Common Drugs and Their Actions, *continued*

CATEGORY	ACTIONS; APPLICATIONS	EXAMPLES GENERIC NAME	TRADE NAME
antiemetics an-tē-e-MET-iks	relieve symptoms of nausea and prevent vomiting (emesis)	ondansetron dimenhydrinate prochlorperazine scopolamine promethezine	Zofran Dramamine Compazine Transderm-Scōp Phenergan
antihistamines an-ti-HIS-ta-mēnz	prevent responses mediated by histamine: allergic and inflammatory reactions	diphenhydramine brompheniramine loratadine cetirizine	Benadryl Dimetane Claritin Zyrtec
antihypertensives an-ti-hī-per-TEN-sivs	lower blood pressure by reducing cardiac output, dilating vessels, or promoting excretion of water by the kidneys; see also calcium channel blockers, beta blockers, and diuretics under cardiac drugs, below	clonidine prazosin minoxidil losartan captopril (ACE inhibitor; see Chapter 9)	Catapres Minipress Loniten Cozaar Capoten
anti-inflammatory drugs an-tē-in-FLAM-a-tō-rē	counteract inflammation and swelling		
corticosteroids kor-ti-kō-STER-oyds	hormones from the cortex of the adrenal gland; used for allergy, respiratory, and blood diseases, injury, and malignancy; suppress the immune system	dexamethasone cortisone prednisone hydrocortisone fluticasone	Decadron Cortone Deltasone Hydrocortone, Cortef Flonase
nonsteroidal anti-inflammatory drugs (NSAIDs) non-ster-OYD-al	reduce inflammation and pain by interfering with synthesis of prostaglandins; also antipyretic	aspirin ibuprofen indomethacin naproxen diclofenac	Motrin, Advil Indocin Naprosyn, Aleve Voltaren
anti-infective agents	kill or prevent the growth of infectious organisms		
antibacterials an-ti-bak-TĒ-rē-als antibiotics an-ti-bī-OT-iks	effective against bacteria	amoxicillin penicillin V erythromycin vancomycin linezolid gentamycin clarithromycin cephalexin sulfisoxazole tetracycline	Polymox Pen-Vee K Erythrocin Vancocin Zyvox Garamycin Biaxin Keflex Gantrisin Achromycin

DISPLAY 8-1 Common Drugs and Their Actions, *continued*

CATEGORY	ACTIONS; APPLICATIONS	EXAMPLES GENERIC NAME	TRADE NAME
		ciprofloxacin (acts on ulcer-causing *Helicobacter pylori*)	Cipro
		isoniazid (INH) (tuberculosis)	Nydrazid
antifungals an-ti-FUNG-gals	effective against fungi	amphotericin B miconazole nystatin fluconazole itraconazole	Fungizone Monistat Nilstat Diflucan Sporanox
antiparasitics an-ti-par-a-SIT-iks	effective against parasites: protozoa, worms	iodoquinol (amebae) quinacrine	Yodoxin Atabrine
antivirals an-ti-VI-rals	effective against viruses	acyclovir amantadine zanamivir (influenza) zidovudine (HIV) indinavir (HIV protease inhibitor)	Zovirax Symmetrel Relenza Retrovir Crixivan
antineoplastics an-ti-ne-o-PLAS-tiks	destroy cancer cells; they are toxic for all cells but have greater effect on cells that are actively growing and dividing; hormones and hormone inhibitors also are used to slow tumor growth	cyclophosphamide doxorubicin methotrexate vincristine tamoxifen (estrogen inhibitor)	Cytoxan Adriamycin Folex Oncovin Nolvadex
cardiac drugs KAR-de-ak			
antiarrhythmics an-te-a-RITH-miks	correct or prevent abnormalities of heart rhythm	quinidine lidocaine digoxin	Quinidex Xylocaine Lanoxin
beta-adrenergic blockers (beta blockers) ba-ta-ad-ren-ER-jik	inhibit sympathetic nervous system; reduce rate and force of heart contractions	propranolol metoprolol atenolol carvedilol	Inderal Lopressor Tenormin Coreg
calcium channel blockers KAL-se-um	dilate coronary arteries, slow heart rate, reduce contractions	diltiazem nifedipine verapamil nitroglycerin isosorbide	Cardizem Procardia Calan Nitrostat Isordil
hypolipidemics hi-po-lip-i-DE-miks	lower cholesterol in patients with high serum	cholestyramine lovastatin	Questran Mevacor

DISPLAY 8-1 Common Drugs and Their Actions, *continued*

CATEGORY	ACTIONS; APPLICATIONS	EXAMPLES GENERIC NAME	TRADE NAME
	levels that cannot be controlled with diet alone; hypocholesterolemics, statins	pravastatin atorvastatin simvastatin	Pravachol Lipitor Zocor
nitrates *NĪ-trāts*	dilate coronary arteries and reduce workload of heart by lowering blood pressure and reducing venous return; antianginal	nitroglycerin isosorbide	Nitrostat Isordil
CNS stimulants	stimulate the central nervous system	methylphenidate amphetamine (chronic use may lead to drug dependence)	Ritalin Adderall, Dexedrine
diuretics *dī-ū-RET-iks*	promote excretion of water, sodium, and other electrolytes by the kidneys; used to reduce edema and blood pressure	bumetanide furosemide mannitol hydrochlorothiazide (HCTZ) triamterene + HCTZ	Bumex Lasix Osmitrol Hydrodiuril Dyazide
gastrointestinal drugs *gas-trō-in-TES-tin-al*			
antidiarrheals *an-ti-di-a-RĒ-als*	treat or prevent diarrhea by reducing intestinal motility or absorbing irritants and soothing the intestinal lining	diphenoxylate loperamide attapulgite atropine	Lomotil Imodium Kaopectate
histamine H$_2$ antagonists *HIS-ta-mēn*	decrease secretion of stomach acid by interfering with the action of histamine at H$_2$ receptors; used to treat ulcers and other gastrointestinal problems	cimetidine ranitidine	Tagamet Zantac
laxatives *LAK-sa-tivs*	promote elimination from the large intestine; types include: stimulants hyperosmotics (retain water) stool softeners bulk-forming agents	bisacodyl lactulose docusate psyllium	Dulcolax Constilac, Chronulac Colace, Surfak Metamucil

DISPLAY 8-1 Common Drugs and Their Actions, *continued*

CATEGORY	ACTIONS; APPLICATIONS	EXAMPLES	
		GENERIC NAME	TRADE NAME
hypnotics *hip-NOT-iks*	induce sleep or dull the senses; see antianxiety agents (below, under psychotropics)		
muscle relaxants *rē-LAK-sants*	depress nervous system stimulation of skeletal muscles; used to control muscle spasms and pain	baclofen carisoprodol methocarbamol	Lioresal Soma Robaxin
psychotropics *sī-kō-TROP-iks*	affect the mind, altering mental activity, mental state, or behavior		
antianxiety agents *an-tē-ang-ZĪ-e-tē*	reduce or dispel anxiety; tranquilizers; anxiolytic agents	lorazepam chlordiazepoxide diazepam hydroxyzine alprazolam buspirone	Ativan Librium Valium Atarax Xanax BuSpar
antidepressants *an-ti-dē-PRES-sants*	relieve depression by raising brain levels of neurotransmitters (chemicals active in the nervous system)	amitriptyline imipramine fluoxetine paroxetine sertraline	Elavil Tofranil Prozac Paxil Zoloft
antipsychotics *an-ti-sī-KOT-iks)*	act on nervous system to relieve symptoms of psychoses	chlorpromazine haloperidol clozapine risperidone olanzapine	Thorazine Haldol Clozaril Risperdal Zyprexa
respiratory drugs			
antitussives *an-ti-TUS-sivs*	suppress coughing	dextromethorphan	Benylin DM
bronchodilators *brong-kō-dī-LĀ-tors*	prevent or eliminate spasm of the bronchi (breathing tubes) by relaxing bronchial smooth muscle; used to treat asthma and bronchitis	albuterol epinephrine metaproterenol salmeterol theophylline montelucast (prevents attacks)	Proventil Sus-Phrine Alupent Serevent Theo-Dur Singulair
expectorants *ek-SPEK-tō-rants*	induce productive coughing to eliminate respiratory secretions	guaifenesin	Robitussin
mucolytics *mū-kō-LIT-iks*	loosen mucus to promote its elimination	acetylcysteine	Mucomyst

DISPLAY 8-1 Common Drugs and Their Actions, *continued*

CATEGORY	ACTIONS; APPLICATIONS	EXAMPLES GENERIC NAME	TRADE NAME
sedatives/hypnotics *SED-a-tivs/hip-NOT-iks*	induce relaxation and sleep; lower (sedative) doses promote relaxation leading to sleep; higher (hypnotic) doses induce sleep; antianxiety agents also used	phenobarbital zolpidem	 Ambien
tranquilizers *tran-kwi-LĪZ-ers*	reduce mental tension and anxiety; see anti-anxiety agents (above, under psychotropics)		

DISPLAY 8-2 Therapeutic Uses of Herbal Medicines

NAME	PART USED	THERAPEUTIC USES
aloe	leaf	treatment of burns and minor skin irritations
black cohosh	root	reduction of menopausal hot flashes
chamomile	flower	anti-inflammatory, gastrointestinal antispasmodic, sedative
echinacea *e-ki-NĀ-shē-a*	all	reduction in severity and duration of colds; may stimulate the immune system; used topically for wound healing
evening primrose oil	seed	source of essential fatty acids important for the health of the cardiovascular system; treatment of premenstrual syndrome (PMS), rheumatoid arthritis, skin disorders
flax	seed	source of fatty acids important in maintaining proper lipids (e.g., cholesterol) in the blood
ginkgo	leaf	improves blood circulation in and function of the brain; improves memory; used to treat dementia; antianxiety agent; protects the nervous system
ginseng	root	stress reduction; lowers blood cholesterol and blood sugar
green tea	leaf	antioxidant; acts against cancer of the gastrointestinal tract and skin; oral antimicrobial agent; reduces dental caries
kava	root	antianxiety agent; sedative
milk thistle	seeds	protects the liver against toxins; antioxidant
saw palmetto	berries	used to treat benign prostatic hyperplasia (BPH)
slippery elm	bark	as lozenge for throat irritation; for gastrointestinal irritation and upset; protects irritated skin
soy	bean	rich source of nutrients; protective estrogenic effects in menopausal symptoms, osteoporosis, cardiovascular disease, cancer prevention
St. John's wort	flower	treatment of anxiety and depression; antibacterial and antiviral properties (note: this product can interact with a variety of drugs)
tea tree oil	leaf	nonirritating antimicrobial; used to heal cuts, skin infections, burns
valerian	root	sedative; sleep aid

DISPLAY 8-3 Routes of Drug Administration

ROUTE	DESCRIPTION
absorption	drug taken into the circulation through the digestive tract or by transfer across another membrane
inhalation *in-ha-LA-shun*	administration though the respiratory system, as by breathing in an aerosol or nebulizer spray
instillation *in-stil-LA-shun*	liquid is dropped or poured slowly into a body cavity or on the surface of the body, such as into the ear or onto the conjunctiva of the eye (Fig. 8-1)
oral *OR-al*	given by mouth; per os (po)
rectal *REK-tal*	administered by rectal suppository or enema
sublingual (SL) *sub-LING-gwal*	administered under the tongue
topical *TOP-i-kal*	applied to the surface of the skin
transdermal *trans-DER-mal*	absorbed through the skin, as from a patch placed on the surface of the skin
injection (Fig. 8-2)	administered by a needle and syringe (Fig. 8-3); described as parenteral (*pa-REN-ter-al*) routes of administration
epidural *ep-i-DUR-al*	injected into the space between the meninges (membranes around the spinal cord) and the spine
intradermal (ID) *in-tra-DER-mal*	injected into the skin
intramuscular (IM) *in-tra-MUS-ku-lar*	injected into a muscle
intravenous *in-tra-VE-nus*	injected into a vein
spinal (intrathecal) *in-tra-THE-kal*	injected through the meninges into the spinal fluid
subcutaneous (SC) *sub-ku-TA-ne-us*	injected beneath the skin; hypodermic

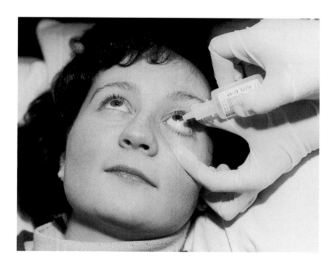

FIGURE 8-1. Instillation of eye drops into the lower conjunctival sac. (Reprinted with permission from Taylor C, Lillis C, LeMone P. Fundamentals of Nursing: The Art and Science of Nursing Care. 4th Ed. Philadelphia: Lippincott Williams & Wilkins, 2001.)

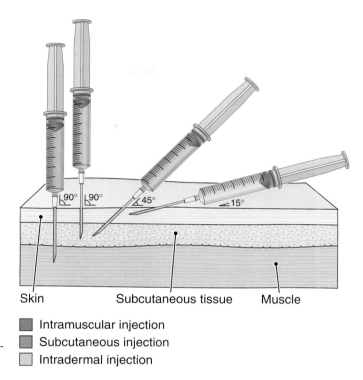

Skin   Subcutaneous tissue   Muscle

FIGURE 8-2. Comparison of the angles of insertion for intramuscular, subcutaneous, and intradermal injections.

☐ Intramuscular injection
☐ Subcutaneous injection
☐ Intradermal injection

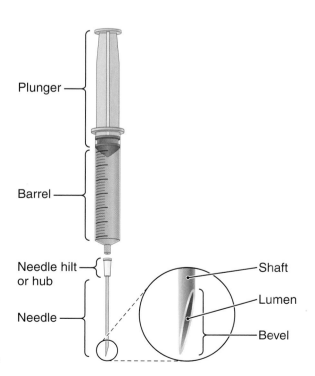

Plunger

Barrel

Needle hilt or hub

Needle

Shaft

Lumen

Bevel

FIGURE 8-3. Parts of a needle and syringe.

DISPLAY 8-4 Drug Preparations

FORM	DESCRIPTION
LIQUID	
aerosol *AR-o-sol*	solution dispersed as a mist to be inhaled
aqueous solution *A-kwē-us*	substance dissolved in water
elixir (elix) *ē-LIK-sar*	a clear, pleasantly flavored and sweetened hydroalcoholic liquid intended for oral use
emulsion *ē-MUL-shun*	a mixture in which one liquid is dispersed but not dissolved in another liquid
lotion *LŌ-shun*	solution prepared for topical use
suspension (susp) *sus-PEN-shun*	fine particles dispersed in a liquid; must be shaken before use
tincture (tinct) *TINK-chur*	substance dissolved in an alcoholic solution
SEMISOLID	
cream *krēm*	a semisolid emulsion used topically
ointment (ung) *OYNT-ment*	drug in a base that keeps it in contact with the skin
SOLID	
capsule (cap) *KAP-sūl*	material in a gelatin container that dissolves easily in the stomach
lozenge *LOZ-enj*	a pleasant-tasting medicated tablet or disk to be dissolved in the mouth, such as a cough drop
suppository (supp) *su-POZ-i-tor-ē*	substance mixed and molded with a base that melts easily when inserted into a body opening
tablet (tab) *TAB-let*	a solid dosage form containing a drug in a pure state or mixed with a nonactive ingredient and prepared by compression or molding; also called a pill

DISPLAY 8-5 Terms Pertaining to Injectable Drugs

TERM	MEANING
ampule *AM-pūl*	a small sealed glass or plastic container used for sterile intravenous solutions (Fig. 8-4)
bolus *BŌ-lus*	a concentrated amount of a diagnostic or therapeutic substance given rapidly intravenously
catheter *KATH-e-ter*	a thin tube that can be passed into a body cavity, organ, or vessel (Fig. 8-5)
syringe *sir-INJ*	an instrument for injecting fluid (see Fig. 8-4)
vial *VĪ-al*	a small glass or plastic container (see Fig. 8-4)

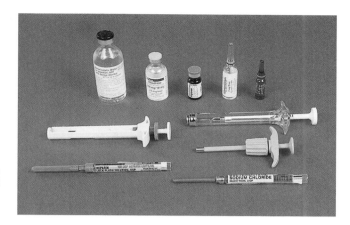

FIGURE 8-4. Ampules, vials, and syringes. (Reprinted with permission from Taylor C, Lillis C, LeMone P. Fundamentals of Nursing: The Art and Science of Nursing Care. 4th Ed. Philadelphia: Lippincott Williams & Wilkins, 2001.)

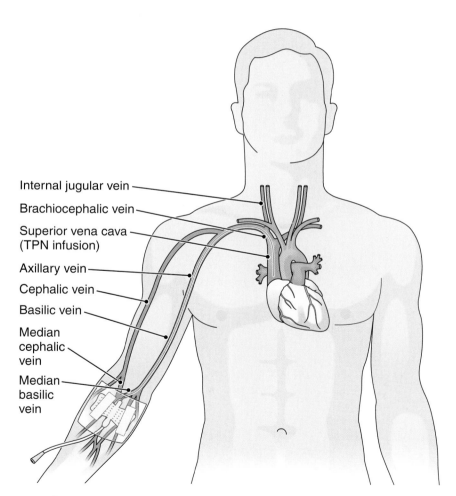

Internal jugular vein

Brachiocephalic vein

Superior vena cava (TPN infusion)

Axillary vein

Cephalic vein

Basilic vein

Median cephalic vein

Median basilic vein

━━━ Peripherally inserted central catheter (PICC)

FIGURE 8-5. Placement of a peripherally inserted central catheter (PICC).

Chapter Review 8-1

Match the following terms and write the appropriate letter to the left of each number:

_____ 1. antitussive   a. promoting excretion of water

_____ 2. diuretic   b. agent that destroys cancer cells

_____ 3. sedative   c. cough suppressant

_____ 4. antiemetic   d. inducing relaxation

_____ 5. antineoplastic   e. relieving nausea

_____ 6. vasodilation   a. extremely high body temperature

_____ 7. adrenergic   b. movement in an opposite direction

_____ 8. psychotropic   c. widening of a vessel

_____ 9. hyperpyrexia   d. sympathomimetic

_____ 10. countertransport   e. acting on the mind

_____ 11. synergy   a. a small glass vial

_____ 12. emulsion   b. an instrument for injecting fluid

_____ 13. ampule   c. a mixture of liquids

_____ 14. expectorant   d. agent that induces coughing

_____ 15. syringe   e. combined action of two or more drugs

_____ 16. tid   a. as needed

_____ 17. qam   b. by mouth

_____ 18. prn   c. without

_____ 19. $\overline{s}$ d. three times a day

_____ 20. po   e. every morning

Multiple choice: Select the best answer and write the letter of your choice to the left of each number.

_____ 21. Another term for trade name is:
    a. indicated name
    b. generic name
    c. prescription name
    d. chemical name
    e. brand name

_____ 22. An analgesic is used to treat:
    a. diarrhea
    b. arrhythmia

      c. psychosis
      d. pain
      e. thrombosis

_____ 23. A drug that is administered topically is:
      a. swallowed
      b. injected
      c. applied to the skin
      d. placed under the tongue
      e. inserted with a catheter

_____ 24. Drug administration by injection is described as:
      a. partial
      b. instilled
      c. encapsulated
      d. a bolus
      e. parenteral

_____ 25. Nitrates, beta blockers, and calcium channel blockers are used to treat disorders of the:
      a. liver
      b. brain
      c. spleen
      d. heart
      e. spinal cord

Fill in the blanks:

26. When a drug has lost its effect at a constant dose, the patient has developed _____.

27. Pharmacokinetics is study of the action and behavior of _____.

28. A hypnogenic agent is one that induces _____.

29. Phytomedicine is the practice of treating with _____.

30. A transdermal route of administration is through the _____.

31. Toxicology is the study of _____.

Define each of the following words:

32. mucolytic _____

33. psychotropic _____

34. bronchodilation _____

35. sublingual _____

Opposites. Write a word that has the opposite meaning of each of the following words:

36. convulsant _____

37. indicated _____

38. act _____

39. coagulant _____

40. vasodilation _____

Word building. Write a word for each of the following definitions:

41. Counteracting fever _____

42. Dissolving blood clots (root *thromb/o*) _____

43. One who prepares, sells, or dispenses drugs _____

44. One who studies poisons _____

Define each of the following abbreviations:

45. Rx _____

46. IM _____

47. USP _____

48. ad lib _____

49. mg _____

50. NSAIDs _____

51. FDA _____

Word analysis. Define each of the following words, and give the meaning of the word parts in each. Use a dictionary if necessary.

52. chronotropic (*kron-ō-TROP-ik*) _____
   a. chron/o _____
   b. trop _____
   c. -ic _____

53. adrenergic (*ad-ren-ER-jik*) _____
   a. adren/o _____
   b. erg/o _____
   c. -ic _____

Case Studies

Case Study 8-1: Cardiac Disease and Crisis

P.L., who has a 4-year history of heart disease, was brought to the emergency room by ambulance with chest pain that radiated down her arm, dyspnea, and syncope. Her routine meds included: Lanoxin to slow and strengthen her heart beat, Inderal to support her heart rhythm, Lipitor to decrease her cholesterol, Catapres to lower her hypertension, nitroglycerin prn for chest pain, Hydro-DIURIL to eliminate fluid and decrease the workload of her heart, Diabinese for her diabetes, and Coumadin to prevent blood clots. She also took Tagamet for her stomach ulcer and several OTC preparations, including an herbal sleeping potion that she mixed in tea, and Metamucil mixed in orange juice every morning for her bowels. Shortly after admission, P.L.'s heart rate deteriorated into full cardiac arrest. Immediate resuscitation was instituted with cardiopulmonary resuscitation (CPR), defibrillation, and a bolus of IV epinephrine. Between shocks she was given a bolus of lidocaine and a bolus of diltiazem plus repeated doses of epinephrine every 5 minutes. P.L. did not respond to resuscitation. On the death certificate, her primary cause of death was listed as cardiac arrest. Multiple secondary diagnoses were listed, including polypharmacy.

Case Study 8-2: Inflammatory Bowel Disease

A.E., a 19-year-old college student, was diagnosed at the age of 13 with Crohn disease, a chronic inflammatory disease that can affect the entire gastrointestinal tract from mouth to anus. A.E.'s disease is limited to his large bowel. During a 9-month period of disease exacerbation, he took oral corticosteroids (prednisone) to reduce the inflammatory response. He experienced many of the drug's side effects, but has been in remission for 4 years. Currently, A.E.'s condition is managed on drugs that reduce inflammation by suppressing the immune response. He takes Pentasa (mesalamine) 250mg 4 caps po bid. Pentasa is of the 5-ASA (acetylsalicylic acid or aspirin) group of anti-inflammatory agents, which work topically on the inner surface of the bowel. It has an enteric coating, which dissolves in the bowel environment. He also takes 6-mercaptopurine (Purinethol) 75 mg po qd and a therapeutic vitamin with breakfast. A.E. may take acetaminophen for pain but must avoid NSAIDs, which will irritate the intestinal mucosa (inner lining) and cause a flare-up of the disease.

Case Study 8-3: Asthma

E.N., a 20-year-old asthmatic woman, visited the preadmission testing unit one week before her cosmetic surgery to meet with the nurse and anesthesiologist. Her current meds included several bronchodilators, which she takes by mouth and by inhalation, and a tranquilizer that she takes when needed for nervousness. She sometimes receives inhalation treatments with Mucomyst, a mucolytic agent. On E.N.'s preoperative note, the nurse wrote:

> Theo-Dur 1 cap tid.
> Flovent inhaler 1 spray (50 mcg) each nostril bid.
> Ativan (lorazepam) 1 mg po bid.
> Albuterol—metered dose inhaler 2 puffs (180 mcg) prn q4-6h for bronchospasm and before exercise.

E.N. stated that she has difficulty with her asthma when she is anxious and when she exercises. She also admitted to occasional use of marijuana and ecstasy, a hallucinogen and mood-altering illegal recreational drug. The anesthesiologist wrote an order for lorazepam 4 mg IV 1 hour preop. The plastic surgeon recommended several herbal products to complement her surgery and her recovery. He ordered a high-potency vitamin 3 tabs with breakfast and dinner to support tissue health and healing. He also prescribed Bromelain, an enzyme from pineapple, to decrease inflammation, 1 po qid 3 days before surgery and postoperatively for 2 weeks. Arnica Montana was prescribed to decrease discomfort, swelling, and bruising; 3 tabs sublingual tid the evening after surgery and for the following 10 days.

CASE STUDY QUESTIONS

Multiple choice: Select the best answer and write the letter of your choice to the left of each number.

_____ 1. P.L.'s nitroglycerine is ordered: prn SL. This means:
   a. as needed, under the tongue
   b. at bedtime, under the tongue
   c. as needed, on the skin
   d. by mouth, on the skin
   e. by mouth, under the skin

Case Studies, continued

_____ 2. P.L. took several OTC preparations. OTC means:
   a. on the cutaneous
   b. off the cuff
   c. over the counter
   d. do not need a prescription
   e. c and d

_____ 3. P.L.'s herbal sleeping potion was mixed into tea and taken at bedtime. The dissolved mixture is called a(n) _____ and is taken at _____.
   a. elixir and QAM
   b. emulsion and bid
   c. suspension and hs
   d. aqueous solution and hs
   e. aqueous solution and QAM

_____ 4. During P.L.'s resuscitation, epinephrine was given in an IV bolus. This means it was administered:
   a. intrathecally in a continuous drip
   b. parenterally in a topical solution
   c. intravenously in a continuous drip
   d. intravenously in a rapid concentrated dose
   e. intrathecally in a rapid concentrated dose

_____ 5. P.L. had a secondary diagnosis of polypharmacy. This means that she:
   a. used more than one drug store
   b. had polyps
   c. used more prescription than OTC drugs
   d. had a toxic dose
   e. used many different drugs

_____ 6. A.E. takes several drugs to prevent or act against his inflammatory response. These agents are called _____ drugs.
   a. contrainflammatory
   b. counterinflammatory
   c. anti-inflammatory
   d. corticosteroids
   e. NSAIDs

_____ 7. A.E. presented with several untoward results or risks from the corticosteroid therapy. These sequelae are called:
   a. contraindications
   b. side effects
   c. antagonistic effects
   d. exacerbations
   e. synergy states

Case Studies, *continued*

_____ 8. A.E. takes four 250-mg capsules of Pentasa po bid. How many capsules does he take in one day?
   a. 2,000
   b. 1,000
   c. 4
   d. 8
   e. 12

_____ 9. A.E. must avoid NSAIDs; therefore, these drugs are _____ in inflammatory bowel disease.
   a. contraindicated
   b. indicated
   c. complementary
   d. synergistic
   e. prescriptive

_____ 10. E.N. used a mucolytic drug when needed. This drug's action is to:
   a. increase secretions
   b. decrease spasm
   c. calm anxiety
   d. decrease mucus secretions
   e. simulate mucus

_____ 11. E.N.'s Flovent inhaler is indicated as 1 spray of 50 mcg in each nostril bid. How many micrograms (mcg) does she get in 1 day?
   a. 100 mcg
   b. 200 mcg
   c. 250 mcg
   d. 500 mcg
   e. 5,000 mcg

_____ 12. The Ativan that E.N. takes for nervousness is a(n) _____ drug.
   a. anxiolytic
   b. potentiating
   c. antiemetic
   d. analgesic
   e. bronchodilator

_____ 13. The anesthesiologist ordered lorazepam (Ativan) to be given IV preop to decrease anxiety and to smooth E.N.'s anesthesia induction. The complementary way that lorazepam and anesthesia work together is called:
   a. antagonistic
   b. complementary medicine
   c. parasympathomimetic
   d. tolerance
   e. synergy

Case Studies, continued

_____ 14. Bromelain and Arnica Montana are herbal products that can be described as all of the following except:
a. phytopharmaceutical
b. alternative
c. herbal
d. complementary
e. chronotropic

_____ 15. Arnica Montana was prescribed 3 tabs SL tid. How many tabs would E.N. take in 1 day?
a. 6
b. 9
c. 12
d. 21
e. 33

_____ 16. Flovent is administered as an inhalant. The form in which the drug is prepared is called a(n) _____.
a. emulsion
b. elixir
c. aerosol
d. suspension
e. unguent

CHAPTER 8 Answer Section

Answers to Chapter Exercises

EXERCISE 8-1

1. -lytic; lysing, destroying, loosening
2. -mimetic; mimicking, simulating
3. -tropic; acting on
4. antipyretic
5. contraindicated
6. anti-inflammatory
7. counterbalance
8. antiseptic
9. contraception
10. hypn/o; sleep
11. tox, toxic/o; poison
12. chem/o; chemical
13. narc/o; stupor
14. pharmac/o; drug
15. narrowing of a blood vessel
16. the study of drugs
17. acting on the gonads (sex glands)
18. working against or counteracting a toxin (poison)

Answers to Chapter Review 8-1

1. c
2. a
3. d
4. e
5. b
6. c
7. d
8. e
9. a
10. b
11. e
12. c
13. a
14. d

15. b
16. d
17. e
18. a
19. c
20. b
21. e
22. d
23. c
24. e
25. d
26. tolerance
27. drugs
28. sleep
29. plants
30. skin
31. toxins, poisons
32. loosening or dissolving mucus
33. acting on the mind
34. widening of a bronchus
35. under the tongue
36. anticonvulsant
37. contraindicated
38. counteract
39. anticoagulant
40. vasoconstriction
41. antipyretic
42. thrombolytic
43. pharmacist
44. toxicologist
45. prescription
46. intramuscular(ly)
47. *United States Pharmacopeia*
48. as desired
49. milligrams
50. nonsteroidal anti-inflammatory drugs
51. Food and Drug Administration
52. acting on rate, as of the heart
    a. time
    b. acting on
    c. pertaining to
53. Activated by or secreting adrenaline (epinephrine)
    a. adrenaline
    b. work
    c. pertaining to

Answers to Case Study Questions

1. a
2. c
3. d
4. d
5. e
6. c
7. b
8. d
9. a
10. d
11. b
12. a
13. e
14. e
15. b
16. c

body *Fluoride* mito

ation pulmonic

ous body dend

jaund

oma ossicle

limbic

RON-ik

hypobari

ortex

Body Systems

In this section, the basics of medical
terminology are applied to the body
systems. Each chapter begins with a
description of normal structure and
function because these form the basis
for all medical studies.

Circulation: The Cardiovascular and Lymphatic Systems

Chapter Contents

Objectives

After study of this chapter you should be able to:

1. Label a diagram of the heart.
2. Trace the path of blood flow through the heart.
3. Trace the path of electrical conduction through the heart.
4. Differentiate among arteries, veins, and capillaries.
5. Name and locate the main components of the lymphatic system.
6. Identify and use the roots pertaining to the cardiovascular and lymphatic systems.
7. List and describe the main disorders that affect the heart and the blood vessels.
8. Define the main medical terms pertaining to the circulatory system.
9. Interpret medical abbreviations referring to the heart and circulation.
10. Analyze case studies concerning the heart and circulation.

Blood circulates throughout the body in the **cardiovascular system**, which consists of the heart and the blood vessels (Fig. 9-1). This system forms a continuous circuit that delivers oxygen and nutrients to all cells and carries away waste products. Also functioning in circulation is the **lymphatic system**, which drains fluid and proteins from the tissues and returns them to the bloodstream.

The Heart

The **heart** is located between the lungs, with its point or **apex** directed toward the left (Fig. 9-2). The thick muscle layer of the heart wall is the **myocardium**. This is lined on the inside with a thin **endocardium** and is covered on the outside with a thin **epicardium**. The heart is contained within a fibrous sac, the **pericardium**.

Each of the upper receiving chambers of the heart is an **atrium** (plural, atria). Each of the lower pumping chambers is a **ventricle** (plural, ventricles). The chambers of the heart are divided by walls, each of which is

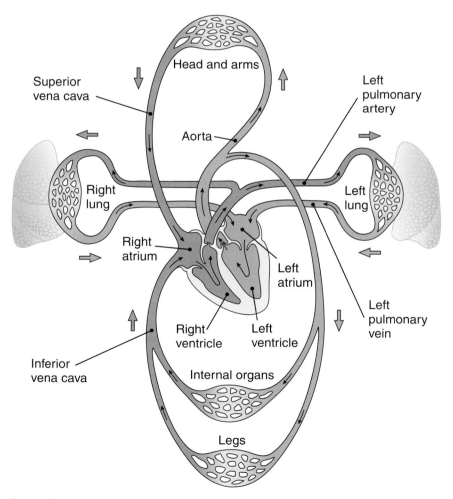

FIGURE 9-1. The cardiovascular system. (Reprinted with permission from Cohen BJ, Wood DL. Memmler's The Human Body in Health and Disease. 9th Ed. Philadelphia: Lippincott Williams & Wilkins, 2000.)

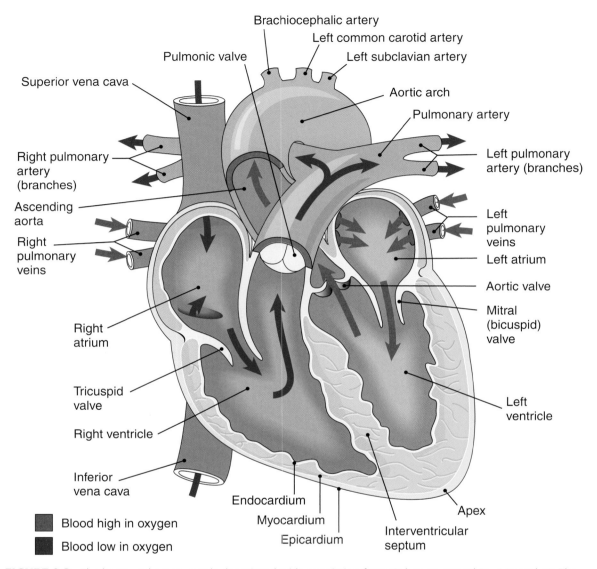

FIGURE 9-2. The heart and great vessels. (Reprinted with permission from Cohen BJ, Wood DL. Memmler's The Human Body in Health and Disease. 9th Ed. Philadelphia: Lippincott Williams & Wilkins, 2000.)

called a **septum.** The interventricular septum separates the two ventricles; the interatrial septum divides the two atria. There is also a septum between the atrium and ventricle on each side.

The heart pumps blood through two circuits. The right side pumps blood to the lungs to be oxygenated through the **pulmonary circuit.** The left side pumps to the remainder of the body through the **systemic circuit.**

Blood Flow Through the Heart

The pathway of blood through the heart is shown by the arrows in Figure 9-2. The right atrium receives blood low in oxygen from all body tissues through the **superior vena cava** and the **inferior vena cava.** The blood then enters the right ventricle and is pumped to the lungs through the **pulmonary artery.** Blood returns from the lungs high in oxygen and enters the left atrium through the **pulmonary veins**. From here it enters the left ventricle and is forcefully pumped into the **aorta** to be distributed to all tissues.

Blood is kept moving in a forward direction by one-way **valves**. The valve in the septum between the right atrium and ventricle is the **tricuspid valve** (meaning three cusps or flaps); the valve in the septum between the left atrium and ventricle is the bicuspid valve (having two cusps), usually called the **mitral valve** (so named because it resembles a bishop's miter). The valves leading into the pulmonary artery and the aorta have three cusps. Each cusp is shaped like a half-moon, so these valves are described as *semilunar valves*. The valve at the entrance to the pulmonary artery is specifically named the **pulmonic valve**; the valve at the entrance to the aorta is the **aortic valve**.

Heart sounds are produced as the heart functions. The loudest of these, the familiar lubb and dupp that can be heard through the chest wall, are produced by alternate closing of the valves. The first heart sound (S_1) is heard when the valves between the chambers close. The second heart sound (S_2) is produced when the valves leading into the aorta and pulmonary artery close. Any sound made as the heart functions normally is termed a **functional murmur**. (The word *murmur* used alone with regard to the heart describes an abnormal sound.)

The Heartbeat

Each contraction of the heart, termed **systole** (*SIS-tō-lē*), is followed by a relaxation phase, **diastole** (*dī-AS-tō-lē*), during which the chambers fill. Each time the heart beats, both atria contract and immediately thereafter both ventricles contract. The wave of increased pressure produced in the **vessels** each time the ventricles contract is the **pulse**.

Contractions are stimulated by a built-in system that regularly transmits electrical impulses through the heart. The components of this conduction system are shown in Figure 9-3. They include the **sinoatrial (SA) node**, called the pacemaker because it sets the rate of the heartbeat, the atrioventricular (AV) node, the **AV bundle** (bundle of His), the left and right **bundle branches**, and **Purkinje** (*pur-KIN-jē*) **fibers**.

Although the heart itself generates the heartbeat, factors such as nervous system stimulation, hormones, and drugs can influence the rate and the force of heart contractions.

Blood Pressure

Blood pressure is the force exerted by blood against the wall of a blood vessel. It is commonly measured in a large artery with an inflatable cuff (Fig. 9-4) known as a blood pressure cuff or blood pressure apparatus, but technically called a **sphygmomanometer**. Both systolic and diastolic pressures are measured and reported as systolic then diastolic separated by a slash, such as 120/80. Pressure is expressed as millimeters of mercury (mm Hg), that is, the height to which the pressure can push a column of mercury in a tube. Blood pressure is a valuable diagnostic measurement that is easily obtained.

The Vascular System

The vascular system consists of:

1. **Arteries** that carry blood away from the heart (Fig. 9-5). **Arterioles** are small arteries that lead into the capillaries.
2. **Capillaries**, the smallest vessels, through which exchanges take place between the blood and the tissues.
3. **Veins** that carry blood back to the heart (Fig. 9-6). The small veins that receive blood from the capillaries and drain into the veins are **venules**.

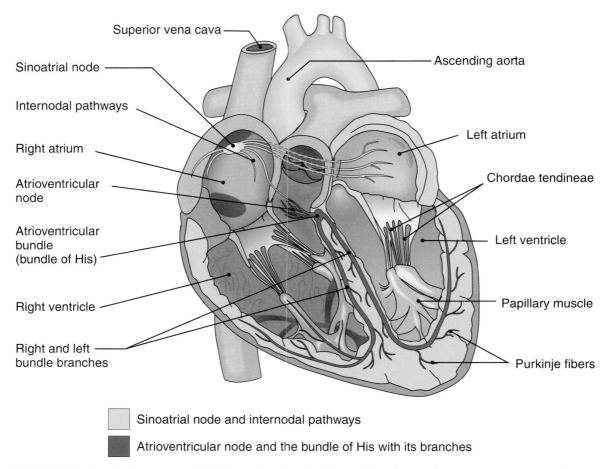

Superior vena cava

Sinoatrial node

Internodal pathways

Right atrium

Atrioventricular node

Atrioventricular bundle (bundle of His)

Right ventricle

Right and left bundle branches

Ascending aorta

Left atrium

Chordae tendineae

Left ventricle

Papillary muscle

Purkinje fibers

Sinoatrial node and internodal pathways

Atrioventricular node and the bundle of His with its branches

FIGURE 9-3. Conduction system of the heart. (Reprinted with permission from Cohen BJ, Wood DL. Memmler's The Human Body in Health and Disease. 9th Ed. Philadelphia: Lippincott Williams & Wilkins, 2000.)

All arteries, except the pulmonary artery (and the umbilical artery in the fetus), carry blood high in oxygen. They are thick-walled, elastic vessels that carry blood under high pressure. All veins, except the pulmonary vein (and the umbilical vein in the fetus), carry blood low in oxygen. Veins have thinner, less elastic walls and tend to give way under pressure. Like the heart, veins have one-way valves that keep blood flowing forward.

Nervous system stimulation can cause the diameter of a vessel to increase (vasodilation) or decrease (vasoconstriction). These changes alter blood flow to the tissues and affect blood pressure.

The Lymphatic System

The **lymphatic system** is a widely distributed system with multiple functions (Fig. 9-7). Its role in circulation is to return excess fluid and proteins from the tissues to the bloodstream. The fluid carried in the lymphatic system is called **lymph**. Lymph drains from the lower part of the body and the upper left side into the

Box 9-1 Name That Structure

An eponym is a name that is based on the name of a person, usually the one who discovered a particular structure, disease, principle, or procedure. Everyday examples are graham cracker, Ferris wheel, and boycott. In the heart, the bundle of His and Purkinje fibers are part of that organ's conduction system. Korotkoff sounds are heard in the vessels when taking blood pressure. Cardiovascular disorders named for people include the tetralogy of Fallot, a combination of four congenital heart defects, Raynaud disease of small vessels, and the cardiac arrhythmia known as Wolff-Parkinson-White syndrome. In treatment, Doppler echocardiography is named for a physicist of the 19th century. The Holter monitor and the Swan-Ganz catheter give honor to their developers.

In other systems, the islets of Langerhans are clusters of cells in the pancreas that secrete insulin. The graafian follicle in the ovary surrounds the developing egg cell. The eustachian tube connects the middle ear to the throat.

Many diseases have eponymic names: Parkinson and Alzheimer, which affect the brain, Graves, a disorder of the thyroid, Addison and Cushing, involving the adrenal cortex, and Down syndrome, a hereditary disorder. The genus and species names of microorganisms often are based on the names of their discoverers, *Escherichia, Salmonella, Pasteurella,* and *Rickettsia* to name a few.

Many reagents, instruments, and procedures are named for their developers. The original name for a radiograph was roentgenograph (*RENT-jen-ō-graf*), named for Wilhelm Röntgen, discoverer of x-rays. A curie is a measure of radiation, derived from the name of Marie Curie, a co-discoverer of radioactivity.

Although eponyms give honor to physicians and scientists of the past, they do not convey any information and may be more difficult to learn. There is a trend to replace these names with more descriptive ones; for example, auditory tube instead of eustachian tube, ovarian follicle for graafian follicle, pancreatic islets for islets of Langerhans, and trisomy 21 for Down syndrome.

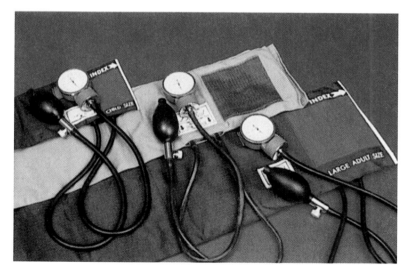

FIGURE 9-4. Blood pressure cuffs in three sizes. Shown are the cuff, the bulb for inflating the cuff, and the manometer for measuring pressure. (Reprinted with permission from Taylor C, Lillis C, LeMone P. Fundamentals of Nursing: The Art and Science of Nursing Care. 4th Ed. Philadelphia: Lippincott Williams & Wilkins, 2001. Photograph courtesy of Ken Kasper.)

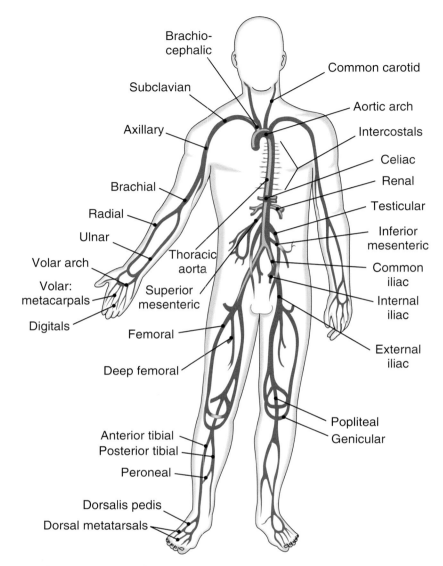

FIGURE 9-5. Principal systemic arteries. (Reprinted with permission from Cohen BJ, Wood DL. Memmler's The Human Body in Health and Disease. 9th Ed. Philadelphia: Lippincott Williams & Wilkins, 2000.)

thoracic duct, which travels upward through the chest and empties into the left subclavian vein near the heart. The **right lymphatic duct** drains the upper right side of the body and empties into the right subclavian vein.

Another function of the lymphatic system is to absorb digested fats from the small intestine (see Chapter 12). These fats are then added to the blood near the heart.

One other major function of the lymphatic system is to protect the body from impurities and invading microorganisms. Along the path of the lymphatic vessels are small masses of lymphoid tissue, the **lymph nodes** (see Fig. 9-7). Their function is to filter the lymph as it passes through. They are concentrated

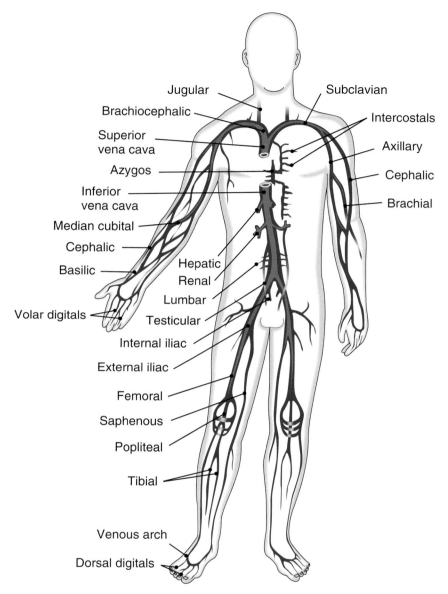

FIGURE 9-6. Principal systemic veins. (Reprinted with permission from Cohen BJ, Wood DL. Memmler's The Human Body in Health and Disease. 9th Ed. Philadelphia: Lippincott Williams & Wilkins, 2000.)

in the cervical (neck), axillary (armpit), mediastinal (chest), and inguinal (groin) regions. The lymph nodes and the remainder of the lymphatic system also play a role in immunity (see Chapter 10). Other organs and tissues of the lymphatic system include the **tonsils**, located in the throat (described in Chapter 11), the **thymus gland** in the chest, and the **spleen** in the upper left region of the abdomen (see Fig. 12-1).

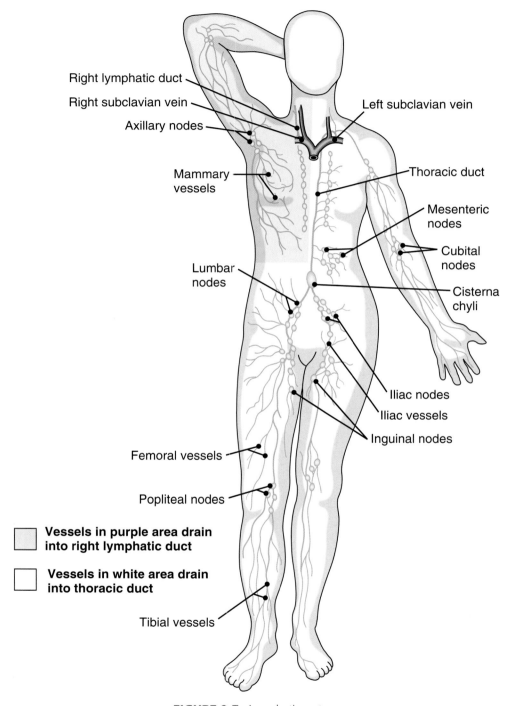

Right lymphatic duct

Right subclavian vein

Axillary nodes

Left subclavian vein

Mammary vessels

Thoracic duct

Mesenteric nodes

Cubital nodes

Lumbar nodes

Cisterna chyli

Iliac nodes

Iliac vessels

Inguinal nodes

Femoral vessels

Popliteal nodes

Vessels in purple area drain into right lymphatic duct

Vessels in white area drain into thoracic duct

Tibial vessels

FIGURE 9-7. Lymphatic system.

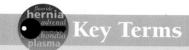 **Key Terms**

NORMAL STRUCTURE AND FUNCTION

Cardiovascular System

aorta *ā-OR-ta*	The largest artery. It receives blood from the left ventricle and branches to all parts of the body (root *aort/o*).
aortic valve *ā-OR-tik*	The semilunar valve at the entrance to the aorta
apex *Ā-peks*	The point of a cone-shaped structure (adjective, apical). The apex of the heart is formed by the left ventricle. It is inferior and pointed toward the left (see Fig. 9-2).
artery	A vessel that carries blood away from the heart. All except the pulmonary and umbilical arteries carry oxygenated blood (root *arter, arteri/o*).
arteriole *ar-TĒ-rē-ōl*	A small artery (root *arteriol/o*)
atrioventricular (AV) node *ā-trē-ō-ven-TRIK-ū-lar*	A small mass in the lower septum of the right atrium that passes impulses from the sinoatrial (SA) node toward the ventricles
AV bundle	A band of fibers that transmits impulses from the atrioventricular (AV) node to the top of the interventricular septum. It divides into the right and left bundle branches, which descend along the two sides of the septum; the bundle of His.
atrium *Ā-trē-um*	An entrance chamber, one of the two upper receiving chambers of the heart (root *atri/o*)
bicuspid valve *bī-KUS-pid*	The valve between the left atrium and the left ventricle; the mitral valve
blood pressure	The force exerted by blood against the wall of a vessel
bundle branches	Branches of the AV bundle that divide to the right and left sides of the interventricular septum
capillary *KAP-i-lar-ē*	A microscopic blood vessel through which materials are exchanged between the blood and the tissues
cardiovascular system *kar-dē-ō-VAS-kū-lar*	The part of the circulatory system that consists of the heart and the blood vessels
diastole *dī-AS-tō-lē*	The relaxation phase of the heartbeat cycle
endocardium *en-dō-KAR-dē-um*	The thin membrane that lines the chambers of the heart and covers the valves
epicardium *ep-i-KAR-dē-um*	The thin outermost layer of the heart wall
functional murmur	Any sound produced as the heart functions normally

Cardiovascular System, *continued*

heart *hart*	The muscular organ with four chambers that contracts rhythmically to propel blood through vessels to all parts of the body (root *cardi/o*)
heart sounds	Sounds produced as the heart functions. The two loudest sounds are produced by alternate closing of the valves and are designated S_1 and S_2.
inferior vena cava *VĒ-na-KĀ-va*	The large inferior vein that brings blood back to the right atrium of the heart from the lower part of the body
mitral valve *MĪ-tral*	The valve between the left atrium and the left ventricle; the bicuspid valve
myocardium *mī-ō-KAR-dē-um*	The thick middle layer of the heart wall composed of cardiac muscle
pericardium *per-i-KAR-dē-um*	The fibrous sac that surrounds the heart
pulmonary artery *PUL-mo-nar-e*	The vessel that carries blood from the right side of the heart to the lungs
pulmonary circuit	The system of vessels that carries blood from the right side of the heart to the lungs to be oxygenated and then back to the left side of the heart
pulmonary veins	The vessels that carry blood from the lungs to the left side of the heart
pulmonic valve *pul-MON-ik*	The semilunar valve at the entrance to the pulmonary artery
pulse	The wave of increased pressure produced in the vessels each time the ventricles contract
Purkinje fibers *pur-KIN-jē*	The terminal fibers of the conducting system of the heart. They carry impulses through the walls of the ventricles.
septum *SEP-tum*	A wall dividing two cavities, such as the chambers of the heart
sinoatrial (SA) node *sī-nō-Ā-trē-al*	A small mass in the upper part of the right atrium that initiates the impulse for each heartbeat; the pacemaker
sphygmomanometer *sfig-mō-man-OM-e-ter*	An instrument for determining arterial blood pressure (root *sphygm/o* means "pulse"); blood pressure apparatus or cuff (see Fig. 9-4)
superior vena cava *VĒ-na-KĀ-va*	The large superior vein that brings deoxygenated blood back to the right atrium from the upper part of the body
systemic circuit *sis-TEM-ik*	The system of vessels that carries oxygenated blood from the left side of the heart to all tissues except the lungs and returns deoxygenated blood to the right side of the heart
systole *SIS-tō-lē*	The contraction phase of the heartbeat cycle

Cardiovascular System, continued

tricuspid valve *trī-KUS-pid*	The valve between the right atrium and the right ventricle
valve	A structure that keeps fluid flowing in a forward direction (root *valv/o, valvul/o*)
vein *vān*	A vessel that carries blood back to the heart. All except the pulmonary and umbilical veins carry blood low in oxygen (root *ven, phleb/o*).
ventricle *VEN-trik-l*	A small cavity. One of the two lower pumping chambers of the heart (root *ventricul/o*).
venule *VEN-ūl*	A small vein
vessel *VES-el*	A tube or duct to transport fluid (root *angi/o, vas/o, vascul/o*)

Lymphatic System

lymph *limf*	The thin plasmalike fluid that drains from the tissues and is transported in lymphatic vessels (root *lymph/o*)
lymph node	A small mass of lymphoid tissue along the path of a lymphatic vessel that filters lymph (root *lymphaden/o*)
lymphatic system *lim-FAT-ik*	The system that drains fluid and proteins from the tissues and returns them to the bloodstream. This system also aids in absorption of fats from the digestive tract and participates in immunity.
right lymphatic duct	The lymphatic duct that drains fluid from the upper right side of the body
spleen	A large reddish-brown organ in the upper left region of the abdomen. It filters blood and destroys old red blood cells (root *splen/o*).
thoracic duct	The lymphatic duct that drains fluid from the upper left side of the body and all of the lower portion of the body
thymus gland *THĪ-mus*	A gland in the upper part of the chest beneath the sternum. It functions in immunity (root *thym/o*).
tonsils *TON-silz*	Small masses of lymphoid tissue located in the region of the throat

Roots Pertaining to the Cardiovascular and Lymphatic Systems

TABLE 9-1 Roots for the Heart

ROOT	MEANING	EXAMPLE	DEFINITION OF EXAMPLE
cardi/o	heart	cardiomyopathy* *kar-dē-ō-mī-OP-a-thē*	any disease of the heart muscle
atri/o	atrium	atriotomy *ā-trē-OT-ō-mē*	surgical incision of an atrium
ventricul/o	cavity, ventricle	supraventricular *SŪ-pra-ven-TRIK-ū-lar*	above a ventricle
valv/o, valvul/o	valve	valvectomy *val-VEK-tō-mē*	surgical removal of a valve

*Preferred over myocardiopathy.

Exercise 9-1

Fill in the blanks:

1. The word cardiogenic (*kar-dē-ō-GEN-ik*) means originating in the
   _____.

2. Interatrial (*in-ter-Ā-trē-al*) means between the _____.

3. The word ventriculotomy (*ven-trik-ū-LOT-ō-mē*) means surgical incision of a(n)
   _____.

4. A valvuloplasty (*val-vū-lō-PLAS-tē*) is plastic repair of a(n) _____.

Write the adjective for each of the following definitions. The proper suffix is given for each.

5. Pertaining to the heart (-ac) _____

6. Pertaining to the myocardium (-al; ending differs from adjective ending for the heart) _____

7. Pertaining to an atrium (-al) _____

8. Pertaining to the pericardium (-al) _____

9. Pertaining to a ventricle (-ar) _____

10. Pertaining to a valve (-ar) _____

Following the example, write a word for each of the following definitions pertaining to the tissues of the heart:

11. Inflammation of the lining of the heart (usually at a valve) _____endocarditis_____

12. Inflammation of the heart muscle _____

13. Inflammation of the fibrous sac around the heart _____

Write a word for each of the following definitions:

14. Study (-logy) of the heart   _____

15. Enlargement (-megaly) of the heart   _____

16. Between (inter-) the ventricles   _____

17. Pertaining to an atrium and a ventricle   _____

18. Surgical incision of a valve   _____

TABLE 9-2 Roots for the Blood Vessels

ROOT	MEANING	EXAMPLE	DEFINITION OF EXAMPLE
angi/o*	vessel	angiopathy *an-jē-OP-a-thē*	any disease of blood vessels
vas/o, vascul/o	vessel, duct	vasodilation *vas-ō-dī-LĀ-shun*	widening of a blood vessel
arter/o, arteri/o	artery	endarterial *end-ar-TĒ-rē-al*	within an artery
arteriol/o	arteriole	arteriolar *ar-tē-rē-Ō-lar*	pertaining to an arteriole
aort/o	aorta	aortoptosis *a-or-top-TŌ-sis*	downward displacement of the aorta
ven/o, ven/i	vein	venous *VĒ-nus*	pertaining to a vein
phleb/o	vein	phlebectasia *fleb-ek-TĀ-zē-a*	dilatation of a vein

*The root *angi/o* usually refers to a blood vessel but is used for other types of vessels as well. *Hemangi/o* refers specifically to a blood vessel.

Exercise 9-2

Fill in the blanks:

1. Vasospasm (*vas-ō-spazm*) means sudden contraction of a(n) _____.

2. Endarterectomy (*end-ar-ter-EK-tō-mē*) is removal of the inner lining of a(n)

   _____.

3. Angioedema (*an-jē-ō-e-DĒ-ma*) is localized swelling caused by changes in

   _____.

4. Aortosclerosis (*ā-or-tō-skle-RŌ-sis*) is hardening of the _____.

5. The term *microvascular* (*mī-krō-VAS-kū-lar*) means pertaining to small

   _____.

6. Arteriolitis is inflammation of an _____.

Define the following words:

7. angiitis (*an-jē-Ī-tis*) (note spelling); also angitis or vasculitis _____

8. cardiovascular (*kar-dē-ō-VAS-kū-lar*) _____

9. arteriorrhexis (*ar-tē-rē-ō-REK-sis*) _____

10. intra-aortic (*in-tra-ā-OR-tik*) _____

11. phlebitis (*fleb-Ī-tis*) _____

Use the ending -*gram* to form a word for a radiograph of each of the following:

12. vessels (use angi/o) _____

13. aorta _____

14. veins _____

Use the root *angi/o* to write a word with each of the following meanings:

15. Surgical removal (-ectomy) of a vessel _____

16. Dilatation (-ectasis) of a vessel _____

17. Formation (-genesis) of a vessel _____

18. Plastic repair of a vessel _____

Use the appropriate root to write a word with each of the following meanings:

19. Narrowing (-stenosis) of the aorta _____

20. Incision of an artery _____

21. Within (intra-) a vein _____

22. Excision of a vein _____

TABLE 9-3 Roots for the Lymphatic System

ROOT	MEANING	EXAMPLE	DEFINITION OF EXAMPLE
lymph/o	lymph, lymphatic system	lymphoid LIM-foyd	resembling lymph or lymphatic tissue
lymphaden/o	lymph node	lymphadenectomy lim-fad-e-NEK-tō-mē	surgical removal of a lymph node
lymphangi/o	lymphatic vessel	lymphangioma lim-fan-jē-Ō-ma	tumor of lymphatic vessels
splen/o	spleen	splenomegaly splē-nō-MEG-a-lē	enlargement of the spleen
thym/o	thymus gland	athymia a-THĪ-mē-a	absence of the thymus gland
tonsill/o	tonsil	tonsillar TON-sil-ar	pertaining to a tonsil

Exercise 9-3

Fill in the blanks:

1. Lymphedema (*limf-e-DĒ-ma*) means swelling caused by obstruction of the flow of
   _____.

2. Lymphadenitis (*lim-fad-e-NĪ-tis*) is inflammation of a(n) _____.

3. A lymphangiogram (*lim-FAN-jē-ō-gram*) is an x-ray image (radiograph) of
   _____.

4. The adjective splenic (*SPLEN-ik*) means pertaining to the _____.

5. Thymectomy (*thī-MEK-tō-mē*) is surgical removal of the _____.

6. Tonsillopathy (*ton-sil-OP-a-thē*) is any disease of the _____.

Identify and define the root in each of the following words:

	Root	Meaning of Root
7. lymphangial (*lim-FAN-jē-al*)	lymphangi/o	lymphatic vessel
8. lymphadenography (*lim-fad-e-NOG-ra-fē*)	_____	_____
9. perisplenitis (*per-i-splē-NĪ-tis*)	_____	_____
10. hypothymism (*hī-pō-THĪ-mizm*)	_____	_____
11. tonsillectomy (*ton-sil-EK-tō-mē*)	_____	_____

Use the appropriate root to write a word with each of the following meanings:

12. Inflammation of lymphatic vessels   _____

13. A tumor (-oma) of lymphatic tissue   _____

14. Any disease (-pathy) of the lymph nodes   _____

15. Pain (-algia) in the spleen   _____

16. Inflammation of a tonsil   _____

Clinical Aspects of the Circulatory System

Atherosclerosis

The accumulation of fatty deposits within the lining of an artery is termed **atherosclerosis** (Fig. 9-8). This type of deposit, called a **plaque**, begins to form when a vessel receives tiny injuries, usually at a point of branching. Plaques gradually thicken and harden with fibrous material, cells, and other deposits, restricting the lumen (opening) of the vessel and reducing blood flow to the tissues, a condition known as **ischemia**. A major risk factor for the development of atherosclerosis is **dyslipidemia**, abnormally high levels or imbalance in **lipoproteins** that are carried in the blood, especially high levels of cholesterol-containing low-density lipoproteins (LDL). Other risk factors for atherosclerosis include smoking, high blood pressure, poor diet, inactivity, stress, and family history of the disorder. Atherosclerosis may involve any arteries, but most of its

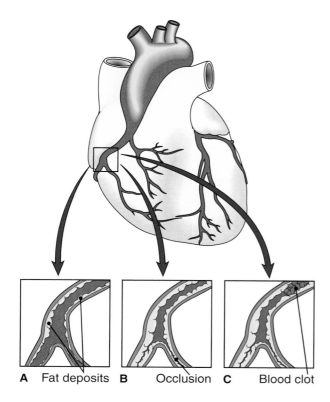

A Fat deposits **B** Occlusion **C** Blood clot

FIGURE 9-8. Coronary atherosclerosis. **(A)** Fat deposits narrow an artery leading to ischemia. **(B)** Blockage (occlusion) of a coronary artery. **(C)** Formation of a blood clot (thrombus) leading to myocardial infarction. (Adapted with permission from Cohen BJ, Wood DL. Memmler's The Human Body in Health and Disease. 9th Ed. Philadelphia: Lippincott Williams & Wilkins, 2000.)

effects are seen in the coronary vessels of the heart, the aorta, the carotid arteries in the neck, and vessels in the brain.

Thrombosis and Embolism

Atherosclerosis predisposes a person to **thrombosis**, the formation of a blood clot within a vessel. The clot, called a **thrombus**, interrupts blood flow to the tissues supplied by that vessel, resulting in necrosis (tissue death). Blockage of a vessel by a thrombus or other mass carried in the bloodstream is an **embolism**, and the mass itself is called an **embolus**. Usually the mass is a blood clot that breaks loose from the wall of a vessel, but it may also be air (as from injection or trauma), fat (as from marrow released after a bone break), bacteria, or other solid materials. Often a venous thrombus will travel through the heart and then lodge in an artery of the lungs, resulting in a life-threatening pulmonary embolism. An embolus from a carotid artery often blocks a cerebral vessel, causing a **cerebrovascular accident (CVA)**, commonly called **stroke** (see Chapter 17).

Aneurysm

An arterial wall weakened by atherosclerosis, malformation, injury, or other causes may balloon out, forming an **aneurysm.** If an aneurysm ruptures, hemorrhage results. Rupture of a cerebral artery is another cause of stroke. The abdominal aorta and carotid arteries are also common sites of aneurysm. In a **dissecting aneurysm** (Fig. 9-9), blood hemorrhages into the thick middle layer of the artery wall, separating the muscle as it spreads and sometimes rupturing the vessel. The aorta is most commonly involved. It may be possible to repair a dissecting aneurysm surgically with a graft.

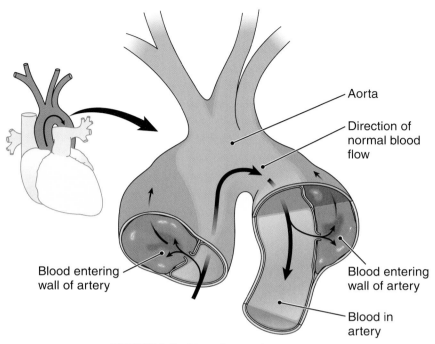

Aorta

Direction of normal blood flow

Blood entering wall of artery

Blood entering wall of artery

Blood in artery

FIGURE 9-9. Dissecting aortic aneurysm.

Hypertension

High blood pressure, or **hypertension** (HTN), is a contributing factor in all of the conditions described above. In simple terms, hypertension is defined as a systolic pressure greater than 140 mm Hg or a diastolic pressure greater than 90 mm Hg. Hypertension causes the left ventricle to enlarge (hypertrophy) as a result of increased work. Some cases of HTN are secondary to other disorders, such as kidney malfunction or endocrine disturbance, but most of the time the causes are unknown, a condition described as primary or essential hypertension.

Changes in diet and life habits are the first line of defense in controlling HTN. Drugs that are used include diuretics to eliminate fluids, vasodilators to relax the blood vessels, and drugs that prevent the formation or action of angiotensin, a substance in the blood that normally acts to increase blood pressure.

Heart Disease

CORONARY ARTERY DISEASE

Coronary artery disease (CAD), which results from atherosclerosis of the vessels that supply blood to the heart muscle, is a leading cause of death in industrialized countries (see Fig. 9-8). An early sign of CAD is the type of chest pain known as **angina pectoris**. This is a feeling of constriction around the heart or pain that may radiate to the left arm or shoulder, usually brought on by exertion. Often there is anxiety, **diaphoresis** (profuse sweating), and **dyspnea** (difficulty in breathing).

CAD is treated by control of exercise and administration of nitroglycerin to dilate coronary vessels. Other drugs may be used to regulate the heartbeat, strengthen the force of heart contraction, or prevent formation of blood clots. Patients with severe cases of CAD may be candidates for **angioplasty,** surgical dilatation of the blocked vessel by means of a catheter, technically called **percutaneous transluminal coronary angioplasty (PTCA)** (Fig. 9-10). If further intervention is required, the blocked vessel may be surgically bypassed with a vascular graft (Fig. 9-11). In this procedure, known as a **coronary artery bypass graft (CABG),** another vessel or a piece of another vessel, usually the saphenous vein of the leg or the left internal mammary artery, is used to carry blood from the aorta to a point past the obstruction in a coronary vessel.

CAD is diagnosed by **electrocardiography** (ECG), study of the electrical impulses given off by the heart as it functions, stress tests, **coronary angiography** (imaging), **echocardiography,** and other tests.

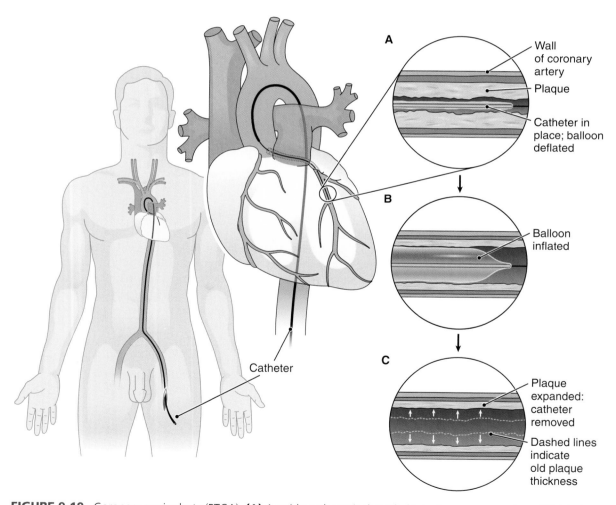

FIGURE 9-10. Coronary angioplasty (PTCA). **(A)** A guide catheter is threaded into the coronary artery. **(B)** A balloon catheter is inserted through the occlusion. **(C)** The balloon is inflated and deflated until plaque is flattened and the vessel is opened.

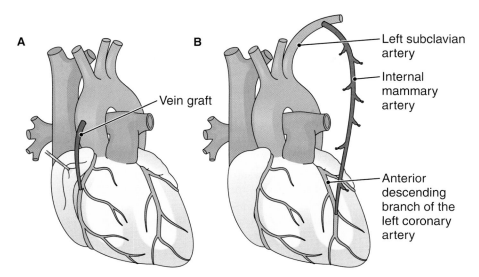

A

B

Vein graft

Left subclavian artery

Internal mammary artery

Anterior descending branch of the left coronary artery

FIGURE 9-11. Coronary artery bypass graft (CABG). **(A)** A segment of the saphenous vein carries blood from the aorta to a part of the right coronary artery that is distal to an occlusion. **(B)** The mammary artery is used to bypass an obstruction in the left anterior descending (LAD) coronary artery.

Degenerative changes in the arteries predispose a person to thrombosis and sudden **occlusion** (obstruction) of a coronary artery. The resultant area of myocardial necrosis is termed an **infarct** (Fig. 9-12), and the process is known as **myocardial infarction** (MI), the "heart attack" that may cause sudden death. Symptoms of MI include pain over the heart (precordial pain) or upper part of the abdomen (epigastric pain) that may extend to the jaw or arms, pallor (paleness), diaphoresis, nausea, and dyspnea. There may be a burning sensation similar to indigestion or heartburn.

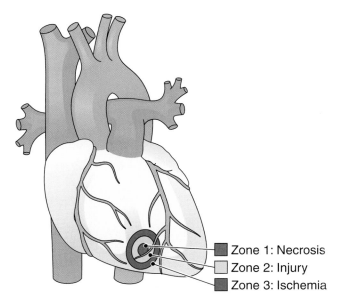

Zone 1: Necrosis
Zone 2: Injury
Zone 3: Ischemia

FIGURE 9-12. Myocardial infarction.

MI is diagnosed by electrocardiography, by measurement of certain enzymes (CK, LDH, AST) released into the blood from the damaged heart muscle and by a variety of other methods described later in this chapter.

Patient outcome is based on the degree of damage and early treatment to dissolve the clot and re-establish normal heart rhythm.

ARRHYTHMIA

Arrhythmia is any irregularity of heart rhythm, such as a higher- or lower-than-average heart rate, extra beats, or an alteration in the pattern of the beat. **Bradycardia** is a slower-than-average rate, and **tachycardia** is a higher-than-average rate. In cases of MI, there is often **fibrillation**, an extremely rapid, ineffective beating of the heart. MI may also result in **heart block**, an interruption in the electrical conduction system of the heart (Fig. 9-13). **Cardioversion** is the general term for restoration of a normal heart rhythm, either by drugs or application of electric current. Several devices are in use for electrical **defibrillation**. If, for any reason, the SA node is not generating a normal heartbeat, an **artificial pacemaker** (Fig. 9-14) may be implanted in the chest to regulate the beat.

HEART FAILURE

The general term **heart failure** refers to any condition in which the heart fails to empty effectively. The resulting increased pressure in the venous system leads to **edema**, often in the lungs (pulmonary edema), and justifies the description congestive heart failure (CHF). Other symptoms of congestive heart failure are **cyanosis**, dyspnea, and **syncope**. Heart failure is one cause of **shock**, a severe disturbance in the circulatory system resulting in inadequate delivery of blood to the tissues. Heart failure is treated with rest, drugs to strengthen heart contractions, diuretics to eliminate fluid, and restriction of salt in the diet.

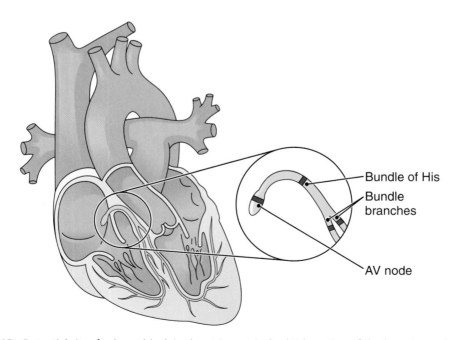

FIGURE 9-13. Potential sites for heart block in the atrioventricular (AV) portion of the heart's conduction system.

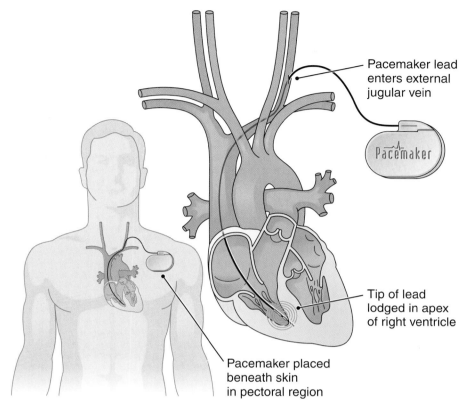

Pacemaker lead
enters external
jugular vein

Pacemaker

Tip of lead
lodged in apex
of right ventricle

Pacemaker placed
beneath skin
in pectoral region

FIGURE 9-14. Placement of a pacemaker.

CONGENITAL HEART DISEASE

A congenital defect is any defect that is present at birth. The most common type of congenital heart defect is a hole in the septum (wall) that separates the atria or the ventricles. The result of a septal defect is that blood is shunted from the left to the right side of the heart and goes back to the lungs instead of out to the body. The heart has to work harder to meet the body's need for oxygen. Symptoms of septal defect include cyanosis (leading to the description "blue baby"), syncope, and **clubbing** of the fingers. Most such congenital defects can be corrected surgically.

Another type of congenital defect is malformation of a heart valve. Failure of a valve to open or close properly is evidenced by a **murmur**, an abnormal sound heard as the heart cycles.

Still other congenital defects result from failure of fetal modifications to convert to their adult form at birth. In **patent ductus arteriosus** (Fig. 9-15), a vessel present in the fetus to bypass the lungs fails to close at birth. Blood can then flow from the aorta to the pulmonary artery and return to the lungs.

RHEUMATIC HEART DISEASE

In **rheumatic heart disease**, infection with a specific type of streptococcus sets up an immune reaction that ultimately damages the heart valves. The infection usually begins as a "strep throat," and most often it is the mitral valve that is involved. Scar tissue fuses the leaflets of the valve, causing a narrowing or **stenosis** that interferes with proper function. People with rheumatic heart disease are subject to repeated infections of the valves and must take antibiotics prophylactically (preventively) before any type of surgery and before even minor invasive

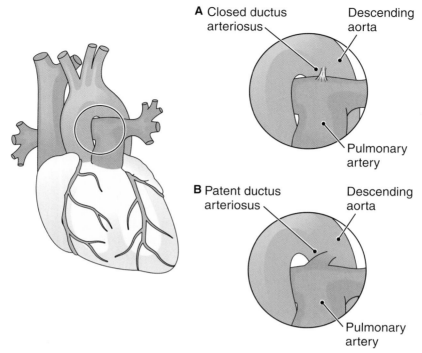

FIGURE 9-15. Patent ductus arteriosus. **(A)** Normal. **(B)** The ductus arteriosus fails to close.

procedures such as dental cleaning. Severe cases of rheumatic heart disease may require surgical correction or even valve replacement. The incidence of rheumatic heart disease has declined with the use of antibiotics.

Disorders of the Veins

A breakdown in the valves of the veins in combination with a chronic dilatation of these vessels results in **varicose veins**. These appear twisted and swollen under the skin, most commonly in the legs. Contributing factors include heredity, obesity, prolonged standing, and pregnancy, which increases pressure in the pelvic veins. This condition can impede blood flow and lead to edema, thrombosis, hemorrhage, or ulceration. Treatment includes the wearing of elastic stockings and, in some cases, surgical removal of the varicosities, after which collateral circulation is established. A varicose vein in the rectum or anal canal is referred to as a **hemorrhoid**.

Phlebitis is any inflammation of the veins and may be caused by infection, injury, poor circulation, or damage to valves in the veins. Such inflammation typically initiates formation of a blood clot, resulting in **thrombophlebitis**. Any veins are subject to thrombophlebitis, but the more serious condition involves the deep veins as opposed to the superficial veins, in the condition termed **deep vein thrombosis** (DVT). The most common sites for DVT are the deep veins of the legs, causing serious reduction in venous drainage from these areas.

Lymphatic Disorders

Changes in the lymphatic system often are related to infection and may consist of inflammation and enlargement of the nodes, called **lymphadenitis**, or inflammation of the vessels, called **lymphangiitis**. Obstruction of lymphatic vessels because of surgical excision or infection results in tissue swelling, or **lymphedema**. Any neoplastic disease involving lymph nodes termed **lymphoma**. These neoplastic disorders affect the white cells found in the lymphatic system, and they are discussed more fully in Chapter 10.

Key Clinical Terms

CARDIOVASCULAR DISORDERS

aneurysm *AN-ū-rizm*	A localized abnormal dilation of a blood vessel, usually an artery, caused by weakness of the vessel wall; may eventually burst
angina pectoris *an-JĪ-na PEK-tō-ris*	A feeling of constriction around the heart or pain that may radiate to the left arm or shoulder, usually brought on by exertion; caused by insufficient blood supply to the heart
arrhythmia *a-RITH-mē-a*	Any abnormality in the rate or rhythm of the heartbeat (literally "without rhythm"; note doubled r). Also called dysrhythmia.
atherosclerosis *ath-er-ō-skle-RŌ-sis*	The development of fatty, fibrous patches (plaques) in the lining of arteries, causing narrowing of the lumen and hardening of the vessel wall. The most common form of arteriosclerosis (hardening of the arteries). Root *ather/o* means "porridge" or "gruel."
bradycardia *brad-ē-KAR-de-a*	A slow heart rate of less than 60 beats per minute
cerebrovascular accident (CVA) *ser-e-brō-VAS-kū-lar*	Sudden damage to the brain resulting from reduction of blood flow. Causes include atherosclerosis, embolism, thrombosis, or hemorrhage from a ruptured aneurysm; commonly called stroke.
clubbing *KLUB-ing*	Enlargement of the ends of the fingers and toes caused by growth of the soft tissue around the nails (see Fig. 7-10). Seen in a variety of diseases in which there is poor peripheral circulation.
cyanosis *sī-a-NŌ-sis*	Bluish discoloration of the skin caused by lack of oxygen
deep vein thrombosis (DVT)	Thrombophlebitis involving the deep veins
diaphoresis *dī-a-fō-RĒ-sis*	Profuse sweating
dissecting aneurysm	An aneurysm in which blood enters the arterial wall and separates the layers. Usually involves the aorta (see Fig. 9-9).
dyslipidemia *dis-lip-i-DĒ-mē-a*	Disorder in serum lipid levels, which is an important factor in development of atherosclerosis. Includes hyperlipidemia (high lipids), hypercholesterolemia (high cholesterol), hypertriglyceridemia (high triglycerides).
dyspnea *DYSP-nē-a*	Difficult or labored breathing (*-pnea*)
edema *e-DĒ-ma*	Swelling of body tissues caused by the presence of excess fluid. Causes include cardiovascular disturbances, kidney failure, inflammation, and malnutrition.
embolism *EM-bō-lizm*	Obstruction of a blood vessel by a blood clot or other matter carried in the circulation

Cardiovascular Disorders, continued

embolus *EM-bō-lus*	A mass carried in the circulation. Usually a blood clot, but may also be air, fat, bacteria, or other solid matter from within or from outside the body.
fibrillation *fi-bri-LĀ-shun*	Spontaneous, quivering, and ineffectual contraction of muscle fibers, as in the atria or the ventricles
heart block	An interference in the conduction system of the heart resulting in arrhythmia (see Fig. 9-13). The condition is classified in order of increasing severity as first-, second-, or third-degree heart block. Block in a bundle branch is designated as a left or right bundle branch block (BBB).
heart failure	A condition caused by the inability of the heart to maintain adequate circulation of blood
hemorrhoid *HEM-ō-royd*	A varicose vein in the rectum
hypertension *hī-per-TEN-shun*	A condition of higher-than-normal blood pressure. Essential (primary, idiopathic) hypertension has no known cause.
infarct *in-FARKT*	An area of localized necrosis (death) of tissue resulting from a blockage or a narrowing of the artery that supplies the area
ischemia *is-KĒ-mē-a*	Local deficiency of blood supply caused by obstruction of the circulation (root *hem/o*)
murmur	An abnormal heart sound
myocardial infarction (MI) *mī-ō-KAR-dē-al* *in-FARK-shun*	Localized necrosis (death) of cardiac muscle tissue resulting from blockage or narrowing of the coronary artery that supplies that area. Myocardial infarction is usually caused by formation of a thrombus (clot) in a vessel (see Fig. 9-12).
occlusion *ō-KLŪ-zhun*	A closing off or obstruction, as of a vessel
patent ductus arteriosus *PĀ-tent DUK-tus* *ar-tēr-ē-Ō-sus*	Persistence of the ductus arteriosus after birth. The ductus arteriosus is a vessel that connects the pulmonary artery to the descending aorta in the fetus to bypass the lungs.
phlebitis *fle-BĪ-tis*	Inflammation of a vein
plaque *plak*	A patch. With regard to the cardiovascular system, a deposit of fatty material and other substances on a vessel wall that impedes blood flow and may block the vessel. Atheromatous plaque.
rheumatic heart disease *rū-MAT-ik*	Damage to heart valves after infection with a type of streptococcus (group A hemolytic streptococcus). The antibodies produced in response to the infection produce scarring of the valves, usually the mitral valve.

Cardiovascular Disorders, continued

shock	Circulatory failure resulting in inadequate supply of blood to the heart. Cardiogenic shock is caused by heart failure; hypovolemic shock is caused by a loss of blood volume; septic shock is caused by bacterial infection.
stenosis *ste-NŌ-sis*	Constriction or narrowing of an opening
stroke	See cerebrovascular accident
syncope *SIN-kō-pē*	A temporary loss of consciousness caused by inadequate blood flow to the brain; fainting
tachycardia *tak-i-KAR-dē-a*	An abnormally rapid heart rate, usually over 100 beats per minute
thrombophlebitis *throm-bō-fle-BĪ-tis*	Inflammation of a vein associated with formation of a blood clot
thrombosis *throm-BŌ-sis*	Development of a blood clot within a vessel
thrombus *THROM-bus*	A blood clot that forms within a blood vessel (root *thromb/o*)
varicose vein *VAR-i-kōs*	A twisted and swollen vein resulting from breakdown of the valves, pooling of blood, and chronic dilatation of the vessel (root *varic/o*); also called varix (VAR-iks) or varicosity (*var-i-KOS-i-tē*)

DIAGNOSIS AND TREATMENT

angioplasty *AN-jē-ō-plas-tē*	A procedure that reopens a narrowed vessel and restores blood flow. Commonly accomplished by surgically removing plaque, inflating a balloon within the vessel, or installing a device (stent) to keep the vessel open.
artificial pacemaker	A battery-operated device that generates electrical impulses to regulate the beating of the heart. It may be external or implanted, may be designed to respond to need, and may have the capacity to prevent tachycardia (see Fig. 9-14).
cardioversion *KAR-dē-ō-ver-zhun*	Correction of an abnormal cardiac rhythm. May be accomplished pharmacologically, with antiarrhythmic drugs, or by application of electric current (see defibrillation).
coronary angiography *an-jē-OG-ra-fē*	Radiographic study of the coronary arteries after introduction of an opaque dye by means of a catheter
coronary artery bypass graft (CABG)	Surgical creation of a shunt to bypass a blocked coronary artery. The aorta is connected to a point past the obstruction with another vessel or a piece of another vessel, usually the saphenous vein of the leg or the left internal mammary artery (see Fig. 9-11).

Diagnosis and Treatment, continued

defibrillation *dē-fib-ri-LĀ-shun*	Use of an electronic device (defibrillator) to stop fibrillation by delivering a brief electric shock to the heart. The shock may be delivered to the surface of the chest or be delivered directly to the heart through wire leads.
echocardiography (ECG) *ek-ō-kar-dē-OG-ra-f ē*	A noninvasive method that uses ultrasound to visualize internal cardiac structures
electrocardiography *ē-lek-trō-kar-dē-OG-ra-f ē*	Study of the electrical activity of the heart as detected by electrodes (leads) placed on the surface of the body. The components of the ECG include the P wave, QRS complex, T wave, ST segment, PR (PQ) interval, and the QT interval (Fig. 9-16). Also abbreviated EKG from the German *electrokardiography*.
lipoprotein *lip-ō-PRŌ-tēn*	A compound of protein with lipid. Lipoproteins are classified according to density as very low density (VLDL), low density (LDL), and high density (HDL). Relatively higher levels of HDLs have been correlated with health of the cardiovascular system.
percutaneous transluminal coronary angioplasty (PTCA)	Dilatation of a sclerotic blood vessel by means of a balloon catheter inserted into the vessel and then inflated to flatten plaque against the artery wall (see Fig. 9-10)

LYMPHATIC DISORDERS

lymphoma *lim-FŌ-ma*	Any neoplastic disease of lymphoid tissue
lymphadenitis *lim-fad-e-NI-tis*	Inflammation and enlargement of lymph nodes, usually as a result of infection
lymphangiitis *lim-fan-jē-Ī-tis*	Inflammation of lymphatic vessels as a result of bacterial infection. Appears as painful red streaks under the skin. (Also spelled lymphangitis.)
lymphedema *lim-fe-DĒ-ma*	Swelling of tissues with lymph caused by obstruction or excision of lymphatic vessels

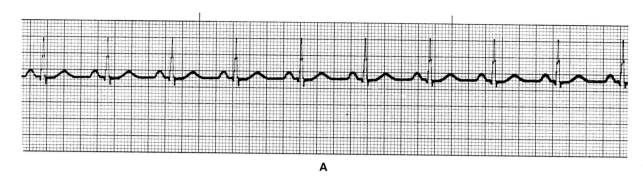

A

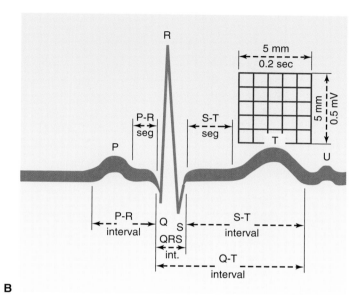

B

FIGURE 9-16. (A) ECG tracing showing normal sinus rhythm. **(B)** Commonly measured components of an ECG tracing. (Reprinted with permission from Smeltzer SC, Bare BG. Brunner & Suddarth's Textbook of Medical-Surgical Nursing. 9th Ed. Philadelphia: Lippincott Williams & Wilkins, 2000.)

Supplementary Terms

NORMAL STRUCTURE AND FUNCTION

apex beat	The pulsing of the heart that can be felt over the apex in the fifth left intercostal space (between the ribs) about 8 to 9 cm from the midline
cardiac output	The amount of blood pumped from the right or left ventricle per minute
ductus arteriosus *DUK-tus ar-tē-rē-O-sus*	A vessel between the pulmonary artery and the aorta that bypasses the lungs in fetal circulation. Failure to close after birth is called patent (*PA-tent*) ductus arteriosus.

Normal Structure and Function, *continued*

foramen ovale *for-Ā-men ō-VAL-ē*	An opening between the two atria that allows blood to bypass the lungs in fetal circulation. Failure to close after birth results in a septal defect.
Korotkoff sounds *ko-rot-KOFS*	Arterial sounds heard with a stethoscope during determination of blood pressure with a cuff
perfusion *per-FŪ-zhun*	The passage of fluid, such as blood, through an organ or tissue
precordium *prē-KOR-dē-um*	The anterior region over the heart and the lower part of the thorax; adjective, precordial
pulse pressure	The difference between systolic and diastolic pressure
sinus rhythm	A normal heart rhythm originating from the sinoatrial (SA) node
stroke volume	The amount of blood ejected by the left ventricle with each beat
Valsalva maneuver *val-SAL-va*	Bearing down, as in childbirth or defecation, by attempting to exhale forcefully with the nose and throat closed. This action has an effect on the cardiovascular system.

SYMPTOMS AND CONDITIONS

bruit *brwē*	An abnormal sound heard in auscultation
cardiac tamponade *tam-pon-ĀD*	Pathologic accumulation of fluid in the pericardial sac. May result from pericarditis or injury to the heart or great vessels.
coarctation of the aorta *kō-ark-TĀ-shun*	Localized narrowing of the aorta
ectopic beat *ek-TOP-ik*	A heartbeat that originates from some part of the heart other than the SA node
extrasystole *eks-tra-SIS-tō-lē*	Premature contraction of the heart that occurs separately from the normal beat and originates from a part of the heart other than the SA node
flutter	Very rapid (200 to 300 beats per minute) but regular contractions, as in the atria or the ventricles
hypotension *hī-po-TEN-shun*	A condition of lower-than-normal blood pressure
intermittent claudication *claw-di-KĀ-shun*	Pain in a muscle during exercise caused by inadequate blood supply. The pain disappears with rest.
mitral valve prolapse	Movement of the cusps of the mitral valve into the left atrium when the ventricles contract
occlusive vascular disease	Arteriosclerotic disease of the vessels, usually peripheral vessels
palpitation *pal-pi-TĀ-shun*	A sensation of abnormally rapid or irregular heartbeat
pitting edema	Edema that retains the impression of a finger pressed firmly into the skin

Symptoms and Conditions, continued

polyarteritis nodosa *nō-DŌ-sa*	Potentially fatal collagen disease causing inflammation of small visceral arteries. Symptoms depend on the organ affected.
Raynaud disease *rā-NŌ*	A disorder characterized by abnormal constriction of peripheral vessels in the arms and legs on exposure to cold
regurgitation *rē-gur-ji-TĀ-shun*	A backward flow, such as the backflow of blood through a defective valve
stasis *STĀ-sis*	Stoppage of normal blood normal flow, as of blood or urine. Blood stasis may lead to dermatitis and ulcer formation.
subacute bacterial endocarditis (SBE)	Growth of bacteria in a heart or valves previously damaged by rheumatic fever
tetralogy of Fallot *fal-Ō*	A combination of four congenital heart abnormalities: pulmonary artery stenosis, interventricular septal defect, displacement of the aorta to the right, right ventricular hypertrophy
thromboangiitis obliterans	Inflammation and thrombus formation resulting in occlusion of small vessels, especially in the legs. Most common in young men and correlated with heavy smoking. Thrombotic occlusion of leg vessels in young men leading to gangrene of the feet. Patients show a hypersensitivity to tobacco. Also called Buerger disease.
vegetation	Irregular outgrowths of bacteria on the heart valves; associated with rheumatic fever
Wolff-Parkinson-White syndrome (WPW)	A cardiac arrhythmia consisting of tachycardia and a premature ventricular beat caused by an alternate conduction pathway

DIAGNOSIS

cardiac catheterization	Passage of a catheter into the heart through a vessel to inject a contrast medium for imaging, diagnosing abnormalities, obtaining samples, or measuring pressure
central venous pressure (CVP)	Pressure in the superior vena cava
cineangiocardiography *sin-e-an-jē-ō-kar-dē-OG-ra-fē*	The photographic recording of fluoroscopic images of the heart and large vessels using motion picture techniques
Doppler echocardiography	An imaging method used to study the rate and pattern of blood flow
enzyme studies	Measurement of serum levels of enzymes that are released in increased amounts from damaged heart tissue. These include CK (creatine kinase), LDH (lactate dehydrogenase), AST (aspartate aminotransferase), and ALT (alanine aminotransferase).
heart scan	Imaging of the heart after injection of a radioactive isotope. The PYP (pyrophosphate) scan using technetium-99m (^{99m}Tc) is used to test for myocardial infarction because the isotope is taken up by damaged tissue. The MUGA (multigated acquisition) scan gives information on heart function.

Diagnosis, continued

Holter monitor	A portable device that can record up to 24 hours of an individual's ECG readings during normal activity
homocysteine *hō-mō-SIS-tēn*	An amino acid that at higher-than-normal levels in the blood is associated with increased risk of cardiovascular disease
phlebotomist *fle-BOT-ō-mist*	Technician who specializes in drawing blood
phonocardiography *fō-nō-kar-dē-OG-ra-fē*	Electronic recording of heart sounds
plethysmography *ple-thiz-MOG-ra-fē*	Measurement of changes in the size of a part based on the amount of blood contained in or passing through it. Impedance plethysmography measures changes in electrical resistance and is used in diagnosis of deep vein thrombosis.
pulmonary wedge pressure (PWP)	Pressure measured by a catheter in a branch of the pulmonary artery. It is an indirect measure of pressure in the left atrium.
stress test	Evaluation of physical fitness by continuous ECG monitoring during exercise. In a thallium stress test, a radioactive isotope of thallium is administered to trace blood flow through the heart during exercise.
Swan-Ganz catheter	A cardiac catheter with a balloon at the tip that is used to measure pulmonary arterial pressure. It is flow-guided through a vein into the right side of the heart and then into the pulmonary artery.
transesophageal echocardiography (TEE)	Use of an ultrasound transducer placed endoscopically into the esophagus to obtain images of the heart
triglycerides *trī-GLIS-er-īdz*	Simple fats that circulate in the bloodstream
ventriculography *ven-trik-ū-LOG-ra-fē*	X-ray study of the ventricles of the heart after introduction of an opaque dye by means of a catheter

TREATMENT AND SURGICAL PROCEDURES

atherectomy *ath-er-EK-tō-mē*	Removal of atheromatous plaque from the lining of a vessel. May be done by open surgery or through the lumen of the vessel.
automated external defibrillator (AED)	Electronic device that detects arrhythmia and automatically delivers a correct programmed shock. These devices, used on the scene of a heart attack, can prevent death.
commissurotomy *kom-i-shur-OT-ō-mē*	Surgical incision of a scarred mitral valve to increase the size of the valve opening
embolectomy *em-bō-LEK-tō-mē*	Surgical removal of an embolus
implantable cardioverter defibrillator (ICD)	A battery-powered device that can shock the heart during fibrillation to restore a normal rhythm. The ICD is implanted under the collarbone. A lead wire is threaded through the pulmonary artery into the right ventricle (Fig. 9-17).

Treatment and Surgical Procedures, continued

intra-aortic balloon pump (IABP)	A mechanical-assist device that consists of an inflatable balloon pump inserted through the femoral artery into the thoracic aorta. It inflates during diastole to improve coronary circulation and deflates before systole to allow blood ejection from the heart.
left ventricular assist device (LVAD)	A pump that takes over the function of the left ventricle in delivering blood into the systemic circuit. These devices are used to assist patients awaiting heart transplantation or those who are recovering from heart failure.
stent	A small metal device in the shape of a coil or slotted tube that is placed inside an artery to keep the vessel open after balloon angioplasty (Fig. 9-18).

MEDICATIONS

angiotensin-converting enzyme (ACE) **inhibitor**	A drug that lowers blood pressure by blocking the formation in the blood of angiotensin II, a substance that normally acts to increase blood pressure
angiotensin II receptor antagonist	A drug that blocks tissue receptors for angiotensin II
antiarrhythmic agent	A drug that regulates the rate and rhythm of the heartbeat
beta-adrenergic blocking agent	Drug that decreases the rate and strength of heart contractions
calcium channel blocker	Drug that controls the rate and force of heart contraction by regulating calcium entrance into the cells
digitalis *dij-i-TAL-is*	A drug that slows and strengthens heart muscle contractions
diuretic *dī-ū-RET-ik*	Drug that eliminates fluid by increasing the output of urine by the kidneys. Lowered blood volume decreases the workload of the heart.
hypolipidemic agent *hī-pō-lip-i-DĒ-mik*	Drug that lowers serum cholesterol
lidocaine *LĪ-dō-kān*	A local anesthetic that is used intravenously to treat cardiac arrhythmias
nitroglycerin *nī-trō-GLIS-er-in*	A drug used in the treatment of angina pectoris to dilate coronary vessels
statins	Drugs that act to lower lipids in the blood. The drug names end with *-statin,* such as lovastatin, pravastatin, atorvastatin.
streptokinase (SK) *strep-tō-KĪ-nas*	An enzyme used to dissolve blood clots
tissue plasminogen activator (tPA)	A drug used to dissolve blood clots. It activates production of a substance (plasmin) in the blood that normally dissolves clots.
vasodilator *vas-ō-dī-LĀ-tor*	A drug that widens blood vessels and improves blood flow

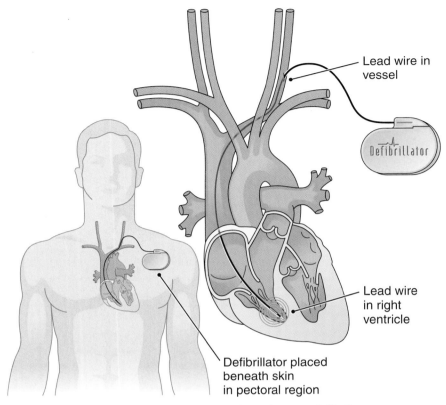

FIGURE 9-17. Implantable cardioverter defibrillator.

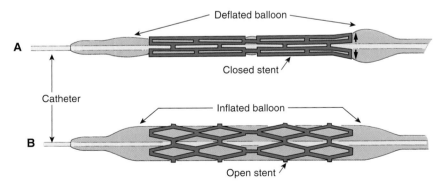

FIGURE 9-18. Intracoronary artery stent. **(A)** Stent closed, before balloon inflation. **(B)** Stent open, balloon inflated. The stent will remain expanded after the balloon is deflated and removed. (Reprinted with permission from Smeltzer SC, Bare BG. Brunner & Suddarth's Textbook of Medical-Surgical Nursing. 9th Ed. Philadelphia: Lippincott Williams & Wilkins, 2000.)

ABBREVIATIONS

ACE	Angiotensin-converting enzyme	**LVAD**	Left ventricular assist device
AED	Automated external defibrillator	**LVEDP**	Left ventricular end-diastolic pressure
AF	Atrial fibrillation	**LVH**	Left ventricular hypertrophy
ALT	Alanine aminotransferase (SGPT)	**MI**	Myocardial infarction
AMI	Acute myocardial infarction	**mm Hg**	Millimeters of mercury
APC	Atrial premature complex	**MR**	Mitral regurgitation, reflux
AR	Aortic regurgitation	**MS**	Mitral stenosis
AS	Aortic stenosis; arteriosclerosis	**MUGA**	Multigated acquisition (scan)
ASCVD	Arteriosclerotic cardiovascular disease	**MVP**	Mitral valve prolapse
ASD	Atrial septal defect	**MVR**	Mitral valve replacement
ASHD	Arteriosclerotic heart disease	**NSR**	Normal sinus rhythm
AST	Aspartate aminotransferase (SGOT)	**P**	Pulse
AT	Atrial tachycardia	**PAC**	Premature atrial contraction
AV	Atrioventricular	**PAP**	Pulmonary arterial pressure
BBB	Bundle branch block (left or right)	**PMI**	Point of maximal impulse
BP	Blood pressure	**PSVT**	Paroxysmal supraventricular tachycardia
bpm	Beats per minute	**PTCA**	Percutaneous transluminal coronary angioplasty
CABG	Coronary artery bypass graft		
CAD	Coronary artery disease	**PVC**	Premature ventricular contraction
CCU	Coronary/cardiac care unit	**PVD**	Peripheral vascular disease
CHD	Coronary heart disease	**PWP**	Pulmonary (artery) wedge pressure
CHF	Congestive heart failure	**PYP**	Pyrophosphate (scan)
C(P)K	Creatine (phospho)kinase	S_1	The first heart sound
CPR	Cardiopulmonary resuscitation	S_2	The second heart sound
CVD	Cardiovascular disease	**SA**	Sinoatrial
CVI	Chronic venous insufficiency	**SBE**	Subacute bacterial endocarditis
CVP	Central venous pressure	**SGOT**	Serum glutamic oxaloacetic trans-aminase (AST)
DOE	Dyspnea on exertion		
DVT	Deep vein thrombosis	**SK**	Streptokinase
ECG (EKG)	Electrocardiogram	**SVT**	Supraventricular tachycardia
HDL	High-density lipoprotein	**99mTc**	Technetium-99m
HTN	Hypertension	**TEE**	Transesophageal echocardiography
IABP	Intra-aortic balloon pump	**tPA**	Tissue plasminogen activator
ICD	Implantable cardioverter defibrillator	**VAD**	Ventricular assist device
IVCD	Intraventricular conduction delay	**VF**	Ventricular fibrillation
JVP	Jugular venous pulse	**VLDL**	Very low density lipoprotein
LAD	Left anterior descending (coronary artery)	**VPC**	Ventricular premature complex
LAHB	Left anterior hemiblock	**VSD**	Ventricular septal defect
LDH	Lactic dehydrogenase	**VT**	Ventricular tachycardia
LDL	Low-density lipoprotein	**VTE**	Venous thromboembolism
LV	Left ventricle	**WPW**	Wolff-Parkinson-White syndrome

Labeling Exercise 9-1

The Cardiovascular System
Write the name of each numbered part on the corresponding line of the answer sheet.

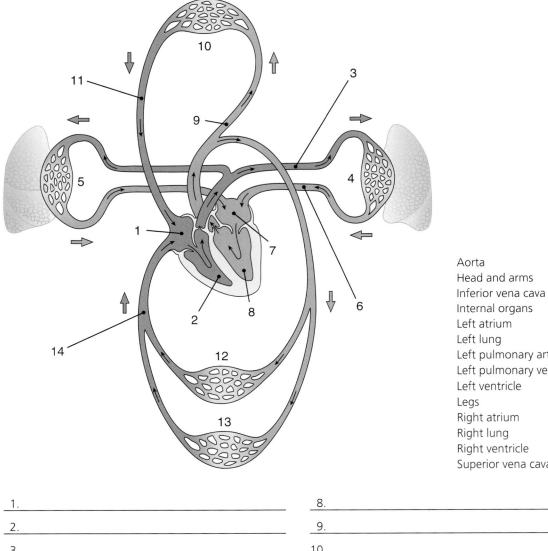

Aorta
Head and arms
Inferior vena cava
Internal organs
Left atrium
Left lung
Left pulmonary artery
Left pulmonary vein
Left ventricle
Legs
Right atrium
Right lung
Right ventricle
Superior vena cava

1. _____	8. _____
2. _____	9. _____
3. _____	10. _____
4. _____	11. _____
5. _____	12. _____
6. _____	13. _____
7. _____	14. _____

Labeling Exercise 9-2

The Heart and Great Vessels

Write the name of each numbered part on the corresponding line of the answer sheet.

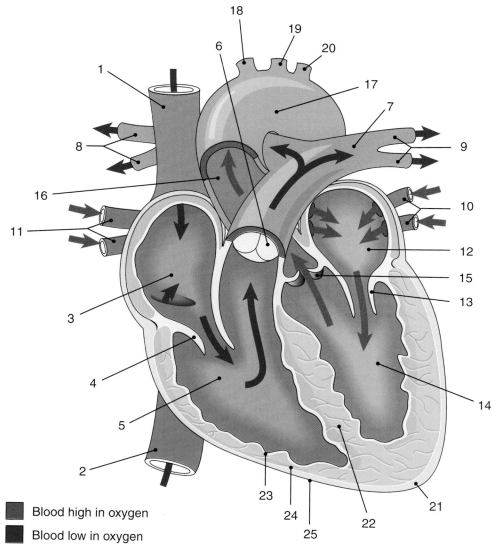

Blood high in oxygen

Blood low in oxygen

Aortic arch	Inferior vena cava	Left pulmonary veins	Right atrium
Aortic valve	Interventricular septum	Left subclavian artery	Right pulmonary artery
Apex	Left atrium	Left ventricle	(branches)
Ascending aorta	Left common carotid	Mitral (bicuspid) valve	Right pulmonary veins
Brachiocephalic artery	artery	Myocardium	Right ventricle
Endocardium	Left pulmonary artery	Pulmonary artery	Superior vena cava
Epicardium	(branches)	Pulmonic valve	Tricuspid valve

1. _____   14. _____

2. _____   15. _____

3. _____   16. _____

4. _____   17. _____

5. _____   18. _____

6. _____   19. _____

7. _____   20. _____

8. _____   21. _____

9. _____   22. _____

10. _____   23. _____

11. _____   24. _____

12. _____   25. _____

13. _____

Chapter Review 9-1

Match the following terms and write the appropriate letter to the left of each number:

_____ 1. tricuspid

_____ 2. pericardium

_____ 3. SA node

_____ 4. apex

_____ 5. lumen

a. central opening of a vessel

b. pacemaker of the heart

c. fibrous sac around the heart

d. lower pointed region of the heart

e. right atrioventricular valve

_____ 6. pulmonic valve

_____ 7. vena cava

_____ 8. thymus

_____ 9. mitral valve

_____ 10. Purkinje fibers

a. lymphoid organ in the chest

b. vessel that empties into the right atrium

c. part of the heart's conduction system

d. valve that regulates blood flow to the lungs

e. left atrioventricular valve

_____ 11. atherosclerosis

_____ 12. aneurysm

_____ 13. ischemia

_____ 14. myocarditis

_____ 15. asystole

a. absence of a heartbeat

b. inflammation of the heart muscle

c. localized dilatation of a blood vessel

d. local deficiency of blood

e. accumulation of fatty deposits in the lining of a blood vessel

_____ 16. thrombosis   a. twisted and swollen vessel

_____ 17. occlusion   b. ineffective quivering of muscle

_____ 18. varix   c. local death of tissue

_____ 19. infarction   d. blockage

_____ 20. fibrillation   e. formation of a blood clot in a vessel

_____ 21. ECG   a. disease of the heart's vessels

_____ 22. CABG   b. defibrillation device

_____ 23. PVC   c. generation of an extra heartbeat

_____ 24. AED   d. study of the electrical activity of the heart

_____ 25. CAD   e. surgery to create a shunt around a blocked vessel

SUPPLEMENTARY TERMS

_____ 26. intermittent claudication   a. drug that lowers serum cholesterol

_____ 27. precordium   b. normal heart rhythm

_____ 28. statin   c. accumulation of fluid in the pericardial sac

_____ 29. cardiac tamponade   d. muscular pain during exercise

_____ 30. sinus rhythm   e. anterior region over the heart

Fill in the blanks:

31. Each lower pumping chamber of the heart is a(n) _____.

32. The heart muscle is the _____.

33. The microscopic vessels through which materials are exchanged between the blood and the tissues are the _____.

34. The largest artery is the _____.

35. Blood returning to the heart from the lungs enters the chamber called the

_____.

36. The lymphoid organ in the abdomen is the _____.

37. At its termination in the abdomen, the aorta divides into the right and left (see Fig. 9-5)

_____.

38. The large vein that drains the head is the (see Fig. 9-6) _____.

39. Microangiopathy (_mī-krō-an-jē-OP-a-thē_) is disease of many small

_____.

40. A phlebotomist (_fle-BOT-ō-mist_) is one who drains blood from a(n)

_____.

41. The term varicoid pertains to a(n) _____.

True-False. Examine each of the following statements. If the statement is true, write T in the first blank. If the statement is false, write F in the first blank and correct the statement by replacing the underlined word in the second blank.

42. The systemic circuit pumps blood to the lungs.   _____ _____

43. An artery is a vessel that carries blood back to the heart.   _____ _____

44. Diastole is the relaxation phase of the heart cycle.   _____ _____

45. The left ventricle pumps blood into the aorta.   _____ _____

46. The brachial artery supplies blood to the leg.   _____ _____

47. The bicuspid valve is also called the mitral valve.   _____ _____

48. Bradycardia is a lower than average heart rate.   _____ _____

Define each of the following terms:

49. Interatrial (in-ter-Ā-trē-al)   _____

50. Avascular (ā-VAS-kū-lar)   _____

51. Atriotomy (ā-trē-OT-ō-mē)   _____

52. Angiostenosis (an-jē-ō-ste-NŌ-sis)   _____

53. Thymectomy (thī-MEK-tō-mē)   _____

54. Lymphangitis (lim-fan-JĪ-tis)   _____

Word building. Write a word for each of the following definitions:

55. Physician who specializes in study and treatment of the heart   _____

56. Suture (-rhaphy) of an artery   _____

57. Radiographic study of the ventricles   _____

58. Stoppage (-stasis) of lymph flow   _____

59. An instrument (-tome) for incising a valve   _____

60. Incision of a lymph node   _____

61. Surgical fixation (-pexy) of the spleen   _____

Word building. Use the root aort/o to write a word with each of the following meanings:

62. Radiograph (-gram) of the aorta   _____

63. Before or in front of (pre-) the aorta   _____

64. Narrowing (-stenosis) of the aorta   _____

65. Any disease (-pathy) of the aorta   _____

66. Downward displacement (-ptosis) of the aorta   _____

Adjectives. Write the adjective form of each of the following words:

67. vein   _____

68. septum   _____

69. atrium _____

70. varix _____

71. spleen _____

72. sclerosis _____

Plurals. Write the plural form of each of the following words:

73. embolus _____

74. stenosis _____

75. apex _____

76. varix _____

77. septum _____

Write the meaning of the following abbreviations as they apply to the cardiovascular system:

78. BBB _____

79. PCTA _____

80. LVH _____

81. BP _____

82. NSR _____

83. CVI _____

Word analysis. Define each of the following words, and give the meaning of the word parts in each. Use a dictionary if necessary.

84. Endarterectomy (*end-ar-ter-EK-tō-mē*) _____
    a. end/o- _____
    b. arteri/o _____
    c. ecto- _____
    d. -tomy _____

85. Telangiectasia (*tel-an-jē-ēk-TĀ-zē-a*) _____
    a. tel- _____
    b. angi/o _____
    c. -ectasia _____

86. Lymphangiophlebitis (*lim-fan-jē-ō-fle-BĪ-tis*) _____
    a. lymph/o _____
    b. angi/o _____
    c. phleb/o _____
    d. -itis _____

Case Studies

Case Study 9-1: PTCA and Echocardiogram

A.L., a 68-year-old woman, was admitted to the CCU with chest pain, dyspnea, diaphoresis, syncope, and nausea. She had taken three sublingual doses of nitroglycerine tablets within a 10-minute time span without relief before dialing 911. A previous stress test and thallium uptake scan suggested cardiac disease.

Her family history was significant for cardiovascular disease. Her father died at the age of 62 of an acute myocardial infarction. Her mother had bilateral carotid endarterectomies and a femoral-popliteal bypass procedure and died at the age of 72 of congestive heart failure. A.L.'s older sister died from a ruptured aortic aneurysm at the age of 65. Her ECG on admission presented tachycardia with a rate of 126 bpm with inverted T waves. A murmur was heard at S_1. Her skin color was dusky to cyanotic on her lips and fingertips. Her admitting diagnosis was possible coronary artery disease, acute myocardial infarction, and valvular disease.

Cardiac catheterization with balloon angioplasty (PTCA) was performed the next day. Significant stenosis of the left anterior descending coronary artery was shown and was treated with angioplasty and stent placement. Left ventricular function was normal.

Echocardiogram, 2 days later, showed normal-sized left and enlarged right ventricular cavities. The mitral valve had normal amplitude of motion. The anterior and posterior leaflets moved in opposite directions during diastole. There was a late systolic prolapse of the mitral leaflet at rest. The left atrium was enlarged. The impression of the study was mitral prolapse with regurgitation. Surgery was recommended.

Case Study 9-2: Mitral Valve Replacement Operative Report

A.L. was transferred to the operating room, placed in a supine position, and given general endotracheal anesthesia. Her pericardium was entered longitudinally through a median sternotomy. The surgeon found that her heart was enlarged with a dilated right ventricle. The left atrium was dilated. Preoperative transesophageal echocardiogram revealed severe mitral regurgitation with severe posterior and anterior prolapse. Extracorporeal circulation was established. The aorta was cross-clamped, and cardioplegic solution (to stop the heartbeat) was given into the aortic root intermittently for myocardial protection.

The left atrium was entered via the interatrial groove on the right, exposing the mitral valve. The middle scallop of the posterior leaflet was resected. The remaining leaflets were removed to the areas of the commissures and preserved for the sliding plasty. The elongated chordae were shortened. The surgeon slid the posterior leaflet across the midline and sutured it in place. A no. 30 annuloplasty ring was sutured in place with interrupted no. 2-0 Dacron suture. The valve was tested by inflating the ventricle with NSS and proved to be competent. The left atrium was closed with continuous no. 4-0 Prolene suture. Air was removed from the heart. The cross-clamp was removed. Cardiac action resumed with normal sinus rhythm. After a period of cardiac recovery and attainment of normothermia, cardiopulmonary bypass was discontinued.

Protamine was given to counteract the heparin. Pacer wires were placed in the right atrium and ventricle. Silicone catheters were placed in the pleural and substernal spaces. The sternum and soft tissue wound was closed. A.L. recovered from her surgery and was discharged 6 days later.

Case Studies, continued

CASE STUDY QUESTIONS

Write the word or phrase from the case study that has the same meaning as each of the following words or phrases:

1. The state of profuse perspiration   _____

2. Under the tongue   _____

3. Test of cardiac function during physical exertion   _____

4. Disease that includes both heart and blood vessel pathology   _____

5. Excision of the inner lining along with atherosclerotic plaque from an artery (plural)   _____

6. An abnormal heart sound   _____

7. Bluish discoloration of the skin; sign of anoxia   _____

8. The noun form of stenotic   _____

9. Between the atria   _____

10. Below the sternum   _____

Multiple choice: Select the best answer and write the letter of your choice to the left of each number.

_____ 11. The word transluminal means:
   a. across a wall
   b. between branches
   c. through an outer layer
   d. through a central opening
   e. across a valve

_____ 12. The term that means backflow, as of blood, is:
   a. infarction
   b. regurgitation
   c. amplitude
   d. prolapse
   e. tourniquet

_____ 13. The term for a narrowing of the bicuspid valve is:
   a. atrial prolapse
   b. pulmonic stenosis
   c. mitral stenosis
   d. mitral prolapse
   e. atrial stenosis

_____ 14. Blowout of a dilated segment of the main artery is:
   a. left anterior diastole
   b. peritoneal infarction

Case Studies, continued

     c. coarctation of the aorta
     d. cardiac tamponade
     e. ruptured aortic aneurysm

_____ 15. Sternotomy is:
     a. incision into the sternum
     b. removal of the sternum
     c. narrowing of the sternum
     d. plastic repair of the sternum
     e. surgical fixation of the sternum

_____ 16. Extracorporeal circulation occurs:
     a. within the brain
     b. within the pericardium
     c. within the body
     d. in the legs
     e. outside the body

_____ 17. Protamine was given to counteract the action of the heparin. This drug action is described as:
     a. antagonistic
     b. synergy
     c. potentiating
     d. similation
     e. addiction

Abbreviations. Define the following abbreviations:

18. CCU _____

19. AMI _____

20. CAD _____

21. LAD _____

22. CHF _____

23. TEE _____

24. MVR _____

Chapter 9 Crossword
Circulation

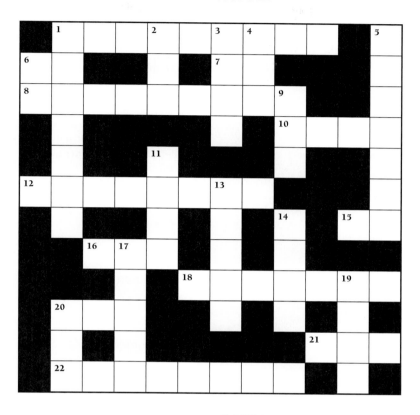

ACROSS

1. A microscopic vessel
6. Pacemaker of the heart: ____ ____ node
7. A route for injection (abbreviation)
8. The right AV valve
10. Vein: combining form
12. Relaxation phase of the heart cycle
15. Hardening of the arteries (abbreviation)
16. Substance used to dissolve blood clots (abbreviation)
18. Pulse: combining form, as in the name of blood pressure apparatus
20. Form of lipoprotein (abbreviation)
21. Heart disease associated with pulmonary edema (abbreviation)
22. Part of the heart's conduction system; it receives impulses from the AV node

DOWN

1. Main artery in the neck
2. Hospital unit that cares for the critically ill (abbreviation)
3. Category of compounds that includes fats: combining form
4. Heart attack (abbreviation)
5. Obstruction circulating in the bloodstream
6. Segment of the ECG tracing
9. Thrombotic condition of the veins (abbreviation)
11. Procedure for dilating an obstructed vessel (abbreviation)
13. Fluid that circulates in the lymphatic system
14. Lymphoid organ in the chest: root
17. Vein: root
19. Units in which blood pressure is measured (abbreviation)
20. Mechanical device to assist the heart, ___ ___ ___ D (abbreviation)

CHAPTER *9* **Answer Section**

Answers to Chapter Exercises

EXERCISE 9-1

1. heart
2. atria
3. ventricle
4. valve
5. cardiac (*KAR-dē-ak*)
6. myocardial (*mī-ō-KAR-dē-al*)
7. atrial (*Ā-trē-al*)
8. pericardial (*per-i-KAR-dē-al*)
9. ventricular (*ven-TRIK-ū-lar*)
10. valvular (*VAL-vū-lar*); also valvar (*VAL-var*)
11. endocarditis (*en-dō-kar-DĪ-tis*)
12. myocarditis (*mī-ō-kar-DĪ-tis*)
13. pericarditis (*per-i-kar-DĪ-tis*)
14. cardiology (*kar-dē-OL-ō-jē*)
15. cardiomegaly (*kar-dē-ō-MEG-a-lē*)
16. interventricular (*in-tra-ven-TRIK-ū-lar*)
17. atrioventricular (*ā-trē-ō-ven-TRIK-ū-lar*)
18. valvotomy (*val-VOT-ō-mē*); also valvulotomy (*val-vū-LOT-ō-mē*)

EXERCISE 9-2

1. vessel
2. artery
3. vessels
4. aorta
5. vessels
6. arteriole
7. inflammation of a vessel or vessels
8. pertaining to the heart and vessels
9. rupture of an artery
10. within the aorta
11. inflammation of a vein
12. angiogram
13. aortogram
14. phlebogram; venogram
15. angiectomy (*an-jē-EK-tō-mē*)
16. angiectasis (*an-jē-EK-ta-sis*); also hemangiectasis (*hē-man-jē-EK-ta-sis*)
17. angiogenesis (*an-jē-ō-JEN-e-sis*)
18. angioplasty (*AN-jē-ō-plas-tē*)
19. aortostenosis (*ā-or-tō-ste-NŌ-sis*)
20. arteriotomy (*ar-tēr-ē-OT-ō-mē*)
21. intravenous (*in-tra-VĒ-nus*)
22. phlebectomy (*fle-BEK-tō-mē*); venectomy (*vē-NEK-tō-mē*)

EXERCISE 9-3

1. lymph
2. lymph node
3. lymphatic vessels
4. spleen
5. thymus gland
6. tonsils
7. lymphangi/o; lymphatic vessel
8. lymphaden/o; lymph node
9. splen/o; spleen
10. thym/o; thymus gland
11. tonsill/o; tonsil
12. lymphangitis (*lim-fan-JĪ-tis*); also lymphangiitis (*lim-fan-jē-Ī-tis*)
13. lymphoma (*lim-FŌ-ma*)
14. lymphadenopathy (*lim-fad-e-NOP-a-thē*)
15. splenalgia (*splē-NAL-jē-a*)
16. tonsillitis (*ton-si-LĪ-tis*)

LABELING EXERCISE 9-1
THE CARDIOVASCULAR SYSTEM

1. right atrium
2. right ventricle
3. left pulmonary artery
4. left lung
5. right lung
6. left pulmonary vein
7. left atrium
8. left ventricle
9. aorta
10. head and arms
11. superior vena cava
12. internal organs
13. legs
14. inferior vena cava

LABELING EXERCISE 9-2
THE HEART AND GREAT VESSELS

1. superior vena cava
2. inferior vena cava
3. right atrium
4. tricuspid valve
5. right ventricle
6. pulmonic valve
7. pulmonary artery
8. right pulmonary artery (branches)
9. left pulmonary artery (branches)

10. left pulmonary veins
11. right pulmonary veins
12. left atrium
13. mitral (bicuspid) valve
14. left ventricle
15. aortic valve
16. ascending aorta
17. aortic arch
18. brachiocephalic artery
19. left common carotid artery
20. left subclavian artery
21. apex
22. interventricular septum
23. endocardium
24. myocardium
25. epicardium

Answers to Chapter Review 9-1

1. e
2. c
3. b
4. d
5. a
6. d
7. b
8. a
9. e
10. c
11. e
12. c
13. d
14. b
15. a
16. e
17. d
18. a
19. c
20. b
21. d
22. e
23. c
24. b
25. a
26. d
27. e
28. a
29. c
30. b
31. ventricle
32. myocardium
33. capillaries
34. aorta
35. left atrium
36. spleen

37. common iliac (*IL-ē-ak*) arteries
38. jugular (*JUG-ū-lar*)
39. vessels
40. vein
41. varicose vein, varix
42. F pulmonary circuit
43. F vein
44. T
45. T
46. F arm
47. T
48. T
49. between the atria
50. without vessels
51. incision of an atrium
52. narrowing of a vessel
53. surgical removal of the thymus
54. inflammation of lymphatic vessels
55. cardiologist
56. arteriorrhaphy
57. ventriculography
58. lymphostasis
59. valvotome; valvulotome
60. lymphadenotomy
61. splenopexy
62. aortogram
63. preaortic
64. aortostenosis
65. aortopathy
66. aortoptosis
67. venous
68. septal
69. atrial
70. varicose
71. splenic; splenetic
72. sclerotic
73. emboli
74. stenoses
75. apices
76. varices
77. septa
78. bundle branch block
79. percutaneous transluminal coronary angioplasty
80. left ventricular hypertrophy
81. blood pressure
82. normal sinus rhythm
83. chronic venous insufficiency
84. Excision of the inner layer of an artery thickened by atherosclerosis
    a. within
    b. artery
    c. out
    d. to cut

85. Permanent dilation of small blood vessels causing small, local red lesions
    a. end
    b. vessel
    c. dilation
86. Inflammation of lymphatic vessels and veins
    a. lymphatic system
    b. vessel
    c. vein
    d. inflammation

Answers to Case Study Questions

1. diaphoresis
2. sublingual
3. stress test
4. cardiovascular disease
5. endarterectomies
6. murmur
7. cyanosis
8. stenosis
9. interatrial
10. substernal
11. d
12. b
13. c
14. e
15. a
16. e
17. a
18. coronary/cardiac care unit
19. acute myocardial infarction
20. coronary artery disease
21. left anterior descending
22. congestive heart failure
23. transesophageal echocardiogram
24. mitral valve replacement

ANSWERS TO CROSSWORD PUZZLE

Circulation

Blood and Immunity

Chapter Contents

Objectives

After study of this chapter you should be able to:

1. Describe the composition of the blood plasma.
2. Describe and give the functions of the three types of blood cells.
3. Label pictures of the blood cells.
4. Explain the basis of blood types.
5. Define immunity.
6. Identify and use roots and suffixes pertaining to the blood and immunity.
7. Identify and use roots pertaining to the chemistry of the blood and other body tissues.
8. List and describe the major disorders of the blood.
9. List and describe the major disorders of the immune system.
10. Describe the major tests used to study blood.
11. Interpret abbreviations used in blood studies.
12. Analyze several case studies involving the blood.

Blood circulates through the vessels, bringing oxygen and nourishment to all cells and carrying away waste products. The total adult blood volume is about 5 liters (5.2 quarts). Whole blood can be divided into two main components: the liquid portion, or **plasma** (55%), and formed elements, or blood cells (45%).

Blood Plasma

Plasma is about 90% water. The remaining 10% contains nutrients, **electrolytes** (dissolved salts), gases, **albumin** (a protein), clotting factors, antibodies, wastes, enzymes, and hormones. A host of these substances are tested for in blood chemistry tests. The pH (relative acidity) of the plasma remains steady at about 7.4.

Blood Cells

The blood cells (Fig. 10-1) are **erythrocytes**, or red blood cells; **leukocytes**, or white blood cells; and **platelets**, also called **thrombocytes**. All blood cells are produced in red bone marrow. Some white blood cells multiply in lymphoid tissue as well.

Erythrocytes

The major function of erythrocytes is to carry oxygen to cells. This oxygen is bound to an iron-containing pigment within the cells called **hemoglobin**. Erythrocytes are small, disk-shaped cells with no nucleus. Their concentration of about 5 million per μL (cubic millimeter) of blood makes them by far the most numerous of the blood cells. The hemoglobin that they carry averages 15 g per deciliter (100 mL) of blood. A red blood cell gradually wears out and dies in about 120 days, so these cells must be constantly replaced. Production of red cells in the bone marrow is regulated by the hormone **erythropoietin** (EPO), which is made in the kidneys.

Leukocytes

White blood cells all show prominent nuclei when stained. They total about 5,000 to 10,000 per μL, but their number may increase during infection. There are five different types of leukocytes, which are identified by the size and appearance of the nucleus and by their staining properties. Granular leukocytes or **granulocytes** have visible granules in the cytoplasm when stained; there are three types of granulocytes: neutrophils, eosinophils, and basophils, named for the kind of stain they take up. **Agranulocytes** do not have visible granules when stained. There are two types of agranulocytes: lymphocytes and monocytes. Characteristics of the different types of white cells are given in Display 10-1.

White blood cells protect against foreign substances. Some engulf foreign material by the process of **phagocytosis**; others function as part of the immune system. In diagnosis it is important to know not only the total number of leukocytes but also the relative number of each type because these numbers can change in different disease conditions. The most numerous white blood cells, neutrophils, are called *polymorphs* because of their various-shaped nuclei. They are also referred to as *segs, polys,* or *PMNs* (polymorphonuclear leukocytes). A **band cell**, also called a *stab* or *staff* cell, is an immature neutrophil with a solid curved nucleus (Fig. 10-2). Large numbers of band cells in the blood indicate an active infection.

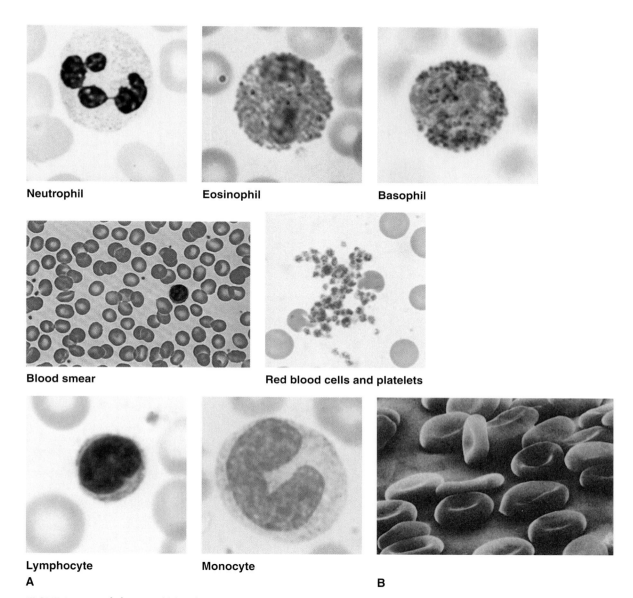

Neutrophil   **Eosinophil**   **Basophil**

Blood smear   **Red blood cells and platelets**

Lymphocyte   **Monocyte**
A   **B**

FIGURE 10-1. **(A)** Normal blood smear and close-up view of individual blood cells. **(B)** Red blood cells as seen by scanning electron microscopy. (Reprinted with permission from Cohen BJ, Wood DL. Memmler's The Human Body in Health and Disease. 9th Ed. Philadelphia: Lippincott Williams & Wilkins, 2000.)

Platelets

The blood platelets (thrombocytes) are fragments of larger cells formed in the bone marrow. They number from 200,000 to 400,000 per μL of blood. Platelets are important in **hemostasis**, the prevention of blood loss, a component of which is the process of blood clotting, also known as **coagulation.**

When a vessel is injured, platelets stick together to form a plug at the site. Substances released from the platelets and from damaged tissue then interact with clotting factors in the plasma to produce a wound-sealing clot. Clotting factors are inactive in the blood until an injury occurs. To protect against unwanted clot formation, 12 different factors must interact before blood coagulates. The final reaction is the conversion of

DISPLAY 10-1 White Blood Cells (Leukocytes)

TYPE OF CELL	RELATIVE PERCENTAGE (ADULT)	FUNCTION
GRANULOCYTES		
neutrophils NŪ-trō-fils	54%–62%	phagocytosis
eosinophils ē-ō-SIN-ō-fils	1%–3%	allergic reactions; defense against parasites
basophils BĀ-sō-fils	less than 1%	allergic reactions
AGRANULOCYTES		
lymphocytes LIM-fō-sītz	25%–38%	immunity
monocytes MON-ō-sītz	3%–7%	phagocytosis

Box 10-1 Acronyms

Acronyms are abbreviations that use the first letters of the words in a name or phrase. They have become very popular because they save time and space in writing as the number and complexity of technical terms increases. Some examples that apply to studies of the blood are CBC (complete blood count), RBC, and WBD for blood cells. Some other common acronyms are CNS (central nervous system), ECG (electrocardiograph), NIH (National Institutes of Health), and STD (sexually transmitted disease).

If the acronym has vowels and lends itself to pronunciation, it may be used as a word in itself, such as AIDS (acquired immunodeficiency syndrome); ELISA (enzyme-linked immunosorbent assay); JAMA (*Journal of the American Medical Association*); NSAID (nonsteroidal antiinflammatory agent), pronounced "en-sayd"; and CABG (coronary artery bypass graft), which inevitably becomes "cabbage." Few people even know that LASER is an acronym that means "light amplification by stimulated emission of radiation."

An acronym usually is introduced the first time a phrase appears in an article and is then used without explanation. If you have spent time searching back through an article in frustration for the meaning of an acronym, you probably wish, as does this author, that all the acronyms used and their meanings would be listed at the beginning of each article.

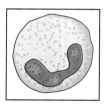

Band cell

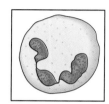

Mature neutrophil

FIGURE 10-2. A band cell (immature neutrophil) as compared with a mature neutrophil.

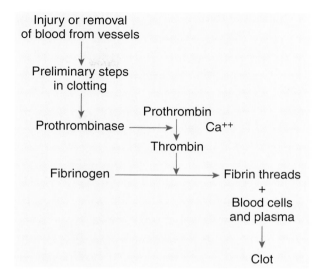

FIGURE 10-3. Main steps in formation of a blood clot. (Reprinted with permission from Cohen BJ, Wood DL. Memmler's The Human Body in Health and Disease. 9th Ed. Philadelphia: Lippincott Williams & Wilkins, 2000.)

fibrinogen to threads of fibrin that trap blood cells and plasma to produce the clot (Fig. 10-3). What remains of the plasma after blood coagulates is **serum**.

Blood Types

Genetically inherited proteins on the surface of red blood cells determine blood type. More than 20 groups of these proteins have now been identified, but the most familiar are the ABO and Rh blood groups. The ABO system includes types A, B, AB, and O. The Rh types are Rh positive (Rh^+) and Rh negative (Rh^-). In giving blood transfusions, it is important to use blood that is the same type as the recipient's blood or a type to which the recipient will not show an immune reaction, as described below. Compatible blood types are determined by **cross-matching**, as illustrated in Figure 10-4. Whole blood may be used to replace a large volume of blood lost, but in most cases requiring blood transfusion, a blood fraction such as packed red cells, platelets, plasma, or specific clotting factors is administered.

The Immune System

Our bodies have an array of defenses against foreign matter. Some of these defenses are nonspecific, that is, they protect against any intruder. Such defenses include the unbroken skin, blood-filtering lymphoid tissue, cilia and mucus that trap foreign material, bactericidal body secretions, and reflexes such as coughing and sneezing.

Specific attacks on disease organisms are mounted by the immune system. The immune response involves complex interactions between components of the lymphatic system and the blood. Any foreign particle may act as an **antigen**, that is, a substance that provokes a response by the immune system. This response comes from two types of lymphocytes that circulate in the blood and lymphatic system. One type, the **T cells** (T lymphocytes), mature in the thymus gland. They are capable of attacking a foreign cell directly, producing *cell-mediated immunity*. **Macrophages**, descendants of monocytes, are important in the function of T cells.

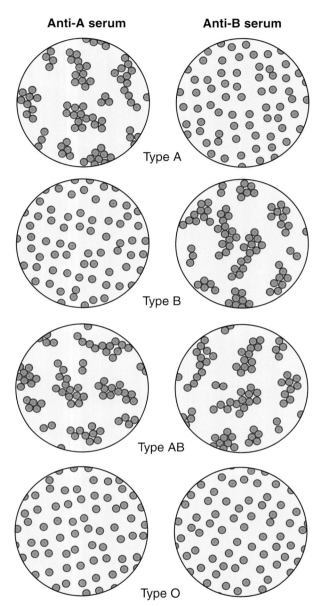

Anti-A serum   **Anti-B serum**

Type A

Type B

Type AB

Type O

FIGURE 10-4. Blood typing. Red cells in type A blood are agglutinated (clumped) by anti-A serum; those in type B blood are agglutinated by anti-B serum. Type AB blood cells are agglutinated by both sera, and type O blood is not agglutinated by either serum. (Reprinted with permission from Cohen BJ, Wood DL. Memmler's The Human Body in Health and Disease. 9th Ed. Philadelphia: Lippincott Williams & Wilkins, 2000.)

Macrophages take in and process foreign antigens. A T cell is activated when it contacts an antigen on the surface of a macrophage in combination with some of the body's own proteins.

The **B cells** (B lymphocytes) mature in lymphoid tissue. When they meet a foreign antigen, they multiply rapidly, transforming into **plasma cells**. These cells produce **antibodies**, also called **immunoglobulins** (Ig), that inactivate an antigen (Fig. 10-5). Antibodies remain in the blood, often providing long-term immunity to the specific organism against which they were formed. Antibody-based immunity is referred to as *humoral immunity*.

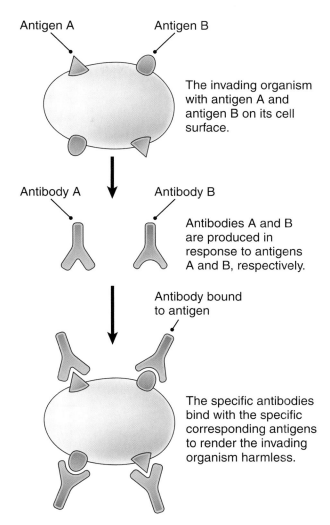

Antigen A   Antigen B

The invading organism with antigen A and antigen B on its cell surface.

Antibody A   Antibody B

Antibodies A and B are produced in response to antigens A and B, respectively.

Antibody bound to antigen

The specific antibodies bind with the specific corresponding antigens to render the invading organism harmless.

FIGURE 10-5. Antibodies are produced by cells of the immune system to bind with specific antigens.

Types of Immunity

Passive immunity involves the transfer of antibodies to an individual either naturally, through the placenta or mother's milk, or artificially, by the administration of an immune serum. Active immunity involves the individual's own response to a disease organism, either through natural contact with the organism or by the administration of an artificially prepared vaccine.

Immunology has long been a very active area of research. The above description is only the barest outline of the events that are known to occur in the immune response, and there is much still to be discovered. Some of the areas of research include autoimmune diseases, in which an individual produces antibodies to his or her own body tissues; hereditary and acquired immune deficiency diseases; the relationship between cancer and immunity; and the development of techniques for avoiding rejection of transplanted tissue.

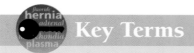

Key Terms

NORMAL STRUCTURE AND FUNCTION

agranulocytes Ā-gran-ū-lō-sītz	White blood cells that do not have visible granules in their cytoplasm. Agranulocytes include lymphocytes and monocytes.
albumin al-BŪ-min	A simple protein found in blood plasma
antibody AN-ti-bod-ē	A protein produced in response to, and interacting specifically with, an antigen
antigen AN-ti-jen	A substance that induces the formation of antibodies
B cell	A lymphocyte that matures in lymphoid tissue and is active in producing antibodies; B lymphocyte (LIM-fō-sīt)
band cell	An immature neutrophil with a nucleus in the shape of a band. Also called a stab or staff cell. Band cell counts are used to trace infections and other diseases (Fig. 10-6).
blood	The fluid that circulates in the cardiovascular system (root hem/o, hemat/o)
coagulation kō-ag-ū-LĀ-shun	Blood clotting
cross-matching	Testing the compatibility of donor and recipient blood in preparation for a transfusion. Donor red cells are mixed with recipient serum, and red cells of the recipient are mixed with donor serum to look for an immunologic reaction. Similar tests are done on tissues before transplantation.
electrolyte ē-LEK-trō-līt	A substance that separates into charged particles (ions) in solution; a salt. Term also applied to ions in body fluids.
erythrocyte e-RITH-rō-sīt	A red blood cell (root erythr/o, erythrocyt/o)
erythropoietin (EPO) e-rith-rō-POY-e-tin	A hormone produced in the kidneys that stimulates red blood cell production in the bone marrow. This hormone is now made by genetic engineering for clinical use.
fibrin FĪ-brin	The protein that forms a clot in the process of blood coagulation
fibrinogen fī-BRIN-ō-jen	The inactive precursor of fibrin
formed elements	The cellular components of blood
granulocytes GRAN-ū-lō-sītz	White blood cells that have visible granules in their cytoplasm. Granulocytes include neutrophils, basophils, and eosinophils.
hemoglobin (Hb, Hgb) HĒ-mō-glō-bin	The iron-containing pigment in red blood cells that transports oxygen
hemostasis hē-mō-STĀ-sis	The stoppage of bleeding

Normal Structure and Function, continued

immunity	The state of being protected against a specific disease (root *immun/o*)
immunoglobulin (Ig) *im-ū-nō-GLOB-ū-lin*	An antibody. Immunoglobulins fall into five classes, each abbreviated with a capital letter: IgG, IgM, IgA, IgD, IgE.
leukocyte *LŪ-kō-sīt*	A white blood cell (root *leuk/o, leukocyt/o*)
lymphocyte *LIM-fō-sīt*	A lymphatic cell; a type of agranular leukocyte (root *lymph/o, lymphocyt/o*)
macrophage *MAK-rō-faj*	A phagocytic cell derived from a monocyte; usually located within the tissues. Macrophages process antigens for T cells.
phagocytosis *fag-ō-sī-TŌ-sis*	The engulfing of foreign material by white blood cells
plasma *PLAZ-ma*	The liquid portion of the blood
plasma cell	A cell that is formed from a B cell and that produces antibodies
platelet *PLĀT-let*	A formed element of the blood that is active in hemostasis; a thrombocyte (root *thrombocyt/o*)
serum *SĒR-um*	The fraction of the plasma that remains after blood coagulation; it is the equivalent of plasma without its clotting factors (plural sera, serums)
T cell	A lymphocyte that matures in the thymus gland and attacks foreign cells directly; T lymphocyte
thrombocyte *THROM-bo-sit*	A blood platelet (root *thrombocyt/o*)

Word Parts Pertaining to Blood and Immunity

TABLE 10-1 Suffixes for Blood

SUFFIX	MEANING	EXAMPLE	DEFINITION OF EXAMPLE
-emia,* -hemia	condition of blood	pachyemia *pak-ē-Ē-mē-a*	thickness (pachy-) of the blood
-penia	decrease in, deficiency of	leukopenia *lū-kō-PĒ-nē-a*	deficiency of leukocytes in the blood
-poiesis	formation, production	hemopoiesis *hē-mō-poy-Ē-sis*	production of blood cells

*A shortened form of the root *hem* plus the suffix -ia.

Exercise 10-1

Define the following terms:

1. hyperalbuminemia (hī-per-al-bū-mi-NĒ-mē-a)   _____ excess albumin in the blood _____

2. hypoproteinemia (hī-pō-prō-tēn-Ē-mē-a)   _____

3. cytopenia (sī-tō-PĒ-nē-a)   _____

4. thrombocytopenia (throm-bō-sī-tō-PĒ-nē-a)   _____

5. erythropoiesis (e-rith-rō-poy-Ē-sis)   _____

Word building. Use the suffix -emia to write a word for each of the following definitions:

6. Presence of pus in the blood   _____

7. Presence of viruses in the blood   _____

8. Presence of toxins in the blood   _____

9. Presence of excess white cells (leuk/o-) in the blood   _____

Many of the words relating to blood cells can be formed either with or without including the root cyt/o, as in erythropenia or erythrocytopenia, leukopoiesis or leukocytopoiesis. The remaining types of blood cells are designated by easily recognized roots such as agranulocyt/o, monocyt/o, granul/o, and so on.

TABLE 10-2 Roots for Blood and Immunity

ROOT	MEANING	EXAMPLE	DEFINITION OF EXAMPLE
myel/o	bone marrow	myelogenous mī-e-LOJ-e-nus	originating in bone marrow
hem/o, hemat/o	blood	hemorrhage HEM-or-ij	profuse flow (-rhage) of blood
erythr/o, erythrocyt/o	red blood cell	erythrocytosis e-rith-rō-sī-TŌ-sis	condition of increased red blood cells
leuk/o, leukocyt/o	white blood cell	leukopoiesis LŪ-kō-poy-Ē-sis	production of white blood cells
lymph/o, lymphocyt/o	lymphocyte	lymphoblast LIM-fō-blast	immature lymphocyte
thromb/o	blood clot	thrombolytic throm-bō-LIT-ik	pertaining to dissolving a blood clot
thrombocyt/o	platelet, thrombocyte	thrombocytopenia throm-bō-sī-tō-PĒ-nē-a	deficiency of platelets in the blood
immun/o	immunity, immune system	immunization im-ū-ni-ZĀ-shun	production of immunity

Exercise 10-2

Identify and define the root in each of the following words:

	Root	Meaning of Root
1. panmyeloid (*pan-MĪ-e-loyd*)	myel/o	bone marrow
2. prothrombin (*prō-THROM-bin*)	_____	_____
3. preimmunization (*prē-im-ū-ni-ZĀ-shun*)	_____	_____
4. ischemia (*is-KĒ-mē-a*)	_____	_____

Fill in the blanks:

5. Erythroclasis (*er-i-THROK-la-sis*) is the breaking (-clasis) of _____.

6. A myeloblast (*MĪ-e-lō-blast*) is an immature cell found in _____.

7. The term thrombocythemia (*throm-bō-sī-THĒ-mē-a*) refers to an increase in the blood in the number of _____.

8. Leukocytosis (*lū-kō-sī-TŌ-sis*) is an increase in the number of _____.

9. An immunocyte (*im-ū-nō-SĪT*) is a cell active in _____.

10. A hemocytometer (*hē-mō-sī-TOM-e-ter*) is a device for counting _____.

11. Lymphokines (*LIM-fō-kīnz*) are chemicals active in immunity that are produced by _____.

Word building. Write a word for each of the following definitions:

12. Tumor of bone marrow _____

13. Immature leukocyte _____

14. Decrease in red blood cells _____

15. Study of blood _____

16. Dissolving (-lysis) of a blood clot _____

17. Formation (-poiesis) of bone marrow _____

The suffix *-osis* added to a root for a type of cell means an increase in that type of cell in the blood. Use this suffix to write a word that has the same meaning as each of the following:

18. Increase in red blood cells — erythrocytosis

19. Increase in monocytes in the blood _____

20. Increase in platelets in the blood _____

21. Increase in granulocytes in the blood _____

22. Increase in lymphocytes in the blood _____

TABLE 10-3 Roots for Chemistry

ROOT	MEANING	EXAMPLE	DEFINITION OF EXAMPLE
azot/o	nitrogen compounds	azoturia az-ō-TŪ-rē-a	increased nitrogen compounds in the urine (-uria)
calc/i	calcium (symbol Ca)	calcareous kal-KAR-ē-us	containing calcium
ferr/o, ferr/i	iron (symbol Fe)	ferric FER-ik	pertaining to or containing iron
sider/o	iron	sideroblast SID-er-ō-blast	an immature red blood cell containing iron granules
kali	potassium (symbol K)	hypokalemia* hī-per-ka-LĒ-mē-a	decrease of potassium in the blood
natri	sodium (symbol Na)	natriuresis nā-trē-ū-RĒ-sis	excretion of sodium in the urine (ur/o)
ox/y	oxygen (symbol O)	hypoxemia hī-pok-SĒ-mē-a	deficiency of oxygen in the blood

*The i in the root is dropped.

Exercise 10-3

Fill in the blanks:

1. Sideroderma (*sid-er-ō-DER-ma*) is the deposit of _____ into the skin.

2. The term normokalemia (*nor-mō-ka-LĒ-mē-a*) refers to a normal blood concentration of

   _____.

3. An oxide (*OKS-īd*) is a compound that contains _____.

4. Ferritin (*FER-i-tin*) is a compound that contains _____.

5. Hypercalcemia (*hī-per-kal-SĒ-mē-a*) is an excess blood level of _____.

Word building. Use the suffix *-emia* to form words with the following meanings:

6. Presence of sodium in the blood _____

7. Presence of nitrogen compounds in the blood _____

8. Presence of calcium in the blood _____

Clinical Aspects: Blood

Anemia

Anemia is defined as a decrease in the amount of hemoglobin in the blood. Anemia may result from too few red blood cells, cells that are too small, or too little hemoglobin in the cells. Cells may be normal in size (normocytic) or abnormal (microcytic or macrocytic), and they may be normal in hemoglobin (normochromic)

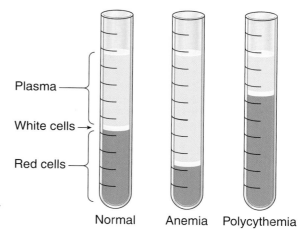

Plasma —

White cells →

Red cells —

Normal   Anemia   Polycythemia

FIGURE 10-6. Hematocrit. The tube on the left shows a normal hematocrit. The middle tube shows that the percentage of red blood cells is low, indicating anemia. The tube on the right shows an excessively high percentage of red blood cells, as seen in polycythemia.

or have too little (hypochromic). Key tests in diagnosing anemia are blood counts, mean corpuscular volume (MCV), and mean corpuscular hemoglobin concentration (MCHC) (Display 10-2). The general symptoms of anemia include fatigue, shortness of breath, heart palpitations, pallor, and irritability. There are many different types of anemia, some of which are caused by underproduction of red cells, others by loss or destruction of cells.

Aplastic anemia results from destruction of the bone marrow and affects all blood cells (pancytopenia). It may be caused by drugs, toxins, viruses, radiation, or bone marrow cancer. Aplastic anemia has a high mortality rate but has been treated successfully with bone marrow transplantation.

DISPLAY 10-2 Common Blood Tests

TEST	ABBREVIATION	DESCRIPTION
red blood cell count	RBC	number of red blood cells per μL (cubic millimeter) of blood
white blood cell count	WBC	number of white blood cells per cubic millimeter of blood
differential count	Diff	relative percentage of the different types of leukocytes
hematocrit (Fig. 10-6)	Ht, Hct, crit	relative percentage of packed red cells in a given volume of blood
packed cell volume	PCV	hematocrit
hemoglobin	Hb, Hgb	amount of hemoglobin in g/dL (100 mL) of blood
mean corpuscular volume	MCV	volume of an average red cell
mean corpuscular hemoglobin	MCH	average weight of hemoglobin in red cells
mean corpuscular hemoglobin concentration	MCHC	average concentration of hemoglobin in red blood cells
erythrocyte sedimentation rate	ESR	rate of settling of erythrocytes per unit of time; used to detect infection or inflammation
complete blood count	CBC	series of tests including cell counts, hematocrit, hemoglobin, and cell volume measurements

Nutritional anemia may result from a deficiency of vitamin B_{12}, folic acid (a B vitamin), or most commonly, iron. A specific form of B_{12} deficiency is **pernicious anemia**. This results from the lack of a substance produced in the stomach, **intrinsic factor** (IF), which aids in the absorption of this vitamin from the intestine. Pernicious anemia must be treated with regular injections of B_{12}. Folic acid deficiency commonly appears in those with poor diet, in pregnant and lactating women, and in those who abuse alcohol. Iron-deficiency anemia result from poor diet, poor absorption of iron, and blood loss. Both folic acid deficiency and iron deficiency respond to dietary supplementation.

In **sideroblastic anemia**, there is adequate iron available, but the iron is not used properly to manufacture hemoglobin. This disorder may be hereditary or acquired, as by exposure to toxins or drugs, or as secondary to another disease. The excess iron precipitates out in immature red cells (normoblasts).

Hemorrhagic anemia results from blood loss. This may be a sudden loss, as from injury, or loss from chronic internal bleeding, as from the digestive tract in cases of ulcers or cancer.

Several hereditary diseases cause hemolysis (rupture) of red cells, resulting in anemia. **Thalassemia** appears in Mediterranean populations. It affects the production of hemoglobin and is designated as α (alpha) or β (beta), according to the part of the molecule affected. Severe β thalassemia is also called **Cooley anemia**. In **sickle cell anemia**, a mutation alters the hemoglobin molecule so that it precipitates when it gives up oxygen and distorts the red blood cells into a crescent shape (Fig. 10-7). The altered cells block small blood vessels and deprive tissues of oxygen, an episode termed *sickle cell crisis*. The misshapen cells are also readily destroyed (hemolyzed). The disease predominates in black populations. Genetic carriers of the defect, those with one normal and one abnormal gene, show sickle cell trait. They usually have no symptoms, except when oxygen is low, such as at high altitudes. They can, however, pass the defective gene to offspring. Sickle cell anemia, as well as many other genetic diseases, can be diagnosed in carriers and in the fetus before birth.

Reticulocyte counts are useful in diagnosing the causes of anemia. Reticulocytes are immature red blood cells that normally appear in a small percentage in the blood. An increase in the number of reticulocytes indicates increased red blood cell formation, as in response to hemorrhage or destruction of red cells. A decrease indicates a failure in red blood cell production, as caused by nutritional deficiency or aplastic anemia.

Coagulation Disorders

The most common cause of coagulation problems is a deficiency in the number of circulating platelets, a condition termed **thrombocytopenia**. Possible causes include aplastic anemia, infections, cancer of the bone mar-

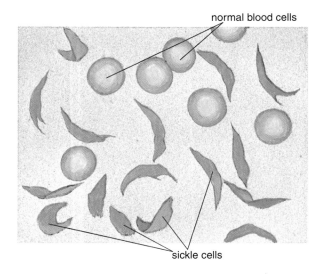

FIGURE 10-7. Sickling of red blood cells in sickle cell anemia. (Reprinted with permission from Cohen BJ, Wood DL. Memmler's The Human Body in Health and Disease. 9th Ed. Philadelphia: Lippincott Williams & Wilkins, 2000.)

row, or agents that destroy bone marrow, such as x-rays or certain drugs. This disorder results in bleeding into the skin and mucous membranes, variously described as **petechiae, ecchymoses,** and **purpura.**

In **disseminated intravascular coagulation** (DIC) there is widespread clotting in the vessels, which obstructs circulation to the tissues. This is followed by diffuse hemorrhages as clotting factors are removed and the coagulation process is impaired. DIC may result from a variety of causes, including infection, cancer, hemorrhage, injury, or allergy.

Hemophilia is a hereditary deficiency of a specific clotting factor. It is a sex-linked disease that is passed from mother to son. There is bleeding into the tissues, especially into the joints (hemarthrosis). Hemophilia must be treated with transfusions of the necessary clotting factor.

Neoplasms

Leukemia is a neoplasm of white blood cells. The rapidly dividing but incompetent white cells accumulate in the tissues and crowd out the other blood cells. The symptoms of leukemia include anemia, fatigue, easy bleeding, **splenomegaly,** and sometimes hepatomegaly (enlargement of the liver). Myelogenous leukemia originates in the bone marrow and involves mainly the granular leukocytes. Lymphocytic leukemia affects B cells and the lymphatic system, causing **lymphadenopathy** and adverse effects on the immune system. Leukemias are further differentiated as acute or chronic based on clinical progress. The acute forms of leukemia are acute lymphoblastic (lymphocytic) leukemia (ALL) and acute myeloblastic (myelogenous) leukemia (AML). Acute leukemia is the most common form of cancer in young children. With treatment, remission rate is high for ALL, but the prognosis in AML is poor for both children and adults. Chronic granulocytic leukemia, also called chronic myelogenous leukemia, affects young to middle-aged adults. Most cases show the **Philadelphia chromosome (Ph),** an inherited anomaly in which part of chromosome 22 shifts to chromosome 9. Chronic lymphocytic leukemia (CLL) appears mostly in the elderly and is the most slowly growing form of the disease.

The causes of leukemia are unknown but may include exposure to radiation or harmful chemicals, hereditary factors, and perhaps virus infection.

Treatment of leukemia includes chemotherapy, radiation therapy, and bone marrow transplantation. One advance in transplantation is the use of umbilical cord blood to replace blood-forming cells in bone marrow. This blood is more readily available than bone marrow and does not have to match as closely to avoid rejection.

Hodgkin disease is a disease of the lymphatic system that may spread to other tissues. It begins with enlarged but painless lymph nodes in the cervical (neck) region and then progresses to other nodes. A feature of Hodgkin disease is giant cells in the lymph nodes called **Reed-Sternberg cells** (Fig. 10-8). There are fever, night

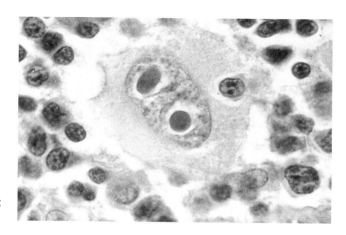

FIGURE 10-8. Reed-Sternberg cell typical of Hodgkin disease. (Reprinted with permission from Rubin E, Farber JL. Pathology. 3rd Ed. Philadelphia: Lippincott Williams & Wilkins, 1999.)

sweats, weight loss, and itching of the skin (pruritus). Persons of any age may be affected, but the disease predominates in young adults and those over age 50. Most cases can be cured with radiation and chemotherapy.

Non-Hodgkin lymphoma (NHL) is also a malignant enlargement of lymph nodes but does not show Reed-Sternberg cells. It is more common than Hodgkin disease and has a higher mortality rate. Cases vary in severity and prognosis. It is most prevalent in the older adult population and in those with AIDS and other forms of immunodeficiency. NHL involves the T or B lymphocytes, and some cases may be related to infection with certain viruses. It requires systemic chemotherapy and, sometimes, bone marrow transplantation.

Multiple **myeloma** is a cancer of the blood-forming cells in bone marrow, mainly the plasma cells that produce antibodies. The disease causes anemia, bone pain, and weakening of the bones. There is a greater susceptibility to infection because of immune deficiency. Abnormally high levels of calcium and protein in the blood often lead to kidney failure. Multiple myeloma is treated with radiation and chemotherapy, but the prognosis is generally poor.

Clinical Aspects: Immunity

Hypersensitivity is a harmful overreaction of the immune system, commonly known as **allergy**. In cases of allergy, a person is more sensitive to a particular antigen than the average individual. Common **allergens** are pollen, animal dander, dust, and foods, but there are many more. A seasonal allergy to inhaled pollens is commonly called "hay fever." Responses may include itching, redness or tearing of the eyes (conjunctivitis), skin rash, asthma, runny nose (rhinitis), sneezing, **urticaria** (hives), and **angioedema**, a reaction similar to hives but involving deeper layers of tissue.

An **anaphylactic reaction** is a severe generalized allergic response that can lead rapidly to death as a result of shock and respiratory distress. It must be treated by immediate administration of **epinephrine** (**adrenaline**), maintenance of open airways, and antihistamines. Common causes of anaphylaxis are drugs, especially penicillin and other antibiotics, vaccines, diagnostic chemicals, foods, and insect venom.

A **delayed hypersensitivity reaction** involves T cells and takes at least 12 hours to develop. A common example is the reaction to contact with plant irritants such as those of poison ivy and poison oak.

The term **immunodeficiency** refers to any failure in the immune system. This may be congenital (present at birth) or acquired and may involve any components of the system. The deficiency may vary in severity but is always evidenced by an increased susceptibility to disease.

AIDS is acquired by infection with **HIV**, which attacks certain T cells. These cells have a specific surface attachment site, the CD4 receptor, for the virus. HIV is spread by sexual contact, use of contaminated needles, blood transfusions, and passage from an infected mother to a fetus. It leaves the host susceptible to opportunistic infections such as pneumonia caused by the protozoon *Pneumocystis carinii;* thrush, a fungal infection of the mouth caused by *Candida albicans;* and infection with *Cryptosporidium,* a protozoon that causes cramps and diarrhea. It also predisposes to **Kaposi sarcoma**, a once-rare form of skin cancer. It may also induce autoimmunity or attack the nervous system.

AIDS is diagnosed and followed by **CD4+ T lymphocyte counts**, which measure the number of cells that have the HIV receptor. A count of less than 200/μL of blood signifies severe immunodeficiency. Antibody levels to HIV and direct viral counts in the blood are also used to track the course of the disease. At present there is no vaccine or cure for AIDS, but some drugs can delay progress of the disease.

A disease that results from an immune response to one's own tissues is classified as an **autoimmune disorder**. The cause may be a failure in the immune system or a reaction to body cells that have been slightly altered by mutation or disease. The list of diseases that are believed to be caused, at least in part, by autoimmunity is long. Some, such as **systemic lupus erythematosus** (SLE), **systemic sclerosis** (scleroderma), and **Sjögren syndrome**, affect tissues in multiple systems. Others target more specific organs or systems. Examples are pernicious anemia, rheumatoid arthritis, Graves disease (of the thyroid), myasthenia gravis (a muscle disease), fibromyalgia syndrome (a musculoskeletal disorder), rheumatic heart disease, and glomerulonephritis (a kidney disease). These diseases are discussed in more detail in other chapters.

Key Clinical Terms

DISORDERS

AIDS	Failure of the immune system caused by infection with HIV (human immunodeficiency virus). The virus infects certain T cells and thus interferes with immunity.
allergen *AL-er-jen*	A substance that causes an allergic response
allergy *AL-er-jē*	Hypersensitivity
anaphylactic reaction *an-a-fi-LAK-tik*	An exaggerated allergic reaction to a foreign substance (root *phylaxis* means "protection"). It may lead to death caused by circulatory collapse, and respiratory distress if untreated. Also called anaphylaxis.
anemia *a-NĒ-mē-a*	A deficiency in the amount of hemoglobin in the blood; may result from blood loss, malnutrition, a hereditary defect, environmental factors, and other causes
angioedema *an-jē-ō-e-DĒ-ma*	A localized edema with large hives (wheals) similar to urticaria but involving deeper layers of the skin and subcutaneous tissue
aplastic anemia *ā-PLAS-tik*	Anemia caused by bone marrow failure resulting in deficient blood cell production, especially of red cells; pancytopenia
autoimmune disorder	A condition in which the immune system produces antibodies against an individual's own tissues (prefix *auto* means "self")
Cooley anemia	A form of thalassemia (hereditary anemia) in which the B (beta) chain of hemoglobin is abnormal
delayed hypersensitivity reaction	An allergic reaction involving T cells that takes at least 12 hours to develop. Examples are various types of contact dermatitis, such as poison ivy or poison oak; the tuberculin reaction (test for TB); and rejections of transplanted tissue.
disseminated intravascular coagulation (DIC)	Widespread formation of clots in the microscopic vessels; may be followed by bleeding as a result of depletion of clotting factors
ecchymosis *ek-i-MŌ-sis*	A collection of blood under the skin caused by leakage from small vessels (root *chym* means "juice")
hemolysis *hē-MOL-i-sis*	The rupture of red blood cells and the release of hemoglobin (adjective, hemolytic)
hemophilia *hē-mō-FIL-ē-a*	A hereditary blood disease caused by lack of a clotting factor and resulting in abnormal bleeding
HIV	The virus that causes AIDS; human immunodeficiency virus
Hodgkin disease	A neoplastic disease of unknown cause that involves the lymph nodes, spleen, liver, and other tissues; characterized by the presence of giant Reed-Sternberg cells

Disorders, continued

hypersensitivity	An immunologic reaction to a substance that is harmless to most people; allergy
immunodeficiency *im-ū-nō-dē-FISH-en-sē*	A congenital or acquired failure of the immune system to protect against disease
intrinsic factor	A substance produced in the stomach that aids in the absorption of vitamin B_{12}, necessary for the manufacture of red blood cells. Lack of intrinsic factor causes pernicious anemia.
Kaposi sarcoma *KAP-ō-sē*	Cancerous lesion of the skin and other tissues, seen most often in patients with AIDS
leukemia *lū-KĒ-mē-a*	Malignant overgrowth of immature white blood cells; may be chronic or acute; may affect bone marrow (myelogenous leukemia) or lymphoid tissue (lymphocytic leukemia)
lymphadenopathy *lim-fad-e-NOP-a-thē*	Any disease of the lymph nodes
lymphoma *lim-FŌ-ma*	Any neoplastic disease of lymphoid tissue, such as Burkitt disease, Hodgkin disease, and others
multiple myeloma *mī-e-LŌ-ma*	A tumor of the blood-forming tissue in bone marrow
non-Hodgkin lymphoma (NHL)	A widespread malignant disease of lymph nodes that involves lymphocytes. It differs from Hodgkin disease in the absence of giant Reed-Sternberg cells (see Fig. 10-8).
Philadelphia chromosome (Ph)	An abnormal chromosome found in the cells of most individuals with chronic granulocytic (myelogenous) leukemia
pernicious anemia *per-NISH-us*	Anemia caused by failure of the stomach to produce intrinsic factor, a substance needed for the absorption of vitamin B_{12}. This vitamin is required for the formation of erythrocytes.
petechiae *pē-TĒ-kē-ē*	Pinpoint, flat, purplish-red spots caused by bleeding within the skin or mucous membrane (singular, petechia)
purpura *PUR-pū-ra*	A condition characterized by hemorrhages into the skin, mucous membranes, internal organs, and other tissues (from Greek word meaning "purple"). Thrombocytopenic purpura is caused by a deficiency of platelets.
sideroblastic anemia *sid-e-rō-BLAS-tik*	Anemia caused by inability to use available iron to manufacture hemoglobin. The excess iron precipitates in normoblasts (developing red blood cells).
Sjögren syndrome *SHŌ-gren*	An autoimmune disease involving dysfunction of the exocrine glands and affecting secretion of tears, saliva, and other body fluids. Deficiency leads to dry mouth, tooth decay, corneal damage, eye infections, and difficulty in swallowing.

Disorders, continued

sickle cell anemia	A hereditary anemia caused by the presence of abnormal hemoglobin. Red blood cells become sickle-shaped and interfere with normal blood flow to the tissues (see Fig. 10-7). Most common in black populations of West African descent.
splenomegaly *splē-nō-MEG-a-lē*	Enlargement of the spleen
systemic lupus erythematosus *LŪ-pus er-i-thē-ma-TŌ-sus*	Inflammatory disease of connective tissue affecting the skin and multiple organs. Patients are sensitive to light and may show a red butterfly-shaped rash over the nose and cheeks.
systemic sclerosis	A diffuse disease of connective tissue that may involve any system causing inflammation, degeneration, and fibrosis. Also called scleroderma because it causes thickening of the skin.
thalassemia *thal-a-SĒ-mē-a*	A group of hereditary anemias mostly found in populations of Mediterranean descent (the name comes from the Greek word for "sea").
thrombocytopenia *throm-bō-sī-tō-PĒ-nē-a*	A deficiency of thrombocytes (platelets) in the blood
urticaria *ur-ti-KAR-ē-a*	A skin reaction consisting of round, raised eruptions (wheals) with itching; hives

DIAGNOSIS AND TREATMENT

adrenaline *a-DREN-a-lin*	See epinephrine
CD4+ T lymphocyte count	A count of the T cells that have the CD4 receptors for the AIDS virus (HIV). A count of less than 200/μL of blood signifies severe immunodeficiency.
epinephrine *ep-i-NEF-rin*	A powerful stimulant produced by the adrenal gland and sympathetic nervous system. Activates the cardiovascular, respiratory, and other systems needed to meet stress. Used as a drug to treat severe allergic reactions and shock. Also called adrenaline.
reticulocyte counts *re-TIK-ū-lō-sīt*	Blood counts of reticulocytes, a type of immature red blood cell; reticulocyte counts are useful in diagnosis to indicate the rate of erythrocyte formation.
Reed-Sternberg cells	Giant cells that are characteristic of Hodgkin disease. They usually have two large nuclei and are surrounded by a halo.

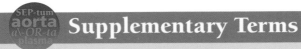

Supplementary Terms

NORMAL STRUCTURE AND FUNCTION

agglutination *a-glū-ti-NĀ-shun*	The clumping of cells or particles in the presence of specific antibodies
bilirubin *bil-i-RŪ-bin*	A pigment derived from the breakdown of hemoglobin. It is eliminated by the liver in bile.
complement *COM-ple-ment*	A group of plasma enzymes that interacts with antibodies
corpuscle *KOR-pus-l*	A small mass or body. A blood corpuscle is a blood cell.
gamma globulin	The fraction of the blood plasma that contains antibodies
hemopoietic stem cell *hē-mō-poy-e-tik*	A primitive bone marrow cell that gives rise to all varieties of blood cells
heparin *HEP-a-rin*	A substance found throughout the body that inhibits blood coagulation; an anticoagulant
megakaryocyte *meg-a-KAR-ē-ō-sīt*	A large bone marrow cell that fragments to release platelets
plasmin *PLAZ-min*	An enzyme that dissolves clots; also called fibrinolysin
thrombin *THROM-bin*	The enzyme derived from prothrombin that converts fibrinogen to fibrin

SYMPTOMS AND CONDITIONS

agranulocytosis *ā-gran-ū-lō-sī-TŌ-sis*	A condition involving decrease in the number of granulocytes in the blood; also called granulocytopenia
erythrocytosis *e-rith-rō-sī-TŌ-sis*	Increase in the number of red cells in the blood; may be normal, such as to compensate for life at high altitudes, or abnormal, such as in cases of pulmonary or cardiac disease
Fanconi syndrome *fan-KŌ-nē*	Congenital aplastic anemia that appears between birth and 10 years of age; may be hereditary or caused by damage before birth, as by a virus
graft-versus-host reaction (GVHR)	An immunologic reaction of transplanted lymphocytes against tissues of the host; a common complication of bone marrow transplantation.
hairy cell leukemia	A form of leukemia in which cells have filaments, making them look "hairy"
hematoma *hē-ma-TŌ-ma*	A localized collection of blood, usually clotted, caused by a break in a blood vessel
hemolytic disease of the newborn (HDN)	Disease that results from incompatibility between the blood of a mother and her fetus, usually involving Rh factor. An Rh-negative mother produces antibody to an Rh-positive fetus that, in later preg-

Symptoms and Conditions, *continued*

	nancies, will destroy the red cells of an Rh-positive fetus. The problem is usually avoided by treating the mother with antibodies to remove the Rh antigen; erythroblastosis fetalis
hemosiderosis *hē-mō-sid-er-Ō-sis*	A condition involving the deposition of an iron-containing pigment (hemosiderin) mainly in the liver and the spleen. The pigment comes from hemoglobin released from disintegrated red blood cells.
idiopathic thrombo-cytopenic purpura (ITP)	A clotting disorder caused by destruction of platelets that usually follows a viral illness. Causes petechiae and hemorrhages into the skin and mucous membranes.
infectious mononucleosis *mon-ō-nū-klē-Ō-sis*	An acute infectious disease caused by Epstein-Barr virus (EBV). Characterized by fever, weakness, lymphadenopathy, hepatosplenomegaly, and atypical lymphocytes (resembling monocytes).
lymphocytosis	An increase in the number of circulating lymphocytes
myelofibrosis *mī-e-lō-fī-BRŌ-sis*	Condition in which bone marrow is replaced with fibrous tissue
neutropenia *nū-trō-PĒ-nē-a*	A decrease in the number of neutrophils with increased susceptibility to infection. Causes include drugs, irradiation, and infection. May be a side effect of treatment for malignancy.
pancytopenia *pan-sī-tō-PĒ-nē-a*	A decrease in all cells of the blood, as in aplastic anemia
polycythemia *pol-ē-sī-THĒ-mē-a*	Any condition in which there is a relative increase in the percent of red blood cells in whole blood. May result from excessive production of red cells because of lack of oxygen, as caused by high altitudes, breathing obstruction, heart failure, or certain forms of poisoning. Apparent polycythemia results from concentration of the blood, as in dehydration.
polycythemia vera *pol-ē-sī-THĒ-mē-a VĒ-ra*	A condition in which overactive bone marrow produces too many red blood cells. These interfere with circulation and promote thrombosis and hemorrhage. Treated by blood removal. Also called erythremia, Vaquez-Osler disease.
septicemia *sep-ti-SĒ-mē-a*	Presence of microorganisms in the blood
spherocytic anemia *sfēr-ō-SIT-ik*	Hereditary anemia in which red blood cells are round instead of disk-shaped and rupture (hemolyze) excessively
thrombotic thrombo-cytopenic purpura (TTP)	An often-fatal disorder in which multiple clots form in blood vessels
von Willebrand disease	A hereditary bleeding disease caused by lack of von Willebrand factor, a substance necessary for blood clotting

DIAGNOSIS *(see also Displays 10-2 and 10-3)*

Bence Jones protein	A protein that appears in the urine of patients with multiple myeloma

Diagnosis, continued

Coombs test	A test for detection of antibodies to red blood cells such as appear in cases of autoimmune hemolytic anemias
electrophoresis *ē-lek-trō-fo-RĒ-sis*	Separation of particles in a liquid by application of an electrical field; used to separate components of blood.
ELISA	Enzyme-linked immunosorbent assay. A highly sensitive immunologic test used to diagnose HIV infection, hepatitis, and Lyme disease, among others.
monoclonal antibody *mon-ō-KLŌ-nal*	A pure antibody produced in the laboratory; used for diagnosis and treatment
pH	A scale that measures the relative acidity or alkalinity of a solution. Represents the amount of hydrogen ion in the solution.
Schilling test *SHIL-ing*	Test used to determine absorption of vitamin B_{12} by measuring excretion of radioactive B_{12} in the urine. Used to distinguish pernicious from nutritional anemia.
seroconversion *sē-rō-con-VER-zhun*	The appearance of antibodies in the serum in response to a disease or an immunization
Western blot assay	A very sensitive test used to detect small amounts of antibodies in the blood
Wright stain	A commonly used blood stain. Figure 10-1 shows blood cells stained with Wright stain.

TREATMENT

anticoagulant *an-ti-kō-AG-ū-lant*	An agent that prevents or delays blood coagulation
antihistamine *an-ti-HIS-ta-mēn*	A drug that counteracts the effects of histamine and is used to treat allergic reactions
apheresis *af-e-RĒ-sis*	A procedure in which blood is withdrawn, a portion is separated and retained, and the remainder is returned to the donor. Apheresis may be used as a suffix with a root meaning the fraction retained, such as plasmapheresis, leukapheresis.
autologous blood *aw-TOL-ō-gus*	A person's own blood. May be donated in advance of surgery and transfused if needed.
cryoprecipitate *krī-ō-prē-SIP-i-tāt*	A sediment obtained by cooling. The fraction obtained by freezing blood plasma contains clotting factors.
desensitization *dē-sen-si-ti-ZĀ-shun*	Treatment of allergy by small injections of the offending allergen. This causes an increase of antibody to destroy the antigen rapidly on contact.
homologous blood *hō-MOL-ō-gus*	Blood from animals of the same species, such as human blood used for transfusion from one person to another. Blood used for transfusions must be compatible with the blood of the recipient.
immunosuppression *im-ū-nō-sū-PRESH-un*	Depression of the immune response. May be correlated with disease but also may be induced therapeutically to prevent rejection in cases of tissue transplantation.
protease inhibitor *PRŌ-tē-ās*	An anti-HIV drug that acts by inhibiting an enzyme the virus needs to multiply

DISPLAY 10-3 Coagulation Tests

TEST	ABBREVIATION	DESCRIPTION
activated partial thromboplastin time	APPT	measures time required for clot formation; used to evaluate clotting factors
bleeding time	BT	measures capacity of platelets to stop bleeding after a standard skin incision
partial thromboplastin time	PTT	evaluates clotting factors; similar to APPT, but less sensitive
prothrombin time	PT, Pro Time	indirectly measures prothrombin; Quick test
thrombin time (thrombin clotting time)	TT (TCT)	measures how quickly a clot forms

ABBREVIATIONS

Ab	Antibody
Ag	Antigen
AIDS	Acquired immunodeficiency syndrome
ALL	Acute lymphoblastic (lymphocytic) leukemia
AML	Acute myeloblastic (myelogenous) leukemia
APPT	Activated partial thromboplastin time
BT	Bleeding time
CBC	Complete blood count
CLL	Chronic lymphocytic leukemia
CML	Chronic myelogenous leukemia
crit	Hematocrit
DIC	Disseminated intravascular coagulation
Diff	Differential count
EBV	Epstein-Barr virus
ELISA	Enzyme-linked immunosorbent assay
EPO	Erythropoietin
ESR	Erythrocyte sedimentation rate
FFP	Fresh frozen plasma
Hb, Hgb	Hemoglobin
HDN	Hemolytic disease of the newborn
Ht, Hct	Hematocrit
HIV	Human immunodeficiency virus
IF	Intrinsic factor
Ig	Immunoglobulin

ITP	Idiopathic thrombocytopenic purpura
lytes	Electrolytes
MCH	Mean corpuscular hemoglobin
MCHC	Mean corpuscular hemoglobin concentration
MCV	Mean corpuscular volume
mEq	Milliequivalent
NHL	Non-Hodgkin lymphoma
PCV	Packed cell volume
pH	Scale for measuring hydrogen ion concentration (acidity)
Ph	Philadelphia chromosome
PMN	Polymorphonuclear (neutrophil)
poly	Neutrophil
polymorph	Neutrophil
PT	Pro time; prothrombin time
PTT	Partial thromboplastin time
RBC	Red blood cell; red blood cell count
seg	Neutrophil
SLE	Systemic lupus erythematosus
T(C)T	Thrombin (clotting) time
TTP	Thrombotic thrombocytopenic purpura
vWF	Von Willebrand factor
WBC	White blood cell; white blood (cell) count

Labeling Exercise 10-1

Blood Cells

Write the name of each numbered part on the corresponding line of the answer sheet.

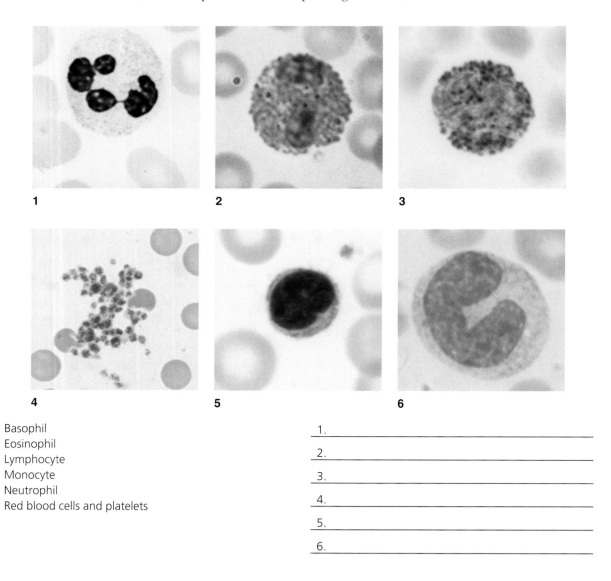

1

2

3

4

5

6

Basophil
Eosinophil
Lymphocyte
Monocyte
Neutrophil
Red blood cells and platelets

1. _____

2. _____

3. _____

4. _____

5. _____

6. _____

Chapter Review 10-1

Match the following terms and write the appropriate letter to the left of each number:

_____ 1. plasma cell   a. stoppage of blood flow

_____ 2. thrombocyte   b. engulfing of foreign particles

_____ 3. electrolyte   c. platelet

_____ 4. hemostasis   d. cell that produces antibodies

_____ 5. phagocytosis   e. substance that separates into ions in solution

_____ 6. leukopoiesis   a. malignant overgrowth of white blood cells

_____ 7. leukemia   b. separation of white blood cells from whole blood

_____ 8. leukapheresis   c. deficiency of white blood cells

_____ 9. leukoblast   d. immature white blood cell

_____ 10. leukopenia   e. formation of white blood cells

_____ 11. azotemia   a. excretion of sodium in the urine

_____ 12. sideroblast   b. compound that contains iron

_____ 13. natriuresis   c. presence of nitrogen compounds in the blood

_____ 14. calcification   d. conversion to calcium salts

_____ 15. ferritin   e. cell that contains iron

_____ 16. ecchymosis   a. hereditary clotting disorder

_____ 17. hemophilia   b. rupture of red blood cells

_____ 18. angioedema   c. collection of blood under the skin

_____ 19. hemolysis   d. allergic skin reaction

_____ 20. systemic sclerosis   e. an autoimmune disease

_____ 21. PMN   a. a form of leukemia

_____ 22. HDN   b. hormone that stimulates red cell formation

_____ 23. ALL   c. measurement of hemoglobin in red cells

_____ 24. MCH   d. neutrophil

_____ 25. EPO   e. disorder caused by Rh incompatibility

SUPPLEMENTARY TERMS

26. bilirubin
27. heparin
28. complement
29. hematoma
30. polycythemia

a. group of enzymes that helps destroy foreign cells
b. increase in RBCs in blood
c. localized collection of blood
d. pigment that comes from hemoglobin
e. anticoagulant

Fill in the blanks:

31. The liquid fraction of the blood is called _____.

32. The iron-containing pigment in red blood cells that carries oxygen is called
    _____.

33. A substance that induces the formation of antibodies is a(n) _____.

34. The cell fragments active in blood clotting are the _____.

35. The substance that forms a blood clot is named _____.

36. Oxyhemoglobin is hemoglobin combined with _____.

37. Disorder involving lack of hemoglobin in the blood _____.

38. A myelotoxin is a poison that affects _____.

The suffixes *-ia*, *-osis*, and *-hemia* all denote an increase in the type of cell indicated by the word root. Define each of the following terms:

39. eosinophilia (*ē-ō-sin-ō-FIL-ē-a*)   _____

40. erythrocytosis (*e-rith-rō-sī-TŌ-sis*)   _____

41. thrombocythemia (*throm-bō-sī-THĒ-mē-a*)   _____

42. neutrophilia (*nū-trō-FIL-ē-a*)   _____

43. monocytosis (*mon-ō-sī-TŌ-sis*)   _____

Word building. Write a word for each of the following definitions:

44. An immature red blood cell   _____

45. A decrease in the number of platelets (thrombocytes) in
    the blood   _____

46. Formation of red blood cells   _____

47. The study of blood   _____

48. Specialist in the study of immunity   _____

49. Immunity to one's own tissues   _____

50. Profuse flow of blood   _____

Adjectives. Use the ending *-ic* to write the adjective form of each of the following words:

51. eosinophil   _____

52. thrombocyte   _____

53. leukemia   _____

54. hemolysis   _____

Define each of the following terms:

55. neutropenia _____

56. hypoxemia _____

57. myeloma _____

58. lymphoblast _____

59. pyemia _____

Word analysis. Define each of the following words, and give the meaning of the word parts in each. Use a dictionary if necessary.

60. Hemocytometer ($h\bar{e}$-$m\bar{o}$-$s\bar{i}$-TOM-e-ter) _____
    a. hem/o _____
    b. cyt/o _____
    c. meter _____

61. Anisocytosis (an-$\bar{i}$-$s\bar{o}$-$s\bar{i}$-$T\bar{O}$-sis) _____
    a. an- _____
    b. iso- _____
    c. cyt/o _____
    d. -sis _____

62. Hemochromatosis ($h\bar{e}$-$m\bar{o}$-$kr\bar{o}$-$m\bar{a}$-$T\bar{O}$-sis) _____
    a. hem/o _____
    b. chromat/o _____
    c. -sis _____

Case Studies

Case Study 10-1: Latex Allergy

M.R., a 36-year-old certified registered nurse anesthetist (CRNA), was diagnosed 7 years ago with latex allergy. She first noticed that she developed contact dermatitis when she wore powdered latex gloves. She soon developed tachycardia, hypotension, bronchospasm, urticaria, and rhinitis with contact or proximity to latex in surgery. She had one frightening episode of anaphylaxis. Her allergy is of the type I hypersensitivity, IgE T-cell-mediated latex allergy, which was diagnosed by both a radioallergosorbent test (RAST) and a skin-prick test.

   M.R. avoids all contact with any natural rubber latex in her home and at work. She can only work in a pediatric OR because they are latex-free, since many children with congenital disorders are latex allergic. She wears a medical alert bracelet, uses a bronchodilator inhaler at the first symptom of bronchospasm, and carries a syringe of epinephrine at all times.

Case Study 10-2: Blood Replacement

C.L., a 16-year-old girl, sustained a ruptured liver when she hit a tree while sledding. Emergency surgery was needed to stop the internal bleeding. During surgery, the ruptured segment of the liver was removed and the laceration was sutured with a heavy, absorbable suture on a large smooth needle. Before surgery, her hemoglobin was 10.2 g/dL, but the reading decreased to 7.6 g/dL before hemostasis was attained. Cell salvage, or autotransfusion, was set up. In this procedure, the free blood was suctioned from her abdomen and mixed with an anticoagulant (heparin). The RBCs were washed in a sterile centrifuge with NSS and transfused back to her through tubing fitted with a filter. She also received 6 units of homologous, leukocyte-reduced whole blood, 5 units of fresh frozen plasma, and 2 units of platelets. During the surgery, the CRNA repeatedly tested her Hgb and Hct as well as prothrombin time and partial thromboplastin time to monitor her clotting mechanisms.

C.L. is B positive. Fortunately, there was enough B-positive blood in the hospital blood bank for her surgery. The lab informed her surgeon that they had 2 units of B-negative and 6 units of O-negative blood, which she could have received safely if she needed more blood during the night. However, her hemoglobin level increased to 12 g/dL, and she was stable during her recovery. She was monitored for DIC and pulmonary emboli.

Case Study 10-3: Myelofibrosis

A.Y., a 52-year-old kindergarten teacher, had myelofibrosis that had been in remission for 25 years. She had seen her hematologist regularly and had had routine blood testing since the age of 27. After several weeks of fatigue, idiopathic joint and muscle aching, weakness, and a frightening episode of syncope, she saw her hematologist for evaluation. Her hemoglobin was 9.0 g/dL and her hematocrit was 29%. Concerned that she was having an exacerbation, her doctor scheduled a bone marrow aspiration, and the results were positive for myelofibrosis.

A.Y. went through a 6-month therapy regimen of iron supplements in the form of ferrous sulfate tablets and received weekly vitamin B_{12} injections. Interferon was given every other week in addition to erythropoiesis therapy, which was unsuccessful. She was treated for presumed aplastic anemia. During treatment, she developed splenomegaly, which compromised her abdominal organs and pulmonary function. She continued to lose weight, and her hemoglobin dropped as low as 6.0 g/dL. Weekly transfusions of packed RBCs did not improve her hemoglobin and hematocrit.

After a regimen of high-dose chemotherapy to shrink the fibers in her bone marrow and a splenectomy, A.Y. received a stem cell transplant. The stems cells were obtained from blood donated by her brother, who was a perfect immunologic match. After a 6-month period of recovery in a protected environment, required because of her immunocompromised state, A.Y. returned home and has been free of disease symptoms for over 1 year.

CASE STUDY QUESTIONS

Multiple choice: Select the best answer and write the letter of your choice to the left of each number.

_____ 1. The natural latex protein in latex gloves may act as a(n):
   a. antibody
   b. allergen
   c. lymphocyte
   d. purpura
   e. immunocyte

_____ 2. Urticaria is commonly called:
   a. rhinitis
   b. dermatitis
   c. hives
   d. ELISA
   e. congenital

_____ 3. The cells involved in a T-cell-mediated allergic response are:
   a. basophils
   b. monocytes
   c. antigen
   d. T lymphocytes
   e. B cells

_____ 4. Anaphylaxis, a life-threatening physiological response, is an extreme form of:
   a. remission
   b. hypersensitivity
   c. hemostasis
   d. exacerbation
   e. homeostasis

_____ 5. The common name for epinephrine is:
   a. heparin
   b. adrenaline
   c. cortisone
   d. apheresis
   e. antihistamine

_____ 6. The removal of part of the liver is called:
   a. partial hepatectomy
   b. hepatomegaly
   c. resection of the liver
   d. a and b
   e. a and c

_____ 7. The unit for measurement of hemoglobin (g/dL) means:
   a. grams in decimal point
   b. grains in a decathlon
   c. drops in 50 cc
   d. grams in 100 cc
   e. grains in deciliter

_____ 8. Heparin, an anticoagulant, is a drug that:
   a. increases the rate of blood clotting
   b. takes the place of fibrin
   c. supports thrombin
   d. interferes with blood clotting
   e. makes blood thinner than water

Case Studies, continued

_____ 9. The RBCs were washed with NSS. This means: the _____ were washed with _____.
a. reticulocytes, heparin
b. red blood cells, nutritional solution
c. red blood cells, normal salt solution (saline)
d. reticulocytes, normal salt solution (saline)
e. red blood cells, heparin

_____ 10. Autotransfusion is transfusion of autologous blood, that is, the patient's own blood. Homologous blood is taken from:
a. another human
b. synthetic chemicals
c. plasma with clotting factors
d. an animal with similar antibodies as humans
e. IV fluid with electrolytes

_____ 11. Patients who lose a significant amount of blood may lose clotting ability. Effective therapy in such cases would be replacement of:
a. IV solution with electrolytes
b. iron supplements
c. platelets
d. heparin
e. packed RBCs

_____ 12. C.L.'s blood type is B positive. The best blood for her to receive is:
a. positive
b. negative
c. AB positive
d. B negative
e. B positive

_____ 13. Myelofibrosis, like aplastic anemia, is a disease in which there is:
a. overgrowth of RBCs
b. destruction of the bone marrow
c. dangerously high hemoglobin and hematocrit
d. absence of bone marrow
e. lymphatic tissue in the bone marrow

_____ 14. Erythropoiesis is:
a. production of blood
b. production of red cells
c. production of plasma
d. destruction of white cells
e. destruction of platelets

Case Studies, continued

_____ 15. The "ferrous" in ferrous sulfate represents:
  a. electrolytes
  b. RBCs
  c. iron
  d. oxygen
  e. B vitamins

_____ 16. Hemoglobin and hematocrit values pertain to:
  a. leukocytes
  b. immune response
  c. granulocytes
  d. red blood cells
  e. fibrinogen

_____ 17. Splenomegaly is:
  a. prolapse of the spleen
  b. movement of the spleen
  c. enlargement of the lymph glands
  d. destruction of the bone marrow
  e. enlargement of the spleen

_____ 18. The stem cells A.Y. received were expected to develop into new:
  a. spleen cells
  b. bone marrow cells
  c. hemoglobin
  d. abdominal organs
  e. cartilage

_____ 19. A.Y.'s health was compromised because the high-dose chemotherapy caused:
  a. immunodeficiency
  b. electrolyte imbalance
  c. anoxia
  d. Rh incompatibility
  e. autoimmunity

Abbreviations. Define the following abbreviations:

20. Ig   _____

21. Hgb _____

22. Hct _____

23. FFP _____

24. PT   _____

25. PTT _____

26. DIC _____

Chapter 10 Crossword
Blood and Immunity

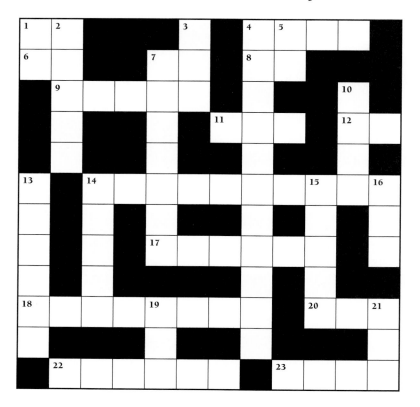

ACROSS

1. Alternate name for antibody (abbreviation)
4. Cold: prefix
6. Chemical symbol for sodium
7. Antibody (abbreviation)
9. Bone marrow: combining form
11. Oxygen-carrying pigment of red cells (abbreviation)
12. Antigen (abbreviation)
14. The substance that is deficient in cases of anemia
17. Most numerous type of white blood cell: combining form
18. Immature form of red blood cell: combining form
20. Type of widespread coagulation disorder (abbreviation)
22. Name used for a hereditary type of anemia
23. A mineral found in the blood (root)

DOWN

1. Prefix meaning "not"
2. Fraction of the blood that contains antibodies: _____ globulin
3. Common blood type system
4. Blood clotting
5. Prescription (abbreviation)
7. Protein found in the blood
10. Potassium: combining form
13. Iron: combining form
14. Blood: root
15. Fluid that brings oxygen and nutrients to the cells
16. New: prefix
19. Form of lymphocytic leukemia (abbreviation)
21. Comprehensive blood study (abbreviation)

CHAPTER 10 Answer Section

Answers to Chapter Exercises

EXERCISE 10-1

1. excess albumin in the blood
2. decreased amount of protein in the blood
3. deficiency of cells in the blood
4. deficiency of lymphocytes in the blood
5. production of erythrocytes
6. pyemia (pī-Ē-mē-a)
7. viremia (vī-RĒ-mē-a)
8. toxemia (tok-SĒ-mē-a)
9. leukemia (lū-KĒ-mē-a)

EXERCISE 10-2

1. myel/o; bone marrow
2. thromb/o; blood clot
3. immun/o; immunity
4. hem/o; blood
5. erythrocytes; red blood cells
6. bone marrow
7. platelets; thrombocytes
8. leukocytes; white blood cells
9. immunity
10. blood cells
11. lymphocytes
12. myeloma (mī-e-LŌ-ma)
13. leukoblast (LŪ-kō-blast)
14. erythropenia (e-rith-rō-PĒ-nē-a); also erythrocytopenia
15. hematology (hē-ma-TOL-ō-jē)
16. thrombolysis (throm-BOL-i-sis)
17. myelopoiesis (mī-e-lō-poy-Ē-sis)
18. erythrocytosis (e-rith-rō-sī-TŌ-sis)
19. monocytosis (mon-ō-sī-TŌ-sis)
20. thrombocytosis (throm-bō-sī-TŌ-sis)
21. granulocytosis (gran-ū-lō-sī-TŌ-sis)
22. lymphocytosis (lim-fō-sī-TŌ-sis)

EXERCISE 10-3

1. iron
2. potassium
3. oxygen
4. iron
5. calcium
6. natremia (na-TRĒ-mē-a)
7. azotemia (az-ō-TĒ-mē-a)
8. calcemia (kal-SĒ-mē-a)

LABELING EXERCISE 10-1 BLOOD CELLS

1. neutrophil
2. eosinophil
3. basophil
4. red blood cells (erythrocytes) and platelets (thrombocytes)
5. lymphocyte
6. monocyte

Answers to Chapter Review 10-1

1. d
2. c
3. e
4. a
5. b
6. e
7. a
8. b
9. d
10. c
11. c
12. e
13. a
14. d
15. b
16. c
17. a
18. d
19. b
20. e
21. d
22. e
23. a
24. c
25. b
26. d
27. e
28. a
29. c
30. b
31. plasma
32. hemoglobin
33. antigen
34. platelets (thrombocytes)
35. fibrin
36. oxygen
37. anemia
38. bone marrow

39. increase in eosinophils in the blood
40. increase in erythrocytes (red blood cells) in the blood
41. increase in thrombocytes (platelets) in the blood
42. increase in neutrophils in the blood
43. increase in monocytes in the blood
44. erythroblast
45. thrombocytopenia
46. erythropoiesis
47. hematology
48. immunologist
49. autoimmunity
50. hemorrhage
51. eosinophilic ($\overline{e}$-$\overline{o}$-sin-$\overline{o}$-FIL-ik)
52. thrombocytic (throm-b$\overline{o}$-SIT-ik)
53. leukemic ($\overline{l}u$-K$\overline{E}$-mik)
54. hemolytic (h$\overline{e}$-m$\overline{o}$-LIT-ik)
55. deficiency in the number of neutrophils in the blood
56. low levels of oxygen in the blood
57. tumor of bone marrow
58. immature lymphocyte
59. presence of pus in the blood
60. device used to count blood cells
    a. blood
    b. cell
    c. instrument for measuring
61. presence in the blood of erythrocytes showing excessive variation in size
    a. not
    b. equal
    c. cell
    d. condition of

62. deposit of iron-containing pigment in tissues causing bronzing of the skin and other symptoms
    a. blood
    b. color
    c. condition of

Answers to Case Study Questions

1. b
2. c
3. d
4. b
5. b
6. e
7. d
8. d
9. c
10. a
11. c
12. e
13. b
14. b
15. c
16. d
17. e
18. b
19. a
20. immunoglobulin
21. hemoglobin
22. hematocrit
23. fresh frozen plasma
24. prothrombin time
25. partial thromboplastin time
26. disseminated intravascular coagulation

ANSWERS TO CROSSWORD PUZZLE

Blood and Immunity

¹I	²G				³A		⁴C	⁵R	Y	O	
⁶N	A		⁷A	B		⁸O	X				
	⁹M	Y	E	L	O		A			¹⁰K	
	M		B		¹¹H	G	B		¹²A	G	
	A		U			U			L		
¹³S		¹⁴H	E	M	O	G	L	O	¹⁵B	I	¹⁶N
I		E		I		A		L			E
D		M	¹⁷N	E	U	T	R	O			O
E		A		I			O				
¹⁸R	E	T	I	C	U	L	O		²⁰D	I	²¹C
O			L		N						B
	²²C	O	O	L	E	Y		²³C	A	L	C

Respiration

Chapter Contents

Objectives

After study of this chapter you should be able to:

1. Explain the roles of oxygen and carbon dioxide in the body and describe how each is carried in the blood.
2. Label a diagram of the respiratory tract and briefly explain the function of each part.
3. Describe the mechanism of breathing, including the roles of the diaphragm and phrenic nerve.
4. Identify and use word parts pertaining to respiration.
5. Discuss the major disorders of the respiratory tract.
6. Define medical terms related to breathing and diseases of the respiratory tract.
7. List and define 10 volumes and capacities commonly used to measure pulmonary function.
8. Interpret abbreviations commonly used in referring to respiration.
9. Analyze several case studies pertaining to diseases that affect respiration.

The main function of the respiratory system is to provide **oxygen** to body cells for energy metabolism and to eliminate **carbon dioxide**, a byproduct of metabolism. Because these gases must be carried to and from the cells in the blood, the respiratory system works closely with the cardiovascular system to accomplish gas exchange.

Exchange of gases between the atmosphere and the blood takes place in the **lungs**, two cone-shaped organs located in the thoracic cavity. A double membrane, the **pleura**, covers the lungs and lines the thoracic cavity. The outer layer that is attached to the wall of the thoracic cavity is the parietal pleura; the inner layer that is attached to the surface of the lungs is the visceral pleura. The very thin, fluid-filled space between the two layers of the pleura is the **pleural space**.

Upper Respiratory Passageways

Air is carried to and from the lungs in a series of tubes in which no gas exchange occurs. Refer to Figure 11-1 as you read the following description of the respiratory tract. Air enters through the **nose**, where it is warmed, filtered, and moistened as it passes over the hair-covered mucous membranes of the nasal cavity. Cilia, microscopic hairlike projections from the cells that line the nose, sweep dirt and foreign material toward the throat for elimination. Material that is eliminated from the respiratory tract by coughing or clearing the throat is called **sputum**.

In the bones of the skull and face near the nose are air-filled cavities lined with mucous membranes that drain into the nasal cavity. These chambers lighten the bones and provide resonance for speech production. Each of these cavities is called a **sinus**, and they are named specifically for the bones in which they are located, such as the sphenoid, ethmoid, and maxillary sinuses. Together, because they are near the nose, these cavities are referred to as the paranasal sinuses (see Fig. 11-1).

Receptors for the sense of smell are located within bony side projections of the nasal cavity called **turbinate bones** or conchae.

Inhaled air passes into the throat, or **pharynx**, where it mixes with air that enters through the mouth and also with food destined for the digestive tract. The pharynx and associated structures are shown in Figure 12-2. The pharynx is divided into three regions: (1) an upper portion, the nasopharynx, behind the nasal cavity; (2) a middle portion, the oropharynx, behind the mouth; and (3) a lower portion, the laryngeal pharynx, behind the larynx. The **palatine tonsils** are on either side of the soft palate in the oropharynx; the pharyngeal tonsils, or **adenoids**, are in the nasopharynx.

Lower Respiratory Passageways and Lungs

The pharynx conducts air into the **trachea**, a tube reinforced with C-shaped rings of cartilage to prevent its collapse (you can feel these rings if you press your fingers gently against the front of your throat). Cilia in the lining of the trachea move impurities up toward the throat, where they can be eliminated by swallowing or by **expectoration**. At the top of the trachea is the **larynx** (Fig. 11-2). The larynx is shaped by nine cartilages, the most prominent of which is the thyroid cartilage at the front that forms the "Adam's apple." The opening between the vocal cords is the **glottis**. The small leaf-shaped cartilage at the top of the larynx is called the **epiglottis**. When one swallows, the epiglottis covers the opening of the larynx and helps to prevent food from entering the respiratory tract.

The larynx contains the **vocal cords**, folds of tissue that are important in speech production (Fig. 11-3). Vibrations produced by air passing over the vocal cords form the basis for voice production, although portions of the throat and mouth are needed for proper articulation of speech.

The trachea is contained in a region known as the **mediastinum,** which consists of the space between the lungs together with the organs contained in this space (see Fig. 11-1). In addition to the trachea, the mediastinum contains the heart, esophagus, large vessels, and other tissues.

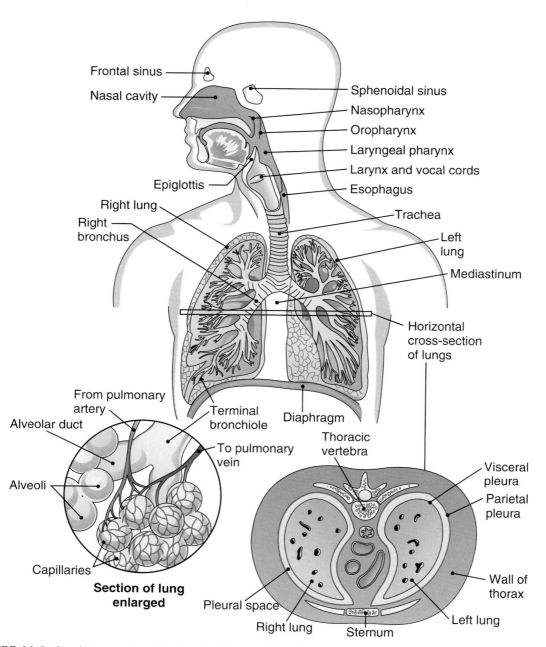

FIGURE 11-1. Respiratory system. (Reprinted with permission from Cohen BJ, Wood DL. Memmler's The Human Body in Health and Disease. 9th Ed. Philadelphia: Lippincott Williams & Wilkins, 2000.)

At its lower end, the trachea divides into a right and a left main stem **bronchus** that enter the lungs. The right bronchus is shorter and wider; it divides into three secondary bronchi that enter the three lobes of the right lung. The left bronchus divides into two branches that supply the two lobes of the left lung. Further divisions produce an increasing number of smaller tubes that supply air to smaller subdivisions of lung tissue. As the air passageways progress through the lungs, the cartilage in the walls gradually disappears and is replaced by smooth (involuntary) muscle.

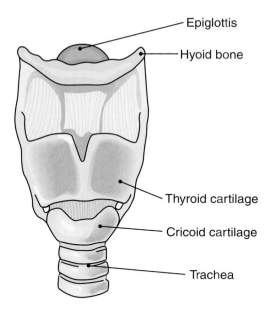

FIGURE 11-2. The larnyx, anterior view. (Reprinted with permission from Cohen BJ, Wood DL. Memmler's The Human Body in Health and Disease. 9th Ed. Philadelphia: Lippincott Williams & Wilkins, 2000.)

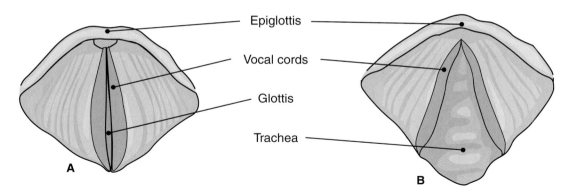

FIGURE 11-3. The vocal cords viewed from above. **(A)** The glottis in closed position. **(B)** The glottis in open position. (Reprinted with permission from Cohen BJ, Wood DL. Memmler's The Human Body in Health and Disease. 9th Ed. Philadelphia: Lippincott Williams & Wilkins, 2000.)

The smallest of the conducting tubes, the **bronchioles**, carry air into the microscopic air sacs, the **alveoli**, through which gases are exchanged between the lungs and the blood. It is through the ultrathin walls of the alveoli and their surrounding capillaries that oxygen diffuses into the blood and carbon dioxide diffuses out of the blood for elimination (see Fig. 11-1).

Breathing

Air is moved into and out of the lungs by the process of breathing, technically called **ventilation**. This consists of a steady cycle of **inspiration** (inhalation) and **expiration** (exhalation), separated by a period of rest. The cycle begins when the **phrenic nerve** stimulates the **diaphragm** to contract and flatten, thus enlarging the chest cavity. The resulting decrease in pressure within the thorax causes air to be pulled into the lungs

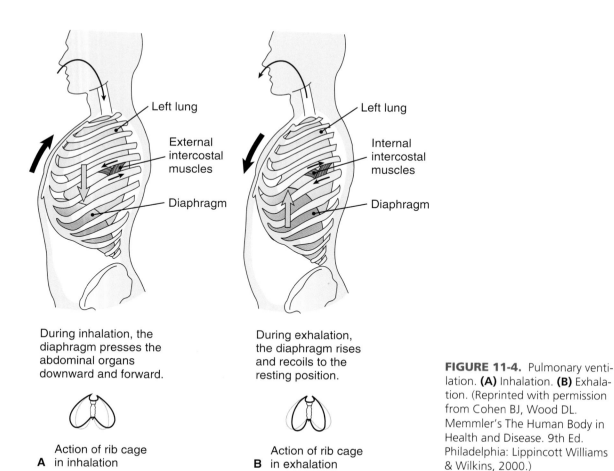

During inhalation, the diaphragm presses the abdominal organs downward and forward.

A Action of rib cage in inhalation

During exhalation, the diaphragm rises and recoils to the resting position.

B Action of rib cage in exhalation

FIGURE 11-4. Pulmonary ventilation. **(A)** Inhalation. **(B)** Exhalation. (Reprinted with permission from Cohen BJ, Wood DL. Memmler's The Human Body in Health and Disease. 9th Ed. Philadelphia: Lippincott Williams & Wilkins, 2000.)

(Fig. 11-4). The intercostal muscles between the ribs aid in inspiration by pulling the ribs up and out. Muscles of the neck and thorax are used in addition for forceful inhalation. The measure of how easily the lungs expand under pressure is **compliance**. Fluid produced within the lung, known as **surfactant**, aids in compliance by reducing surface tension within the alveoli. Expiration occurs as the breathing muscles relax, the lungs spring back to their original size, and air is forced out. Muscles of the rib cage and abdomen can be called on for forceful exhalation.

Breathing is normally regulated unconsciously by centers in the brainstem. These centers adjust the rate and rhythm of breathing according to changes in the composition of the blood, especially the concentration of carbon dioxide.

Gas Transport

Oxygen is carried in the blood bound to hemoglobin in red blood cells. The oxygen is released to the cells as needed. Carbon dioxide is carried in several ways but is mostly converted to an acid called carbonic acid. The amount of carbon dioxide that is exhaled is important in regulating the acidity or alkalinity of the blood, based on the amount of carbonic acid that is formed. Dangerous shifts in blood pH can result from too much or too little carbon dioxide being exhaled.

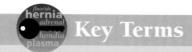

Key Terms

NORMAL STRUCTURE AND FUNCTION

adenoids *AD-e-noyds*	Lymphoid tissue located in the nasopharynx; the pharyngeal tonsils
alveoli *al-VĒ-ō-lī*	The tiny air sacs in the lungs through which gases are exchanged between the atmosphere and the blood in respiration (singular, alveolus). An alveolus, in general, is a small hollow or cavity, and the term is also used to describe the bony socket for a tooth.
bronchiole *BRONG-kē-ōl*	One of the smaller subdivisions of the bronchial tubes (root *bronchiol*)
bronchus *BRONG-kus*	One of the larger air passageways in the lungs. The bronchi begin as two branches of the trachea and then subdivide within the lungs (plural, bronchi) (root *bronch*).
carbon dioxide (CO$_2$)	A gas produced by energy metabolism in cells and eliminated through the lungs
carbonic acid *kar-BON-ik*	An acid formed by carbon dioxide when it dissolves in water; H$_2$CO$_3$
compliance *kom-PLĪ-ans*	A measure of how easily the lungs expand under pressure. Compliance is reduced in many types of respiratory disorders.
diaphragm *DĪ-a-fram*	The dome-shaped muscle under the lungs that flattens during inspiration (root *phren/o*)
epiglottis *ep-i-GLOT-is*	A leaf-shaped cartilage that covers the larynx during swallowing to prevent food from entering the trachea
expectoration *ek-spek-to-RĀ-shun*	The act of coughing up material from the respiratory tract; also the material thus released; sputum
expiration *ek-spi-RĀ-shun*	The act of breathing out or expelling air from the lungs; exhalation
glottis *GLOT-is*	The opening between the vocal cords
hemoglobin *HĒ-mō-glō-bin*	The iron-containing pigment in red blood cells that transports oxygen
inspiration *in-spi-RĀ-shun*	The act of drawing air into the lungs; inhalation
larynx *LAR-inks*	The enlarged upper end of the trachea that contains the vocal cords (root *laryng/o*)
lung	A cone-shaped spongy organ of respiration contained within the thorax (roots *pneum, pulm*)
mediastinum *mē-dē-as-TĪ-num*	The space between the lungs together with the organs contained in this space
nose *NŌZ*	The organ of the face used for breathing and for housing receptors for the sense of smell; includes an external portion and an internal nasal cavity (roots *nas/o, rhin/o*)

Normal Structure and Function, *continued*

oxygen (O₂) OK-si-jen	The gas needed by cells to release energy from food in metabolism
palatine tonsils PAL-a-tīn	The paired masses of lymphoid tissue located on either side of the oropharynx; usually meant when the term *tonsils* is used alone
pharynx FAR-inks	The throat; a common passageway for food entering the esophagus and air entering the larynx (root *pharyng/o*)
phrenic nerve FREN-ik	The nerve that activates the diaphragm (root *phrenic/o*)
pleura PLŪR-a	A double-layered membrane that covers the lungs (visceral pleura) and lines the thoracic cavity (parietal pleura) (root *pleur/o*)
pleural space	The thin, fluid-filled space between the two layers of the pleura; pleural cavity
sinus SĪ-nus	A cavity or channel; the paranasal sinuses are located near the nose and drain into the nasal cavity
sputum SPŪ-tum	The substance released by coughing or clearing the throat. It may contain a variety of material from the respiratory tract.
surfactant sur-FAK-tant	A substance that decreases surface tension within the alveoli and eases expansion of the lungs
trachea TRĀ-kē-a	The air passageway that extends from the larynx to the bronchi (root *trache/o*)
turbinate bones TUR-bi-nat	The bony projections in the nasal cavity that contain receptors for the sense of smell. Also called conchae (KON-kē).
ventilation	The movement of air into and out of the lungs
vocal cords VŌ-kal	Membranous folds on either side of the larynx that are important in speech production. Also called vocal folds.

Word Parts Pertaining to Respiration

TABLE 11-1 Suffixes for Respiration

SUFFIX	MEANING	EXAMPLE	DEFINITION OF EXAMPLE
-pnea	breathing	orthopnea or-THOP-nē-a	difficulty in breathing except in an upright (-ortho) position
-oxia*	level of oxygen	hypoxia hī-POK-sē-a	decreased amount of oxygen in the tissues
-capnia*	level of carbon dioxide	hypercapnia hī-per-KAP-nē-a	increased carbon dioxide in the tissues
-phonia	voice	dysphonia dis-FŌ-nē-a	difficulty in speaking

*When referring to levels of oxygen and carbon dioxide in the blood, the suffix *-emia* is used, as in hypoxemia, hypercapnemia.

Exercise 11-1

Use the suffix *-pnea* to build a word with each of the following meanings:

1. painful or difficult breathing _____ dyspnea _____

2. easy, normal (eu-) breathing _____

3. lack of (a-) of breathing _____

4. rapid rate of breathing _____

Use the ending *-pneic* to write the adjective form of each of the above words:

5. _____ dyspneic _____

6. _____

7. _____

8. _____

Use the suffixes in Table 11-1 to write a word for each of the following definitions:

9. lack of (an-) oxygen in the tissues _____

10. decreased carbon dioxide in the tissues _____

11. normal levels (eu-) of carbon dioxide in the tissues _____

12. lack of voice _____

TABLE 11-2 Roots for the Respiratory Passageways

ROOT	MEANING	EXAMPLE	DEFINITION OF EXAMPLE
nas/o	nose	nasal NĀ-zal	pertaining to the nose
rhin/o	nose	rhinorrhea rī-NŌ-rē-a	discharge from the nose
pharyng/o	pharynx	pharyngeal* fa-RIN-jē-al	pertaining to the pharynx
laryng/o	larynx	laryngoscopy lar-ing-GOS-kō-pē	endoscopic examination of the larynx
trache/o	trachea	tracheotome trā-kē-ō-TŌM	instrument used to incise the trachea
bronch/o, bronch/i	bronchus	bronchogenic brong-kō-GEN-ik	originating in a bronchus
bronchiol	bronchiole	bronchiolectasis brong-kē-ō-LEK-ta-sis	dilatation of the bronchioles

*Note addition of e before adjective ending -al.

Exercise 11-2

Write a word for each of the following definitions:

1. near the nose — paranasal

2. inflammation of the pharynx _____

3. pertaining to the larynx (see pharynx in Table 11-2) _____

4. endoscopic examination of a bronchus _____

5. inflammation of the bronchioles _____

6. narrowing of a bronchus _____

7. plastic repair of the larynx _____

8. surgical incision of the trachea _____

Define the following words (note the adjectival endings):

9. intranasal (*in-tra-NĀ-zal*) — within the nose

10. bronchiolar (*brong-KĒ-ō-lar*) _____

11. bronchiectasis (*brong-kē-EK-ta-sis*) _____

12. peribronchial (*per-i-BRONG-kē-al*) _____

13. endotracheal (*en-dō-TRĀ-kē-al*) _____

14. nasopharyngeal (*nā-zō-fa-RIN-jē-al*) _____

TABLE 11-3 Roots for the Lungs and Breathing

ROOT	MEANING	EXAMPLE	DEFINITION OF EXAMPLE
phren/o	diaphragm	phrenic *FREN-ik*	pertaining to the diaphragm
phrenic/o	phrenic nerve	phrenicotripsy *fren-i-kō-TRIP-sē*	crushing of the phrenic nerve
pleur/o	pleura	pleurodesis *plū-ROD-e-sis*	fusion of the pleura
pulm/o, pulmon/o	lungs	intrapulmonary *in-tra-PUL-mō-ner-ē*	within the lungs
pneumon/o	lung	pneumonectomy *nū-mō-NEK-tō-mē*	surgical removal of a lung or lung tissue (pneumectomy and pulmonectomy also used)
pneum/o, pneumat/o	air, gas; also respiration, lung	pneumatocardia *nū-ma-tō-KAR-dē-a*	presence of air in the heart
spir/o	breathing	spirometer *spī-ROM-e-ter*	instrument for measuring breathing volumes

Exercise 11-3

Define the following words:

1. pneumonitis (nū-mō-NĪ-tis) _____
2. pleuropulmonary (plūr-ō-PUL-mō-ner-ē) _____
3. pneumoplasty (NŪ-mō-plas-tē) _____
4. pleuralgia (plū-RAL-jē-a) _____
5. pulmonology (pul-mō-NOL-ō-jē) _____
6. pneumatic (nū-MAT-ik) _____

Write a word for each of the following definitions:

7. between (inter) the pleura _____
8. below the diaphragm _____
9. surgical incision of the phrenic nerve _____
10. any disease of the lungs (pneumon/o) _____
11. record of breathing volumes _____
12. surgical puncture of the pleural space _____

Clinical Aspects of Respiration

Pulmonary function is affected by conditions that cause resistance to air flow through the respiratory tract or that limit expansion of the chest. These may be conditions that affect the respiratory system directly, such as infection, injury, allergy, **aspiration** (inhalation) of foreign bodies, or cancer. They also may be conditions that result from disturbances in other systems, such as in the skeletal, muscular, cardiovascular, or nervous systems.

As noted above, changes in ventilation can affect the acidity and alkalinity of the blood. If too much carbon dioxide is exhaled by **hyperventilation**, the blood tends to become too alkaline, a condition termed **alkalosis**. If too little carbon dioxide is exhaled as a result of **hypoventilation**, the blood tends to become too acidic, a condition termed **acidosis**.

Infections

Pneumonia is caused by several different microorganisms, most commonly bacteria and viruses. Viral pneumonia is more diffuse and is commonly caused by influenza virus, adenovirus and, in young children, respiratory syncytial virus (RSV). Bacterial agents are most commonly *Streptococcus pneumoniae* and *Klebsiella pneumoniae*. Bronchopneumonia (bronchial pneumonia) begins in terminal bronchioles, which become clogged with exudate and form consolidated (solidified) patches. Lobar pneumonia is an acute disease that involves one or more lobes of the lung (Fig. 11-5). Pneumonia usually can be treated successfully in otherwise healthy people, but in debilitated patients it is a leading cause of death. Immunocompromised patients, such as those with AIDS, are often subject to a form of pneumonia called *Pneumocystis carinii* pneumonia (PCP), which is caused by a protozoon.

The term *pneumonia* is also applied to inflammation of the lungs caused by noninfectious causes, such as asthma, allergy, or inhalation of irritants. In these cases, however, the more general term **pneumonitis** is often used.

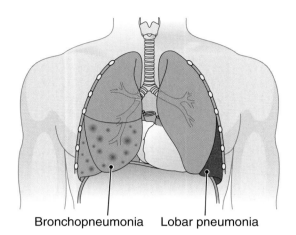

Bronchopneumonia   Lobar pneumonia

FIGURE 11-5. Distribution of lung involvement in bronchial and lobar pneumonia. In bronchopneumonia (*left*), patchy areas of consolidation occur. In lobar pneumonia, an entire lobe is consolidated.

The incidence of **tuberculosis** (TB) has increased in recent years, along with the increase of AIDS and the appearance of antibiotic resistance in the organism that causes the disease, *Mycobacterium tuberculosis* (MTB). (This organism, because of its staining properties, also is referred to as AFB, meaning *acid-fast bacillus*.) The name tuberculosis comes from the small lesions, or tubercles, that appear with the infection. The symptoms of TB include fever, weight loss, weakness, cough and, as a result of damage to blood vessels in the lungs, **hemoptysis**, the coughing up of sputum containing blood. Sputum analysis is used to isolate, stain, and identify infectious organisms. Accumulation of exudate in the alveoli may result in consolidation of lung tissue. The **tuberculin test** is used to test for tuberculosis infection. The test material that is used, tuberculin, is made from byproducts of the tuberculosis organism. PPD (purified protein derivative) is the form of tuberculin commonly used.

Influenza is a viral disease of the respiratory tract. Different strains of the influenza virus have caused serious epidemics throughout history.

Emphysema

Emphysema is a chronic disease associated with overexpansion and destruction of the alveoli. Common causes are exposure to cigarette smoke and other forms of pollution as well as chronic infection. Emphysema is the main disorder included under the heading of **chronic obstructive pulmonary disease** (COPD) (also called COLD, chronic obstructive lung disease). Other conditions included in this category are asthma, chronic **bronchitis**, and **bronchiectasis**.

BOX 11-1 Don't Breathe a Word

Some laypersons' terms for respiratory symptoms and conditions are so old-fashioned and quaint that you might see them today only in Victorian novels. Catarrh (ka-TAR) is an old word for an upper respiratory infection with much mucus production. Quinsy (KWIN-zē) referred to a sore throat or tonsillar abscess. Consumption was tuberculosis, and dropsy referred to generalized edema. The grip meant influenza, which we more often abbreviate as "flu."

Some unscientific words are still in use. These include whooping cough for pertussis, croup for laryngeal spasm, cold sore for a herpes lesion, and phlegm for sputum.

Many informal terms are used instead of scientific words by the general public. Health professionals should be familiar with the slang or colloquialisms that are used to describe symptoms so that they can better communicate with their patients.

Asthma

Attacks of **asthma** result from narrowing of the bronchial tubes. This constriction, along with edema (swelling) of the bronchial linings and accumulation of mucus, results in wheezing, extreme **dyspnea** (difficulty in breathing), and **cyanosis**. Asthma is most common in children. Although its causes are uncertain, a main factor is irritation caused by allergy. Heredity may also play a role. Treatment of asthma includes removal of allergens, administration of bronchodilators to widen the airways, and administration of steroids.

Pneumoconiosis

Chronic irritation and inflammation caused by inhalation of dust particles is termed **pneumoconiosis**. This is an occupational hazard seen mainly in people involved in the mining and stoneworking industries. Different forms of pneumoconiosis are named for the specific type of dust inhaled: silicosis (silica or quartz), anthracosis (coal dust), asbestosis (asbestos fibers).

Although the term pneumoconiosis is limited to conditions caused by inhalation of inorganic dust, lung irritation may also result from inhalation of organic dusts, such as textile or grain dusts.

Disorders of the Pleura

Pleurisy, also called pleuritis, is an inflammation of the pleura, usually associated with infection. Pain is the common symptom of pleurisy. Because this pain is intensified by breathing or coughing, as the inflamed membranes move, breathing becomes rapid and shallow. Analgesics and anti-inflammatory drugs are used to treat the symptoms of pleurisy.

As a result of injury, infection, or weakness in the pleural membrane, substances may accumulate between the layers of the pleura. When air or gas collects in this space, the condition is termed **pneumothorax** (Fig. 11-6). Compression may result in collapse of the lung, termed **atelectasis**.

In **pleural effusion**, other materials accumulate in the pleural space (Fig. 11-7). Depending on the substances involved, these are described as **empyema** (pus), also termed **pyothorax; hemothorax** (blood); or **hydrothorax** (fluid). Causes of these conditions include injury, infection, heart failure, and pulmonary embolism. **Thoracentesis**, needle puncture of the chest to remove fluids (Fig. 11-8), or fusion of the pleural membranes (pleurodesis) may be required.

Lung Cancer

Lung cancer is the leading cause of cancer-related deaths in both men and women. The incidence of this form of cancer has increased steadily over the past 50 years, especially in women. Cigarette smoking is a major risk factor in this as well as other forms of cancer. The most common form of lung cancer is squamous carcinoma, originating in the lining of the bronchi (bronchogenic). Lung cancer usually cannot be detected early, and it metastasizes rapidly. The overall survival rate is low.

Methods used to diagnose lung cancer include radiographic studies, computed tomography (CT) scans, and examination of sputum for cancer cells. A **bronchoscope** can be used to examine the airways and to collect tissue samples for study. Surgical or needle biopsies may also be taken.

Respiratory Distress Syndrome (RDS)

Respiratory distress syndrome of the newborn, also called *hyaline membrane disease*, occurs in premature infants and is the most common cause of death in this group. It results from a lack of surfactant in the lungs, which reduces compliance. **Acute respiratory distress syndrome** (ARDS), also known as *shock lung*, may result from trauma, allergic reactions, infection, and other causes. It involves edema that can lead to respiratory failure and death if untreated.

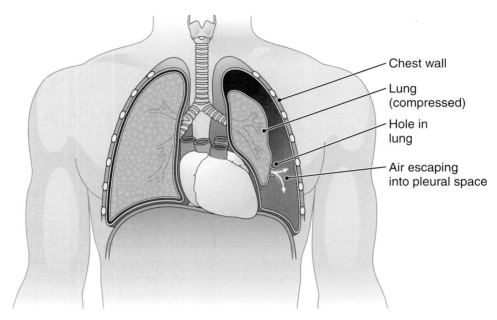

FIGURE 11-6. Pneumothorax. Injury to lung tissue allows air to leak into the pleural space and put pressure on the lung.

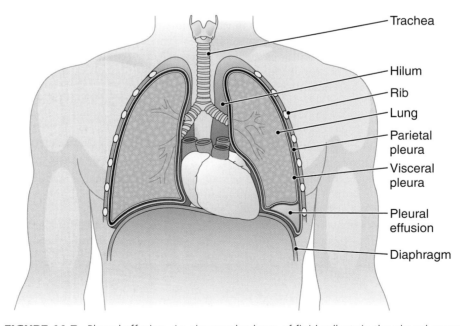

FIGURE 11-7. Pleural effusion. An abnormal volume of fluid collects in the pleural space.

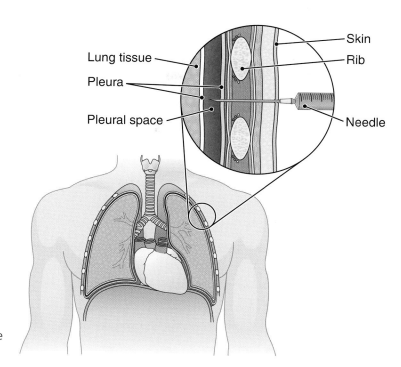

FIGURE 11-8. Thoracentesis. A needle is inserted into the pleural space.

Cystic Fibrosis

Cystic fibrosis (CF) is the most common fatal hereditary disease among white children. The flawed gene that causes CF affects glandular secretions by altering chloride transport across cell membranes. Thickening of bronchial secretions leads to infection and other respiratory disorders. Other mucus-secreting glands, sweat glands, and glands of the pancreas are also involved, causing electrolyte imbalance and digestive disturbances.

CF is diagnosed by the increased amounts of sodium and chloride in the sweat, and the gene that results in CF can be identified by DNA analysis. There is no cure at present for CF. Patients are treated to relieve their symptoms, such as by postural drainage, aerosol mists, bronchodilators, antibiotics, and mucolytic agents, which dissolve mucus.

Diagnosis

In addition to chest radiographs, CT scans, and magnetic resonance imaging (MRI) scans, methods for diagnosing respiratory disorders include **lung scans**, bronchoscopy, and tests of pleural fluid removed by thoracentesis. **Arterial blood gases** (ABGs) are used to evaluate gas exchange in the lungs by measuring carbon dioxide, oxygen, bicarbonate, and pH in an arterial blood sample. **Pulse oximetry** is routinely used to measure the oxygen saturation of arterial blood by means of a simple apparatus, an oximeter, placed on a thin part of the body, usually the finger or the ear (Fig. 11-9).

Pulmonary function tests are used to assess breathing, usually by means of a **spirometer**. They measure the volumes of air that can be moved into or out of the lungs with different degrees of effort. Often used to monitor treatment in cases of allergy, asthma, emphysema, and other respiratory conditions, they are also used to measure progress in cessation of smoking. The main volumes and capacities measured in these tests are given in Display 11-1. A capacity is the sum of two or more volumes.

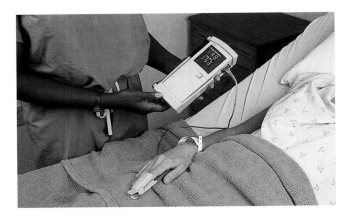

FIGURE 11-9. Pulse oximetry is used to measure oxygen saturation of arterial blood. (Reprinted with permission from Taylor C, Lillis C, LeMone P. Fundamentals of Nursing: The Art and Science of Nursing Care. 4th Ed. Philadelphia: Lippincott Williams & Wilkins, 2001. Copyright © B. Proud)

DISPLAY 11-1 Volumes and Capacities (Sums of Volumes) Used in Pulmonary Function Tests

VOLUME OR CAPACITY	DEFINITION
tidal volume (TV)	amount of air breathed into or out of the lungs in quiet, relaxed breathing
residual volume (RV)	amount of air that remains in the lungs after maximum exhalation
expiratory reserve volume (ERV)	amount of air that can be exhaled after a normal exhalation
inspiratory reserve volume (IRV)	amount of air that can be inhaled above a normal inspiration
total lung capacity (TLC)	total amount of air that can be contained in the lungs after maximum inhalation
inspiratory capacity (IC)	amount of air that can be inhaled after normal exhalation
vital capacity (VC)	amount of air that can be expelled from the lungs by maximum exhalation after maximum inhalation
functional residual capacity (FRC)	amount of air remaining in the lungs after normal exhalation
forced expiratory volume (FEV)	volume of gas exhaled with maximum force within a given interval of time; the time interval is shown as a subscript, such as FEV_1 (1 second), FEV_3 (3 seconds)
forced vital capacity (FVC)	the volume of gas exhaled as rapidly and completely as possible after a complete inhalation

Key Clinical Terms

DISORDERS

acidosis *as-i-DŌ-sis*	Abnormal acidity of body fluids. Respiratory acidosis is caused by abnormally high levels of carbon dioxide in the body.
acute respiratory distress syndrome (ARDS)	Pulmonary edema that can lead rapidly to fatal respiratory failure; causes include trauma, aspiration into the lungs, viral pneumonia, and drug reactions; shock lung

Disorders, *continued*

alkalosis *al-ka-LŌ-sis*	Abnormal alkalinity of body fluids. Respiratory alkalosis is caused by abnormally low levels of carbon dioxide in the body.
aspiration *as-pi-RĀ-shun*	The accidental inhalation of food or other foreign material into the lungs. Also used to mean the withdrawal of fluid from a cavity by suction.
asthma *AZ-ma*	A disease characterized by dyspnea and wheezing caused by spasm of the bronchial tubes or swelling of their mucous membranes
atelectasis *at-e-LEK-ta-sis*	Incomplete expansion of a lung or part of a lung; lung collapse. May be present at birth (as in respiratory distress syndrome) or be caused by bronchial obstruction or compression of lung tissue (prefix *atel/o* means "imperfect").
bronchiectasis *brong-kē-EK-ta-sis*	Chronic dilatation of a bronchus or bronchi
bronchitis *brong-KĪ-tis*	Inflammation of a bronchus
chronic obstructive pulmonary disease (COPD)	Any of a group of chronic, progressive, and debilitating respiratory diseases, which includes emphysema, asthma, bronchitis, and bronchiectasis
cyanosis *sī-a-NŌ-sis*	Bluish discoloration of the skin caused by lack of oxygen in the blood (adjective, cyanotic)
cystic fibrosis (CF) *SIS-tik fī-BRŌ-sis*	An inherited disease that affects the pancreas, respiratory system, and sweat glands. Characterized by mucus accumulation in the bronchi causing obstruction and leading to infection.
dyspnea *dysp-NĒ-a*	Difficult or labored breathing, sometimes with pain; "air hunger"
emphysema *em-fi-SĒ-ma*	A chronic pulmonary disease characterized by enlargement and destruction of the alveoli
empyema *em-pī-Ē-ma*	Accumulation of pus in a body cavity, especially the pleural space; pyothorax
hemoptysis *hē-MOP-ti-sis*	The spitting of blood from the mouth or respiratory tract (*ptysis* means "spitting")
hemothorax *hē-mō-THOR-aks*	Presence of blood in the pleural space
hydrothorax *hī-drō-THOR-aks*	Presence of fluid in the pleural space
hyperventilation	Increased rate and depth of breathing; increase in the amount of air entering the alveoli
hypoventilation	Decreased rate and depth of breathing; decrease in the amount of air entering the alveoli

Disorders, continued

influenza in-flū-EN-za	An acute, contagious respiratory infection causing fever, chills, headache, and muscle pain
pleural effusion	Accumulation of fluid in the pleural space. The fluid may contain blood (hemothorax) or pus (pyothorax or empyema).
pleurisy PLŪR-i-sē	Inflammation of the pleura; pleuritis. A symptom of pleurisy is sharp pain on breathing.
pneumoconiosis nū-mō-kō-nē-Ō-sis	Disease of the respiratory tract caused by inhalation of dust particles. Named more specifically by the type of dust inhaled, such as silicosis, anthracosis, asbestosis.
pneumonia nū-MŌ-nē-a	Inflammation of the lungs generally caused by infection. May involve the bronchioles and alveoli (bronchopneumonia) or one or more lobes of the lung (lobar pneumonia).
pneumonitis nū-mō-NĪ-tis	Inflammation of the lungs; may follow infection or be caused by asthma, allergy, or inhalation of irritants
pneumothorax nū-mō-THOR-aks	Accumulation of air or gas in the pleural space. May result from injury or disease or may be produced artificially to collapse a lung.
pyothorax pī-ō-THOR-aks	Accumulation of pus in the pleural space; empyema
respiratory distress syndrome (RDS)	A respiratory disorder that affects premature infants born without enough surfactant in the lungs. It is treated with respiratory support and administration of surfactant.
tuberculosis tū-ber-kū-LŌ-sis	An infectious disease caused by the tubercle bacillus, *Mycobacterium tuberculosis.* Often involves the lungs but may involve other parts of the body as well.

DIAGNOSIS

arterial blood gases (ABGs)	The concentrations of gases, specifically oxygen and carbon dioxide, in arterial blood. Reported as the partial pressure (P) of the gas in arterial (a) blood, such as Pao_2 or $Paco_2$. These measurements are important in measuring acid-base balance.
bronchoscope BRONG-kō-skōp	An endoscope used to examine the tracheobronchial passageways. Also allows access for biopsy of tissue to removal of a foreign object (see Fig. 7-3).
lung scan	Study based on the accumulation of radioactive isotope in lung tissue. A *ventilation scan* measures ventilation after inhalation of radioactive material. A *perfusion scan* measures blood supply to the lungs after injection of radioactive material. Also called a pulmonary scintiscan.
pulse oximetry ok-SIM-e-trē	Determination of the oxygen saturation of arterial blood by means of a photoelectric apparatus (oximeter), usually placed on the finger or the ear; reported as Spo_2 in percent (see Fig. 11-9).

Diagnosis, *continued*

pulmonary function tests	Tests done to assess breathing, usually by spirometry
spirometer *spī-ROM-e-ter*	An apparatus used to measure breathing volumes and capacities; record of test is a spirogram
thoracentesis *thor-a-sen-TĒ-sis*	Surgical puncture of the chest for removal of air or fluids, such as may accumulate after surgery or as a result of injury, infection, or cardiovascular problems. Also called thoracocentesis (see Fig. 11-8).
tuberculin test *tū-BER-kū-lin*	A skin test for tuberculosis. Tuberculin, the test material made from products of the tuberculosis organism, is injected below the skin or inoculated with a four-pronged device (tine test).

Supplementary Terms

NORMAL STRUCTURE AND FUNCTION

carina *ka-RI-na*	A projection of the lowest tracheal cartilage that forms a ridge between the two bronchi. Used as a landmark for endoscopy. Any ridge or ridgelike structure (from a Latin word that means "keel").
hilum *HĪ-lum*	A depression in an organ where vessels and nerves enter; also called hilus
nares *NĀ-rēz*	The external openings of the nose; the nostrils (singular, naris)
nasal septum	The partition that divides the nasal cavity into two parts (root *sept/o* means "septum")

SYMPTOMS AND CONDITIONS

anoxia *an-OK-sē-a*	Lack or absence of oxygen in the tissues; often used incorrectly to mean hypoxia
asphyxia *as-FIK-sē-a*	Condition caused by inadequate intake of oxygen; suffocation (literally "lack of pulse")
Biot respirations *bē-Ō*	Deep, fast breathing interrupted by sudden pauses; seen in spinal meningitis and other disorders of the central nervous system
bronchospasm *BRONG-kō-spazm*	Narrowing of the bronchi because of spasm of the smooth muscle in their walls; common in cases of asthma and bronchitis
Cheyne-Stokes respiration *chān-stokes*	A repeating cycle of gradually increased and then decreased respiration followed by a period of apnea; caused by depression of the breathing centers of the nervous system; seen in cases of coma and in terminally ill patients
cor pulmonale *kor pul-mō-NĀ-lē*	Enlargement of the right ventricle of the heart because of disease of the lungs or their blood vessels

Symptoms and Conditions, continued

coryza *kō-RĪ-za*	Acute inflammation of the nasal passages with profuse nasal discharge
croup *krūp*	A childhood disease usually caused by a viral infection that involves inflammation and obstruction of the upper airway. Croup is characterized by a barking cough, difficulty breathing, and laryngeal spasm.
deviated septum	A shifted nasal septum; may require surgical correction
epiglottitis *ep-i-glo-TĪ-tis*	Inflammation of the epiglottis that may lead to obstruction of the upper airway. Commonly seen in cases of croup (also spelled *epiglottiditis*).
epistaxis *ep-i-STAK-sis*	Hemorrhage from the nose; nosebleed (Greek *-staxis* means "dripping")
fremitus *FREM-i-tus*	A vibration, especially as felt through the chest wall on palpation
Kussmaul respiration *KOOS-mawl*	Rapid and deep gasping respiration without pause; characteristic of severe acidosis
pleural friction rub	A sound heard on auscultation that is produced by the rubbing together of the two layers of the pleura; a common sign of pleurisy
rale *rahl*	Abnormal chest sounds heard when air enters small airways or alveoli containing fluid; usually heard during inspiration (plural, rales [*rahlz*])
rhonchi *RONG-kī*	Abnormal chest sounds produced in airways with accumulated fluids; more noticeable during expiration (singular, rhonchus)
stridor *STRĪ-dor*	A harsh, high-pitched sound caused by obstruction of an upper air passageway
tussis *TUS-is*	A cough. An antitussive drug is one that relieves or prevents coughing.
wheeze	A whistling or sighing sound caused by narrowing of a respiratory passageway

DISORDERS

miliary tuberculosis *MIL-ē-ar-ē*	Acute generalized form of tuberculosis with formation of minute tubercles that resemble millet seeds
pertussis *per-TUS-is*	An acute, infectious disease characterized by a cough ending in a whooping inspiration; whooping cough
small cell carcinoma	A highly malignant type of bronchial tumor involving small, undifferentiated cells; "oat cell" carcinoma
sudden infant death syndrome *(SIDS)*	The sudden and unexplained death of an apparently healthy infant; crib death

DIAGNOSIS

Mantoux test *man-TOO*	A test for tuberculosis in which PPD (tuberculin) is injected into the skin. The test does not differentiate active from inactive cases.

Diagnosis, continued

mediastinoscopy *mē-dē-as-ti-NOS-kō-pē*	Examination of the mediastinum by means of an endoscope inserted through an incision above the sternum
plethysmograph *ple-THIZ-mō-graf*	An instrument that measures changes in gas volume and pressure during respiration
pneumotachometer *nū-mō-tak-OM-e-ter*	A device for measuring air flow
thoracoscopy *thor-a-KOS-kō-pē*	Examination of the pleural cavity through an endoscope; pleuroscopy
tine test	A test for tuberculosis in which PPD (tuberculin) is introduced into the skin with a multipronged device. The test does not differentiate active from inactive cases.

TREATMENT

aerosol therapy	Treatment by inhalation of a drug or water in spray form
continuous positive airway pressure (CPAP)	Use of a mechanical respirator to maintain pressure throughout the respiratory cycle in a patient who is breathing spontaneously
extubation	Removal of a previously inserted tube
intermittent positive pressure breathing (IPPB)	Use of a ventilator to inflate the lungs at intervals under positive pressure during inhalation
intermittent positive pressure ventilation (IPPV)	Use of a mechanical ventilator to force air into the lungs while allowing for passive exhalation
nasal cannula *KAN-ū-la*	A two-pronged plastic device inserted into the nostrils for delivery of oxygen (Fig. 11-10)
orthopneic position *or-thop-NĒ-ik*	An upright or semiupright position that aids breathing
positive end-expiratory pressure (PEEP)	Use of a mechanical ventilator to increase the volume of gas in the lungs at the end of exhalation, thus improving gas exchange
postural drainage *POS-tū-ral*	Use of body position to drain secretions from the lungs by gravity. The patient is placed so that secretions will move passively into the larger airways for elimination.
thoracic gas volume **(TGV, V_{TG})**	The volume of gas in the thoracic cavity calculated from measurements made with a body plethysmograph

SURGERY

adenoidectomy *ad-e-noyd-EK-tō-mē*	Surgical removal of the adenoids
intubation *in-tū-BĀ-shun*	Insertion of a tube into a hollow organ, such as into the larynx or trachea for entrance of air (Fig. 11-11). Patients may be intubated during surgery for administration of anesthesia or to maintain an airway. Endotracheal intubation may be used as an emergency measure when airways are blocked.

Surgery, continued

lobectomy *lō-BEK-tō-mē*	Surgical removal of a lobe of the lung or of another organ
pneumoplasty *NŪ-mō-plas-tē*	Plastic surgery of the lung. In *reduction pneumoplasty*, nonfunctional portions of the lung are removed, as in cases of advanced emphysema.
tracheotomy	Incision of the trachea through the neck, usually to establish an airway in cases of tracheal obstruction
tracheostomy	Surgical creation of an opening into the trachea to form an airway or to prepare for the insertion of a tube for ventilation (Fig. 11-12), also the opening thus created

DRUGS

antihistamine *an-ti-HIS-ta-mēn*	Agent that prevents responses mediated by histamine, such as allergic and inflammatory reactions
antitussive *an-ti-TUS-iv*	Drug that prevents or relieves coughing
bronchodilator *brong-kō-DĪ-lā-tor*	Drug that relieves bronchial spasm and widens the bronchi
decongestant *dē-kon-JES-tant*	Agent that reduces congestion or swelling
expectorant *ek-SPEK-tō-rant*	Agent that aids in removal of bronchopulmonary secretions
isoniazid (INH) *ī-sō-NĪ-a-zid*	Drug used to treat tuberculosis
mucolytic *mū-kō-LIT-ik*	Agent that loosens mucus to aid in its removal

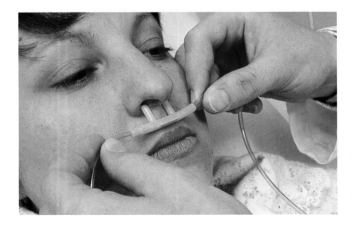

FIGURE 11-10. A nasal cannula. (Reprinted with permission from Taylor C, Lillis C, LeMone P. Fundamentals of Nursing: The Art and Science of Nursing Care. 4th Ed. Philadelphia: Lippincott Williams & Wilkins, 2001.)

Intranasal intubation

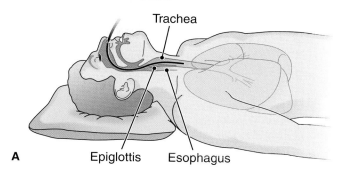

Oral intubation

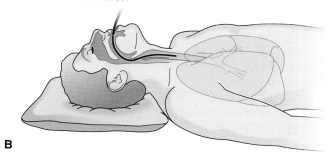

FIGURE 11-11. Endotracheal intubation.
(A) Nasal endotracheal catheter in proper position. **(B)** Oral endotracheal intubation.

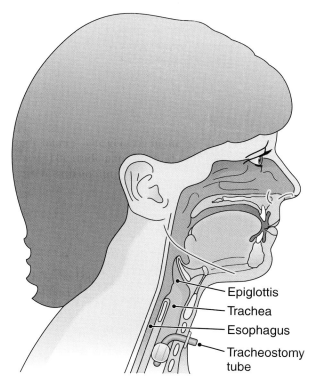

FIGURE 11-12. A tracheostomy tube in place.

ABBREVIATIONS

ABG(s)	Arterial blood gas(es)	**O$_2$**	Oxygen
AFB	Acid-fast bacillus (usually *Myco-bacterium tuberculosis*)	**Paco$_2$**	Arterial partial pressure of carbon dioxide
ARDS	Acute respiratory distress syndrome; shock lung	**Pao$_2$**	Arterial partial pressure of oxygen
ARF	Acute respiratory failure	**PCP**	*Pneumocystis carinii* pneumonia
BS	Breath sounds	**PEEP**	Positive end-expiratory pressure
C	Compliance	**PEFR**	Peak expiratory flow rate
CF	Cystic fibrosis	**PFT**	Pulmonary function test(s)
CO$_2$	Carbon dioxide	**PIP**	Peak inspiratory pressure
COLD	Chronic obstructive lung disease	**PND**	Paroxysmal nocturnal dyspnea
COPD	Chronic obstructive pulmonary disease	**PPD**	Purified protein derivative (tuberculin)
CPAP	Continuous positive airway pressure	**R**	Respiration
CXR	Chest radiograph, chest x-ray	**RDS**	Respiratory distress syndrome
ERV	Expiratory reserve volume	**RLL**	Right lower lobe (of lung)
FEV	Forced expiratory volume	**RML**	Right middle lobe (of lung)
FRC	Functional residual capacity	**RSV**	Respiratory syncytial virus
FVC	Forced vital capacity	**RUL**	Right upper lobe (of lung)
IC	Inspiratory capacity	**RV**	Residual volume
INH	Isoniazid	**SIDS**	Sudden infant death syndrome
IPPB	Intermittent positive pressure breathing	**Spo$_2$**	Oxygen percent saturation
IPPV	Intermittent positive pressure ventilation	**TB**	Tuberculosis
		T & A	Tonsils and adenoids; tonsillectomy and adenoidectomy
IRV	Inspiratory reserve volume	**TGV**	Thoracic gas volume
LLL	Left lower lobe (of lung)	**TLC**	Total lung capacity
LUL	Left upper lobe (of lung)	**TV**	Tidal volume
MEFR	Maximal expiratory flow rate	**URI**	Upper respiratory infection
MMFR	Maximum midexpiratory flow rate	**VC**	Vital capacity
		V$_{TG}$	Thoracic gas volume

Labeling Exercise 11-1

The Respiratory System

Write the name of each numbered part on the corresponding line of the answer sheet.

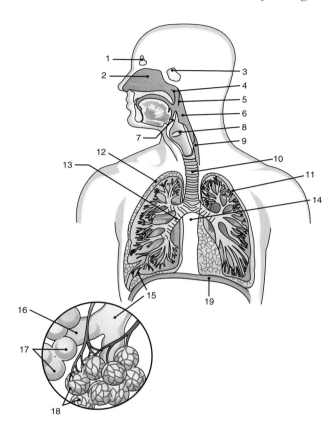

Alveolar duct
Alveoli
Capillaries
Diaphragm
Epiglottis
Esophagus
Frontal sinus
Laryngeal pharynx
Larynx and vocal cords
Left lung
Mediastinum
Nasal cavity
Nasopharynx
Oropharynx
Right bronchus
Right lung
Sphenoidal sinus
Terminal bronchiole
Trachea

1. _____

2. _____

3. _____

4. _____

5. _____

6. _____

7. _____

8. _____

9. _____

10. _____

11. _____

12. _____

13. _____

14. _____

15. _____

16. _____

17. _____

18. _____

19. _____

Chapter Review 11-1

Match the following terms and write the appropriate letter to the left of each number:

_____ 1. aspiration   a. decreased rate and depth of breathing

_____ 2. hypopnea   b. accidental inhalation of foreign material into the lungs

_____ 3. apnea   c. substance that reduces surface tension

_____ 4. surfactant   d. a measure of how easily the lungs expand

_____ 5. compliance   e. cessation of breathing

_____ 6. atelectasis   a. incomplete expansion of lung tissue

_____ 7. concha   b. space and organs between the lungs

_____ 8. glottis   c. expectoration

_____ 9. mediastinum   d. opening between the vocal cords

_____ 10. sputum   e. turbinate bone

_____ 11. COPD   a. volume used in pulmonary function tests

_____ 12. URI   b. respiratory condition seen most often in newborns

_____ 13. FEV   c. a lobe of the lung

_____ 14. LUL   d. respiratory infection of the upper airways

_____ 15. RDS   e. chronic respiratory obstructive condition

SUPPLEMENTARY TERMS

_____ 16. tussis   a. abnormal chest sound

_____ 17. asphyxia   b. cough

_____ 18. rale   c. suffocation

_____ 19. coryza   d. nosebleed

_____ 20. epistaxis   e. inflammation of nasal passages

_____ 21. nares   a. high sound caused by obstruction

_____ 22. croup   b. device used to measure air flow

_____ 23. stridor   c. nostrils

_____ 24. pneumotachometer   d. childhood disease with barking cough

_____ 25. fremitus   e. vibration felt through the chest wall

Fill in the blanks:

26. The dome-shaped muscle under the lungs that flattens during inspiration is the

_____ .

27. The turbinate bones contain receptors for the sense of _____.

28. The double membrane that covers the lungs and lines the thoracic cavity is the

_____.

29. The scientific name for the throat is the _____.

30. The small air sacs in the lungs through which gases are exchanged between the atmosphere and the blood are the _____.

31. The trachea divides into the right and left main stem _____.

32. The vocal cords are located in the _____.

33. A pneumotropic virus is one that invades the _____.

34. The tonsils located in the nasopharynx are commonly called _____.

35. The term *acid-fast bacillus* (AFB) is commonly applied to the organism that causes

_____.

36. A person suffering from orthopnea can breathe comfortably only in a position that is

_____.

SUPPLEMENTARY TERMS

37. The amount of air moved into or out of the lungs in quiet breathing is the

_____.

38. A mucolytic agent dissolves _____.

39. The partition between the two portions of the nasal cavity is the nasal

_____.

40. The amount of air that remains in the lungs after maximal exhalation is the

_____.

Word building. Write a word for each of the following definitions:

41. surgical puncture (-centesis) of the pleurae _____

42. creation of an opening into the trachea _____

43. inflammation of the throat _____

44. inflammation of the bronchioles _____

45. spasm of a bronchus _____

46. hernia of the pleura _____

47. incision of the phrenic nerve _____

The word *thorax* (chest) is used as an ending in compound words that mean the accumulation of substances in the pleural space. Define each of the following terms:

48. pneumothorax   accumulation of air or gas in the pleural space

49. hemothorax _____

50. pyothorax _____

51. hydrothorax _____

Define each of the following words:

52. hypoxemia _____

53. adenoidectomy _____

54. bradypnea _____

55. pneumonitis _____

56. bronchiectasis _____

57. subpulmonary _____

58. rhinoplasty _____

59. pharyngoxerosis _____

Identify and define the root in each of the following words:

	Root	**Meaning of Root**
60. respiration	_____	_____
61. pulmonology	_____	_____
62. empyema	_____	_____
63. phrenodynia	_____	_____
64. pneumonopathy	_____	_____

Opposites. Write a word that has the opposite meaning of each of the following words:

65. hypercapnia _____

66. inspiration _____

67. tachypnea _____

68. intubation _____

69. hypopnea _____

Adjectives. Write the adjective form for each of the following words:

70. alveolus _____

71. pharynx _____

72. pleura _____

73. nose _____

74. trachea _____

75. bronchus _____

Plurals. Write the plural form for each of the following words:

76. naris _____

77. bronchiole _____

78. alveolus _____

79. concha   _____

80. bronchus   _____

Word analysis. Define each of the following words, and give the meaning of the word parts in each. Use a dictionary if necessary.

81. hemoptysis   _____
    a. hem/o   _____
    b. ptysis   _____

82. atelectasis   _____
    a. atel/o-   _____
    b. -ectasis   _____

83. epiglottis   _____
    a. epi-   _____
    b. glottis   _____

Case Studies

Case Study 11-1: Preoperative Testing in a Patient With Asthma

A.D., 15 years old, was seen in the preadmission testing unit in preparation for her elective spinal surgery. She has a history of mild asthma since age 4, with at least one attack per week. In an acute attack, she will have mild dyspnea, diffuse wheezing, yet an adequate air exchange that responds to bronchodilators. She was sent to pulmonary health services for a consult with a specialist and pulmonary function studies to clear her for surgery. The anesthesiologist reviewed the pulmonologist's report.

Her prebronchodilator spirometry showed a mild reduction in vital capacity but with a moderate to severe decrease in FEV_1 and FEV_1/FVC ratio. After bronchodilator administration, there was a mild but insignificant improvement in FEV_1. The postbronchodilator FEV_1 was 55% of predicted and was considered moderately abnormal. The flow volume loops and spirographic curves were consistent with airflow obstruction.

Case Study 11-2: Giant Cell Sarcoma of the Lung

L.E., a 68-year-old man, was admitted to the pulmonary unit with chest pain on inspiration, dyspnea, and diaphoresis. He had smoked $1\frac{1}{2}$ packs of cigarettes per day for 52 years and had quit 3 months ago. L.E. was retired from the advertising industry and admitted to occasional alcohol use. He was treated for primary giant cell sarcoma of the left lung 3 years ago with a lobectomy of the left lung followed by radiation and chemotherapy.

Physical examination was unremarkable except for a thoracotomy scar in the left hemithorax, decreased breath sounds, and dullness to percussion of the left base. There was no hemoptysis. Radionucleotide bone scan showed increased activity in the left upper posterior hemithorax. Chest and upper abdomen CT scan showed findings compatible with recurrent sarcoma of the left hemithorax. Abnormal mediastinal nodes were evident. Thoracentesis was attempted but did not yield fluid. L.E. was scheduled for a left thoracoscopy, mediastinoscopy, and biopsy.

Case Studies, continued

Case Study 11-3: Terminal Dyspnea

N.A., a 76-year-old woman, was in the ICU in the terminal stage of multisystem organ failure. She had been admitted to the hospital for bacterial pneumonia, which had not resolved with antibiotic therapy. She had a 20-year history of COPD. She was not conscious and was unable to breathe on her own. Her ABGs were abnormal, and she was diagnosed with refractory ARDS. The decision was made to support her breathing with endotracheal intubation and mechanical ventilation. After 1 week and several unsuccessful attempts to wean her from the ventilator, the pulmonologist suggested a permanent tracheostomy and family consideration of continuing or withdrawing life support. Her physiologic status met the criteria of remote or no chance for recovery.

N.A.'s family discussed her condition and decided not to pursue aggressive life-sustaining therapies. N.A. was assigned DNR status. After the written orders were read and signed by the family, the endotracheal tube, feeding tube, pulse oximeter, and ECG electrodes were removed and a morphine IV drip was started with prn boluses ordered to promote comfort and relieve pain and other symptoms of dying. The family sat with N.A. for many hours while her breaths became shallow with Cheyne-Stokes respirations. She died surrounded by her family, joined by the hospital chaplain.

CASE STUDY QUESTIONS

Multiple choice: Select the best answer and write the letter of your choice to the left of each number.

_____ 1. The root *spir/o*, as in *spirometry*, means:
   a. turbulence
   b. breathing
   c. twisted
   d. air quality
   e. saturation

_____ 2. The root *pulmon*, as in *pulmonary*, means:
   a. chest
   b. air
   c. lung
   d. breath sound
   e. blood vessel

_____ 3. Hemoptysis is:
   a. drooping eyelids
   b. discoloration of skin
   c. blue nail beds
   d. spitting of blood
   e. acute leukemia

_____ 4. Dyspnea could NOT be described as:
   a. difficulty breathing
   b. eupnea
   c. air hunger
   d. orthopnea
   e. Cheyne-Stokes respirations

Case Studies, continued

_____ 5. Pulse oximetry is used to measure:
   a. partial pressure of oxygen in the blood
   b. tidal volume
   c. end-tidal CO_2
   d. oxygen saturation of blood
   e. positive end-expiratory pressure

_____ 6. An endotracheal tube is placed:
   a. under the trachea
   b. beyond the carina
   c. within the bronchus
   d. around the airway
   e. within the trachea

Write the word in the case histories with each of the following meanings:

7. Removal of a lobe   _____

8. Profuse sweating   _____

9. Surgical puncture of the chest   _____

10. A drug that enlarges the lumen of the bronchi   _____

11. Endoscopic examination of the chest cavity   _____

12. Half of the chest   _____

13. Movement of air into and out of the lungs   _____

14. A lung infection   _____

15. Whistling breath sounds due to narrowing of   _____
    the breathing passageways

16. Endoscopic examination of the space between the lungs _____

Abbreviations. Define the following abbreviations:

17. COPD _____

18. FEV _____

19. FVC _____

20. ABG _____

21. ARDS _____

22. DNR _____

Chapter 11 Crossword
The Respiratory System

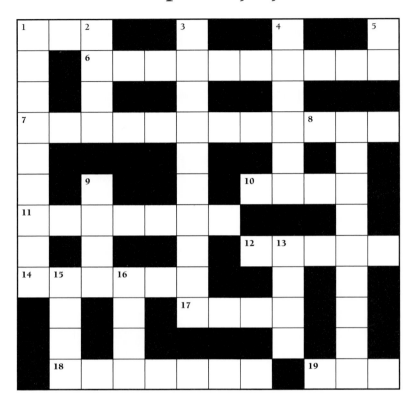

ACROSS

1. Drug used to treat tuberculosis (abbreviation)
6. Portion of the throat behind the mouth
7. Instrument used to examine the larynx
10. Blood: combining form
11. RDS may appear in a newborn, also called a(n)
12. Rapid: prefix
14. Respiratory disease involving constriction of the bronchial tubes
17. An organ of respiration
18. Abnormal chest sounds
19. Diagnostic imaging test (abbreviation)

DOWN

1. Infectious disease of the respiratory tract
2. The abbreviation qh means every _____
3. Pertaining to the cartilage above the larynx
4. The tube between the throat and the bronchi: root
5. Diagnosis (abbreviation)
8. Accumulation of pus in the pleural space
9. After, behind: prefix
13. Vessel: root
15. Breathing: root
16. Under, below, decreased: prefix

CHAPTER 11 Answer Section

Answers to Chapter Exercises

EXERCISE 11-1

1. dyspnea (*DISP-nē-a*)
2. eupnea (*ŪP-nē-a*)
3. apnea (*AP-nē-a*)
4. tachypnea (*tak-ip-NĒ-a*)
5. dyspneic (*disp-NĒ-ik*)
6. eupneic (*ūp-NĒ-ik*)
7. apneic (*AP-nē-ik*)
8. tachypneic (*tak-ip-NĒ-ik*)
9. anoxia (*an-OK-sē-a*)
10. hypocapnia (*hī-pō-KAP-nē-a*)
11. eucapnia (*ū-KAP-nē-a*)
12. aphonia (*a-FŌ-nē-a*)

EXERCISE 11-2

1. paranasal (*par-a-NA-zal*)
2. pharyngitis (*far-in-JĪ-tis*)
3. laryngeal (*la-RIN-jē-al*)
4. bronchoscopy (*brong-KOS-kō-pe*)
5. bronchiolitis (*brong-kē-ō-LĪ-tis*)
6. bronchostenosis (*brong-ko-ste-NŌ-sis*)
7. laryngoplasty (*la-RING-gō-plas-tē*)
8. tracheotomy (*trā-kē-OT-ō-mē*)
9. within the nose
10. pertaining to a bronchiole
11. dilatation of the bronchi
12. around the bronchi
13. within the trachea
14. pertaining to the nose and pharynx

EXERCISE 11-3

1. inflammation of the lungs
2. pertaining to the pleura and lungs
3. plastic repair of the lungs
4. pain in the pleura
5. study of the lungs
6. pertaining to air or gas
7. interpleural (*in-ter-PLŪ-ral*)
8. subphrenic (*sub-FREN-ik*)
9. phrenicotomy (*fren-i-KOT-ō-mē*)
10. pneumonopathy (*nu-mō-NOP-a-thē*)
11. spirogram (*SPĪ-rō-gram*)
12. pleurocentesis (*plū-rō-sen-TĒ-sis*)

LABELING EXERCISE 11-1
RESPIRATORY SYSTEM

1. frontal sinus
2. nasal cavity
3. sphenoidal sinus
4. nasopharynx
5. oropharynx
6. laryngeal pharynx
7. epiglottis
8. larynx and vocal cords
9. esophagus
10. trachea
11. left lung
12. right lung
13. right bronchus
14. mediastinum
15. terminal bronchiole
16. alveolar duct
17. alveoli
18. capillaries
19. diaphragm

Answers to Chapter Review 11-1

1. b
2. a
3. e
4. c
5. d
6. a
7. e
8. d
9. b
10. c
11. e
12. d
13. a
14. c
15. b
16. b
17. c
18. a
19. e
20. d
21. c
22. d
23. a
24. b
25. e

26. diaphragm
27. smell
28. pleura
29. pharynx
30. alveoli
31. bronchi
32. larynx
33. lungs
34. adenoids
35. tuberculosis
36. upright
37. tidal volume
38. mucus
39. septum
40. residual volume
41. pleurocentesis (plū-rō-sen-TĒ-sis)
42. tracheostomy (tra-kē-OS-tō-mē)
43. pharyngitis (far-in-JĪ-tis)
44. bronchiolitis (brong-kē-ō-LĪ-tis)
45. bronchospasm (brong-kō-spazm)
46. pleurocele (PLŪ-rō-sēl)
47. phrenicotomy (fren-i-KOT-ō-mē)
48. accumulation of air or gas in the pleural space
49. accumulation of blood in the pleural space
50. accumulation of pus in the pleural space
51. accumulation of fluid in the pleural space
52. deficiency of oxygen in the blood
53. excision of the adenoids
54. slow rate of respiration
55. inflammation of the lungs
56. dilatation of the bronchi
57. below the lungs
58. plastic repair of the nose
59. dryness of the throat
60. spir/o; breathing
61. pulmon/o; lung
62. py/o; pus
63. phren/o; diaphragm
64. pneumon/o; lung
65. hypocapnia
66. expiration
67. bradypnea
68. extubation
69. hyperpnea

70. alveolar
71. pharyngeal
72. pleural
73. nasal
74. tracheal
75. bronchial
76. nares
77. bronchioles
78. alveoli
79. conchae
80. bronchi
81. spitting blood
   a. blood
   b. spitting
82. incomplete expansion of the alveoli
   a. incomplete
   b. expansion, dilation
83. the cartilage that covers the larynx during swallowing
   a. over, upon
   b. the space between the vocal cords

Answers to Case Study Questions
1. b
2. c
3. d
4. b
5. d
6. e
7. lobectomy
8. diaphoresis
9. thoracotomy
10. bronchodilator
11. thoracoscopy
12. hemithorax
13. ventilation
14. pneumonia
15. wheezing
16. mediastinoscopy
17. chronic obstructive pulmonary disease
18. forced expiratory volume
19. forced vital capacity
20. arterial blood gas
21. adult respiratory distress syndrome
22. do not resuscitate

ANSWERS TO CROSSWORD PUZZLE

The Respiratory System

1 I	N	2 H		3 E		4 T		5 D
N		6 O	R	O	P	H	A	R	Y	N	X
F		U			I		A			
7 L	A	R	Y	N	G	O	S	C	8 P	E
U				L		H		Y		
E		9 P		O		10 H	E	M	O	
11 N	E	O	N	A	T	E			T	
Z		S		T		12 T	13 A	C	H	Y
14 A	15 S	T	16 H	M	A		N		O	
	P		Y		17 L	U	N	G		R	
	I		P					I		A	
	18 R	H	O	N	C	H	I		19 C	X	R

Digestion

Chapter Contents

Objectives

After study of this chapter you should be able to:

1. Explain the function of the digestive system.
2. Label a diagram of the digestive tract, and describe the function of each part.
3. Label a diagram of the accessory organs, and explain the role of each in digestion.
4. Identify and use the roots pertaining to the digestive system.
5. Describe the major disorders of the digestive system.
6. Define medical terms used in reference to the digestive system.
7. Interpret abbreviations used in referring to the gastrointestinal system.
8. Analyze case studies concerning gastroenterology.

The function of the digestive system (Fig. 12-1) is to prepare food for intake by body cells. Nutrients must be broken down by mechanical and chemical means into molecules that are small enough to be absorbed into the circulation. Within cells, the nutrients are used for energy and for rebuilding vital cell components. Digestion takes place in the digestive tract proper, also called the alimentary canal or gastrointestinal (GI) tract. Also contributing to the digestive process are several accessory organs that release secretions into the small intestine. Food is moved through the digestive tract by **peristalsis**, wavelike contractions of the organ walls. Peristalsis also moves undigested waste material out of the body.

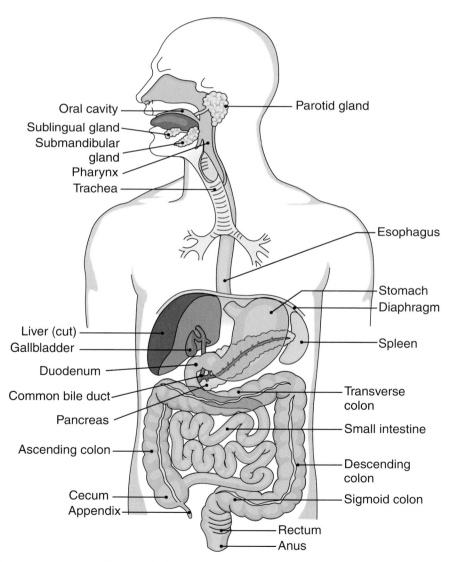

FIGURE 12-1. Digestive system. (Reprinted with permission from Cohen BJ, Wood DL. Memmler's The Human Body in Health and Disease. 9th Ed. Philadelphia: Lippincott Williams & Wilkins, 2000.)

The Mouth to the Small Intestine

Digestion begins in the **mouth** (Fig. 12-2), where food is chewed into small bits by the teeth (Fig. 12-3). In the process of chewing, or **mastication**, the tongue and the **palate**, the roof of the mouth, help to break up the food and mix it with **saliva**, a secretion that moistens the food and begins the digestion of starch. The moistened food is then passed into the pharynx (throat) and through the **esophagus** into the **stomach**. Here

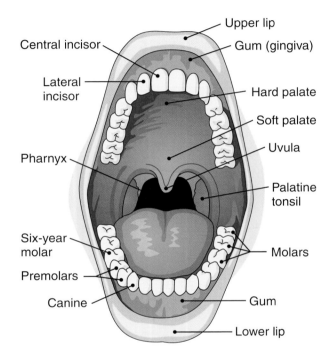

FIGURE 12-2. The mouth, showing the teeth, pharynx, and tonsils. (Reprinted with permission from Cohen BJ, Wood DL. Memmler's The Human Body in Health and Disease. 9th Ed. Philadelphia: Lippincott Williams & Wilkins, 2000.)

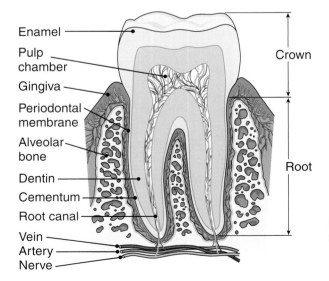

FIGURE 12-3. A molar tooth. (Reprinted with permission from Cohen BJ, Wood DL. Memmler's The Human Body in Health and Disease. 9th Ed. Philadelphia: Lippincott Williams & Wilkins, 2000.)

it is further broken down by churning of the stomach as it is mixed with the enzyme pepsin and with powerful hydrochloric acid (HCl), both of which break down proteins.

The partially digested food passes through the lower portion of the stomach, the **pylorus**, into the first part of the small intestine, the **duodenum**. As the food continues through the **jejunum** and **ileum**, the remaining sections of the small intestine, digestion is completed. The substances active in digestion in the small intestine include enzymes from the intestine itself and secretions from the accessory organs of digestion. The digested nutrients, as well as water, minerals, and vitamins, are absorbed into the circulation, aided by small projections in the lining of the small intestine called **villi**.

The Accessory Organs

The accessory organs of digestion are illustrated in Figure 12-4. The **liver** is a large gland with many functions. A major part of its activity is to process blood brought to it by a special circulatory pathway called the **hepatic portal system**. Its role in digestion is the secretion of **bile**, which breaks down fats. Bile is stored in the **gallbladder** until needed. The common hepatic duct from the liver and the cystic duct from the gallbladder merge to form the **common bile duct**, which empties into the duodenum. The **pancreas** produces a mixture of digestive enzymes that is delivered into the duodenum through the pancreatic duct.

The Large Intestine

Undigested food, water, and digestive juices pass into the large **intestine**. This part of the digestive tract begins in the lower right region of the abdomen with a small pouch, the **cecum**, to which the **appendix** is attached. The large intestine continues as the **colon**, a name that is often used to mean the large intestine because the colon constitutes such a large portion of that organ. The colon travels upward along the right side of the abdomen as the ascending colon, crosses below the stomach as the transverse colon, then continues down the left side of the abdomen as the descending colon. As food is pushed through the colon, water is reabsorbed and stool or **feces** is formed. This waste material passes into the S-shaped **sigmoid colon** and is stored in the **rectum** until eliminated through the **anus**.

BOX 12-1 Homonyms

Homonyms are words that sound alike but have different meanings. One must know the context in which they are used to tell what meaning is meant. For example, the ilium is the upper portion of the pelvis, but the ileum is the last portion of the small intestine. Different adjectives are preferred for each, iliac for the first and ileal for the second.

The word meiosis refers to the type of cell division that halves the chromosomes to form the gametes, but miosis means abnormal contraction of the pupil. Both words come from the Greek word that means a decrease.

Similar-sounding names lead to some funny misspellings. The large bone of the upper arm is the humerus, but this bone is often written as humorous. The vagus nerve (cranial nerve X) is named with a root that means "wander," as in the words vague and vagabond, because this nerve branches to many of the internal organs. Students often write the name as if it had some relation to the famous gambling city in Nevada.

Homonyms may have a more serious side as well. Drug names may sound or look so similar that clinicians confuse them, leading to some dangerous situations.

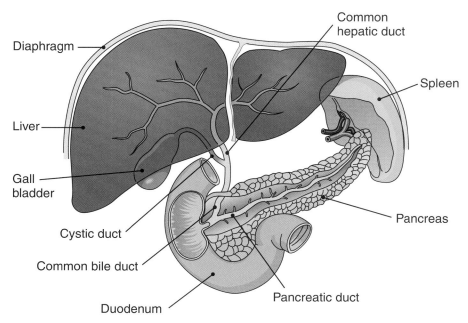

FIGURE 12-4. Accessory organs of digestion. (Reprinted with permission from Cohen BJ, Wood DL. Memmler's The Human Body in Health and Disease. 9th Ed. Philadelphia: Lippincott Williams & Wilkins, 2000.)

Key Terms

NORMAL STRUCTURE AND FUNCTION

anus $\bar{A}$-nus	The distal opening of the digestive tract (root *an/o*)
appendix a-PEN-diks	An appendage; usually means the narrow tube attached to the cecum, the vermiform (wormlike) appendix
bile $b\bar{i}l$	The fluid secreted by the liver that aids in the digestion and absorption of fats (roots *chol/e, bili*)
cecum S$\bar{E}$-kum	A blind pouch at the beginning of the large intestine (root *cec/o*)
colon K$\bar{O}$-lon	The major portion of the large intestine; extends from the cecum to the rectum and is formed by ascending, transverse, and descending portions (root *col/o, colon/o*)
common bile duct	The duct that carries bile into the duodenum; formed by the union of the cystic duct and the common hepatic duct (root *choledoch/o*)
duodenum $d\bar{u}$-$\bar{o}$-D$\bar{E}$-num	The first portion of the small intestine (root *duoden/o*)

Normal Structure and Function, *continued*

esophagus *e-SOF-a-gus*	The muscular tube that carries food from the pharynx to the stomach. The opening of the esophagus into the stomach is controlled by the lower esophageal sphincter (LES) (root *esphag/o*).
feces *FĒ-sēz*	The waste material eliminated from the intestine (adjective, fecal); stool
gallbladder	A sac on the undersurface of the liver that stores bile (root *cholecyst/o*)
hepatic portal system	A special pathway of the circulation that brings blood directly from the abdominal organs to the liver for processing (also called simply the *portal system*). The vessel that enters the liver is the hepatic portal vein (portal vein).
ileum *IL-ē-um*	The terminal portion of the small intestine (root *ile/o*)
intestine *in-TES-tin*	The portion of the digestive tract between the stomach and the anus. It consists of the small intestine and large intestine. It functions in digestion, absorption, and elimination of waste (root *enter/o*).
jejunum *je-JŪ-num*	The middle portion of the small intestine (root *jejun/o*)
liver *LIV-er*	The large gland in the upper right part of the abdomen. In addition to many other functions, it secretes bile for digestion of fats (root *hepat/o*).
mastication *mas-ti-KĀ-shun*	Chewing
pancreas *PAN-krē-as*	A large, elongated gland behind the stomach. It produces hormones that regulate sugar metabolism and also produces digestive enzymes (root *pancreat/o*).
palate *PAL-at*	The roof of the mouth; the partition between the mouth and nasal cavity; consists of an anterior portion formed by bone, the hard palate, and a posterior portion formed of tissue, the soft palate (root *palat/o*)
peristalsis *per-i-STAL-sis*	Wavelike contractions of the walls of an organ
pylorus *pī-LOR-us*	The distal opening of the stomach into the duodenum. The opening is controlled by a ring of muscle, the pyloric sphincter (root *pylor/o*).
rectum *REK-tum*	The distal portion of the large intestine. It stores and eliminates undigested waste (root *rect/o, proct/o*).
saliva *sa-LĪ-va*	The clear secretion released into the mouth that moistens food and contains an enzyme that digests starch. It is produced by three pairs of glands: the parotid, submandibular, and sublingual glands (see Fig. 12-1) (root *sial/o*).
stomach *STUM-ak*	A muscular saclike organ below the diaphragm that stores food and secretes juices that digest proteins (root *gastr/o*)
villi *VIL-Ī*	Tiny projections in the lining of the small intestine that absorb digested foods into the circulation (singular, villus)

Roots Pertaining to Digestion

TABLE 12-1 Roots for the Mouth

ROOT	MEANING	EXAMPLE	DEFINITION OF EXAMPLE
or/o	mouth	perioral per-ē-OR-al	around the mouth
stoma, stomat/o	mouth	stomatitis stō-ma-TĪ-tis	inflammation of the mouth
gnath/o	jaw	prognathous PROG-na-thus	having a projecting jaw
labi/o	lip	labiodental lā-bē-ō-DEN-tal	pertaining to the lip and teeth (dent/o)
bucc/o	cheek	buccoversion buk-kō-VER-zhun	turning toward the cheek
dent/o, dent/i	tooth, teeth	dentifrice DEN-ti-fris	a substance used to clean the teeth
odont/o	tooth, teeth	periodontist per-ē-ō-DON-tist	dentist who treats the tissues around the teeth
gingiv/o	gum (gingiva)	gingivectomy jin-ji-VEK-tō-mē	excision of gum tissue
lingu/o	tongue	sublingual sub-LING-gwal	under the tongue
gloss/o	tongue	glossopharyngeal glos-ō-fa-RIN-gē-al	pertaining to the tongue and pharynx
sial/o	saliva, salivary gland, salivary duct	sialogram sī-AL-ō-gram	radiograph of the salivary glands and ducts
palat/o	palate	palatorrhaphy pal-at-OR-a-fē	suture of the palate

Exercise 12-1

Use the adjective suffix *-al* to write a word that has the same meaning as each of the following:

1. pertaining to the mouth   _____oral_____

2. pertaining to the teeth   _____

3. pertaining to the gums   _____

4. pertaining to the tongue   _____

5. pertaining to the cheek   _____

6. pertaining to the lip   _____

Fill in the blanks:

7. Micrognathia (*mī-krō-NĀ-thē-a*) is excessive smallness of the _____.

8. Hemiglossal (*hem-ī-GLOS-al*) means pertaining to one half of the

    _____.

9. Stomatosis (*stō-ma-TŌ-sis*) is any disease condition of the _____.

10. The oropharynx is the part of the pharynx that is located behind the

    _____.

11. A sialolith (*sī-AL-ō-lith*) is a stone formed in a _____ gland or duct.

12. Orthodontics (*or-thō-DON-tiks*) is the branch of dentistry that deals with straightening (ortho-) of the

    _____.

13. Xerostomia (*zē-rō-STŌ-mē-a*) is dryness of the _____.

Define each of the following words:

14. orolingual (*or-o-LING-gwal*)   _____

15. palatine (*PAL-a-tīn*)   _____

16. gingivitis (*jin-ji-VĪ-tis*)   _____

17. glossolabial (*glos-ō-LĀ-bē-al*)   _____

18. extrabuccal (*ex-tra-BUK-al*)   _____

TABLE 12-2 Roots for the Digestive Tract (Except the Mouth)

ROOT	MEANING	EXAMPLE	DEFINITION OF EXAMPLE
esophag/o	esophagus	esophageal* *e-sof-a-JĒ-al*	pertaining to the esophagus
gastr/o	stomach	gastroparesis *gas-trō-pa-RĒ-sis*	partial paralysis of the stomach
pylor/o	pylorus	pylorostenosis *pī-lor-ō-ste-NŌ-sis*	narrowing of the pylorus
enter/o	intestine	dysentery *DIS-en-ter-ē*	infectious disease of the intestine
duoden/o	duodenum	duodenoscopy *du-o-de-NOS-ko-pe*	endoscopic examination of the duodenum
jejun/o	jejunum	jejunotomy *je-jū-NOT-ō-mē*	incision of the jejunum
ile/o	ileum	ileectomy *il-ē-EK-tō-mē*	excision of the ileum
cec/o	cecum	cecoptosis *sē-kop-TŌ-sis*	downward displacement of the cecum
col/o, colon/o	colon	colocentesis *kō-lō-sen-TĒ-sis*	surgical puncture of the colon
sigmoid/o	sigmoid colon	sigmoidoscope *sig-MOY-dō-skōp*	an endoscope for examining the sigmoid colon

TABLE 12-2 Roots for the Digestive Tract, *continued*

ROOT	MEANING	EXAMPLE	DEFINITION OF EXAMPLE
rect/o	rectum	rectocele *REK-tō-sēl*	hernia of the rectum
proct/o	rectum	proctopexy *PROK-tō-pek-sē*	surgical fixation of the rectum
an/o	anus	transanal *ā-nō-REK-tal*	through the anus

*Note addition of e before -al.

Exercise 12-2

Use the adjective suffix -*ic* to write a word that means each of the following:

1. pertaining to the intestine   enteric

2. pertaining to the stomach   _____

3. pertaining to the colon   _____

4. pertaining to the pylorus   _____

Use the adjective suffix -*al* to write a word that means each of the following:

5. pertaining to the duodenum   duodenal

6. pertaining to the cecum   _____

7. pertaining to the jejunum   _____

8. pertaining to the ileum   _____

9. pertaining to the rectum   _____

10. pertaining to the anus   _____

Write a word for each of the following definitions:

11. surgical fixation of the stomach   _____

12. endoscopic examination of the esophagus   _____

13. plastic repair of the pylorus   _____

14. inflammation of the ileum   _____

15. surgical creation of an opening into the duodenum   _____

16. surgical creation of an opening into the ileum   _____

17. study of the stomach and intestines   _____

Use the root *col/o* to write a word for each of the following definitions:

18. inflammation of the colon _____

19. surgical fixation of the colon _____

20. surgical creation of an opening into the colon _____

21. irrigation (-clysis) of the colon _____

Use the root *colon/o* to write a word for each of the following definitions:

22. any disease of the colon _____

23. endoscopic examination of the colon _____

Two organs of the digestive tract or even two parts of the same organ may be surgically connected by a passage (anastomosis) after removal of damaged tissue. Such a procedure is named for the connected organs plus the ending *-stomy*. Use two roots plus the suffix *-stomy* to write a word that has the same meaning as each of the following definitions:

24. surgical creation of a passage between the esophagus and stomach _____esophagogastrostomy_____

25. surgical creation of a passage between the stomach and intestine _____

26. surgical creation of a passage between the stomach and the jejunum _____

27. surgical creation of a passage between the duodenum and the ileum _____

28. surgical creation of a passage between the sigmoid colon and the rectum (proct/o) _____

TABLE 12-3 Roots for the Accessory Organs

ROOT	MEANING	EXAMPLE	DEFINITION OF EXAMPLE
hepat/o	liver	hepatocyte *HEP-a-tō-sīt*	a liver cell
bili	bile	biliary *BIL-ē-ar-ē*	pertaining to the bile or bile ducts
chol/e, chol/o	bile, gall	cholelith *KŌ-lē-lith*	gallstone, biliary calculus
cholecyst/o	gallbladder	cholecystorrhaphy *kō-lē-sis-TOR-a-fē*	suture of the gallbladder
cholangi/o	bile duct	cholangiogram *kō-LAN-jē-ō-gram*	radiograph of the bile ducts
choledoch/o	common bile duct	choledochal *kō-LED-o-kal*	pertaining to the common bile duct
pancreat/o	pancreas	pancreatolysis *pan-krē-a-TOL-i-sis*	dissolving of the pancreas

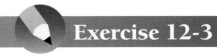

Exercise 12-3

Use the suffix *-ic* to write a word for each of the following definitions:

1. pertaining to the liver   _____

2. pertaining to the gallbladder   _____

3. pertaining to the pancreas   _____

Use the suffix *-graphy* to write a word for each of the following definitions:

4. radiographic study of the bile ducts   _____

5. radiographic study of the liver   _____

6. radiographic study of the gallbladder   _____

7. radiographic study of the pancreas   _____

Use the suffix *-lithiasis* to write a word for each of the following definitions:

8. condition of having a stone in the common bile duct   _____

9. condition of having a stone in the pancreas   _____

Fill in the blanks:

10. The word biligenesis (*bil-i-JEN-e-sis*) means the formation of _____.

11. Choledochotomy (*kō-led-o-KOT-o-mē*) is incision of the _____.

12. Hepatomegaly (*hep-a-tō-MEG-a-lē*) is enlargement of the _____.

13. A word that means inflammation of the liver is _____.

14. A pancreatotropic (*pan-krē-at-ō-TROP-ik*) substance acts on the _____.

15. Cholangitis is inflammation of a(n) _____.

Clinical Aspects of Digestion

Gastrointestinal Tract

INFECTION

A variety of organisms can infect the gastrointestinal tract, from viruses and bacteria to protozoa and worms. Some produce short-lived upsets with **gastroenteritis, nausea, diarrhea**, and **emesis** (vomiting). Others, such as typhoid, cholera, and dysentery, are more serious, even fatal.

ULCERS

An ulcer is a lesion of the skin or a mucous membrane marked by inflammation and tissue damage. Ulcers caused by the damaging action of gastric, or peptic, juices on the lining of the GI tract are termed **peptic ulcers**. Most peptic ulcers appear in the first portion of the duodenum. The origins of such ulcers are not completely known, although infection with a bacterium, *Helicobacter pylori*, has been identified as a major cause. Heredity and stress may be factors as well as chronic inflammation and exposure to damaging drugs, such as

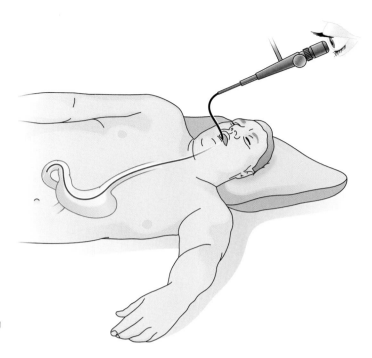

FIGURE 12-5. Patient undergoing gastroscopy.

aspirin, or to irritants in food and drink. Current treatment includes the administration of antibiotics to eliminate *H. pylori* infection and use of drugs that block the action of histamine, which stimulates gastric secretion. Ulcers may lead to hemorrhage or to perforation of the digestive tract wall.

Ulcers can be diagnosed by **endoscopy** (Fig. 12-5) and by radiographic study of the GI tract using a contrast medium, usually barium sulfate. A **barium study** can reveal a variety of GI disorders in addition to ulcers, including tumors and obstructions. A barium swallow is used for study of the pharynx and esophagus; an upper GI series examines the esophagus, stomach, and small intestine.

CANCER

The most common sites for cancer of the GI tract are the colon and rectum. Together these colorectal cancers rank among the most frequent causes of cancer deaths in the United States in both men and women. A diet low in fiber and calcium and high in fat is a major risk factor in colorectal cancer. Heredity is also a factor, as is chronic inflammation of the colon (colitis). **Polyps** (growths) in the intestine often become cancerous and should be removed. Polyps can be identified and even removed by endoscopy.

One sign of colorectal cancer is bleeding into the intestine, which can be detected by testing the stool for blood. Because this blood may be present in very small amounts, it is described as **occult** ("hidden") **blood**. Colorectal cancers are staged according to **Dukes classification**, ranging from A to C according to severity.

The interior of the intestine can be observed with various endoscopes named for the specific area in which they are used, such as proctoscope (rectum), sigmoidoscope (sigmoid colon) (Fig. 12-6), colonoscope (colon).

In some cases of cancer, and for other reasons as well, it may be necessary to surgically remove a portion of the GI tract and create a **stoma** (opening) on the abdominal wall for elimination of waste. Such **ostomy** surgery (Fig. 12-7) is named for the organ involved, such as ileostomy (ileum) or colostomy (colon). When a connection **(anastomosis)** is formed between two organs of the tract, both organs are included in naming, such as gastroduodenostomy (stomach and duodenum) or coloproctostomy (colon and rectum).

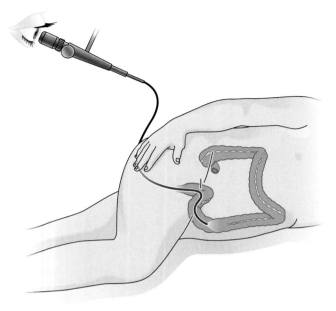

FIGURE 12-6. Sigmoidoscopy. The flexible fiberoptic endoscope is advanced past the proximal sigmoid colon and then into the descending colon.

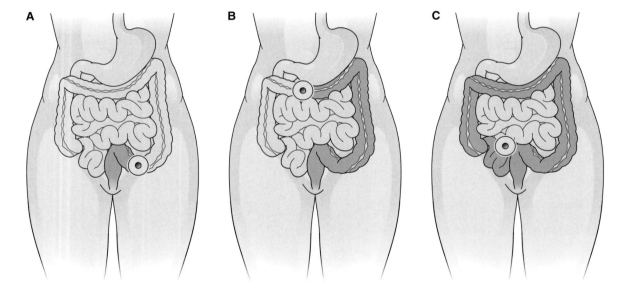

FIGURE 12-7. Location of various colostomies. The shaded portions represent the sections of the bowel that have been removed or are inactive. **(A)** Sigmoid colostomy. **(B)** Transverse colostomy. **(C)** Ileostomy.

OBSTRUCTIONS

A hernia is the protrusion of an organ through an abnormal opening. The most common type is an inguinal hernia, described in Chapter 14 (see Fig. 14-4). In a **hiatal hernia**, part of the stomach moves upward into the chest cavity through the space (hiatus) in the diaphragm where the esophagus passes through (see Fig. 6-5). Often this condition produces no symptoms, but it may result in chest pain, **dysphagia** (difficulty in swallowing), or reflux of stomach contents into the esophagus.

In **pyloric stenosis**, the opening between the stomach and small intestine is too narrow. This usually occurs in infants and in male more often than in female subjects. A sign of pyloric stenosis is projectile vomiting. Surgery may be needed to correct it.

Other types of obstruction include **intussusception** (Fig. 12-8), slipping of a part of the intestine into a part below it; **volvulus**, twisting of the intestine (see Fig. 12-8); and **ileus**, intestinal obstruction often caused by lack of peristalsis. **Hemorrhoids** are varicose veins in the rectum associated with pain, bleeding, and, in some cases, prolapse of the rectum.

APPENDICITIS

Appendicitis results from infection of the appendix, often secondary to its obstruction. Surgery is necessary to avoid rupture and **peritonitis**, infection of the peritoneal cavity.

DIVERTICULITIS

Diverticula are small pouches in the wall of the intestine, most commonly in the colon. If these pouches are present in large number the condition is termed **diverticulosis**, which has been attributed to a diet low in fiber. Collection of waste and bacteria in these sacs leads to **diverticulitis**, which is accompanied by pain and sometimes bleeding. Diverticula can be seen by radiographic studies of the lower GI tract using barium as a contrast medium, a so-called barium enema (Fig. 12-9). Although there is no cure, diverticulitis is treated with diet, stool softeners, and drugs to reduce motility (antispasmodics).

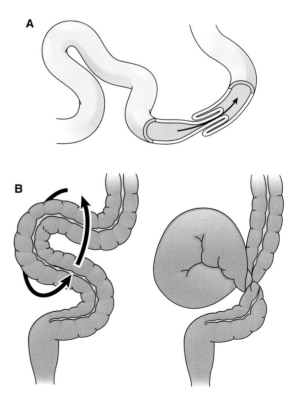

FIGURE 12-8. Intestinal obstruction. **(A)** Intussusception. **(B)** Volvulus, showing counterclockwise twist.

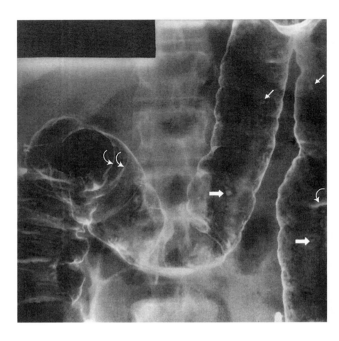

FIGURE 12-9. Lower gastrointestinal series (barium enema) showing lesions of enteritis (*straight arrows*) and thickened mucosa (*curved arrows*). (Reprinted with permission from Erkonen WE, Smith WL. Radiology 101: Basics and Fundamentals of Imaging. Philadelphia: Lippincott Williams & Wilkins, 1998.)

INFLAMMATORY BOWEL DISEASE

Two similar diseases are included under the heading of inflammatory bowel disease (IBD): **Crohn disease** and **ulcerative colitis**, both of which occur mainly in adolescents and young adults. Crohn disease is a chronic inflammation of segments of the intestinal wall, usually in the ileum, causing pain, diarrhea, abscess, and often formation of an abnormal passageway, or **fistula**. Ulcerative colitis involves a continuous inflammation of the lining of the colon and usually the rectum.

Accessory Organs

HEPATITIS

In the United States and other industrialized countries, **hepatitis** is most often caused by viral infection. More than six types of hepatitis virus have now been identified. The most common is hepatitis A virus (HAV), which is spread by fecal–oral contamination, often by food handlers, and in crowded, unsanitary conditions. It may also be acquired by eating contaminated food, especially seafood. Hepatitis B virus (HBV) is spread by blood and other body fluids. It may be transmitted sexually, by sharing needles used for injection, and by close interpersonal contact. Infected individuals may become carriers of the disease. Most patients recover, but the disease may be serious, even fatal, and may lead to liver cancer. Hepatitis C is spread through blood and blood products or by close contact with an infected person. Hepatitis D, the delta virus, is highly pathogenic but only infects those already infected with hepatitis B. Hepatitis E, like HAV, is spread by contaminated food and water. It has caused epidemics in Asia, Africa, and Mexico. Hepatitis G is believed to be spread through contact with blood of an infected person. Vaccines are available for hepatitis A and B.

The name *hepatitis* simply means "inflammation of the liver," but this disease also causes necrosis (death) of liver cells. Hepatitis also may be caused by other infections and by drugs and toxins. Liver function tests performed on blood serum are important in diagnosis.

Jaundice, or **icterus**, is a symptom of hepatitis and other diseases of the liver and biliary system. It appears as yellowness of the skin, whites of the eyes, and mucous membranes caused by the presence of bile pigments, mainly **bilirubin**, in the blood.

CIRRHOSIS

Cirrhosis is a chronic liver disease characterized by **hepatomegaly**, edema, **ascites**, and jaundice. As the disease progresses there is **splenomegaly**, internal bleeding, and brain damage caused by changes in the composition of the blood. A complication of cirrhosis is increased pressure in the portal system that brings blood from the abdominal organs to the liver, a condition called **portal hypertension**. The main cause of cirrhosis is the excess consumption of alcohol.

GALLSTONES

Cholelithiasis refers to the presence of stones in the gallbladder or bile ducts, which is usually associated with **cholecystitis**, inflammation of the gallbladder. Most of these stones are composed of cholesterol, an ingredient of bile. Gallstones form more commonly in women than in men, especially in women on oral contraceptives and in those who have had several pregnancies. The condition is characterized by biliary **colic** (pain) in the right upper quadrant (RUQ), nausea, and vomiting. Drugs may be used to dissolve gallstones, but often the cure is removal of the gallbladder in a **cholecystectomy**. This procedure was originally performed through a major abdominal incision, but now the gallbladder is almost always removed laparoscopically through a small incision in the abdomen.

Ultrasonography and radiography are used for diagnosis of gallstones. **Endoscopic retrograde cholangiopancreatography (ERCP)** (Fig. 12-10) is a technique for viewing the pancreatic and bile ducts and for performing certain techniques to relieve obstructions. Contrast medium is injected into the biliary system from the duodenum and radiographs are taken.

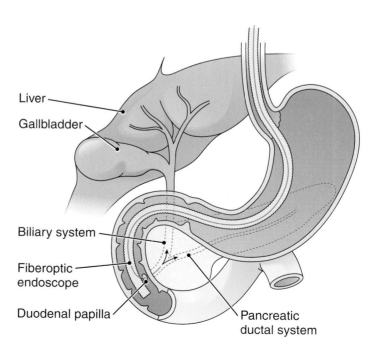

Liver
Gallbladder
Biliary system
Fiberoptic endoscope
Duodenal papilla
Pancreatic ductal system

FIGURE 12-10. Endoscopic retrograde cholangiopancreatography (ERCP). A contrast medium is injected into the pancreatic and bile ducts in preparation for radiography.

PANCREATITIS

Pancreatitis, or inflammation of the pancreas, may result from alcohol abuse, drug toxicity, bile obstruction, infections, and other causes. Blood tests in acute pancreatitis show increased levels of the enzymes amylase and lipase. Glucose and bilirubin levels may also be elevated. Often the disease subsides with only treatment of the symptoms.

Key Clinical Terms

DISORDERS

appendicitis *a-pen-di-SĪ-tis*	Inflammation of the appendix
ascites *a-SĪ-tēz*	Accumulation of fluid in the abdominal cavity; a form of edema. May be caused by heart disease, lymphatic or venous obstruction, cirrhosis, or changes in plasma composition.
bilirubin *bil-i-RŪ-bin*	A pigment released in the breakdown of hemoglobin from red blood cells; mainly excreted by the liver in bile
cholecystitis *kō-lē-sis-TĪ-tis*	Inflammation of the gallbladder
cholelithiasis *kō-lē-li-THĪ-a-sis*	The condition of having stones in the gallbladder; also used to refer to stones in the common bile duct
cirrhosis *sir-RŌ-sis*	Chronic liver disease with degeneration of liver tissue
colic *KOL-ik*	Acute abdominal pain, such as biliary colic caused by gallstones in the bile ducts
Crohn disease *krōn*	A chronic inflammatory disease of the gastrointestinal tract usually involving the ileum
diarrhea *dī-a-RĒ-a*	The frequent passage of watery bowel movements
diverticulitis *dī-ver-tik-ū-LĪ-tis*	Inflammation of diverticula (small pouches) in the wall of the digestive tract, especially in the colon
diverticulosis *dī-ver-tik-ū-LŌ-sis*	The presence of diverticula, especially in the colon
dysphagia *dis-FĀ-jē-a*	Difficulty in swallowing
emesis *EM-e-sis*	Vomiting
fistula *FIS-tū-la*	An abnormal passageway between two organs or from an organ to the body surface, such as between the rectum and anus (anorectal fistula)

Disorders, continued

gastroenteritis *gas-trō-en-ter-Ī-tis*	Inflammation of the stomach and intestine
hemorrhoids *HEM-ō-roydz*	Varicose veins in the rectum associated with pain, bleeding, and sometimes prolapse of the rectum
hepatitis *hep-a-TĪ-tis*	Inflammation of the liver; commonly caused by a viral infection
hepatomegaly *hep-a-tō-MEG-a-lē*	Enlargement of the liver
hiatal hernia *hī-Ā-tal*	A protrusion of the stomach through the opening (hiatus) in the diaphragm through which the esophagus passes (see Fig. 6-5)
icterus *IK-ter-us*	Jaundice
ileus *IL-ē-us*	Intestinal obstruction. May be caused by lack of peristalsis (adynamic, paralytic ileus) or by contraction (dynamic ileus). Intestinal matter and gas may be relieved by passage of a tube for drainage.
intussusception *in-tu-su-SEP-shun*	Slipping of one part of the intestine into another part below it. Occurs mainly in male infants in the ileocecal region (see Fig. 12-8). May be fatal if untreated for more than 1 day.
jaundice *JAWN-dis*	A yellowish color of the skin, mucous membranes, and whites of the eye caused by bile pigments in the blood (from French *jaune* meaning "yellow"). The main pigment is bilirubin, a byproduct of the breakdown of red blood cells.
nausea *NAW-zha*	An unpleasant sensation in the upper abdomen that often precedes vomiting. Typically occurs in digestive upset, motion sickness, and sometimes early pregnancy.
occult blood	Blood present in such small amounts that it can be detected only microscopically or chemically; in the feces, a sign of intestinal bleeding (*occult* means "hidden")
pancreatitis *pan-krē-a-TĪ-tis*	Inflammation of the pancreas
peptic ulcer *PEP-tik UL-ser*	A lesion in the mucous membrane of the esophagus, stomach, or duodenum caused by the action of gastric juice
peritonitis *per-i-tō-NĪ-tis*	Inflammation of the peritoneum, the membrane that lines the abdominal cavity and covers the abdominal organs. May result from perforation of an ulcer, rupture of the appendix, or infection of the reproductive tract, among other causes.
polyp *POL-ip*	A tumor that grows on a stalk and bleeds easily
portal hypertension	An abnormal increase in pressure in the hepatic portal system. May be caused by cirrhosis, infection, thrombosis, or tumors.

Disorders, continued

pyloric stenosis	Narrowing of the opening between the stomach and the duodenum; pylorostenosis
splenomegaly *splē-nō-MEG-a-lē*	Enlargement of the spleen
ulcerative colitis *UL-ser-a-tiv kō-LĪ-tis*	Chronic ulceration of the colon of unknown cause
volvulus *VOL-vū-lus*	Twisting of the intestine resulting in obstruction. Usually involves the sigmoid colon and occurs most often in children and in the elderly. May be caused by congenital malformation, foreign body, or adhesion. Failure to treat immediately may result in death (see Fig. 12-8).

DIAGNOSIS AND TREATMENT

anastomosis *a-nas-to-MŌ-sis*	A passage or communication between two vessels or organs. May be normal or pathologic, or may be created surgically.
barium study	Use of barium sulfate as a liquid contrast medium for fluoroscopic or radiographic study of the digestive tract. Can show obstruction, tumors, ulcers, hiatal hernia, and motility disorders, among others.
cholecystectomy *kō-lē-sis-TEK-tō-mē*	Surgical removal of the gallbladder
Dukes classification	A system for staging colorectal cancer based on degree of penetration of the bowel wall and lymph node involvement; severity is graded from A to C
endoscopy *en-DOS-kō-pē*	Use of a fiberoptic endoscope for direct visual examination. GI studies include esophagogastroduodenoscopy, proctosigmoidoscopy (rectum and distal colon), and colonoscopy (all regions of the colon) (see Fig. 12-5).
ERCP	Endoscopic retrograde cholangiopancreatography; a technique for viewing the pancreatic and bile ducts and for performing certain techniques to relieve obstructions. Contrast medium is injected into the biliary system from the duodenum and radiographs are taken (see Fig. 12-9).
ostomy *OS-tō-mē*	An opening into the body; generally refers to an opening created for elimination of body waste. Also refers to the operation done to create such an opening (see stoma).
stoma *STŌ-ma*	A surgically created opening to the body surface or between two organs (literally "mouth")

Supplementary Terms

NORMAL STRUCTURE AND FUNCTION

bolus *BŌ-lus*	A mass, such as the rounded mass of food that is swallowed
cardia *KAR-dē-a*	The part of the stomach near the esophagus, named for its closeness to the heart
chyme *kīm*	The semiliquid partially digested food that moves from the stomach into the small intestine
defecation *def-e-KĀ-shun*	The evacuation of feces from the rectum
deglutition *deg-lū-TISH-un*	Swallowing
duodenal bulb	The part of the duodenum near the pylorus; the first bend (flexure) of the duodenum
duodenal papilla	The raised area where the common bile duct and pancreatic duct enter the duodenum (see Fig. 12-10); papilla of Vater (*FA-ter*)
greater omentum *ō-MEN-tum*	A fold of the peritoneum that extends from the stomach over the abdominal organs
hepatic flexure	The right bend of the colon, forming the junction between the ascending colon and the transverse colon (see Fig. 12-1)
ileocecal valve *il-ē-ō-SĒ-kal*	A valvelike structure between the ileum of the small intestine and the cecum of the large intestine
mesentery *MES-en-ter-ē*	The portion of the peritoneum that folds over and supports the intestine
mesocolon *mes-ō-KŌ-lon*	The portion of the peritoneum that folds over and supports the colon
papilla of Vater	See duodenal papilla
peritoneum *per-i-tō-NĒ-um*	The serous membrane that lines the abdominal cavity and supports the abdominal organs
rugae *RŪ-jē*	The large folds in the lining of the stomach seen when the stomach is empty
sphincter of Oddi *OD-ē*	The ring of muscle at the opening of the common bile duct into the duodenum
splenic flexure	The left bend of the colon, forming the junction between the transverse colon and the descending colon (see Fig. 12-1)
uvula *Ū-vū-la*	A hanging fleshy mass. Usually means the mass that hangs from the soft palate (see Fig. 12-2).

DISORDERS

achalasia *ak-a-LĀ-zē-a*	Failure of a smooth muscle to relax, especially the lower esophageal sphincter, so that food is retained in the esophagus
achlorhydria *ā-klor-HĪ-drē-a*	Lack of hydrochloric acid in the stomach; opposite is hyperchlorhydria
anorexia *an-ō-REK-sē-a*	Loss of appetite. Anorexia nervosa is a psychologically induced refusal or inability to eat (adjective, anorectic, anorexic).
aphagia *a-FĀ-jē-a*	Refusal or inability to eat; inability to swallow or difficulty in swallowing
aphthous ulcer *AF-thus*	A small ulcer in the mucous membrane of the mouth
bulimia *bū-LIM-ē-a*	Excessive, insatiable appetite. A disorder characterized by overeating followed by induced vomiting, diarrhea, or fasting.
cachexia *ka-KEK-sē-a*	Profound ill health, malnutrition, and wasting
caries *KA-rē*	Tooth decay
celiac disease *SĒ-lē-ak*	A disease characterized by the inability to absorb foods containing gluten
cheilosis *kī-LŌ-sis*	Cracking at the corners of the mouth, often caused by B vitamin deficiency (root *cheil/o* means "lip")
cholestasis *kō-lē-STA-sis*	Stoppage of bile flow
constipation *con-sti-PĀ-shun*	Infrequency or difficulty in defecation and the passage of hard, dry feces
dyspepsia *dis-PEP-sē-a*	Poor or painful digestion
eructation *e-ruk-TĀ-shun*	Belching
familial adenomatous polyposis (FAP)	A heredity condition in which multiple polyps form in the colon and rectum, predisposing to colorectal cancer
flatulence *FLAT-ū-lens*	Condition of having gas or air in the GI tract
flatus *FLĀ-tus*	Gas or air in the gastrointestinal tract; gas or air expelled through the anus
gastroesophageal reflux disease (GERD)	Backflow of gastric contents into the esophagus. May result in inflammation and damage to the esophagus; heartburn.
hematemesis *hē-ma-TEM-e-sis*	Vomiting of blood

Disorders, continued

irritable bowel syndrome (IBS)	A chronic stress-related disease characterized by diarrhea, constipation, and pain associated with rhythmic contractions of the intestine. Mucous colitis; spastic colon.
megacolon *meg-a-KŌ-lon*	An extremely dilated colon. Usually congenital but may occur in acute ulcerative colitis.
melena *MEL-ē-na*	Black tarry feces resulting from blood in the intestines. Common in newborns. May also be a sign of gastrointestinal bleeding.
obstipation *ob-sti-PĀ-shun*	Extreme constipation
pernicious anemia *per-NISH-us*	A form of anemia caused by failure of the stomach to secrete a substance (intrinsic factor) needed for the absorption of vitamin B_{12}
pilonidal cyst *pī-lō-NĪ-dal*	A dermal cyst in the region of the sacrum, usually at the top of the cleft between the buttocks. May become infected and begin to drain.
regurgitation *rē-gur-ji-TĀ-shun*	A backward flowing, such as the backflow of undigested food

DIAGNOSIS AND TREATMENT

appendectomy *ap-en-DEK-tō-mē*	Surgical removal of the appendix
Billroth operations	Gastrectomy with anastomosis of the stomach to the duodenum (Billroth I) or to the jejunum (Billroth II) (Fig. 12-11)
gavage *ga-VAHZH*	Process of feeding through a nasogastric tube into the stomach
lavage *la-VAJ*	Washing out of a cavity; irrigation
manometry *man-OM-e-trē*	Measurement of pressure; pertaining to the GI tract, measurement of pressure in the portal system as a sign of obstruction
Murphy sign	Inability to take a deep breath when fingers are pressed firmly below the right arch of the ribs (below the liver). Signifies gallbladder disease.
nasogastric (NG) **tube**	Tube that is passed through the nose into the stomach (Fig. 12-12). May be used for emptying the stomach, administering medication, giving liquids, or sampling stomach contents.
parenteral hyperalimentation	Complete intravenous feeding for one who cannot take in food. Total parenteral nutrition (TPN).
percutaneous endoscopic gastrostomy (PEG) **tube**	Tube inserted into the stomach for long-term feeding (Fig. 12-13)
vagotomy *vā-GOT-ō-mē*	Interruption of impulses from the vagus nerve to reduce stomach secretions in the treatment of gastric ulcer. Originally done surgically but may also be done with drugs.

DRUGS

antacid *ant-AS-id*	Agent that counteracts acidity, usually gastric acidity
antidiarrheal *an-ti-dī-a-RĒ-al*	Treats or prevents diarrhea by reducing intestinal motility or absorbing irritants and soothing the intestinal lining
antiemetic *an-tē-e-MET-ik*	Agent that relieves or prevents nausea and vomiting
antiflatulent *an-ti-FLAT-ū-lent*	Agent that prevents or relieves flatulence
antispasmodic *an-ti-spas-MOD-ik*	Agent that relieves spasm, usually of smooth muscle
emetic *e-MET-ik*	An agent that causes vomiting
histamine H₂ antagonist	Drug that decreases secretion of stomach acid by interfering with the action of histamine at H_2 receptors. Used to treat ulcers and other gastrointestinal problems.
laxative *LAK-sa-tiv*	Promotes elimination from the large intestine. Types include stimulants, substances that retain water (hyperosmotics), stool softeners, and bulk-forming agents.

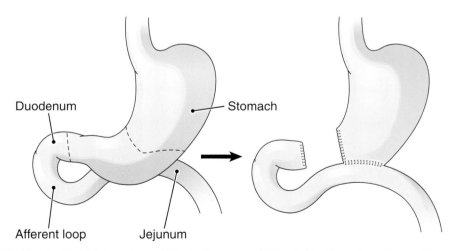

FIGURE 12-11. Gastrojejunostomy (Billroth II operation). The *dotted lines* show the portion removed

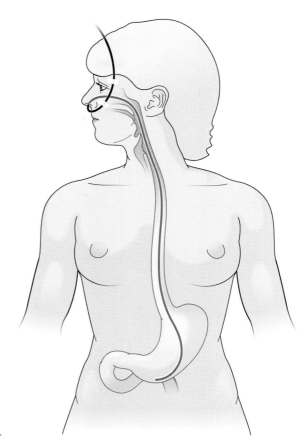

FIGURE 12-12. A nasogastric (NG) tube in place.

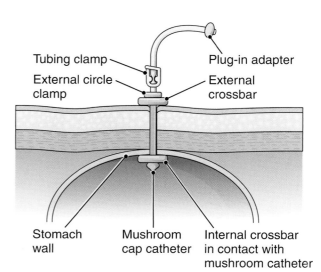

FIGURE 12-13. Percutaneous endoscopic gastrostomy (PEG) tube in place in the stomach.

ABBREVIATIONS

BE	Barium enema (for radiographic study of the colon)	**HDV**	Hepatitis D virus
		HEV	Hepatitis E virus
BM	Bowel movement	**HCl**	Hydrochloric acid
CBD	Common bile duct	**IBD**	Inflammatory bowel disease
ERCP	Endoscopic retrograde cholangio-pancreatography	**IBS**	Inflammatory bowel syndrome
		NG	Nasogastric (tube)
FAP	Familial adenomatous polyposis	**N & V**	Nausea and vomiting
GERD	Gastroesophageal reflux disease	**N/V/D**	Nausea, vomiting, and diarrhea
GI	Gastrointestinal	**ponv**	Postoperative nausea and vomiting
HAV	Hepatitis A virus	**TPN**	Total parenteral nutrition
HBV	Hepatitis B virus	**UGI**	Upper gastrointestinal (radiograph series)
HCV	Hepatitis C virus		

Labeling Exercise 12-1

The Digestive System

Write the name of each numbered part on the corresponding line of the answer sheet.

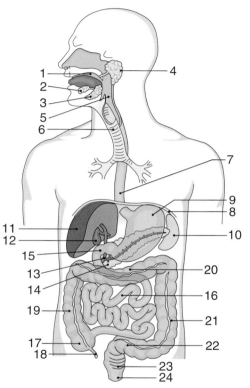

Anus
Appendix
Ascending colon
Cecum
Common bile duct
Descending colon
Diaphragm
Duodenum
Esophagus
Gallbladder
Liver
Oral cavity
Pancreas
Parotid gland
Pharynx
Rectum
Sigmoid colon
Small intestine
Spleen
Stomach
Sublingual gland
Submandibular gland
Trachea
Transverse colon

1. _____	13. _____
2. _____	14. _____
3. _____	15. _____
4. _____	16. _____
5. _____	17. _____
6. _____	18. _____
7. _____	19. _____
8. _____	20. _____
9. _____	21. _____
10. _____	22. _____
11. _____	23. _____
12. _____	24. _____

Labeling Exercise 12-2

Accessory Organs of Digestion

Write the name of each numbered part on the corresponding line of the answer sheet.

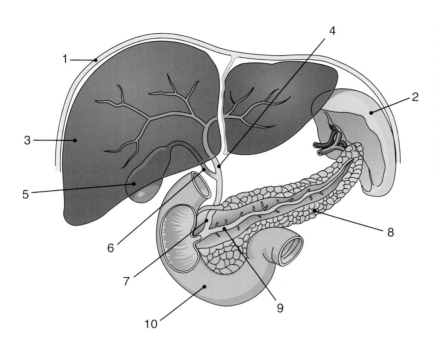

Common bile duct
Common hepatic duct
Cystic duct
Diaphragm
Duodenum
Gallbladder
Liver
Pancreas
Pancreatic duct
Spleen

1. _____   6. _____

2. _____   7. _____

3. _____   8. _____

4. _____   9. _____

5. _____   10. _____

Chapter Review 12-1

Match the following terms and write the appropriate letter to the left of each number:

_____	1. polysialia	a.	pertaining to the lip
_____	2. gingiva	b.	gum
_____	3. agnathia	c.	absence of the jaw
_____	4. hypoglossal	d.	excess secretion of saliva
_____	5. labial	e.	sublingual

_____	6. choledochal	a.	jaundice
_____	7. lithiasis	b.	pertaining to the common bile duct
_____	8. cholangiectasis	c.	crushing of a biliary calculus
_____	9. icterus	d.	condition of having stones
_____	10. cholelithotripsy	e.	dilation of a bile duct

_____	11. gastropathy	a.	narrowing of the pylorus
_____	12. pylorostenosis	b.	substance that induces vomiting
_____	13. gastrocele	c.	hernia of the stomach
_____	14. pylorospasm	d.	any disease of the stomach
_____	15. emetic	e.	sudden contraction of the pylorus

_____	16. cecopexy	a.	stoppage of bile flow
_____	17. proctocele	b.	hernia of the rectum
_____	18. cholestasis	c.	surgical fixation of the cecum
_____	19. proctorrhaphy	d.	surgical puncture of the colon
_____	20. colocentesis	e.	surgical repair of the rectum

SUPPLEMENTARY TERMS

_____	21. cachexia	a.	malnutrition and wasting
_____	22. caries	b.	chewing
_____	23. deglutition	c.	tooth decay
_____	24. gavage	d.	swallowing
_____	25. mastication	e.	feeding through a tube

_____ 26. bolus   a. inability to eat

_____ 27. cardia   b. partially digested food

_____ 28. peritoneum   c. part of the stomach near the esophagus

_____ 29. aphagia   d. a mass, as of food

_____ 30. chyme   e. serous membrane in the abdomen

Fill in the blanks:

31. The palatine tonsils are located on either side of the _____.

32. Stomatosis is any disease condition of the _____.

33. Dentin is the main substance of the _____.

34. Glossorrhaphy is suture of the _____.

35. From its name you might guess that the buccinator muscle is in the

_____.

36. An enterovirus is a virus that infects the _____.

37. A wave of contractions in an organ wall, such as the contractions that move material through the digestive tract, is called _____.

38. The blind pouch at the beginning of the colon is the _____.

39. The anticoagulant heparin is found throughout the body, but it is named for its presence in the

_____.

40. The substance cholesterol is named for its chemical composition (sterol) and for its presence in

_____.

41. The organ that produces bile is the _____.

42. The organ that stores bile is the _____.

True-False. Examine each of the following statements. If the statement is true, write T in the first blank. If the statement is false, write F in the first blank and correct the statement by replacing the underlined word in the second blank.

43. The epigastrium is the region of the abdomen above the stomach.   _____ _____

44. The first portion of the small intestine is the jejunum.   _____ _____

45. The cystic duct carries bile to and from the gallbladder.   _____ _____

46. Cirrhosis is a disease of the esophagus.   _____ _____

47. The appendix is attached to the ileum.   _____ _____

48. The common hepatic duct and the cystic duct merge to form the common bile duct.   _____ _____

49. Enteropathy is any disease of the intestine.   _____ _____

50. The hepatic portal system carries blood to the spleen.   _____ _____

Word building. Write a word for each of the following definitions:

51. a dentist who specializes in straightening of the teeth   _____

52. surgical repair of the palate   _____

53. surgical excision of the stomach   _____

54. inflammation of the pancreas   _____

55. pertaining to the ileum and cecum   _____

56. hernia of the rectum   _____

57. surgical creation of a passage between the stomach and the duodenum   _____

58. medical specialist who treats diseases of the stomach and intestine   _____

59. surgical creation of an opening into the colon   _____

60. inflammation of the ileum   _____

61. within (intra-) the liver   _____

Plurals. Write the plural form of each of the following words:

62. diverticulum   _____

63. gingiva   _____

64. calculus   _____

65. anastomosis   _____

Write the meaning of each of the following abbreviations:

66. IBD _____

67. TPN _____

68. HAV _____

69. GI _____

70. HCl _____

71. ERCP _____

72. PEG (tube) _____

73. GERD _____

Word analysis. Define each of the following words, and give the meaning of the word parts in each. Use a dictionary if necessary.

74. parenteral (*par-EN-ter-al*) _____
    a. par(a)- _____
    b. enter/o _____
    c. -al   _____

75. cholecystectomy _____
    a. chol/e _____
    b. cyst/o _____
    c. ec- _____
    d. -tomy _____

76. myenteric (*m-i-en-TER-ik*) _____
    a. my/o _____
    b. enter/o _____
    c. -ic _____

Case Studies

Case Study 12-1: Cholecystectomy

G.L., a 42-year-old obese Caucasian woman, entered the hospital with nausea and vomiting, flatulence and eructation, a fever of 100.5°F, and continuous right upper quadrant and subscapular pain. Examination on admission showed rebound tenderness in the RUQ with a positive Murphy sign. Her skin, nails, and conjunctivae were yellowish, and she complained of frequent clay-colored stools. Her leukocyte count was 16,000. An ERCP and ultrasound of the abdomen suggested many small stones in her gallbladder and possibly the common bile duct. Her diagnosis was cholecystitis with cholelithiasis.

A laparoscopic cholecystectomy was attempted, with an intraoperative cholangiogram and common bile duct exploration. Because of G.L.'s size and some unexpected bleeding, visualization was difficult and the procedure was converted to an open approach. Small stones and granular sludge were irrigated from her common duct, and the gallbladder was removed. She had a T-tube inserted into the duct for bile drainage; this tube was removed on the second postoperative day. She had an NG tube in place before and during the surgery, which was also removed on day two. She was discharged on the fifth postoperative day with a prescription for prn pain medication and a low-fat diet.

Case Study 12-2: Surgical Pathology Report

Gross Description: The specimen is received in formalin labeled "ruptured duodenal diverticula" and consists of enteric tissue measuring approximately 6.3 × 2.8 × 0.7 cm. The serosal surface is markedly dull in appearance and fibrotic. The mucosal surface is hemorrhagic. Representative sections are taken for microscopic examination.

Microscopic Description: Sectioned slide shows segments of duodenal tissues with areas of gangrenous change in the bowel wall, and acute and chronic inflammatory infiltrates. There are chronic and focal acute inflammatory cell infiltrates with hemorrhage in the mesenteric fatty tissue. There are areas of acute inflammatory exudates noted in the fatty tissue. Histopathologic changes are consistent with ruptured duodenal diverticula.

Case Study 12-3: Colonoscopy With Biopsy

S.M., a 24-year-old man, had a recent history of lower abdominal pain with frequent loose mucoid stools. He described symptoms of occasional dysphagia, dyspepsia, nausea, and aphthous ulcers of his tongue and buccal mucosa. A previous barium enema showed some irregularities in the sigmoid and rectal segments of his large bowel. Stool samples for culture, ova, and parasites were negative. His tentative diagnosis was irritable bowel syndrome.

He followed a lactose-free, low-residue diet and took Imodium to reduce intestinal motility. His gastroenterologist recommended a colonoscopy. After a 2-day regimen of soft to clear liquid diet, laxatives, and an enema the morning of the procedure, he reported to the endoscopy unit. He was transported to the procedure room. ECG electrodes, a pulse oximeter sensor, and a blood pressure cuff were applied for monitoring, and an IV was inserted in S.M.'s right arm. An IV bolus of Demerol and a bolus of Versed were given, and S.M. was positioned on his left side. The colonoscope was gently inserted through the anal sphincter and advanced proximally. S.M. was instructed to take a deep breath when the scope approached the splenic flexure and the hepatic flexure to facilitate comfortable passage.

The physician was able to advance past the ileocecal valve, examining the entire length of the colon. Ulcerated granulomatous lesions were seen throughout the colon, with a concentration in the sigmoid segment. Many biopsy specimens were taken. The mucosa of the distal ileum was normal. Pathology examination of the biopsy samples was expected to establish a diagnosis of IBD.

CASE STUDY QUESTIONS

Multiple choice: Select the best answer and write the letter of your choice to the left of each number.

_____ 1. Flatulence and eructation represent:
   a. regurgitation of chyme
   b. distention of the esophagus
   c. passage of gas or air from the GI tract
   d. muscular movement of the alimentary tract
   e. sounds heard only by abdominal auscultation

_____ 2. Murphy sign is tested for:
   a. under the ribs on the left
   b. near the spleen
   c. in the lower right abdomen
   d. under the ribs on the right
   e. in the lower left abdomen

_____ 3. The NG tube is inserted through the _____ and terminates in the _____:
   a. nose/stomach
   b. nostril/gallbladder
   c. glottis/nephron
   d. anus/cecum
   e. Nissen/glottis

_____ 4. Enteric tissue is found in the:
   a. gallbladder
   b. stomach
   c. esophagus
   d. liver
   e. intestine

Case Studies, continued

_____ 5. The mucosal surface of a digestive organ is the:
   a. outer surface
   b. medulla
   c. cortex
   d. inner surface
   e. central opening

_____ 6. Diverticula are:
   a. small pouches in the wall of the colon
   b. communications between two organs
   c. ducts in the liver
   d. intestinal obstructions
   e. polyps in the intestine

_____ 7. Dysphagia and dyspepsia are difficulty or pain with:
   a. chewing and intestinal motility
   b. speaking and motility
   c. swallowing and digestion
   d. breathing and absorption
   e. swallowing and nutrition

_____ 8. The buccal mucosa is in the:
   a. nostril, medial side
   b. mouth, inside of the cheek
   c. greater curvature of the stomach
   d. lesser curvature near the duodenum
   e. base of the tongue

_____ 9. A gastroenterologist is a physician who specializes in study of:
   a. respiration and pathology
   b. mouth and teeth
   c. stomach, intestines, and related structures
   d. musculoskeletal system
   e. nutritional and weight loss diets

_____ 10. The splenic and hepatic flexures are bends in the colon near the:
   a. liver and splanchnic vein
   b. common bile duct and biliary tree
   c. spleen and appendix
   d. spleen and liver
   e. mesenteric vessels and liver

_____ 11. Intestinal motility refers to:
   a. chewing
   b. peristalsis
   c. absorption
   d. antiemetics
   e. ascites

Case Studies, continued

_____ 12. A colonoscopy is:
  a. a radiograph of the small intestine
  b. an endoscopic study of the esophagus
  c. an upper endoscopy with biopsy
  d. a type of barium enema
  e. an endoscopic examination of the large bowel

_____ 13. The ileocecal valve is:
  a. part of a colonoscope
  b. at the distal ileum
  c. near the appendix
  d. a and b
  e. b and c

Write the meaning of each of the following abbreviations:

14. ERCP _____

15. RUQ _____

16. NG _____

17. IBD _____

Give the word or words in the case studies with each of the following meanings:

18. pertaining to the first part of the small intestine   _____

19. pertaining to the membrane that supports the intestine   _____

20. localized   _____

21. fluid that escapes from blood vessels as a result of inflammation   _____

22. presence of hidden or microscopic blood   _____

23. jaundice   _____

24. drug that treats nausea and vomiting   _____

25. stones in the gallbladder   _____

26. endoscopic surgery of the gallbladder   _____

27. inflammation of the gallbladder   _____

28. radiographic study of the gallbladder and biliary system   _____

29. ring of muscle that regulates the distal opening of the colon   _____

30. surgical excision of tissue for pathology examination   _____

Chapter 12 Crossword
Digestion

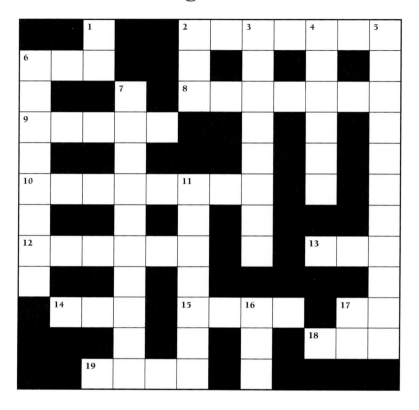

ACROSS

2. Pertaining to the jaw
6. Major portion of the large intestine: root
8. Mouth: combining form
9. Tooth: combining form
10. Small appendage to the cecum
12. Stomach: combining form
13. Inflammatory condition of the bowel (abbreviation)
14. Parenteral hyperalimentation (abbreviation)
15. Technique for viewing the accessory ducts (abbreviation)
17. Two, twice: prefix
18. Blind pouch at the beginning of the large intestine: root
19. Last portion of the small intestine: combining form

DOWN

1. 1/1000 of 1 liter (abbreviation)
2. Results in flatulence
3. Loss of appetite
4. Pertaining to the opening in the diaphragm that the esophagus passes through
5. Pertaining to the gallbladder
6. Bile duct: root
7. Enteric
11. First portion of the small intestine: combining form
16. Duct that carries bile into the intestine (abbreviation)
17. Down, without, removal: prefix

CHAPTER 12 **Answer Section**

Answers to Chapter Exercises

EXERCISE 12-1

1. oral (*OR-al*); stomal (*STŌ-mal*)
2. dental (*DEN-tal*)
3. gingival (*JIN-ji-val*)
4. lingual (LING-gwal); glossal (*GLOS-sal*)
5. buccal (*BUK-al*)
6. labial (*LĀ-bē-al*)
7. jaw
8. tongue
9. mouth
10. mouth
11. salivary
12. teeth
13. mouth
14. pertaining to the mouth and tongue
15. pertaining to the palate
16. inflammation of the gums
17. pertaining to the tongue and lip
18. outside the cheek

EXERCISE 12-2

1. enteric (*en-TER-ik*)
2. gastric (*GAS-trik*)
3. colic (*KOL-ik*); also colonic (*kō-LON-ik*)
4. pyloric (*p-i-LOR-ik*)
5. duodenal (*dū-ō-DĒ-nal*)
6. cecal (*SĒ-kal*)
7. jejunal (*je-JUN-al*)
8. ileal (*IL-ē-al*); also ileac (IL-ē-ak)
9. rectal (*REK-tal*)
10. anal (*Ā-nal*)
11. gastropexy (*GAS-trō-pek-sē*)
12. esophagoscopy (*e-sof-a-GOS-kō-pē*)
13. pyloroplasty (*pi-LOR-ō-plas-tē*)
14. ileitis (*il-ē-Ī-tis*)
15. duodenostomy (*dū-ō-de-NOS-tō-mē*)
16. ileostomy (*il-ē-OS-tō-mē*)
17. gastroenterology (*gas-trō-en-ter-OL-ō-jē*)
18. colitis (*kō-LĪ-tis*)
19. colopexy (*KŌ-lō-pek-sē*)
20. colostomy (*kō-LOS-tō-mē*)
21. coloclysis (*kō-lō-KLĪ-sis*)
22. colonopathy (*kō-lō-NOP-a-thē*)
23. colonoscopy (*kō-lon-OS-kō-pē*)
24. esophagogastrostomy (*e-sof-a-gō-gas-TROS-tō-mē*)
25. gastroenterostomy (*gas-trō-en-ter-OS-tō-mē*)
26. gastrojejunostomy (*gas-trō-je-jū-NOS-tō-mē*)
27. duodenoileostomy (*dū-ō-dē-nō-il-ē-OS-tō-mē*)
28. sigmoidoproctostomy (*sig-moy-dō-prok-TOS-tō-mē*)

EXERCISE 12-3

1. hepatic (*he-PAT-ik*)
2. cholecystic (*kō-lē-SIS-tik*)
3. pancreatic (*pan-krē-AT-ik*)
4. cholangiography (*kō-lan-jē-OG-ra-fē*)
5. hepatography (*hep-a-TOG-ra-fē*)
6. cholecystography (*kō-lē-sis-TOG-ra-fē*)
7. pancreatography (*pan-krē-a-TOG-ra-fē*)
8. choledocholithiasis (*kō-led-o-kō-li-THĪ-a-sis*)
9. pancreatolithiasis (*pan-krē-a-tō-li-THĪ-a-sis*)
10. bile
11. common bile duct
12. liver
13. hepatitis
14. pancreas
15. bile duct

LABELING EXERCISE 12-1
THE DIGESTIVE SYSTEM

1. oral cavity
2. sublingual gland
3. submandibular gland
4. parotid gland
5. pharynx
6. trachea
7. esophagus
8. diaphragm
9. stomach
10. spleen
11. liver
12. gallbladder
13. common bile duct
14. pancreas
15. duodenum
16. small intestine
17. cecum
18. appendix
19. ascending colon
20. transverse colon
21. descending colon
22. sigmoid colon
23. rectum
24. anus

LABELING EXERCISE 12-2 ACCESSORY ORGANS OF DIGESTION

1. diaphragm
2. spleen
3. liver
4. common hepatic duct
5. gallbladder
6. cystic duct
7. common bile duct
8. pancreas
9. pancreatic duct
10. duodenum

Answers to Chapter Review 12-1

1. d
2. b
3. c
4. e
5. a
6. b
7. d
8. e
9. a
10. c
11. d
12. a
13. c
14. e
15. b
16. c
17. b
18. a
19. e
20. d
21. a
22. c
23. d
24. e
25. b
26. d
27. c
28. e
29. a
30. b
31. palate
32. mouth
33. teeth
34. tongue
35. cheek
36. intestine
37. peristalsis
38. cecum
39. liver
40. bile
41. liver
42. gallbladder
43. T
44. F duodenum
45. T
46. F liver
47. F cecum
48. T
49. T
50. F liver
51. orthodontist
52. palatorrhaphy
53. gastrectomy
54. pancreatitis
55. ileocecal
56. rectocele; proctocele
57. gastroduodenostomy
58. gastroenterologist
59. colostomy
60. ileitis
61. intrahepatic
62. diverticula
63. gingivae
64. calculi
65. anastomoses
66. inflammatory bowel disease
67. total parenteral nutrition
68. hepatitis A virus
69. gastrointestinal
70. hydrochloric acid
71. endoscopic retrograde cholangiopancreatography
72. percutaneous endoscopic gastrostomy (tube)
73. gastroesophageal reflux disease
74. referring to any route other than the alimentary canal
    a. beside
    b. intestine
    c. pertaining to
75. surgical removal of the gallbladder
    a. gall, bile
    b. bladder
    c. out
    d. to cut
76. pertaining to the muscular coat of the intestine
    a. muscle
    b. intestine
    c. pertaining to

Answers to Case Study Questions

1. c
2. d
3. a
4. e
5. d

6. a
7. c
8. b
9. c
10. d
11. b
12. e
13. e
14. endoscopic retrograde cholangiopancreatography
15. right upper quadrant
16. nasogastric
17. inflammatory bowel disease
18. duodenal

19. mesenteric
20. focal
21. exudate
22. occult blood
23. icterus
24. antiemetic
25. cholelithiasis
26. laparoscopic cholecystectomy
27. cholecystitis
28. cholangiogram
29. sphincter
30. biopsy

ANSWERS TO CROSSWORD PUZZLE

Digestion

The Urinary System

Chapter Contents

Objectives

After study of this chapter you should be able to:

1. Label a diagram of the urinary tract and follow the flow of urine through the body.
2. Label a diagram of the kidney.
3. Identify the portions of the nephron and explain how each functions in urine formation.
4. Explain the relationship between the kidney and the blood circulation.
5. Identify and use the roots pertaining to the urinary system.
6. Describe the major disorders of the urinary system.
7. Define medical terms commonly used in reference to the urinary system.
8. Interpret abbreviations used in reference to the urinary system.
9. Analyze several case studies pertaining to urinary disorders.

The urinary system consists of two kidneys, two ureters, the urinary bladder, and a urethra (Fig. 13-1). This system forms and eliminates urine, which contains metabolic waste products. The kidneys, the organs of excretion, also regulate the composition, volume, and acid–base balance (pH) of body fluids. Thus they are of critical importance in maintaining the state of internal balance known as homeostasis. In addition, they produce two substances that act on the circulatory system. **Erythropoietin** (EPO) is a hormone that stimulates the production of red blood cells in the bone marrow. **Renin** is an enzyme that functions to raise blood pressure. It does so by activating a blood component called **angiotensin**, which causes constriction of the blood vessels. The drugs known as ACE inhibitors (angiotensin-converting enzyme inhibitors) lower blood pressure by interfering with the production of angiotensin.

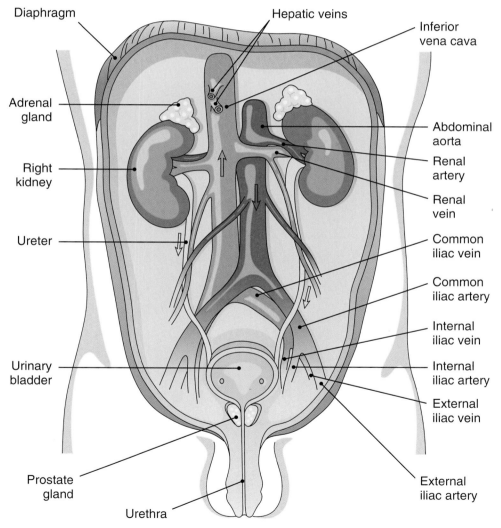

FIGURE 13-1. Male urinary system, with blood vessels. (Reprinted with permission from Cohen BJ, Wood DL. Memmler's The Human Body in Health and Disease. 9th Ed. Philadelphia: Lippincott Williams & Wilkins, 2000.)

The Kidneys

The **kidneys** are located behind the peritoneum in the lumbar region. On the top of each kidney rests an adrenal gland. Each kidney is encased in a capsule of fibrous connective tissue overlaid with fat. An outermost layer of connective tissue supports the kidney and anchors it to the body wall.

If you look inside the kidney, you will see that it has an outer region, the **renal cortex**, and an inner region, the **renal medulla** (Fig. 13-2). The medulla is divided into triangular sections, each called a **pyramid**. The pyramids have a lined appearance because they are made up of the loops and collecting tubules of the nephrons, the functional units of the kidney. Each collecting tubule empties into a urine-collecting area called a **calyx** (from the Latin word meaning "cup"). Several of these smaller minor calyces merge to form a major calyx. The major calyces then unite to form the **renal pelvis**, the upper funnel-shaped portion of the ureter.

The Nephrons

The tiny working units of the kidneys are the **nephrons** (Fig. 13-3). Each of these microscopic structures is basically a single tubule coiled and folded into various shapes. At the beginning of the tubule is the cup-shaped **Bowman capsule**, which is part of the blood-filtering device of the nephron. The tubule then folds into the proximal convoluted tubule, straightens out to form the loop of Henle, coils again into the distal convoluted tubule, and then finally straightens out to form a collecting tubule.

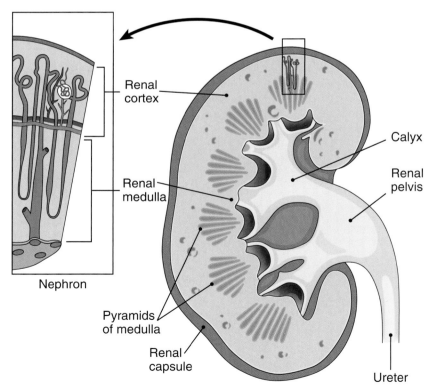

FIGURE 13-2. Longitudinal section through the kidney showing its internal structure, and an enlarged diagram of a nephron. There are more than 1 million nephrons in each kidney. (Reprinted with permission from Cohen BJ, Wood DL. Memmler's The Human Body in Health and Disease. 9th Ed. Philadelphia: Lippincott Williams & Wilkins, 2000.)

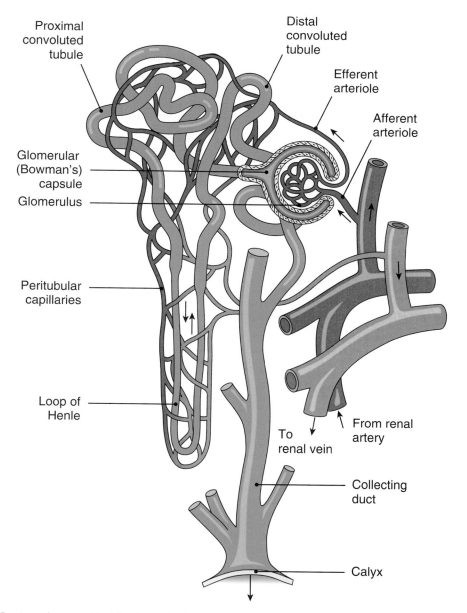

FIGURE 13-3. A nephron and its blood supply. (Reprinted with permission from Cohen BJ, Wood DL. Memmler's The Human Body in Health and Disease. 9th Ed. Philadelphia: Lippincott Williams & Wilkins, 2000.)

Blood Supply to the Kidney

Blood enters the kidney through a renal artery, a short branch of the abdominal aorta. This vessel subdivides into smaller vessels as it branches throughout the kidney tissue, until finally blood is brought into the glomerular (Bowman's) capsule and circulated through a cluster of capillaries, called a **glomerulus**, within the capsule.

Blood leaves the kidney by a series of vessels that finally merge to form the renal vein, which empties into the inferior vena cava.

Urine Formation

As blood flows through the glomerulus, blood pressure forces materials through the glomerular wall and through the wall of the glomerular capsule into the nephron. The fluid that enters the nephron, the **glomerular filtrate**, consists mainly of water, electrolytes, soluble wastes, nutrients, and toxins. The main waste material is **urea**, the nitrogenous (nitrogen-containing) byproduct of protein metabolism. The filtrate should not contain any cells or proteins such as albumin. The waste material and the toxins must be eliminated, but most of the water, electrolytes, and nutrients must be returned to the blood or we would rapidly starve and dehydrate. This return process, termed **tubular reabsorption**, occurs through the peritubular capillaries that surround the nephron. As the filtrate flows through the nephron, other processes further regulate its composition and pH. The concentration of the filtrate is also adjusted under the effects of the pituitary hormone **antidiuretic hormone (ADH)**. Finally, the filtrate, now called **urine**, flows into the collecting tubules to be eliminated.

Removal of Urine

Urine is drained from the renal pelvis and carried by the **ureter** to the **urinary bladder** (Fig. 13-4). Urine is stored in the bladder until fullness stimulates a reflex contraction of the bladder muscle and expulsion of urine through the **urethra**. The female urethra is short (4 cm; 1.5 in) and carries only urine. The male urethra is longer (20 cm; 8 in) and carries both urine and semen.

The voiding (release) of urine, technically called **micturition** or **urination**, is regulated by two sphincters (circular muscles) that surround the urethra. The upper sphincter, just below the bladder, functions involuntarily; the lower sphincter is under conscious control.

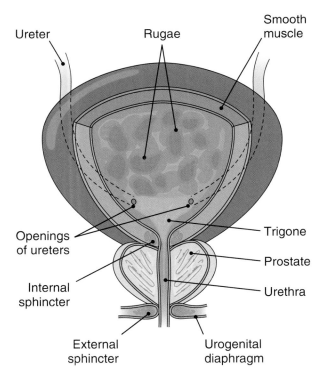

FIGURE 13-4. Interior of the urinary bladder, shown in a male subject. The trigone is a triangle in the floor of the bladder marked by the openings of the ureters and the urethra. (Reprinted with permission from Cohen BJ, Wood DL. Memmler's The Human Body in Health and Disease. 9th Ed. Philadelphia: Lippincott Williams & Wilkins, 2000.)

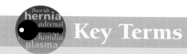

Key Terms

NORMAL STRUCTURE AND FUNCTION

Antidiuretic hormone (ADH) *an-ti-dī-ū-RET-ik*	A hormone released from the pituitary gland that causes reabsorption of water in the kidneys, thus concentrating the urine
angiotensin *an-jē-ō-TEN-sin*	A substance that increases blood pressure; activated in the blood by renin, an enzyme produced by the kidneys
calyx *KĀ-liks*	A cuplike cavity in the pelvis of the kidney; also calix (plural, calyces) (root *cali, calic*)
erythropoietin (EPO) *e-rith-rō-POY-e-tin*	A hormone produced by the kidneys that stimulates red blood cell production in the bone marrow
glomerular capsule *glō-MER-ū-lar KAP-sūl*	The cup-shaped structure at the beginning of the nephron that surrounds the glomerulus and receives material filtered out of the blood
glomerular filtrate *glō-MER-ū-lar FIL-trāt*	The fluid and dissolved materials that filter out of the blood and enter the nephron at the Bowman capsule
glomerulus *glō-MER-ū-lus*	The cluster of capillaries within the glomerular capsule (plural, glomeruli) (root *glomerul/o*)
kidney *KID-nē*	An organ of excretion (root *ren/o, nephr/o*); the two kidneys filter the blood and form urine, which contains the waste products of metabolism and other substances as needed to regulate the water and electrolyte balance and the pH of body fluids
micturition *mik-tū-RISH-un*	The voiding of urine; urination
nephron *NEF-ron*	A microscopic functional unit of the kidney; working with blood vessels, the nephron filters the blood and balances the composition of urine
renal cortex *RĒ-nal KOR-tex*	The outer portion of the kidney
renal medulla *me-DUL-la*	The inner portion of the kidney; contains portions of the nephrons and tubules that transport urine toward the renal pelvis
renal pelvis *PEL-vis*	The expanded upper end of the ureter that receives urine from the kidney (root *pyel/o*, from the Greek word for pelvis, meaning "basin")
renal pyramid *PIR-a-mid*	A triangular structure in the medulla of the kidney composed of the loops and collecting tubules of the nephrons
renin *RĒ-nin*	An enzyme produced by the kidneys that activates angiotensin in the blood

Normal Structure and Function, *continued*

tubular reabsorption *TŪB-ū-lar rē-ab-SORP-shun*	The return of substances from the glomerular filtrate to the blood through the peritubular capillaries
urea *ū-RĒ-a*	The main nitrogenous (nitrogen-containing) waste product in the urine
ureter *Ū-rē-ter*	The tube that carries urine from the kidney to the bladder (root *ureter/o*)
urethra *ū-RĒ-thra*	The tube that carries urine from the bladder to the outside of the body (root *urethr/o*)
urinary bladder *Ū-ri-nar-ē BLAD-der*	The organ that stores and eliminates urine excreted by the kidneys (root *cyst/o, vesic/o*)
urination *ū-ri-NĀ-shun*	The voiding of urine; micturition
urine *Ū-rin*	The fluid excreted by the kidneys. It consists of water, electrolytes, urea, other metabolic wastes, and pigment. A variety of other substances may appear in urine in cases of disease (root *ur/o*).

Box 13-1 Words That Serve Double Duty

Some words appear in more than one body system to represent different structures. The medulla of the kidney is the inner portion of the organ. Other organs, such as the adrenal gland, ovary, and lymph nodes, may also be divided into a central medulla and outer cortex. But *medulla* means "marrow," and this term is also applied to the bone marrow, to the spinal cord, and to the part of the brain that connects with the spinal cord, the medulla oblongata.

A ventricle is a chamber. There are ventricles in the brain and in the heart. The word *fundus* means the back part or base of an organ. The uterus has a fundus, the upper rounded portion farthest from the cervix, and so does the stomach. The fundus of the eye, examined for signs of diabetes and glaucoma, is the innermost layer where the retina is located. A macula is a spot. There is a macula in the eye, which is the point of sharpest vision. There is also a macula in the ear, which contains receptors for equilibrium.

In interpreting medical terminology, it is often important to know the context in which a word is used.

Roots Pertaining to the Urinary System

TABLE 13-1 Roots for the Kidney

ROOT	MEANING	EXAMPLE	DEFINITION OF EXAMPLE
ren/o	kidney	infrarenal *in-fra-RĒ-nal*	below the kidney
nephr/o	kidney	nephrosis *nef-RŌ-sis*	any noninflammatory disease condition of the kidney
glomerul/o	glomerulus	juxtaglomerular *juks-ta-glō-MER-ū-lar*	near the glomerulus
pyel/o	renal pelvis	pyeloplasty *pī -e-lō-PLAS-tē*	plastic repair of the renal pelvis
cali-, calic-	calyx	calicectasis *kal-i-SEK-ta-sis*	dilatation of a renal calyx

Exercise 13-1

Use the root *ren/o* to write a word that has the same meaning as each of the following definitions:

1. near (para-) the kidney   _____ pararenal _____

2. above (supra-) the kidney   _____

3. between the kidneys   _____

4. around the kidneys   _____

5. behind (post-) the kidney   _____

Use the root *nephr/o* to write a word that has the same meaning as each of the following definitions:

6. inflammation of the kidney   _____

7. any disease of the kidney   _____

8. softening of the kidney   _____

9. surgical removal of the kidney   _____

10. study of the kidney   _____

Use the appropriate root to write a word that has the same meaning for each of the following definitions:

11. inflammation of a glomerulus   _____

12. excision of a renal calyx   _____

13. radiograph of the renal pelvis   _____

14. dilatation of the renal pelvis   _____

15. hardening of a glomerulus   _____

16. radiographic study (-graphy) of the kidney   _____

17. inflammation of the renal pelvis and kidney   _____

TABLE 13-2 Roots for the Urinary Tract (Except the Kidney)

ROOT	MEANING	EXAMPLE	DEFINITION OF EXAMPLE
ur/o	urine, urinary tract	urosepsis ū-rō-SEP-sis	generalized infection that originates in the urinary tract
urin/o	urine	urination ū-ri-NĀ-shun	discharge of urine
ureter/o	ureter	ureterostenosis ū-rē-ter-ō-ste-NŌ-sis	narrowing of the ureter
cyst/o	urinary bladder	cystotomy sis-TOT-ō-mē	incision of the bladder
vesic/o	urinary bladder	intravesical in-tra-VES-i-kal	within the urinary bladder
urethr/o	urethra	urethroscopy ū-rē-THROS-kō-pē	endoscopic examination of the urethra

 Exercise 13-2

Use the root *ur/o* to write a word that has the same meaning as each of the following definitions:

1. radiography of the urinary tract   _____

2. a urinary calculus (stone)   _____

3. study of the urinary tract   _____

4. presence of urinary waste products in the blood (-emia) _____

The root *ur/o-* is used in the suffix *–uria*, which means "condition of urine or of urination." Use *-uria* to write a word that has the same meaning as each of the following definitions:

5. presence of proteins in the urine   _____ proteinuria _____

6. lack of urine   _____

7. formation of excess (poly-) urine   _____

8. painful or difficult urination   _____

9. presence of pus in the urine   _____

10. presence of cells in the urine   _____

11. presence of blood (hemat/o) in the urine   _____

12. urination during the night (noct/i)   _____

The suffix *-uresis* means "urination." Use *-uria* to write a word that has the same meaning as each of the following definitions:

13. increased excretion of urine   _____diuresis_____

14. lack of urination   _____

15. excretion of sodium (natri-) in the urine   _____

16. excretion of potassium (kali-) in the urine   _____

The adjective endings for the above words is *-uretic*, as in *diuretic* (pertaining to diuresis) and *natriuretic* (pertaining to the excretion of sodium in the urine). Fill in the blanks:

17. Urinalysis (*ū-ri-NAL-i-sis*) is the laboratory study of _____.

18. Hydroureter (*hī-drō-ū-RĒ-ter*) is fluid distension of a(n) _____.

19. A urethrotome (*ū-RĒ-thrō-tōm*) is an instrument for cutting the _____.

20. The word cystic (*SIS-tik*), as applied to the urinary system, pertains to the

_____.

21. The word vesical (*VES-i-kal*) pertains to the _____.

Use the appropriate root to write a word for each of the following definitions:

22. inflammation of the urethra   _____

23. a ureteral calculus   _____

24. surgical creation of an opening in the ureter   _____

25. surgical fixation of the urethra   _____

Use the root *cysto/o* to write a word that has the same meaning as each of the following definitions:

26. inflammation of the urinary bladder   _____

27. surgical fixation of the urinary bladder   _____

28. an instrument for examining the inside of the bladder   _____

29. hernia of the bladder   _____

Use the root *vesic/o* to write a word that has the same meaning as each of the following definitions:

30. in front of (pre-) the bladder   _____

31. pertaining to the urethra and bladder   _____

Define each of the following terms:

32. transurethral (*trans-ū-RĒ-thral*)   _____

33. cystostomy (*sis-TOS-tō-mē*)   _____

34. ureterotomy (*ū-rē-ter-OT-ō-mē*)   _____

35. cystalgia (*sis-TAL-jē-a*)   _____

36. uropoiesis (*ū-rō-poy-Ē-sis*)   _____

Clinical Aspects of the Urinary System

Infections

Organisms that infect the urinary tract generally enter through the urethra and ascend toward the bladder. Although urinary tract infections (UTIs) do occur in males, they appear more commonly in females. Infection of the urinary bladder produces **cystitis**. The infecting organisms are usually colon bacteria carried in feces, particularly *Escherichia coli*. Cystitis is more common in females than in males because the female urethra is shorter than the male urethra and the opening is closer to the anus. Poor toilet habits and **urinary stasis** are contributing factors. In the hospital, UTIs may result from procedures involving the urinary system, especially **catheterization**, in which a tube is inserted into the bladder to withdraw urine (Fig. 13-5). Less frequently, UTIs originate in the blood and descend through the urinary system.

An infection that involves the kidney and renal pelvis is termed **pyelonephritis**. As in cystitis, signs of this condition include **dysuria**, painful or difficult urination, and the presence of bacteria and pus in the urine, **bacteriuria** and **pyuria**, respectively.

Urethritis is inflammation of the urethra, generally associated with sexually transmitted diseases such as gonorrhea and chlamydial infections (see Chapter 14).

Glomerulonephritis

Although the name simply means inflammation of the kidney and glomeruli, **glomerulonephritis** is a specific disorder that occurs after an immunologic reaction. It is usually a response to infection in another system, commonly a streptococcal infection of the respiratory tract or a skin infection. It may also accompany autoimmune diseases such as lupus erythematosus. The symptoms are hypertension, edema, and **oliguria**, the passage of small amounts of urine. This urine is highly concentrated. Because of damage to kidney tissue, blood and proteins escape into the nephrons, causing **hematuria**, blood in the urine, and **proteinuria**, protein in the urine. Blood cells may also form into small molds of the kidney tubule, called **casts**, which can be found in the urine.

Most patients recover fully from glomerulonephritis, but in some cases, especially among the elderly, the disorder may lead to chronic renal failure (CRF) or end-stage renal disease (ESRD). In such cases, urea and other nitrogen-containing compounds accumulate in the blood, a condition termed **uremia**. These compounds affect the central nervous system, causing irritability, loss of appetite, stupor, and other symptoms. There is also electrolyte imbalance and **acidosis**.

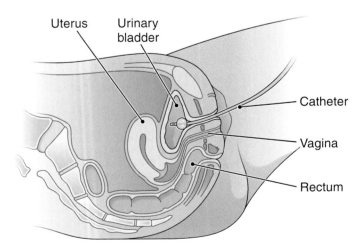

FIGURE 13-5. An indwelling (Foley) catheter in place in the female bladder.

Acute Renal Failure

Injury, shock, exposure to toxins, infections, and other renal disorders may cause damage to the nephrons, resulting in acute renal failure (ARF). There is rapid loss of kidney function with oliguria and accumulation of nitrogenous wastes in the blood. Failure of the kidneys to eliminate potassium leads to **hyperkalemia**, along with other electrolyte imbalances and acidosis. When destruction (necrosis) of kidney tubules is involved, the condition may be referred to as acute tubular necrosis (ATN).

Renal failure may lead to a need for kidney **dialysis** or, ultimately, **renal transplantation**. Dialysis refers to the movement of substances across a semipermeable membrane; it is a method used for removing harmful or unnecessary substances from the body when the kidneys are impaired or have been removed (Fig. 13-6). In **hemodialysis**, blood is cleansed by passage over a membrane surrounded by fluid (dialysate) that draws out unwanted substances. In **peritoneal dialysis**, fluid is introduced into the peritoneal cavity. The fluid is periodically withdrawn along with waste products and replaced (Fig. 13-7). The exchange may be done at intervals throughout the day in continuous ambulatory peritoneal dialysis (CAPD) or during the night in continuous cyclic peritoneal dialysis (CCPD).

Urinary Stones

Urinary lithiasis (condition of having stones) may be related to infection, irritation, diet, or hormone imbalances that lead to an increased level of calcium in the blood. Most urinary stones, or calculi, are formed of calcium salts, but they may be composed of other materials as well. Causes of stone formation include dehydration, infection, abnormal pH of urine, urinary stasis, and metabolic imbalances. The stones generally form in the kidney and may move to the bladder (Fig. 13-8). This results in great pain, termed **renal colic**, and obstruction that can promote infection and cause **hydronephrosis** (collection of urine in the renal pelvis). Because they are radiopaque, stones can usually be seen on simple radiographs of the abdomen. Stones may dissolve and pass out of the body on their own. If not, they may be removed surgically, in a **lithotomy**, or by

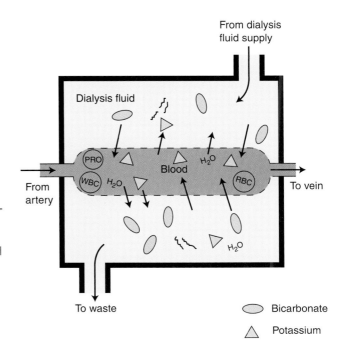

FIGURE 13-6. Schematic diagram of a hemodialysis system. A cellophane membrane separates the blood compartment and dialysis solution compartment. This membrane is porous enough to allow all of the constituents except the plasma proteins and blood cells to diffuse between the two compartments. (Reprinted with permission from Porth CM. Pathophysiology: Concepts in Altered Health States. 6th Ed. Philadelphia: Lippincott Williams & Wilkins, 2002.)

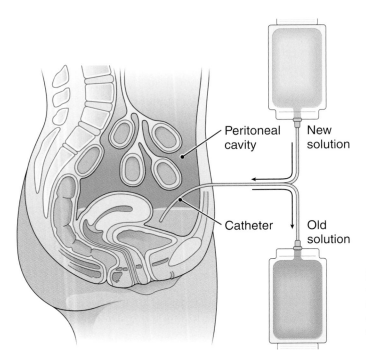

Peritoneal cavity

New solution

Catheter

Old solution

FIGURE 13-7. Peritoneal dialysis. A semipermeable membrane richly supplied with small blood vessels lines the peritoneal cavity. With dialysate dwelling in the peritoneal cavity, waste products diffuse from the network of blood vessels into the dialysate.

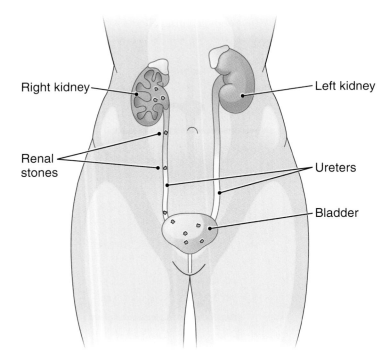

Right kidney

Left kidney

Renal stones

Ureters

Bladder

FIGURE 13-8. Various sites of calculus formation in the urinary tract.

using an endoscope. External shock waves are used to crush stones in the urinary tract in a procedure called extracorporeal (outside the body) shock wave **lithotripsy** (crushing of stones).

Cancer

Carcinoma of the bladder has been linked to occupational exposure to chemicals, parasitic infections, and cigarette smoking. A key symptom is sudden, painless hematuria. Often the cancer can be seen by viewing the lining of the bladder with a **cystoscope** (Fig. 13-9). This instrument can also be used to biopsy tissue for study. If treatment is not effective in permanently removing the tumor, a **cystectomy** (removal of the bladder) may be necessary. In this case, the ureters must be vented elsewhere, such as directly to the surface of the body through the ileum in an **ileal conduit** (Fig. 13-10), or to some other portion of the intestine.

Cancer may also involve the kidney and renal pelvis. Additional means for diagnosing cancer and other disorders of the urinary tract include ultrasound, computed tomography scans, and radiographic studies such as **intravenous urography** (Fig. 13-11), also called **intravenous pyelography**, and **retrograde pyelography**.

Urinalysis

Urinalysis (UA) is a simple and widely used method for diagnosing disorders of the urinary tract. It may also reveal disturbances in other systems when abnormal byproducts are eliminated in the urine. In a routine urinalysis, the urine is grossly examined for color and turbidity (a sign of bacteria); **specific gravity** (a measure of concentration) and pH are recorded; test are performed for chemical components such as glucose, ketones, and hemoglobin; and the urine is examined microscopically for cells, crystals, or casts. In more detailed tests, drugs, enzymes, hormones, and other metabolites may be analyzed and bacterial cultures may be performed.

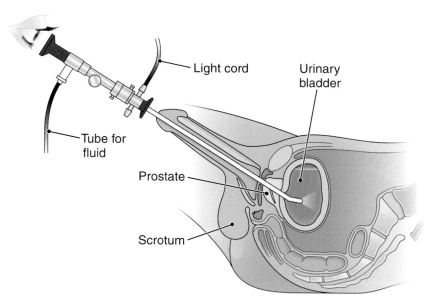

FIGURE 13-9. Cystoscopy. A lighted cystoscope is introduced into the bladder of a male subject. Sterile fluid is used to inflate the bladder.

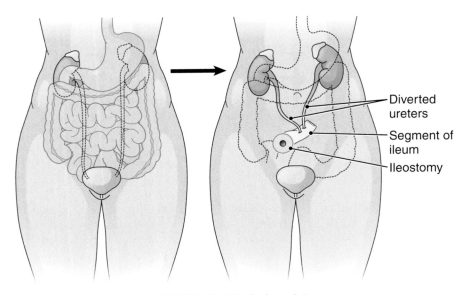

FIGURE 13-10. Ileal conduit.

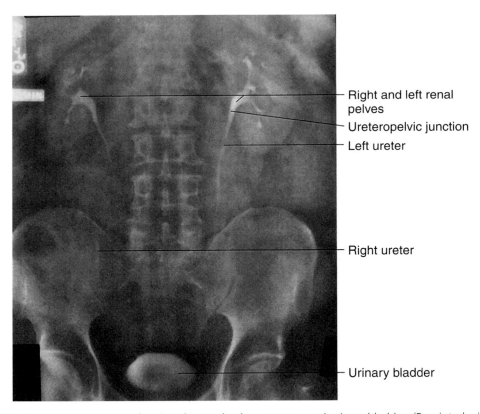

FIGURE 13-11. Intravenous urogram showing the renal pelves, ureters, and urinary bladder. (Reprinted with permission from Erkonen WE, Smith WL. Radiology 101: Basics and Fundamentals of Imaging. Philadelphia: Lippincott Williams & Wilkins, 1998.)

Key Clinical Terms

DISORDERS

acidosis
as-i-DŌ-sis
Excessive acidity of body fluids

bacteriuria
bak-tē-rē-Ū-rē-a
Presence of bacteria in the urine

cast
A solid mold of a renal tubule found in the urine

cystitis
sis-TĪ-tis
Inflammation of the urinary bladder, usually as a result of infection

dysuria
dis-Ū-rē-a
Painful or difficult urination

glomerulonephritis
glō-mer-ū-lō-nef-RĪ-tis
Inflammation of the kidney primarily involving the glomeruli. The acute form usually occurs after an infection elsewhere in the body; the chronic form varies in cause and usually leads to renal failure.

hematuria
hē-mat-Ū-rē-a
Presence of blood in the urine

hydronephrosis
hī-drō-nef-RŌ-sis
Collection of urine in the renal pelvis caused by obstruction; causes distention and atrophy of renal tissue. Also called nephrohydrosis or nephrydrosis.

hyperkalemia
hī-per-ka-LĒ-mē-a
Excess amount of potassium in the blood

oliguria
ol-ig-Ū-rē-a
Elimination of small amounts of urine

proteinuria
prō-tē-NŪ-rē-a
Presence of protein, mainly albumin, in the urine

pyelonephritis
pī-e-lō-ne-FRĪ-tis
Inflammation of the renal pelvis and kidney, usually as a result of infection

pyuria
pī-Ū-rē-a
Presence of pus in the urine

renal colic
KOL-ik
Radiating pain in the region of the kidney associated with the passage of a stone

uremia
ū-RĒ-mē-a
Presence in the blood of toxic levels of nitrogen-containing substances, mainly urea, as a result of renal insufficiency

urethritis
ū-rē-THRĪ-tis
Inflammation of the urethra, usually as a result of infection

urinary stasis
STĀ-sis
Stoppage or stagnation of the flow of urine

DIAGNOSIS AND TREATMENT

catheterization
kath-e-ter-i-ZĀ-shun
Introduction of a tube into a passage, such as through the urethra into the bladder for withdrawal of urine

Diagnosis and Treatment, continued

cystoscope *SIS-tō-skōp*	An instrument for examining the inside of the urinary bladder. Also used for removing foreign objects, for surgery, and for other forms of treatment.
dialysis *dī-AL-i-sis*	Separation of substances by passage through a semipermeable membrane. Dialysis is used to rid the body of unwanted substances when the kidneys are impaired or missing. The two forms of dialysis are hemodialysis and peritoneal dialysis.
hemodialysis *hē-mō-dī-AL-i-sis*	Removal of unwanted substances from the blood by passage through a semipermeable membrane
intravenous pyelography (IVP)	Intravenous urography
intravenous urography (IVU)	Radiographic visualization of the urinary tract after intravenous administration of a contrast medium that is excreted in the urine; also called excretory urography or intravenous pyelography, although the latter is less accurate because the procedure shows more than just the renal pelvis
lithotripsy *LITH-ō-trip-sē*	Crushing of a stone
peritoneal dialysis *per-i-tō-NĒ-al*	Removal of unwanted substances from the body by introduction of a dialyzing fluid into the peritoneal cavity followed by removal of the fluid
retrograde pyelography	Pyelography in which the contrast medium is injected into the kidneys from below, by way of the ureters
specific gravity (SG)	The weight of a substance compared with the weight of an equal volume of water. The specific gravity of normal urine ranges from 1.015 to 1.025. This value may increase or decrease in disease.
urinalysis *ū-ri-NAL-i-sis*	Laboratory study of the urine. Physical and chemical properties and microscopic appearance are included.

SURGERY

cystectomy *sis-TEK-tō-mē*	Surgical removal of all or part of the urinary bladder
ileal conduit *IL-ē-al KON-dū-it*	Diversion of urine by connection of the ureters to an isolated segment of the ileum. One end of the segment is sealed, and the other drains through an opening in the abdominal wall (see Fig. 13-10).
lithotomy *lith-OT-ō-mē*	Incision of an organ to remove a stone (calculus)
renal transplantation	Surgical implantation of a donor kidney into a patient

Supplementary Terms

NORMAL STRUCTURE AND FUNCTION

aldosterone *al-DOS-ter-ōn*	A hormone secreted by the adrenal gland that regulates electrolyte excretion by the kidneys
clearance	The volume of plasma that can be cleared of a substance by the kidneys per unit of time; renal plasma clearance
creatinine *krē-AT-in-in*	A nitrogen-containing byproduct of muscle metabolism. An increase in creatinine in the blood is a sign of renal failure.
detrusor muscle *dē-TRŪ-sor*	The muscle in the bladder wall
diuresis *dī-ū-RĒ-sis*	Increased excretion of urine
glomerular filtration rate (GFR)	The amount of filtrate formed per minute by the nephrons of both kidneys
maximal transport capacity (Tm)	The maximum rate at which a given substance can be transported across the renal tubule; tubular maximum
renal corpuscle *KOR-pus-l*	The glomerular capsule and the glomerulus considered as a unit; the filtration device of the kidney
trigone *TRĪ-gōn*	A triangle at the base of the bladder formed by the openings of the two ureters and the urethra (see Fig. 13-4)

SYMPTOMS AND CONDITIONS

anuresis *an-ū-RĒ-sis*	Lack of urination
anuria *an-Ū-re-a*	Lack of urine formation
azotemia *az-ō-TĒ-mē-a*	Presence of an increased amount of nitrogenous waste, especially urea, in the blood
azoturia *az-ō-TŪ-rē-a*	Presence of an increased amount of nitrogen-containing compounds, especially urea, in the urine
cystocele *SIS-tō-sēl*	Herniation of the bladder into the vagina (see Fig. 15-17); vesicocele
dehydration *dē-hī-DRĀ-shun*	Excessive loss of body fluids
diabetes insipidus *dī-a-BĒ-tēz in-SIP-id-us*	A condition caused by inadequate production of antidiuretic hormone resulting in excessive excretion of dilute urine and extreme thirst
enuresis *en-ū-RĒ-sis*	Involuntary urination, usually at night; bed-wetting

Symptoms and Conditions, continued

epispadias *ep-i-SPĀ-dē-as*	A congenital condition in which the urethra opens on the dorsal surface of the penis as a groove or cleft; anaspadias
glycosuria *glī-kō-SŪ-rē-a*	Presence of glucose in the urine, as in cases of diabetes mellitus
horseshoe kidney	A congenital union of the lower poles of the kidneys, resulting in a horseshoe-shaped organ (Fig. 13-12)
hydroureter *hī-drō-ū-RĒ-ter*	Distention of the ureter with urine caused by obstruction
hypoproteinemia *hī-pō-prō-tē-NĒ-mē-a*	Decreased amount of protein in the blood; may result from loss of protein because of kidney damage
hypospadias *hī-pō-SPĀ-dē-as*	A congenital condition in which the urethra opens on the undersurface of the penis or into the vagina (Fig. 13-13)
hypovolemia *hī-pō-vō-LĒ-mē-a*	A decrease in blood volume
incontinence *in-KON-tin-ens*	Inability to retain urine. Incontinence may originate with a neurologic disorder, trauma to the spinal cord, weakness of the pelvic muscles, urinary retention, or impaired bladder function. Term also applies to inability to retain semen or feces.
neurogenic bladder *nū-rō-JEN-ik*	Any bladder dysfunction that results from a central nervous system lesion
nocturia *nok-TŪ-rē-a*	Excessive urination at night (*noct/o* means "night")
pitting edema	Edema in which the skin, when pressed firmly with the finger, will maintain the depression produced
polycystic kidney disease	A hereditary condition in which the kidneys are enlarged and contain many cysts
polydipsia *pol-i-DIP-sē-a*	Excessive thirst
polyuria *pol-ē-Ū-rē-a*	Elimination of large amounts of urine, as in diabetes mellitus
retention of urine	Accumulation of urine in the bladder because of an inability to urinate
staghorn calculus	A kidney stone that fills the renal pelvis and calyces to give a "staghorn" appearance (Fig. 13-14)
ureterocele *ū-RĒ-ter-ō-sēl*	A cystlike dilation of the ureter near its opening into the bladder. Usually results from a congenital narrowing of the ureteral opening (Fig. 13-15).
urinary frequency	A need to urinate often without an increase in average output
urinary urgency	Sudden need to urinate

Symptoms and Conditions, continued

water intoxication *in-tok-si-KĀ-shun*	Excess intake or retention of water with decrease in sodium concentration. May result from excess drinking, excess ADH, or replacement of a large amount of body fluid with pure water. Causes an imbalance in the cellular environment with edema and other disturbances.
Wilms tumor	A malignant tumor of the kidney that usually appears in children before the age of 5 years

DIAGNOSIS

anion gap	A measure of electrolyte imbalance
blood urea nitrogen (BUN)	Nitrogen in the blood in the form of urea. An increase in BUN indicates an increase in nitrogenous waste products in the blood and renal failure.
clean-catch specimen	A urine sample obtained after thorough cleansing of the urethral opening and collected in midstream to minimize the chance of contamination
cystometrography *sis-tō-me-TROG-ra-fē*	A study of bladder function in which the bladder is filled with fluid or air and the pressure exerted by the bladder muscle at varying degrees of filling is measured. The tracing recorded is a cystometrogram.
protein electrophoresis (PEP)	Laboratory study of the proteins in urine; used to diagnose multiple myeloma, systemic lupus erythematosus, lymphoid tumor
urinometer *ū-ri-NOM-e-ter*	Device for measuring the specific gravity of urine

TREATMENT

diuretic *dī-ū-RET-ik*	A substance that increases the excretion of urine; pertaining to diuresis
indwelling Foley catheter	A urinary tract catheter with a balloon at one end that prevents the catheter from leaving the bladder (see Fig. 13-5)
lithotrite *LITH-ō-trīt*	Instrument for crushing a bladder stone

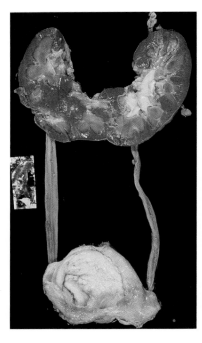

FIGURE 13-12. Horseshoe kidney. The kidneys are fused at the poles. (Reprinted with permission from Rubin E, Farber JL. Pathology. 3rd Ed. Philadelphia: Lippincott Williams & Wilkins, 1999.)

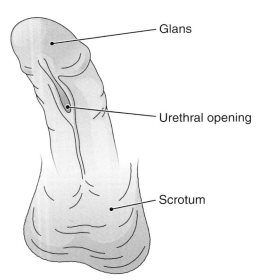

Glans

Urethral opening

Scrotum

FIGURE 13-13. Hypospadias. Ventral view of penis.

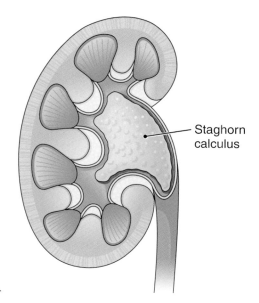

FIGURE 13-14. Staghorn calculus.

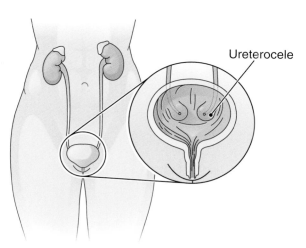

FIGURE 13-15. Ureterocele. The ureter bulges into the bladder with resultant hydroureter and hydronephrosis.

ABBREVIATIONS

ADH	Antidiuretic hormone		**GFR**	Glomerular filtration rate
ARF	Acute renal failure		**GU**	Genitourinary
ATN	Acute tubular necrosis		**IVP**	Intravenous pyelography
BUN	Blood urea nitrogen		**IVU**	Intravenous urography
CAPD	Continuous ambulatory peritoneal dialysis		**K**	Potassium
			KUB	Kidney-ureter-bladder (radiography)
CCPD	Continuous cyclic peritoneal dialysis		**Na**	Sodium
CMG	Cystometrography; cystometrogram		**PEP**	Protein electrophoresis
CRF	Chronic renal failure		**SG**	Specific gravity
EPO	Erythropoietin		**Tm**	Maximal transport capacity
ESRD	End-stage renal disease		**UA**	Urinalysis
ESWL	Extracorporeal shock wave lithotripsy		**UTI**	Urinary tract infection

Labeling Exercise 13-1

Urinary System, With Blood Vessels

Write the name of each numbered part on the corresponding line of the answer sheet.

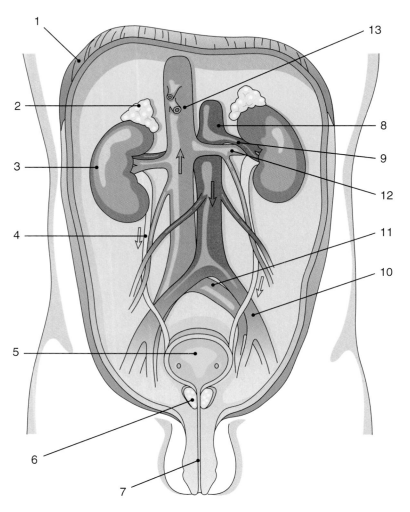

Abdominal aorta
Adrenal gland
Common iliac artery
Common iliac vein
Diaphragm
Inferior vena cava
Prostate gland
Renal artery
Renal vein
Right kidney
Ureter
Urethra
Urinary bladder

1. _____	8. _____
2. _____	9. _____
3. _____	10. _____
4. _____	11. _____
5. _____	12. _____
6. _____	13. _____
7. _____	

Labeling Exercise 13-2

Longitudinal Section Through the Kidney

Write the name of each numbered part on the corresponding line of the answer sheet.

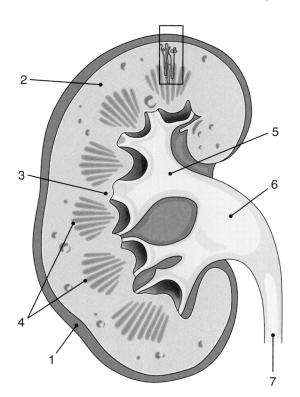

Calyx
Pyramids of medulla
Renal capsule
Renal medulla
Renal pelvis
Renal cortex
Ureter

1. _____

2. _____

3. _____

4. _____

5. _____

6. _____

7. _____

Labeling Exercise 13-3

Interior of the Urinary Bladder

Write the name of each numbered part on the corresponding line of the answer sheet.

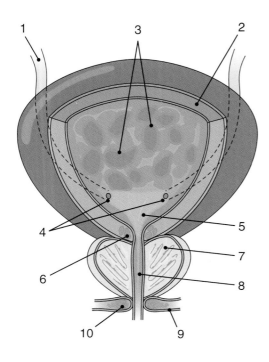

1. _____

2. _____

3. _____

4. _____

5. _____

6. _____

7. _____

8. _____

9. _____

10. _____

External sphincter   Smooth muscle
Internal sphincter   Trigone
Openings of ureters   Ureter
Prostate   Urethra
Rugae   Urogenital diaphragm

Chapter Review 13-1

Match the following terms and write the appropriate letter to the left of each number:

_____ 1. albuminuria

_____ 2. pyuria

_____ 3. chromaturia

_____ 4. oliguria

_____ 5. cyturia

a. abnormal color of urine

b. pus in the urine

c. elimination of small amounts of urine

d. cells in the urine

e. proteinuria

_____ 6. adrenal

_____ 7. intrarenal

_____ 8. prerenal

_____ 9. renovascular

_____ 10. hepatorenal

a. pertaining to the blood vessels of the kidneys

b. within the kidneys

c. pertaining to the liver and kidneys

d. before or in front of the kidneys

e. near the kidney

_____ 11. nocturia

_____ 12. erythropoietin

_____ 13. uropenia

_____ 14. kaliuresis

_____ 15. renin

a. excretion of potassium in the urine

b. deficiency of urine

c. excessive urination during the night

d. enzyme that increases blood pressure

e. hormone that stimulates red cell production

_____ 16. micturition

_____ 17. acystia

_____ 18. stasis

_____ 19. catheterization

_____ 20. lithotomy

a. congenital absence of the bladder

b. urination

c. introduction of a tube

d. incision to remove a stone

e. stagnation, as of urine

SUPPLEMENTARY TERMS

_____ 21. trigone

_____ 22. azoturia

_____ 23. enuresis

_____ 24. glycosuria

_____ 25. polydipsia

a. presence of nitrogenous waste in the urine

b. excessive thirst

c. bed-wetting

d. triangular area in the base of the bladder

e. presence of glucose in the urine

_____ 26. creatinine

a. drug that increases urination

_____ 27. diabetes insipidus

b. a nitrogenous byproduct of metabolism

_____ 28. epispadias

c. inability to retain urine

_____ 29. incontinence

d. congenital misplacement of the ureteral opening

_____ 30. diuretic

e. condition caused by lack of ADH

Fill in the blanks:

31. A microscopic working unit of the kidney is called a(n) _____.

32. The cluster of capillaries within the glomerular capsule is the _____.

33. The inner portion of the kidney is the _____.

34. Laboratory study of the urine is a(n) _____.

35. The tube that carries urine from the kidney to the bladder is the _____.

36. The main nitrogenous waste product in urine is _____.

37. A solid mold of the renal tubule found in the urine is a(n) _____.

Define each of the following words:

38. reniform (*REN-i-form*)   _____

39. nephrotropic (*nef-rō-TROP-ik*)   _____

40. juxtaglomerular (*juks-ta-glō-MER-ū-lar*)   _____

41. urethritis (*ū-rē-THRĪ-tis*)   _____

42. caliceal (*kal-i-SĒ-al*) (note addition of e)   _____

43. urethrostenosis (*ū-rē-thrō-ste-NŌ-sis*)   _____

44. dysuria (*dis-Ū-rē-a*)   _____

Word building. Write a word for each of the following definitions:

45. any disease of the kidney (nephr/o)   _____

46. radiograph of the bladder (cyst/o) and urethra   _____

47. incision of the bladder (cyst/o)   _____

48. inflammation of the urinary bladder   _____

49. inflammation of the renal pelvis and the kidney   _____

50. surgical removal of a kidney (nephr/o)   _____

51. plastic repair of a ureter and renal pelvis   _____

52. surgical creation of an opening between a ureter and
    the sigmoid colon   _____

53. dilatation of the renal pelvis and calices   _____

Opposites. Write a word that has the opposite meaning of each of the following words:

54. hydration   _____

55. hypovolemia   _____

56. diuretic _____

57. hypernatremia _____

58. uresis _____

Adjectives. Write the adjective form of each of the following words:

59. vesica (bladder) _____

60. urology _____

61. uremia _____

62. diuresis _____

63. calyx _____

64. nephrosis _____

65. ureter _____

66. urethra _____

Plurals. Write the plural form of each of the following words:

67. glomerulus _____

68. calyx _____

69. pelvis _____

Write the meaning of each of the following abbreviations:

70. IVP _____

71. ADH _____

72. EPO _____

73. BUN _____

74. UTI _____

75. GFR _____

76. UA _____

Word analysis. Define each of the following words, and give the meaning of the word parts in each. Use a dictionary if necessary.

77. cystometrography (*sis-tō-me-TROG-ra-fē*) _____
    a. cyst/o _____
    b. metr/o _____
    c. -graphy _____

78. ureteroneocystostomy (*ū-rē-ter-ō-nē-ō-sis-TOS-tō-mē*) _____
    a. ureter/o _____
    b. neo- _____
    c. cyst/o _____
    d. -stomy _____

Case Studies

Case Study 13-1: Renal Calculi

A.A., a 48-year-old woman, was admitted to the in-patient unit from the ER with severe right flank pain unresponsive to analgesics. Her pain did not decrease with administration of 100 mg of IV meperidine. She had a 3-month history of chronic UTI. Six months ago she had been prescribed calcium supplements for low bone density. Her gynecologist warned her that calcium could be a problem for people who are "stone-formers." A.A. was unaware that she might be at risk. An IV urogram showed a right staghorn calculus. The diagnosis was further confirmed by a renal ultrasound. A renal flow scan showed normal perfusion and no obstruction. Kidney function was 37% on the right and 63% on the left. While the pain became intermittent, A.A. had no hematuria, dysuria, frequency, urgency, or nocturia. Urinalysis revealed no albumin, glucose, bacteria, or blood; there was evidence of cells, crystals, and casts.

A.A. was transferred to surgery for a cystoscopic ureteral laser lithotripsy, insertion of a right retrograde ureteral catheter, and right percutaneous nephrolithotomy. A ureteral calculus was fragmented with the pulsed-dye laser. Most of the staghorn was removed from the renal pelvis with no remaining stone in the renal calices. She was discharged 2 days later and ordered to strain her urine for the next week for evidence of stones.

Case Study 13-2: End-Stage Renal Disease

M.C., a 20-year-old part-time college student, has had chronic glomerulonephritis since age 7. He has been managed at home with CAPD for the last 16 months as he awaits a kidney transplant. His doctor advised him to go immediately to the ER when he complained of chest pain, shortness of breath, and oliguria. On admission, M.C. was placed on oxygen and given a panel of blood tests and an ECG to rule out an acute cardiac episode. His hemoglobin was 8.2 and hematocrit was 26%. He had bilateral lung rales. ABGs were: pH, 7.0; $PaCO_2$, 28; PaO_2, 50; HCO_3, 21. His BUN, serum creatinine, and BUN/creatinine ratio were abnormally high. His ECG and liver enzyme studies were normal. His admission diagnosis was ESRD, fluid overload, and metabolic acidosis. He was typed and crossed for blood; tested for HIV, hepatitis B antigen, and sexually transmitted disease; and sent to hemodialysis. A bed was reserved for him on the transplant unit.

Case Study 13-3: Set-Up for Cystoscopy

Renovations had been completed recently in the new surgical suite, and J.O., a surgical technologist, set up the two new adjoining "cysto" rooms. Each room had a new cystoscopy bed with padded knee crutches for lithotomy position, a drainage drawer for irrigation solution collection, and radiology capability. The instrument storage carts were stocked with rigid and flexible cystoscopes, sheaths with obturators, and resectoscopes with assorted fulgurating loops, connectors, guide wires, laser fibers, and fiberoptic light cords. Sterile storage closets held assorted urethral and ureteral catheters, irrigation tubing and syringes, collection bags, biopsy needles and forceps, basic soft tissue instruments, and dressing supplies.

An electrosurgery machine was placed in each room. Cysto no. 1 had the CMG machine and urinometer. Cysto no. 2 had a Nd:YAG (neodymium:yttrium-aluminum-garnet) and a liquid tunable pulsed-dye laser machine. Each room had a machine to collect and decontaminate the liquid waste, instead of the former floor drains.

Case Studies, continued

The substerile room between Cysto no. 1 and no. 2 had a steam sterilizer, a peracetic acid processor/sterilizer, and glutaraldehyde soaking pans under a ventilation hood to high level-disinfect the instruments between cases. A warming closet contained blankets and sterile PSS, H_2O, and glycine for bladder irrigation during the procedures. J.O. wished there was room left for an ESWL system.

CASE STUDY QUESTIONS

Multiple choice: Select the best answer and write the letter of your choice to the left of each number.

_____ 1. The term perfusion means:
    a. size
    b. shape
    c. passage of fluid
    d. surrounding tissue
    e. metabolism

_____ 2. M.C.'s chronic glomerulonephritis means that he has had:
    a. long-term kidney stones
    b. an acute bout of kidney infection
    c. short-term bladder inflammation
    d. a long-term kidney infection
    e. dysuria for 13 years

_____ 3. Renal dialysis can be performed by shunting venous blood through a dialysis machine and returning the blood to the patient's arterial system. This procedure is called:
    a. hemodialysis
    b. arterio/venous transplant
    c. CAPD
    d. phlebotomy
    e. glomerular filtration rate

_____ 4. A surgical endoscope that can enter and visualize the bladder is a(n) _____, whereas a scope that cuts tissue is called a(n) _____.
    a. cystoscope, resectoscope
    b. resectoscope, fulgurating loop
    c. urinometer, obturator with sheath
    d. cystoscope, scissorscope
    e. urethrascope, ureteralscope

_____ 5. A transurethral approach for examination or surgery always begins with inserting a catheter or scope:
    a. through the ureter
    b. alongside of the urethra
    c. between the ureters
    d. through the urethra
    e. below the perineum

Case Studies, continued

Write a term from the case studies with each of the following meanings:

6. intravenous injection of contrast dye and radiographic study of the urinary tract
   _____

7. production of a reduced amount of urine _____

8. getting up to go to the bathroom at night _____

9. crushing a stone in the ureter with a laser _____

10. kidney replacement _____

11. surgical incision for removal of a stone _____

Abbreviations. Define the following abbreviations:

12. UTI _____

13. CAPD _____

14. BUN _____

15. ESRD _____

16. HIV _____

17. CMG _____

18. PSS _____

19. ESWL _____

Chapter 13 Crossword
Urinary System

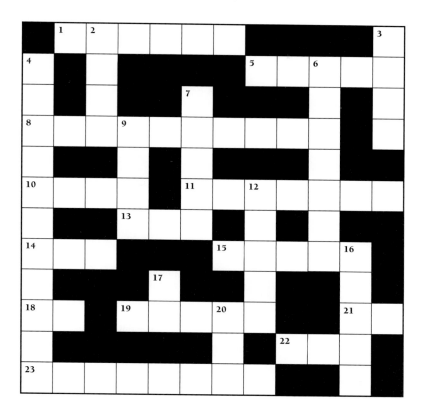

ACROSS

1. Tube that carries urine from the kidney to the bladder
5. Water; fluid: combining form
8. Cluster of capillaries in Bowman capsule
10. Few; scant: prefix
11. Microscopic functional unit of the kidney
13. Drug that reduces blood pressure, ____ inhibitor
14. Hormone that stimulates red cell production: abbreviation
15. Pertaining to the kidney
18. Measure of the weight of a substance as compared to water: abbreviation
19. Urinary bladder: combining form
21. Maximum amount of a substance that can be reabsorbed: abbreviation
22. Pituitary hormone that regulates water reabsorption: abbreviation
23. Excessive urination at night

DOWN

2. Kidney: combining form
3. Organism often involved in urinary tract infections, *E.* ____
4. Substance produced in response to renin that increases blood pressure
6. Painful or difficult urination
7. The fluid excreted by the kidneys
9. Large or abnormally large: prefix
12. Renal pelvis: combining form
16. Calculus (stone): combining form
17. Pus: root
20. Three: prefix

CHAPTER **13 Answer Section**

Answers to Chapter Exercises

EXERCISE 13-1

1. pararenal (*par-a-RĒ-nal*)
2. suprarenal (*sū-pra-RĒ-nal*)
3. interrenal (*in-ter-RĒ-nal*)
4. perirenal (*per-i-RĒ-nal*); circumrenal (*sir-kum-RĒ-nal*)
5. postrenal (*post-RĒ-nal*)
6. nephritis (*nef-RĪ-tis*)
7. nephropathy (*nef-ROP-a-thē*)
8. nephromalacia (*nef-rō-ma-LĀ-shē-a*)
9. nephrectomy (*nef-REK-tō-mē*)
10. nephrology (*ne-FROL-ō-jē*)
11. glomerulitis (*glō-mer-ū-LĪ-tis*)
12. calicectomy (*kal-i-SEK-tō-mē*)
13. pyelogram (*PĪ-e-lō-gram*)
14. pyelectasis (*pi-e-LEK-ta-sis*)
15. glomerulosclerosis (*glo-mer-ū-lō-skle-RŌ-sis*)
16. renography (*rē-NOG-ra-fē*); nephrography (*nef-ROG-ra-fē*)
17. pyelonephritis (*pi-e-lō-nef-RĪ-tis*)

EXERCISE 13-2

1. urography (*ū-ROG-ra-fē*)
2. urolith (*Ū-rō-lith*)
3. urology (*ū-ROL-ō-jē*)
4. uremia (*ū-RĒ-mē-a*)
5. proteinuria (*prō-tē-NŪ-rē-a*)
6. anuria (*an-Ū-rē-a*)
7. polyuria (*pol-ē-Ū-rē-a*)
8. dysuria (*dis-Ū-rē-a*)
9. pyuria (*pi-Ū-rē-a*)
10. cyturia (*si-TŪ-rē-a*)
11. hematuria (*hē-ma-TŪ-rē-a*)
12. nocturia (*nok-TŪ-rē-a*)
13. diuresis (*di-u-RĒ-sis*)
14. anuresis (*an-ū-RĒ-sis*)
15. natriuresis (*nā-trē-ū-RĒ-sis*)
16. kaliuresis (*kā-lē-ū-RĒ-sis*)
17. urine
18. ureter
19. urethra
20. urinary bladder
21. urinary bladder
22. urethritis (*ū-rē-THRĪ-tis*)
23. ureterolith (*ū-RĒ-ter-ō-lith*)
24. ureterostomy (*ū-rē-ter-OS-tō-mē*)
25. urethropexy (*ū-RĒ-thrō-pek-sē*)
26. cystitis (*sis-TĪ-tis*)
27. cystopexy (*SIS-tō-pek-sē*)
28. cystoscope (*SIS-tō-skōp*)
29. cystocele (*SIS-tō-sēl*); also vesicocele (*VES-i-kō-sēl*)
30. prevesical (*prē-VES-i-kal*)
31. urethrovesical (*ū-rē-thrō-VES-i-kal*)
32. through the urethra
33. surgical creation of an opening in the bladder
34. surgical incision of the ureter
35. pain in the urinary bladder
36. formation of urine

LABELING EXERCISE 13-1 URINARY SYSTEM, WITH BLOOD VESSELS

1. diaphragm
2. adrenal gland
3. right kidney
4. ureter
5. urinary bladder
6. prostate gland
7. urethra
8. abdominal aorta
9. renal artery
10. common iliac artery
11. common iliac vein
12. renal vein
13. inferior vena cava

LABELING EXERCISE 13-2 LONGITUDINAL SECTION THROUGH THE KIDNEY

1. renal capsule
2. renal cortex
3. renal medulla
4. pyramids of medulla
5. calyx
6. renal pelvis
7. ureter

LABELING EXERCISE 13-3 INTERIOR OF THE URINARY BLADDER

1. ureter
2. smooth muscle
3. rugae
4. openings of ureters

5. trigone
6. internal sphincter
7. prostate
8. urethra
9. urogenital diaphragm
10. external sphincter

Answers to Chapter Review 13-1

1. e
2. b
3. a
4. c
5. d
6. e
7. b
8. d
9. a
10. c
11. c
12. e
13. b
14. a
15. d
16. b
17. a
18. e
19. c
20. d
21. d
22. a
23. c
24. e
25. b
26. b
27. e
28. d
29. c
30. a
31. nephron
32. glomerulus
33. medulla
34. urinalysis
35. ureter
36. urea
37. cast
38. like or resembling a kidney
39. acting on the kidney
40. near the glomerulus
41. inflammation of the urethra
42. pertaining to a calyx
43. narrowing of a urethra
44. painful or difficult urination
45. nephropathy
46. cystourethrogram

47. cystotomy
48. cystitis
49. pyelonephritis
50. nephrectomy
51. ureteropyeloplasty
52. ureterosigmoidostomy
53. pyelocaliectasis; pyelocaliectasis
54. dehydration
55. hypervolemia
56. antidiuretic
57. hyponatremia
58. anuresis
59. vesical
60. urologic
61. uremic
62. diuretic
63. caliceal
64. nephrotic
65. ureteral
66. urethral
67. glomeruli
68. calyces
69. pelves
70. intravenous pyelography
71. antidiuretic hormone
72. erythropoietin
73. blood urea nitrogen
74. urinary tract infection
75. glomerular filtration rate
76. urinalysis
77. test that measures and records bladder function
    a. urinary bladder
    b. measure
    c. act of recording data
78. surgical creation of a new passage between a ureter and the bladder
    a. ureter
    b. new
    c. bladder
    d. surgical creation of an opening

Answers to Case Study Questions

1. c
2. d
3. a
4. a
5. d
6. IV urogram
7. oliguria
8. nocturia
9. ureteral laser lithotripsy
10. kidney transplant
11. lithotomy
12. urinary tract infection

The Male Reproductive System

Chapter Contents

Objectives

After study of this chapter you should be able to:

1. Label a diagram of the male reproductive tract and describe the function of each part.
2. Describe the contents and functions of semen.
3. Identify and use roots pertaining to the male reproductive system.
4. Describe the main disorders of the male reproductive system.
5. Interpret abbreviations used in referring to the reproductive system.
6. Analyze several case studies concerning the male reproductive system.

he function of the **gonads** (sex glands) in both males and females is to produce the reproductive cells, the **gametes**, and to produce hormones. The gametes are generated by **meiosis**, a process of cell division that halves the chromosome number from 46 to 23. When male and female gametes unite in fertilization, the original chromosome number is restored. The sex hormones aid in the manufacture of the gametes, function in pregnancy and lactation, and also produce the secondary sex characteristics such as the typical size, shape, body hair, and voice that we associate with the male and female genders.

The reproductive tract develops in close association with the urinary tract. In females, the two systems become completely separate, whereas the male reproductive and urinary tracts share a common passage, the urethra. Thus, the two systems are referred to together as the genitourinary (GU) or urogenital (UG) tract, and urologists are called on to treat disorders of the male reproductive system as well as of the urinary system.

The Testes

The male germ cells, the **spermatozoa** (sperm cells), are produced in the paired **testes** (singular, testis) that are suspended outside of the body in the **scrotum** (Fig. 14-1). Although the testes develop in the abdominal cavity, they normally descend through the **inguinal canal** into the scrotum before birth or shortly

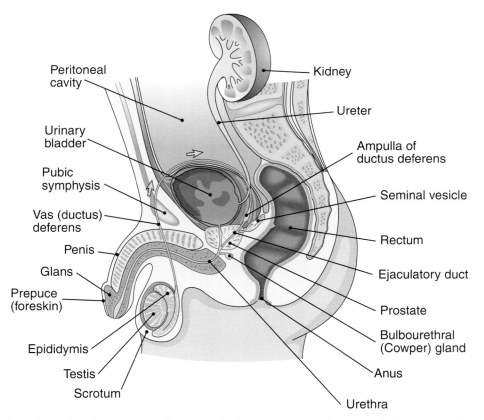

FIGURE 14-1. Male genitourinary system. The *arrows* indicate the course of sperm cells through the duct system. (Reprinted with permission from Cohen BJ, Wood DL. Memmler's The Human Body in Health and Disease. 9th Ed. Philadelphia: Lippincott Williams & Wilkins, 2000.)

thereafter. From puberty on, spermatozoa form continuously within the testes in coiled seminiferous tubules (Fig. 14-2). Their development requires the aid of special **Sertoli cells** and male sex hormones, or **androgens**, mainly **testosterone**. These hormones are manufactured in **interstitial cells** located between the tubules. In both males and females, the gonads are stimulated by the hormones **follicle stimulating hormone (FSH)** and **luteinizing hormone (LH)**, released from the anterior **pituitary gland** beneath the brain. Although these hormones are the same in both males and females, LH is called **interstitial cell-stimulating hormone (ICSH)** in males.

Transport of Spermatozoa

After their manufacture, sperm cells are stored in a much-coiled tube on the surface of each testis, the **epididymis** (see Figs. 14-1 and 14-2). Here they remain until ejaculation propels them into a series of ducts that lead out of the body. The first of these is the **vas (ductus) deferens**. This duct ascends through the inguinal canal into the abdominal cavity and travels behind the bladder. A short continuation, the **ejaculatory duct**, delivers the spermatozoa to the urethra as it passes through the prostate gland below the bladder. Finally, the cells, now mixed with other secretions, travel in the **urethra** through the **penis** to be released. The penis is the male organ that transports both urine and semen. It enlarges at the tip to form the **glans penis**, which is covered by loose skin, the **prepuce** or foreskin. Surgery to remove the foreskin is **circumcision**. This may be performed for medical reasons, but is most often performed electively in male infants for reasons of hygiene, cultural preferences, or religion.

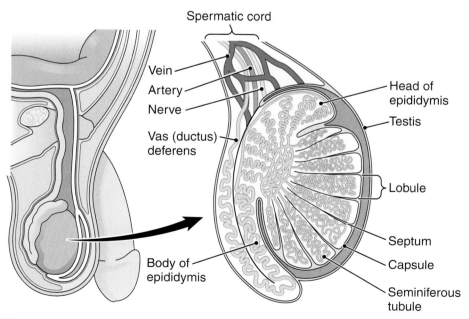

FIGURE 14-2. Structure of the testis, also showing the epididymis and spermatic cord. (Reprinted with permission from Cohen BJ, Wood DL. Memmler's The Human Body in Health and Disease. 9th Ed. Philadelphia: Lippincott Williams & Wilkins, 2000.)

BOX 14-1 Which Is It?

Some of the work of learning medical terminology is made more difficult by the fact that many structures and processes are known by two or even more names. This duplication may occur because different names have been assigned at different times or places or because the name is in a state of transition to another name and the new one has not been universally accepted.

The tube that leads from the testis to the urethra in males was originally called the vas deferens, vas being a general term for vessel. To distinguish this tube from a blood vessel, efforts have been made to change the name to ductus deferens. The original name has lingered, however, because the surgical procedure used to

sterilize a man is still called a vasectomy and not a "ductusectomy."

Similar inconsistencies appear in other systems. Dorsal is also posterior; ventral could be anterior. Human growth hormone is also called somatotropin. LH (luteinizing hormone) is called ICSH (interstitial cell-stimulating hormone) in the male.

In the nervous system, the little swellings at the ends of axons that contain neurotransmitters are variously called end-feet, end-bulbs, terminal knobs, terminal feet, and even more. In the woman, the tube that carries the ovum from the ovary to the uterus is referred to as the oviduct, or maybe the Fallopian tube. . . or the uterine tube. . . or. . . .

Formation of Semen

Semen is the thick, whitish fluid in which spermatozoa are transported. It contains, in addition to sperm cells, secretions from three types of accessory glands. The first of these, the paired **seminal vesicles**, release their secretions into the ejaculatory duct. The second, the **prostate gland**, secretes into the first part of the urethra beneath the bladder. As men age, enlargement of the prostate gland may compress the urethra and cause urinary problems. The two **bulbourethral** (Cowper) **glands** secrete into the urethra just below the prostate gland. Together these glands produce a slightly alkaline mixture that nourishes and transports the sperm cells and also protects them by neutralizing the acidity of the female vaginal tract.

NORMAL STRUCTURE AND FUNCTION

androgen AN-drō-jen	Any hormone that produces male characteristics; root *andelo* means "male"
bulbourethral gland bul-bō-ū-RĒ-thral	A small gland beside the urethra below the prostate that secretes part of the seminal fluid. Also called Cowper gland.
circumcision ser-kum-SI-zhun	Surgical removal of the end of the prepuce (foreskin)

Normal Structure and Function, *continued*

ejaculation *ē-jak-ū-LĀ-shun*	Ejection of semen from the male urethra
ejaculatory duct *ē-JAK-ū-la-tōr-ē*	The duct formed by union of the ductus deferens and the duct of the seminal vesicle; it carries spermatozoa and seminal fluid into the urethra
epididymis *ep-i-DID-i-mis*	A coiled tube on the surface of the testis that stores sperm until ejaculation (root *epididym/o*)
follicle stimulating hormone (FSH)	A hormone secreted by the anterior pituitary that acts on the gonads. In the male, FSH stimulates development of sperm cells.
gamete *GAM-ēt*	A mature reproductive cell, the spermatozoon in the male and the ovum in the female
glans penis *glanz PĒ-nis*	The bulbous end of the penis
gonad *GŌ-nad*	A sex gland; testis or ovary
interstitial cell-stimulating hormone (ICSH)	A hormone secreted by the pituitary that acts on the gonads. In the male, it stimulates production of testosterone. Also called luteinizing hormone (LH).
inguinal canal *ING-gwin-al*	The channel through which the testis descends into the scrotum in the male
interstitial cells *in-ter-STISH-al*	Cells located between the seminiferous tubules of the testes that produce hormones, mainly testosterone. Also called cells of Leydig.
luteinizing hormone (LH) *LŪ-tē-in-Ī-zing*	A hormone secreted by the anterior pituitary that acts on the gonads; also called interstitial cell-stimulating hormone (ICSH) in males
meiosis *mī-Ō-sis*	The type of cell division that forms the gametes; it results in cells with 23 chromosomes, half the number found in other body cells (from Greek word meaning "diminution")
pituitary gland *pi-TŪ-i-tar-ē*	An endocrine gland at the base of the brain
penis *PĒ-nis*	The male organ of copulation and urination; adjective, penile
prepuce *PRĒ-pūs*	The fold of skin over the glans penis; the foreskin
prostate gland *PROS-tāt*	A gland that surrounds the urethra below the bladder in males and contributes secretions to the semen (root *prostat/o*)
scrotum *SKRŌ-tum*	A double pouch that contains the testes (root *osche/o*)
semen	The thick secretion that transports spermatozoa (root *semin, sperm/i, spermat/o*)

Normal Structure and Function, continued

seminal vesicle *SEM-i-nal VES-i-kl*	A saclike gland behind the bladder that contributes secretions to the semen (root *vesicul/o*)
Sertoli cells *ser-TŌ-lēz*	Cells in the seminiferous tubules that aid in the development of spermatozoa
spermatozoa *sper-ma-tō-ZŌ-a*	Mature male sex cells (singular, spermatozoon) (root *sperm/i*, *spermat/o*)
testis *TES-tis*	The male reproductive gland (plural, testes) (see Fig. 14-2); also called testicle (root *test/o*)
testosterone *tes-TOS-ter-ōn*	The main male sex hormone
urethra *ū-RĒ-thra*	The duct that carries urine out of the body and also transports semen in the male
vas deferens *DEF-er-enz*	The duct that conveys spermatozoa from the epididymis to the ejaculatory duct. Also called ductus deferens.

Roots Pertaining to Male Reproduction

TABLE 14-1 Roots Pertaining to Male Reproduction

ROOT	MEANING	EXAMPLE	DEFINITION OF EXAMPLE
test/o	testis, testicle	testicular *tes-TIK-ū-lar*	pertaining to a testicle
orchi/o, orchid/o	testis	anorchism *an-OR-kizm*	absence of a testis
semin	semen	inseminate *in-SEM-i-nāt*	to introduce semen into a woman
sperm/i, spermat/o	semen, spermatozoa	oligospermia *ol-i-gō-SPER-mē-a*	deficiency of spermatozoa
epididym/o	epididymis	epididymitis *ep-i-did-i-MĪ-tis*	inflammation of the epididymis
vas/o	vas deferens; also vessel	vasorrhaphy *vas-OR-a-fē*	suture of the vas deferens
vesicul/o	seminal vesicle	vesiculography *ve-sik-ū-LOG-ra-fē*	radiographic study of the seminal vesicles
prostat/o	prostate	prostatometer *pros-ta-TOM-e-ter*	instrument for measuring the prostate
osche/o	scrotum	oscheoma *os-kē-Ō-ma*	tumor of the scrotum

Exercise 14-1

Define each of the following words:

1. seminal (*SEM-i-nal*)   _____

2. testopathy (*test-TOP-a-thē*)   _____

3. orchialgia (*or-kē-AL-jē-a*)   _____

4. epididymectomy (*ep-i-did-i-MEK-tō-mē*)   _____

5. prostatic (*pros-TAT-ik*)   _____

6. oscheal (*OS-kē-al*)   _____

7. orchiepididymitis (*or-kē-ep-i-did-i-MĪ-tis*)   _____

Use the root *orchi/o* to write a word that has the same meaning as each of the following definitions. Each is also written with the root *orchid/o.*

8. surgical fixation of a testis   _____

9. plastic repair of a testis   _____

10. incision of a testis   _____

Use the root *spermat/o* to write a word that has the same meaning as each of the following definitions:

11. a sperm-forming cell   _____

12. destruction (-lysis) of sperm   _____

13. formation (-genesis) of spermatozoa   _____

14. excessive discharge (-rhea) of semen   _____

15. condition of having sperm in the urine (-uria)   _____

The ending *-spermia* means "condition of sperm or semen." Add a prefix to *-spermia* to form a word that has the same meaning as each of the following definitions:

16. presence of blood in the semen   _____

17. presence of pus in the semen   _____

18. lack of semen   _____

19. secretion of excess (poly-) semen   _____

Write a word that has the same meaning as each of the following definitions:

20. inflammation of a seminal vesicle   _____

21. excision of the vas deferens   _____

22. plastic repair of the scrotum   _____

23. excision of the prostate gland   _____

24. radiograph (x-ray) of a seminal vesicle   _____

25. surgical creation of an opening in the vas deferens   _____

26. incision of the epididymis   _____

Clinical Aspects of the Male Reproductive System

Infection

Most infections of the male reproductive tract are **sexually transmitted diseases** (STDs), listed in Display 14-1. The most common STD in the United States is caused by the bacterium *Chlamydia trachomatis,* which, in males, mainly causes **urethritis**. This same organism also causes lymphogranuloma venereum, an STD associated with lymphadenopathy, which is rare in the United States. Both forms of these chlamydial infections respond to treatment with antibiotics.

Gonorrhea is caused by *Neisseria gonorrhoeae,* the gonococcus (GC). Infection usually centers in the urethra, causing urethritis with burning, a purulent discharge, and dysuria. Untreated, the disease can spread through the reproductive system. Gonorrhea is treated with antibiotics, but there has been rapid development of resistance to these drugs by gonococci.

Another common STD is herpes infection, caused by a virus. Other STDs are discussed in Chapter 15.

Mumps is a non–sexually transmitted viral disease that can infect the testes and lead to sterility. Other microorganisms can infect the reproductive tract as well, causing urethritis, **prostatitis, orchitis,** or **epididymitis**.

Benign Prostatic Hyperplasia

As men age, the prostate gland commonly enlarges, a condition known as **benign prostatic hyperplasia** (BPH). Although not cancerous, this overgrown tissue can press on the urethra near the bladder and interfere with urination. Urinary retention, infection, and other complications may follow if an obstruction is not corrected.

Medications for increasing urinary flow rate by relaxing smooth muscle in the prostate and bladder neck are used to treat the symptoms of BPH. Drugs that interfere with testosterone activity in the prostate may slow

DISPLAY 14-1 Sexually Transmitted Diseases

DISEASE	ORGANISM	DESCRIPTION
BACTERIAL		
chlamydial infection	*Chlamydia trachomatis* types D to K	Ascending infection of reproductive and urinary tracts. May spread to pelvis in women, causing pelvic inflammatory disease (PID).
lymphogranuloma venereum	*Chlamydia trachomatis* type L	General infection with swelling of inguinal lymph nodes; scarring of genital tissue
gonorrhea	*Neisseria gonorrhoeae;* gonococcus (GC)	Inflammation of reproductive and urinary tracts. Urethritis in men. Vaginal discharge and inflammation of the cervix (cervicitis) in women, leading to pelvic inflammatory disease (PID). Possible systemic infection. May spread to newborns. Treated with antibiotics.
bacterial vaginosis	*Gardnerella vaginalis*	Vaginal infection with foul-smelling discharge

DISPLAY 14-1 Sexually Transmitted Diseases, *continued*

DISEASE	ORGANISM	DESCRIPTION
syphilis	*Treponema pallidum* (a spirochete)	Primary stage: chancre (lesion); secondary stage: systemic infection and syphilitic warts; tertiary stage: degeneration of other systems. Cause of abortions, stillbirths, and fetal deformities. Treated with antibiotics.
VIRAL		
acquired immune deficiency syndrome (AIDS)	human immunodeficiency virus (HIV)	An often fatal disease that infects T cells of the immune system, weakening the host and leading to other diseases
genital herpes	*Herpes simplex*	Painful lesions of the genitalia. In women, may be a risk factor in cervical carcinoma. Often fatal infections of newborns. No cure at present.
hepatitis B	hepatitis B virus (HBV)	Causes inflammation of the liver, which may be acute or may develop into a chronic carrier state. Linked to liver cancer.
condyloma acuminatum (genital warts)	human papilloma virus (HPV)	Benign genital warts. In women, predisposes to cervical dysplasia and carcinoma.
PROTOZOAL		
trichomoniasis	*Trichomonas vaginalis*	Vaginitis. Green, frothy discharge with itching; pain on intercourse (dyspareunia); and painful urination (dysuria).

progress of the disorder. An herbal remedy that seems to act in this same manner is an extract of the berries of the saw palmetto, a low-growing palm tree. Saw palmetto has been found to delay the need for surgery in some cases of BPH.

In advanced cases of BPH, removal of the prostate, or **prostatectomy**, may be required. When this is performed through the urethra, the procedure is called a transurethral resection of the prostate (TURP) (Fig. 14-3). The prostate may also be cut in a transurethral incision of the prostate (TUIP) to reduce pressure on the urethra (see Fig. 14-3). Other forms of energy, such as a laser beam or heat, have also been used to destroy prostatic tissue. BPH is diagnosed by digital rectal examination (DRE) or imaging studies.

Cancer of the Prostate

Cancer of the prostate is the most common malignancy in men in the United States. Only lung cancer and colon cancer cause more cancer-related deaths in men who are past middle age. Prostatic cancer may metastasize rapidly and is difficult to remove surgically. Other methods of treatment include radiation; measures to reduce male hormones (androgens), which stimulate prostatic growth; and chemotherapy. In cases of prostatic cancer, a protein produced by prostate cells increases in the blood. This prostate-specific antigen (PSA) is used, along with rectal examinations, to screen for prostate cancer and to assess the results of treatment.

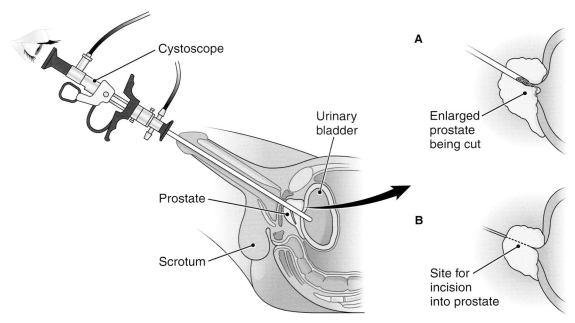

FIGURE 14-3. Prostate surgery procedures. **(A)** Transurethral resection of the prostate (TURP). Portions of the prostate are removed at the bladder opening. **(B)** Transurethral incision of the prostate (TUIP). One or two incisions are made in the prostate to reduce pressure on the urethra.

Cryptorchidism

It is fairly common that one or both testes will fail to descend into the scrotum by the time of birth. This condition is termed **cryptorchidism**, literally hidden (crypt/o) testis (orchid/o). The condition usually corrects itself within the first year of life. If not, it must be corrected surgically to avoid sterility and an increased risk of cancer.

Infertility

An inability or a diminished ability to reproduce is termed **infertility**. Its causes may be hereditary, hormonal, disease-related, or the result of exposure to chemical or physical agents. The most common causes of infertility are STDs. A total inability to produce offspring may be termed **sterility**. Men may be voluntarily sterilized by cutting and sealing the vas deferens on both sides in a **vasectomy** (see Fig. 15-4).

ERECTILE DYSFUNCTION

Erectile dysfunction, also called **impotence**, is the male lack of ability to perform intercourse because of failure to initiate or maintain an erection until ejaculation. The disorder may be broadly characterized as psychogenic, in which case it is caused by emotional factors, or organic, caused by some physical problem such as an anatomic defect or circulatory problem. More specifically, neurogenic impotence results from a disorder of the nervous system, such as a central nervous system lesion, paralysis, or neurologic damage complicating diabetes. Erectile dysfunction may also be a side effect of drug treatment.

Drugs that are used to treat erectile dysfunction work by dilating arteries in the penis to increase blood flow to that organ. One highly prescribed drug of this sort is sildenafil (trade name, Viagra). Penile vacuum pumps and penile prostheses are nondrug approaches to therapy for erectile dysfunction.

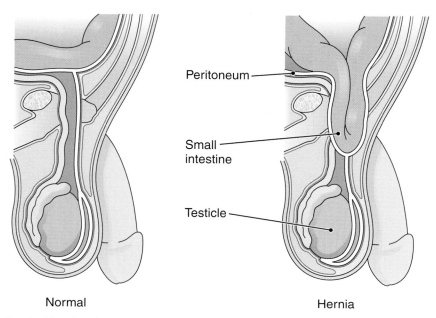

Peritoneum

Small intestine

Testicle

Normal   Hernia

FIGURE 14-4. Inguinal hernia. The hernial sac is a continuation of the peritoneum. The intestine or other abdominal contents can protrude into the hernial sac.

Inguinal Hernia

The inguinal canal, through which the testis descends, may represent a weakness in the abdominal wall that can lead to a hernia. In the most common form of **inguinal hernia** (Fig. 14-4), an abdominal organ, usually the intestine, enters the inguinal canal and may extend into the scrotum. This is an indirect or external inguinal hernia. In a direct or internal inguinal hernia, the organ protrudes through the abdominal wall into the scrotum. If blood supply to the organ is cut off, the hernia is said to be *strangulated*. Surgery to correct a hernia is a **herniorrhaphy**.

Key Clinical Terms

DISORDERS

benign prostatic hyperplasia (BPH)	Nonmalignant enlargement of the prostate; frequently develops with age; also called benign prostatic hypertrophy
cryptorchidism *krip-TOR-kid-izm*	Failure of the testis to descend into the scrotum
epididymitis *ep-i-did-i-MĪ-tis*	Inflammation of the epididymis. Common causes are UTIs and STDs.
erectile dysfunction *e-REK-tĭl dis-FUNK-shun*	A lack of ability to perform intercourse in the man because of failure to initiate or maintain an erection until ejaculation; impotence

Disorders, continued

impotence *IM-pō-tens*	Erectile dysfunction
infertility *in-fer-TIL-i-tē*	Decreased capacity to produce offspring
inguinal hernia *ING-gwin-al*	Protrusion of the intestine or other abdominal organ through the inguinal canal (see Fig. 14-3) or through the wall of the abdomen into the scrotum
orchitis *or-KĪ-tis*	Inflammation of a testis. May be caused by injury, mumps virus, or other infections.
prostatitis *pros-ta-TĪ-tis*	Inflammation of the prostate gland. Often appears with UTI, STD, and a variety of other stresses.
sexually transmitted disease (STD)	Disease spread through sexual activity (see Display 14-1)
sterility	Complete inability to produce offspring
urethritis *ū-rē-THRĪ-tis*	Inflammation of the urethra; often caused by gonorrhea and chlamydial infections

SURGERY

herniorrhaphy *her-nē-OR-a-fē*	Surgical repair of a hernia
prostatectomy *pros-ta-TEK-tō-mē*	Surgical removal of the prostate
vasectomy *va-SEK-tō-mē*	Excision of the vas deferens. Usually done bilaterally to produce sterility (see Fig. 15-4). May be accomplished through the urethra (transurethral resection).

Supplementary Terms

NORMAL STRUCTURE AND FUNCTION

coitus *KŌ-i-tus*	Sexual intercourse
emission *ē-MISH-un*	The discharge of semen
erection *ē-REK-shun*	The stiffening or hardening of the penis or the clitoris, usually because of sexual excitement

Normal Structure and Function, *continued*

genitalia *jen-i-TĀL-ē-a*	The organs concerned with reproduction, divided into internal and external components
insemination *in-sem-i-NĀ-shun*	Introduction of semen into a woman's vagina
orgasm *OR-gazm*	A state of physical and emotional excitement, especially that which occurs at the climax of sexual intercourse
phallus *FAL-us*	The penis
puberty *PŪ-ber-tē*	Period during which the ability for sexual reproduction is attained and secondary sex characteristics begin to develop
spermatic cord	The cord that suspends the testis; composed of the vas deferens, vessels, and nerves

DISORDERS

balanitis *bal-a-NĪ-tis*	Inflammation of the glans penis and mucous membrane beneath it (root *balan/o* means "glans penis")
bladder neck obstruction (BNO)	Blockage of urine flow at the outlet of the bladder. The common cause is benign prostatic hyperplasia.
hydrocele *HĪ-drō-sēl*	The accumulation of fluid in a saclike cavity, especially within the covering of the testis or spermatic cord (Fig. 14-5)
phimosis *fi-MŌ-sis*	Narrowing of the opening of the prepuce so that the foreskin cannot be pushed back over the glans penis
priapism *PRĪ-a-pizm*	Abnormal, painful, continuous erection of the penis, as may be caused by damage to specific regions of the spinal cord
seminoma *sem-i-NŌ-ma*	A tumor of the testis
spermatocele *SPER-ma-tō-sēl*	An epididymal cyst containing spermatozoa (see Fig. 14-5)
varicocele *VAR-i-kō-sēl*	Enlargement of the veins of the spermatic cord (see Fig. 14-5)

ABBREVIATIONS

AIDS	Acquired immunodeficiency syndrome	**FSH**	Follicle stimulating hormone
BNO	Bladder neck obstruction	**GC**	Gonococcus
BPH	Benign prostatic hyperplasia (hypertrophy)	**GU**	Genitourinary
		HBV	Hepatitis B virus
DRE	Digital rectal examination	**HIV**	Human immunodeficiency virus

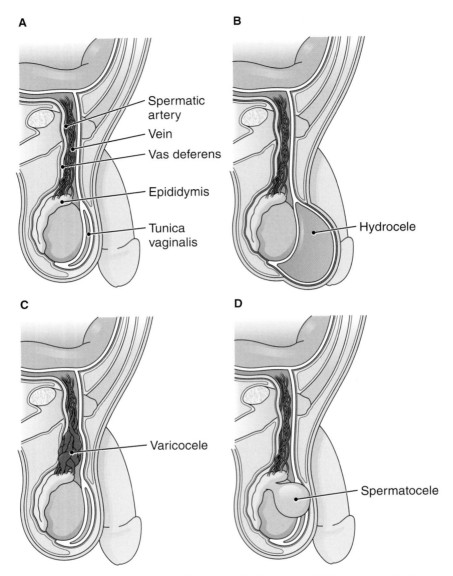

A

Spermatic artery

Vein

Vas deferens

Epididymis

Tunica vaginalis

B

Hydrocele

C

Varicocele

D

Spermatocele

FIGURE 14-5. Scrotal abnormalities. **(A)** Normal. **(B)** Hydrocele. **(C)** Varicocele. **(D)** Spermatocele.

ABBREVIATIONS

ICSH	Interstitial cell-stimulating hormone	**TUIP**	Transurethral incision of prostate
LH	Luteinizing hormone	**TURP**	Transurethral resection of prostate
NGU	Nongonococcal urethritis	**VD**	Venereal disease (sexually transmitted disease)
PSA	Prostate-specific antigen		
STD	Sexually transmitted disease	**VDRL**	Venereal disease research laboratory (test for syphilis)
TPUR	Transperineal urethral resection		
TSE	Testicular self-examination		

Labeling Exercise 14-1

Male Genitourinary System

Write the name of each numbered part on the corresponding line of the answer sheet.

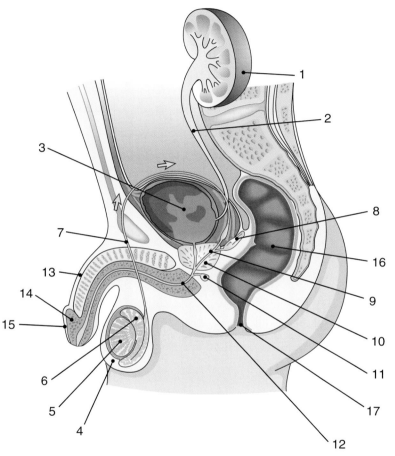

Anus
Bulbourethral (Cowper) gland
Vas (ductus) deferens
Ejaculatory duct
Epididymis
Glans penis
Kidney
Penis
Prepuce
Prostate
Rectum
Scrotum
Seminal vesicle
Testis
Ureter
Urethra
Urinary bladder

1. _____	10. _____
2. _____	11. _____
3. _____	12. _____
4. _____	13. _____
5. _____	14. _____
6. _____	15. _____
7. _____	16. _____
8. _____	17. _____
9. _____	

Chapter Review 14-1

Match the following terms and write the appropriate letter to the left of each number:

_____ 1. gonad

_____ 2. glans

_____ 3. epididymis

_____ 4. androgen

_____ 5. prostate

a. coiled tube on the surface of the testis

b. any male sex hormone

c. gland located below the bladder in the male

d. end of the penis

e. sex gland

_____ 6. FSH

_____ 7. anorchism

_____ 8. oligospermia

_____ 9. vasectomy

_____ 10. oscheoma

a. excision of the ductus deferens

b. pituitary hormone active in reproduction

c. tumor of the scrotum

d. deficiency of spermatozoa

e. absence of a testis

SUPPLEMENTARY TERMS

_____ 11. emission

_____ 12. balanitis

_____ 13. hydrocele

_____ 14. phimosis

_____ 15. seminoma

a. narrowing of the foreskin opening

b. inflammation of the glans penis

c. tumor of the testis

d. discharge of semen

e. accumulation of fluid in a saclike cavity

_____ 16. insemination

_____ 17. coitus

_____ 18. genitalia

_____ 19. spermatic cord

_____ 20. spermatocele

a. epididymal cyst

b. introduction of semen into a woman's vagina

c. sexual intercourse

d. organs of reproduction

e. structure that suspends the testis

Fill in the blanks:

21. The common passage for urine and semen in the male is the _____.

22. The male gonad is the _____.

23. The sac that holds the testis is the _____.

24. The thick fluid that transports spermatozoa is _____.

25. The main male sex hormone is _____.

26. Orchitis is inflammation of the _____.

Define each of the following terms:

27. orchialgia (*or-kē-AL-jē-a*) _____

28. hemospermia (*hē-mō-SPER-mē-a*) _____

29. prostatometer (*pros-ta-TOM-e-ter*) _____

30. vesiculotomy (*ve-sik-ū-LOT-ō-mē*) _____

Word building. Write a word for each of the following definitions:

31. surgical creation of an opening between two parts of a cut
    ductus deferens (done to reverse a vasectomy) _____

32. stone in the scrotum _____

33. surgical incision of the prostate _____

34. inflammation of a seminal vesicle _____

35. surgical fixation of the testis _____

36. plastic repair of the scrotum _____

Write the adjective form of each of the following words:

37. semen _____

38. prostate _____

39. penis _____

40. urethra _____

41. scrotum _____

Write the meaning of each of the following abbreviations:

42. STD _____

43. BPH _____

44. GC _____

45. PSA _____

46. TURP _____

47. BNO _____

Word analysis. Define each of the following words, and give the meaning of the word parts in each. Use a dictionary if necessary.

48. cryptorchidism (*krip-TOR-kid-izm*) _____
    a. crypt- _____
    b. orchid/o _____
    c. -ism _____

49. vasovesiculitis (*vas-ō-ve-sik-ū-LĪ-tis*) _____
    a. vas/o _____
    b. vesicul/o _____
    c. -itis _____

Case Studies

Case Study 14-1: Herniorrhaphy and Vasectomy

E.D., a 48-year-old married dock worker with three children, developed inguinal bulging and pain on exertion when he lifted heavy objects. An occupational health service advised a surgical referral. The surgeon diagnosed E.D. with bilateral direct inguinal hernias and suggested that he not delay surgery, although he was not at high risk for a strangulated hernia. E.D. asked the surgeon if he could also be sterilized at the same time. He was scheduled for bilateral inguinal herniorrhaphy and elective vasectomy.

During the herniorrhaphy procedure an oblique incision was made in each groin. The incision continued through the muscle layers by either resecting or splitting the muscle fibers. The spermatic vessels and vas deferens were identified, separated, and gently retracted. The spermatic cord was examined for an indirect hernia. Repair began with suturing the defect in the rectus abdominis muscles, transverse fascia, cremaster muscle, external oblique aponeurosis, and Scarpa fascia with heavy-gauge synthetic nonabsorbable suture material.

The vasectomy began with the identification of the vas deferens through the scrotal skin. An incision was made, and the vas was gently dissected and retracted through the opening. Each vas was clamped with a small hemostat, and a 1-cm length was resected. Both cut ends were coagulated with electrosurgery and tied independently with a fine-gauge absorbable suture material. The testicles were examined, and the scrotal incision was closed with an absorbable suture material.

Case Study 14-2: Benign Prostatic Hyperplasia with TURP

C.S., a 62-year-old businessman, saw a urologist with complaints of decreased force of urine stream and ejaculation, hesitancy, and sensation of incomplete bladder emptying. He claimed he had taken prostate-health herbal supplements without any real benefit for 2 years before making the appointment. He denied dysuria, hematuria, or flank pain. He has no history of UTI, epididymitis, prostatitis, renal disease, or renal calculi. Rectal examination revealed a 50-g prostate with slight firmness in the right prostatic lobe. Bladder ultrasound showed no intravesical lesions or prostate protrusion into the bladder base. C.S. was diagnosed with benign prostatic hyperplasia with bladder neck obstruction and was scheduled for a TURP.

Case Study 14-3: Circumcision

S.G., a 12-year-old Jewish Russian immigrant, was preparing for his bar mitzvah. He had not been circumcised on the eighth day after his birth, as is Jewish tradition, because he had been unable to practice his religion within the former soviet system. On recommendation of his rabbi, his family brought him to a urologist for referral and surgery. On examination, the phallus and meatus were normal and without lesions. S.G. had no signs of discharge, phimosis, or balanitis. Surgery for an adult circumcision was scheduled along with the attendance of a mohel, a Jewish ritual circumciser.

S.G. was positioned in the supine position after administration of general anesthesia. His penis and scrotum were prepped with an antimicrobial solution and draped in sterile sheets. The surgeon and mohel scrubbed in and donned sterile gowns and gloves. The mohel chanted several prayers in Hebrew before and after making the first small cut below the foreskin, enough to draw blood. The urologist completed the resection of the redundant foreskin and approximated the circumferential incisions with fine-gauge absorbable suture material. After the incision was dressed with petrolatum gauze, and S.G. recovered enough to be returned to his room, the mohel met with him and his family to continue the sacred rite with prayer and ceremonial wine.

Case Studies, continued

CASE STUDY QUESTIONS

Multiple choice: Select the best answer and write the letter of your choice to the left of each number.

_____ 1. The term for male sterilization surgery is:
    a. herniorrhaphy
    b. circumcision
    c. vagotomy
    d. vasectomy
    e. vasovasotomy

_____ 2. An oblique surgical incision follows what direction?
    a. slanted or angled
    b. superior to inferior
    c. lateral
    d. circumferential
    e. elliptical

_____ 3. When the ends of the vas were coagulated with electrosurgery, they were:
    a. probed
    b. dilated
    c. sealed
    d. sutured
    e. clamped

_____ 4. A urologist is a physician who treats health and disease conditions of the:
    a. male reproductive system
    b. urinary system
    c. digestive system
    d. a and b
    e. b and c

_____ 5. A person with painful, blood-tinged, scanty urination would be described with:
    a. hematocrit, dyspnea, oliguria
    b. dystonia, hematuria, oliguria
    c. dysuria, hematuria, oliguria
    d. oliguria, hematogenesis, dystonia
    e. dyspnea, hematuria, polyuria

_____ 6. Another name for the foreskin is the:
    a. prepuce
    b. phimosis
    c. phallus
    d. glans
    e. balan

Case Studies, continued

_____ 7. The circumferential incisions followed a direction:
   a. inferior to the scrotum
   b. suprapubic and transverse
   c. around the penis
   d. lateral to the prostate
   e. medial to the inguinal canal

Write a term from the case studies with each of the following meanings:

8. surgical repair of a weak abdominal muscle in the groin area on both sides

   _____

9. entrapment of a loop of bowel in a hernia _____

10. inflammation of the prostate gland _____

11. within the urinary bladder _____

12. inflammation of the glans penis _____

13. narrowing of the distal opening of the foreskin _____

Abbreviations. Define the following abbreviations:

14. BPH _____

15. TURP _____

16. BNO _____

17. UTI _____

Chapter 14 Crossword
Male Reproductive System

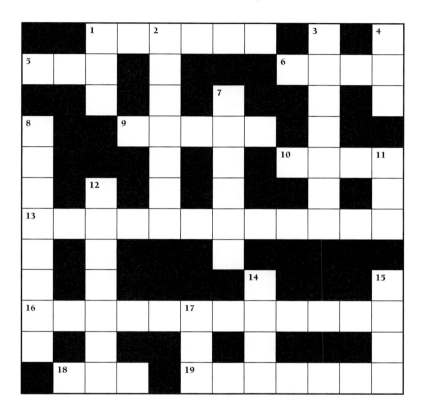

ACROSS

1. The male gonad
5. Abnormal, painful, difficult: prefix
6. Pertaining to condition of urine: suffix
9. A reproductive organ
10. Stone or calculus: root
13. Male gamete or sex cell
16. Main male sex hormone
18. Protein associated with prostate cancer: abbreviation
19. Semen or spermatozoa: root

Down

1. Self-examination of the testis: abbreviation
2. Sac that holds the testis
3. Testis: combining form
4. Ductus deferens: root
7. A reproductive or germ cell
8. Gland that contributes to semen
11. High blood pressure: abbreviation
12. Type of cell division that forms the gametes
14. Hernia or localized dilation: suffix
15. Male reproductive gland: root
17. Condition of: suffix

CHAPTER 14 Answer Section

Answers to Chapter Exercises

EXERCISE 14-1

1. pertaining to semen
2. any disease of a testis
3. pain in a testis
4. excision of the epididymis
5. pertaining to the prostate
6. pertaining to the scrotum
7. inflammation of the testis and epididymis
8. orchiopexy (*or-kē-ō-PEK-sē*); also orchidopexy (*or-ki-dō-PEK-sē*)
9. orchioplasty (*OR-kē-ō-plas-tē*); also orchidoplasty (*OR-ki-dō-pek-sē*)
10. orchiotomy (*or-kē-OT-ō-mē*); also orchidotomy (*or-ki-DOT-ō-mē*)
11. spermatocyte (*sper-MA-tō-sīt*)
12. spermatolysis (*sper-ma-TOL-i-sis*)
13. spermatogenesis (*sper-ma-tō-JEN-e-sis*)
14. spermatorrhea (*sper-ma-to-RĒ-a*)
15. spermaturia (*sper-ma-TŪ-rē-a*)
16. hemospermia (*hē-mō-SPER-mē-a*); also hematospermia (*hem-at-ō-SPER-mē-a*)
17. pyospermia (*pī-ō-SPER-mē-a*)
18. aspermia (*a-SPER-mē-a*)
19. polyspermia (*pol-ē-SPER-mē-a*)
20. vesiculitis (*ve-sik-ū-LĪ-tis*)
21. vasectomy (*va-SEK-tō-mē*)
22. oscheoplasty (*OS-kē-ō-plas-tē*)
23. prostatectomy (*pros-ta-TEK-tō-mē*)
24. vesiculogram (*ve-SIK-ū-lō-gram*)
25. vasostomy (*vas-OS-tō-mē*)
26. epididymotomy (*ep-i-did-i-MOT-ō-mē*)

LABELING EXERCISE 14-1: MALE GENITOURINARY SYSTEM

1. kidney
2. ureter
3. urinary bladder
4. scrotum
5. testis
6. epididymis
7. vas (ductus) deferens
8. seminal vesicle
9. ejaculatory duct
10. prostate
11. bulbourethral (Cowper) gland
12. urethra
13. penis
14. glans penis
15. prepuce (foreskin)
16. rectum
17. anus

Answers to Chapter Review 14-1

1. e
2. d
3. a
4. b
5. c
6. b
7. e
8. d
9. a
10. c
11. d
12. b
13. e
14. a
15. c
16. b
17. c
18. d
19. e
20. a
21. urethra
22. testis
23. scrotum
24. semen
25. testosterone
26. testis
27. pain in the testis
28. presence of blood in the semen
29. instrument for measuring the prostate
30. incision of the seminal vesicle
31. vasovasostomy
32. oscheolith
33. prostatotomy
34. vesiculitis
35. orchiopexy
36. oscheoplasty
37. seminal
38. prostatic
39. penile
40. urethral
41. scrotal

42. sexually transmitted disease
43. benign prostatic hyperplasia (hypertrophy)
44. gonococcus
45. prostate-specific antigen
46. transurethral resection of the prostate
47. bladder neck obstruction
48. undescended testes
    a. hidden
    b. testis
    c. condition of
49. inflammation of the ductus deferens and seminal vesicle
    a. vas (ductus) deferens
    b. seminal vesicle
    c. inflammation

3. c
4. d
5. c
6. a
7. c
8. bilateral inguinal herniorrhaphy
9. strangulated hernia
10. prostatitis
11. intravesical
12. balanitis
13. phimosis
14. benign prostatic hyperplasia
15. transurethral resection of the prostate
16. bladder neck obstruction
17. urinary tract infection

Answers to Case Study Questions

1. d
2. a

ANSWERS TO CROSSWORD PUZZLE

Male Reproductive System

The Female Reproductive System; Pregnancy and Birth

Chapter Contents

Objectives

After study of this chapter you should be able to:

1. Label a diagram of the female reproductive tract and describe the function of each part.
2. Describe the structure and function of the mammary glands.
3. Outline the events in the menstrual cycle.
4. Outline the major events that occur in the first 2 months after fertilization.
5. Describe the structure and function of the placenta.
6. Describe the three stages of childbirth.
7. List the hormonal and nervous controls over lactation.
8. Identify and use roots pertaining to the female reproductive system, pregnancy, and birth.
9. Describe the main disorders of the female reproductive system and reproductive function.
10. Interpret abbreviations used in referring to reproduction.
11. Analyze several case studies concerning the female reproductive system, pregnancy, and birth.

The Female Reproductive System

The Ovaries

The female gonads are the paired **ovaries** (singular, ovary) that are held by ligaments in the pelvic cavity on either side of the uterus (Fig. 15-1). It is within the ovaries that the female gametes, the eggs or **ova** (singular, ovum), develop. Every month several ova ripen, each within a cluster of cells called a **graafian follicle**. At the time of ovulation, usually only one ovum is released from the ovary and the remainder of the ripening ova degenerate. The follicle remains behind and continues to function for about 2 weeks if there is no fertilization of the ovum and for about 2 months if the ovum is fertilized.

The Oviducts, Uterus, and Vagina

After ovulation, the ovum travels into an **oviduct** (also called the uterine tube or **fallopian tube**), one of the two tubes attached to the upper lateral portions of the uterus (see Fig. 15-1). These tubes arch above the ovaries and have fingerlike projections (fimbriae) that sweep the released ovum into the oviduct. If fertilization occurs, it usually takes place in the oviduct.

The **uterus** is the organ that nourishes the developing offspring. It is pear-shaped, with an upper rounded fundus, a triangular cavity, and a lower narrow **cervix** that projects into the vagina. The innermost layer of the uterine wall, the **endometrium**, has a rich blood supply. It receives the fertilized ovum and becomes part of the placenta during pregnancy. The endometrium is shed during the menstrual period if no fertilization occurs. The muscle layer of the uterine wall is the **myometrium**.

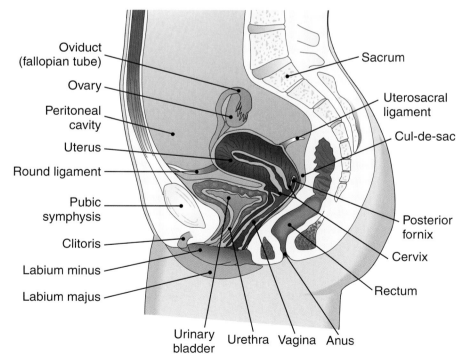

FIGURE 15-1. Female reproductive system, as seen in sagittal section. (Reprinted with permission from Cohen BJ, Wood DL. Memmler's The Human Body in Health and Disease. 9th Ed. Philadelphia: Lippincott Williams & Wilkins, 2000.)

The **vagina** is a muscular tube that receives the penis during intercourse, functions as a birth canal, and transports the menstrual flow out of the body (see Fig. 15-1).

The External Genital Organs

All of the external female genital organs together are called the **vulva** (Fig. 15-2). This includes the large outer **labia majora** and small inner **labia minora** that enclose the openings of the vagina and the urethra. The **clitoris**, anterior to the urethral opening, is similar in origin to the penis and responds to sexual stimulation.

In both male and female, the region between the thighs, from the external genital organs to the anus, is the **perineum**. During childbirth, an incision may be made between the vagina and the anus to facilitate birth and prevent the tearing of tissue, a procedure called an *episiotomy*. (This procedure is actually a perineotomy, as the root *episi/o* means "vulva.")

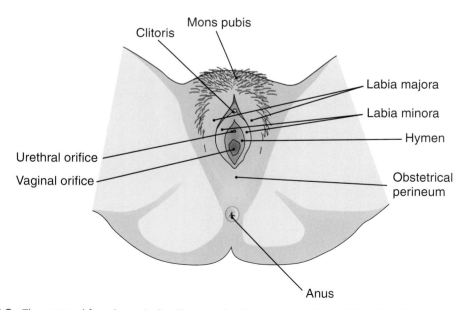

FIGURE 15-2. The external female genitalia. (Reprinted with permission from Cohen BJ, Wood DL. Memmler's The Human Body in Health and Disease. 9th Ed. Philadelphia: Lippincott Williams & Wilkins, 2000.)

The Mammary Glands

The **mammary glands**, or breasts, are composed mainly of glandular tissue and fat (Fig. 15-3). Their purpose is to provide nourishment for the newborn. The milk secreted by the glands is carried in ducts to the nipple.

The Menstrual Cycle

Reproductive activity in the female normally begins during puberty with **menarche**, the first menstrual period. Each month, the menstrual cycle is controlled, like reproductive activity in the male, by hormones from the anterior pituitary gland. Follicle stimulating hormone (**FSH**) begins the cycle by causing the ovum to ripen in the graafian follicle. The follicle secretes **estrogen**, a hormone that starts development of the endometrium in preparation for the fertilized egg. A second pituitary hormone, luteinizing hormone (**LH**), triggers **ovulation** and conversion of the follicle to the **corpus luteum**. This structure, left behind in the ovary, secretes **progesterone** and estrogen, which further the growth of the endometrium. If no fertilization occurs, hormone levels decline, and the endometrium sloughs off in the process of **menstruation**.

The average menstrual cycle lasts 28 days, with the first day of menstruation taken as day 1 and ovulation occurring on about day 14. Throughout the cycle, estrogen and progesterone feed back to the pituitary to regulate the production of FSH and LH. Hormonal methods of birth control act by supplying estrogen and progesterone, which inhibit the pituitary and prevent ovulation, while not interfering with menstruation.

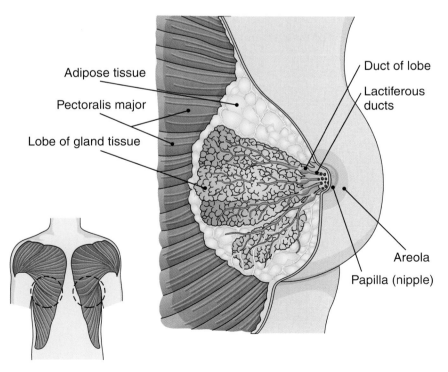

FIGURE 15-3. Section of the breast. (Reprinted with permission from Cohen BJ, Wood DL. Memmler's The Human Body in Health and Disease. 9th Ed. Philadelphia: Lippincott Williams & Wilkins, 2000.)

Menopause

Menopause is the cessation of monthly menstrual cycles. This generally occurs between the ages of 45 and 55 years. Levels of reproductive hormones decline, and egg cells in the ovaries gradually degenerate. Some women experience unpleasant symptoms, such as hot flashes, headaches, insomnia, mood swings, and urinary problems. There is also some atrophy of the reproductive tract with vaginal dryness. Most importantly, decline in estrogen is associated with weakening of the bones (osteoporosis).

Hormone replacement therapy (HRT), usually consisting of estrogen in combination with progestin, has been recommended to alleviate menopausal symptoms. Replacement hormones also seem to reduce loss of bone tissue associated with aging. Recent concerns about the safety of HRT, however, have caused reconsideration of this therapy beyond the early postmenopausal years. As always, exercise and a balanced diet with adequate calcium are important in maintaining health. Addition of soybeans to the diet, as found in products such as soy nuts, tofu, and soybean oil, has been recommended for the protective estrogen-like compounds they contain. There are also nonhormonal drugs available to build bone mass if needed.

Contraception

Contraception is the use of artificial methods to prevent fertilization of the ovum or its implantation in the uterus. Methods can be used to block sperm penetration of the uterus (condom, diaphragm), prevent implantation (intrauterine device [IUD]), or prevent ovulation (hormonal methods). Surgical sterilization for the male is a vasectomy; for the female, surgical sterilization is a **tubal ligation**, in which the fallopian tubes are cut and tied on both sides (Fig. 15-4). The preferred method for performing this surgery is through the abdominal wall with a laparoscope (Fig. 15-5).

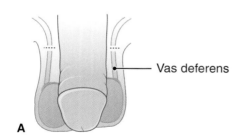

Vas deferens

A

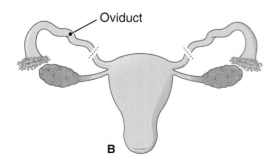

Oviduct

B

FIGURE 15-4. Sterilization. **(A)** Vasectomy. **(B)** Tubal ligation.

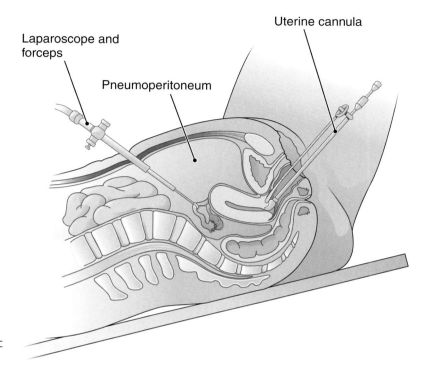

Laparoscope and forceps

Pneumoperitoneum

Uterine cannula

FIGURE 15-5. Laparoscopic sterilization.

Pregnancy and Birth

Fertilization and Early Development

If an ovulated egg cell is penetrated by a sperm cell, **fertilization** (Fig. 15-6) results. After this union, the nuclei of the sperm and egg cells fuse, restoring the chromosome number to 46 and forming a **zygote**. As the zygote travels through the oviduct toward the uterus, it divides rapidly. Within 6 to 7 days, the fertilized egg reaches the uterus and implants into the endometrium, and the **embryo** begins to develop.

During the first 8 weeks of growth, all of the major body systems are established. Embryonic tissue produces **human chorionic gonadotropin (HCG)**, a hormone that keeps the corpus luteum functional in the ovary to maintain the endometrium. (The presence of HCG in urine is the basis for the most commonly used tests for pregnancy.) After 2 months, placental hormones take over this function and the corpus luteum degenerates. At this time the embryo becomes a **fetus**.

The Placenta

During development, the fetus is nourished by the **placenta**, an organ formed from the outermost layer of the embryo, the **chorion**, and the innermost layer of the uterus, the endometrium (Fig. 15-7). Here, exchanges take place between the bloodstreams of the mother and the fetus through fetal capillaries.

The **umbilical cord** contains the blood vessels that link the fetus to the placenta. Fetal blood is carried to the placenta in two umbilical arteries. While traveling through the placenta, the blood picks up nutrients and oxygen and gives up carbon dioxide and metabolic waste. Restored blood is carried from the placenta to the fetus in a single umbilical vein.

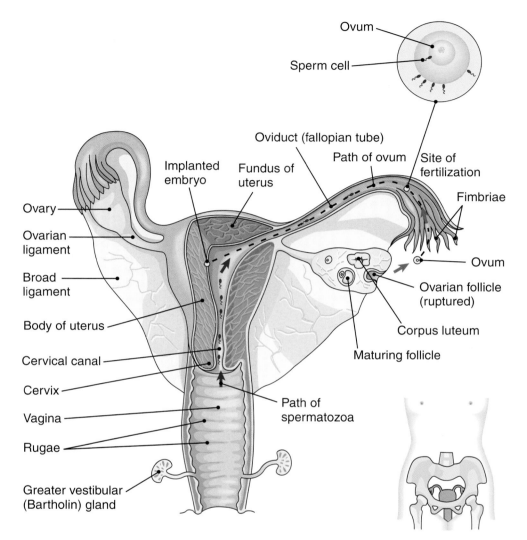

FIGURE 15-6. Female reproductive system showing fertilization. (Reprinted with permission from Cohen BJ, Wood DL. Memmler's The Human Body in Health and Disease. 9th Ed. Philadelphia: Lippincott Williams & Wilkins, 2000.)

Although the bloodstreams of the mother and the fetus do not mix, and all exchanges take place through capillaries, some materials do manage to get through the placenta in both directions. For example, some viruses, drugs, and other harmful substances are known to pass from the mother to the fetus; fetal proteins can enter the mother's blood and cause immunologic reactions.

During **gestation** (the period of development), the fetus is cushioned and protected by fluid contained in the **amniotic sac** (amnion) (Fig. 15-8), commonly called the bag of waters. This sac ruptures at birth.

Fetal Circulation

The fetus has several adaptations that serve to bypass the lungs, which are not needed to oxygenate the blood. When blood coming from the placenta enters the right atrium, the **foramen ovale**, a small hole in the septum between the atria, allows some of the blood to go directly into the left atrium, thus bypassing the pulmonary artery. Further, blood pumped out of the right ventricle can shunt directly into the aorta through a short ves-

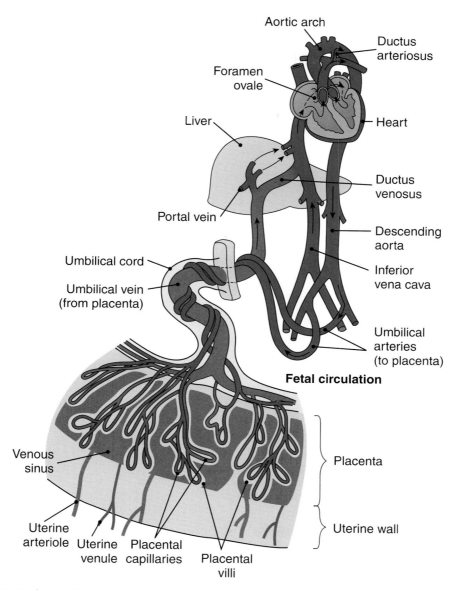

FIGURE 15-7. Fetal circulation and placenta. Color shows relative oxygen content of blood. (Reprinted with permission from Cohen BJ, Wood DL. Memmler's The Human Body in Health and Disease. 9th Ed. Philadelphia: Lippincott Williams & Wilkins, 2000.)

sel, the **ductus arteriosus**, which connects the pulmonary artery with the descending aorta (see Fig. 15-7). Both of these passages close off at birth when the pulmonary circuit is established. Their failure to close hampers the work of the heart and may require medical attention.

Childbirth

The length of pregnancy, from fertilization of the ovum to birth, is about 38 weeks or 266 days. In practice, it is calculated as approximately 280 days or 40 weeks from the first day of the last menstrual period (LMP).

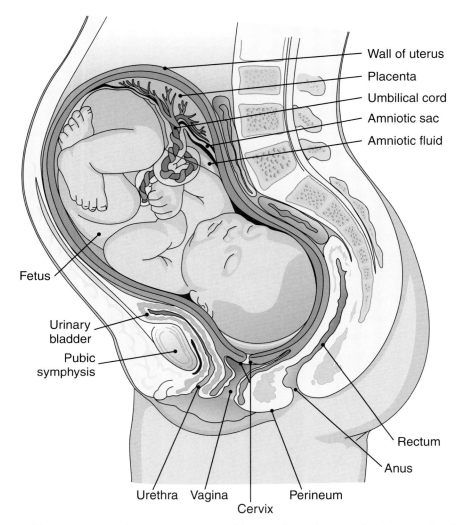

FIGURE 15-8. Midsagittal section of a pregnant uterus with intact fetus. (Reprinted with permission from Cohen BJ, Wood DL. Memmler's The Human Body in Health and Disease. 9th Ed. Philadelphia: Lippincott Williams & Wilkins, 2000.)

For study purposes, pregnancy is divided into 3-month periods (trimesters), during which defined changes can be observed in the fetus.

Childbirth or **parturition** occurs in three stages: (1) onset of regular uterine contractions and dilation of the cervix; (2) expulsion of the fetus; (3) delivery of the placenta and fetal membranes. The third stage is followed by contraction of the uterus and control of bleeding. The factors that start labor are not completely understood, but it is clear that the hormone **oxytocin** from the posterior pituitary gland and other hormones called **prostaglandins** are involved.

The term **gravida** refers to a pregnant woman. A prefix may be added to show the number of pregnancies, such as primigravida, meaning a woman pregnant for the first time, or a number may be used, such as gravida 1, gravida 2, and so forth. The term **para** refers to a woman who has given birth. This means the production of a viable infant (500 g or more or over 20 weeks' gestation) regardless of whether the infant is alive at birth or whether the birth is single or multiple. Again, prefixes or numerals are used to indicate the number of such pregnancies.

Lactation

The secretion of milk from the breasts, called **lactation**, is started by the hormone prolactin from the anterior pituitary gland, as well as hormones from the placenta. The release of milk is then stimulated by suckling. For the first few days after delivery, only **colostrum** is produced. This has a slightly different composition than milk, but like the milk, it has protective antibodies.

Key Terms

NORMAL STRUCTURE AND FUNCTION

Female Reproductive System

cervix *SER-viks*	Neck. Usually means the lower narrow portion (neck) of the uterus; cervix uteri (*U-ter-ī*) (root *cervic/o*).
clitoris *KLIT-o-ris*	A small erectile body in front of the urethral opening that is similar in origin to the penis (root *clitor/o, clitorid/o*)
contraception *kon-tra-SEP-shun*	The prevention of pregnancy
corpus luteum *KOR-pus LŪ-tē-um*	The small yellow structure that develops from the graafian follicle after ovulation and secretes progesterone and estrogen
endometrium *en-dō-MĒ-trē-um*	The inner lining of the uterus
estrogen *ES-trō-jen*	A group of hormones that produces female characteristics and prepares the uterus for the fertilized egg. The most active of these is estradiol.
fallopian tube *fa-LŌ-pē-an*	See oviduct
follicle stimulating hormone (FSH)	A hormone secreted by the anterior pituitary that acts on the gonads. In the female, it stimulates ripening of the eggs in the ovary.
graafian follicle *GRAF-ē-an*	The cluster of cells in which the ovum ripens in the ovary. Also called ovarian follicle.
human chorionic gonadotropin (HCG) *kor-ē-ON-ik* *GŌ-na-dō-trō-pin*	A hormone secreted by the embryo early in pregnancy that maintains the corpus luteum so that it will continue to secrete hormones; also abbreviated hCG
labia majora *LĀ-bē-a ma-JOR-a*	The two large folds of skin that form the sides of the vulva (root *labi/o* means "lip"); singular, *labium majus*

Normal Structure and Function, *continued*

labia minora *LĀ-bē-a mī-NOR-a*	The two small folds of skin within the labia majora; singular, *labium minus*
luteinizing hormone (LH) *LŪ-tē-in-ī-zing*	A hormone secreted by the anterior pituitary that acts on the gonads. In the female, it stimulates ovulation and formation of the corpus luteum.
mammary gland *MAM-a-rē*	A specialized gland capable of secreting milk in the female; the breast (root *mamm/o, mast/o*)
menarche *men-AR-kē*	The first menstrual period, which normally occurs during puberty
menopause *MEN-ō-pawz*	Cessation of menstrual cycles in the female
menstruation *men-strū-Ā-shun*	The cyclic discharge of blood and mucosal tissues from the lining of the nonpregnant uterus (root *men/o, mens*)
myometrium *mī-ō-MĒ-trē-um*	The muscular wall of the uterus
ovary *Ō-va-rē*	A female gonad (root *ovari/o, oophor/o*)
oviduct *Ō-vi-dukt*	A tube extending from the upper lateral portion of the uterus that carries the ovum to the uterus. Also called fallopian or uterine tube (root *salping/o*).
ovulation *ov-ū-LĀ-shun*	The release of a mature ovum from the ovary (from *ovule*, meaning "little egg")
ovum *Ō-vum*	The female gamete or reproductive cell (plural, *ova*) (root *oo, ov/o*)
perineum *per-i-NĒ-um*	The region between the thighs from the external genitals to the anus (root *perine/o*)
progesterone *prō-JES-ter-ōn*	A hormone produced by the corpus luteum and the placenta that maintains the endometrium for pregnancy
tubal ligation *lī-GĀ-shun*	Surgical constriction of the oviducts to produce sterilization (see Figs. 15-4 and 15-5)
uterus *Ū-ter-us*	The organ that receives the fertilized egg and maintains the developing offspring during pregnancy (root *uter/o, metr, hyster/o*)
vagina *va-JĪ-na*	The muscular tube between the cervix and the vulva (root *vagin/o, colp/o*)
vulva *VUL-va*	The external female genital organs (root *vulv/o, episi/o*)

Pregnancy and Birth

amniotic sac *am-nē-OT-ik*	The membranous sac filled with fluid that holds the fetus; also called amnion (root *amnio*)

Pregnancy and Birth, continued

chorion *KOR-ē-on*	The outermost layer of the embryo that, with the endometrium, forms the placenta (adjective, chorionic)
colostrum *kō-LOS-trum*	Breast fluid that is secreted in the first few days after giving birth, before milk is produced
ductus arteriosus *DUK-tus ar-tēr-ē-Ō-sus*	A fetal blood vessel that connects the pulmonary artery with the descending aorta, thus allowing blood to bypass the lungs
embryo *EM-brē-ō*	The stage in development between the zygote and the fetus, extending from the second to the eighth week of growth in the uterus (adjective, embryonic) (root *embry/o*)
fertilization *fer-ti-li-ZĀ-shun*	The union of an ovum and a spermatozoon
fetus *FĒ-tus*	The developing child in the uterus from the third month to birth (adjective, fetal) (root *fet/o*)
foramen ovale *fō-RĀ-men ō-VĀ-lē*	A small hole in the septum between the atria in the fetal heart that allows blood to pass directly from the right to the left side of the heart
gestation *jes-TĀ-shun*	The period of development from conception to birth
gravida *GRAV-i-da*	Pregnant woman
lactation *lak-TĀ-shun*	The secretion of milk from the mammary glands
neonate *NĒ-ō-nāt*	Newborn
oxytocin *ok-sē-TŌ-sin*	A pituitary hormone that stimulates contractions of the uterus. It also stimulates release ("letdown") of milk from the breasts.
para	Woman who has produced a viable infant. Multiple births are considered as single pregnancies.
parturition *par-tū-RI-shun*	Childbirth; labor (root *toc/o, nat/i*)
placenta *pla-SEN-ta*	The organ, composed of fetal and maternal tissues, that nourishes and maintains the developing fetus
prostaglandins *PROS-ta-glan-dinz*	A group of hormones with varied effects, including the stimulation of uterine contractions
umbilical cord *um-BIL-i-kal*	The structure that connects the fetus to the placenta. It contains vessels that carry blood between the mother and the fetus.
zygote *ZĪ-gōt*	The fertilized ovum

Roots Pertaining to the Female Reproductive System

TABLE 15-1 Roots for Female Reproduction and the Ovaries

ROOT	MEANING	EXAMPLE	DEFINITION OF EXAMPLE
gyn/o, gynec/o*	woman	gynecology gī-ne-KOL-ō-jē	study of diseases of women
men/o, mens	month, menstruation	premenstrual prē-MEN-strū-al	before a menstrual period
oo	ovum, egg cell	oocyte Ō-ō-sīt	cell that gives rise to an ovum
ov/o	ovum, egg cell	ovulation ov-ū-LĀ-shun	release of an ovum from the ovary
ovari/o	ovary	ovarian ō-VAR-ē-an	pertaining to an ovary
oophor/o	ovary	oophorotomy ō-of-ō-ROT-ō-mē	incision of an ovary

*This root may also be pronounced with a soft g, as in *jin-e-KOL-ō-jē*.

Exercise 15-1

Define each of the following words:

1. gynecopathy (*ji-ne-KOP-a-thē*) _____

2. intermenstrual (*in-ter-MEN-strū-al*) _____

3. oogenesis (*ō-ō-JEN-e-sis*) _____

4. ovulatory (*OV-ū-la-tō-rē*) _____

5. ovariorrhexis (*ō-var-ē-ō-REK-sis*) _____

6. oophoritis (*ō-of-ō-RĪ-tis*) _____

Write a word that has the same meaning as each of the following definitions:

7. a physician who specializes in the study of diseases of women _____

8. pertaining to an absence of ovulation _____

9. profuse bleeding (-rhagia) at the time of menstruation _____

The word *menorrhea* means "menstruation." Add a prefix to menorrhea to form a word with each of the following meanings:

10. absence of menstruation _____

11. painful or difficult menstruation _____

12. scanty menstrual flow _____

Use the root *ovari/o* to write a word that has the same meaning as each of the following definitions:

13. hernia of the ovary _____

14. surgical fixation of the ovary _____

15. surgical puncture of an ovary _____

Use the root *oophor/o* to write a word that has the same meaning as each of the following definitions:

16. excision of an ovary _____

17. malignant tumor of the ovary _____

TABLE 15-2 Roots for the Oviducts, Uterus, and Vagina

ROOT	MEANING	EXAMPLE	DEFINITION OF EXAMPLE
salping/o	oviduct, tube	salpingectomy *sal-pin-JEK-tō-mē*	excision of an oviduct
uter/o	uterus	uterine *Ū-ter-in*	pertaining to the uterus
metr/o, metr/i	uterus	metrorrhagia *mē-trō-RĀ-jē-a*	abnormal uterine bleeding
hyster/o	uterus	hysteroscopy *his-ter-OS-kō-pē*	endoscopic examination of the uterus
cervic/o	cervix, neck	endocervical *en-dō-SER-vi-kal*	pertaining to the lining of the cervix
vagin/o	vagina	vaginoplasty *vaj-i-nō-PLAS-tē*	plastic repair of the vagina
colp/o	vagina	colpocele *KOL-pō-sēl*	hernia of the vagina

Exercise 15-2

Define each of the following terms:

1. salpingoplasty (*sal-PING-gō-plas-tē*) _____

2. hysterectomy (*his-ter-EK-tō-mē*) _____

3. metrostenosis (*mē-trō-ste-NŌ-sis*) _____

4. uterovesical (*ū-ter-ō-VES-i-kl*) _____

5. vaginometer (*vaj-i-NOM-e-ter*) _____

6. colpodynia (*kol-pō-DIN-ē-a*) _____

Write a word that has the same meaning as each of the following definitions:

7. surgical fixation of an oviduct   _____

8. radiographic study of the oviduct   _____

The root *salping/o* is taken from the word *salpinx*, which means "tube." Add a prefix to salpinx to write a word that has the same meaning as each of the following definitions:

9. Presence of pus in an oviduct   _____

10. Collection of fluid in an oviduct   _____

Note how the roots *salping/o* and *oophor/o* are combined to form *salpingo-oophoritis* (inflammation of an oviduct and ovary). Write a word with the following meaning:

11. surgical removal of an oviduct and ovary   _____

Use the roots indicated to write a word that has the same meaning as each of the following definitions:

12. within (intra-) the uterus (uter/o)   _____

13. radiograph of the uterus (hyster/o) and oviducts   _____

14. surgical fixation of the uterus (hyster/o)   _____

15. prolapse of the uterus (metr/o)   _____

16. softening of the uterus (metr/o)   _____

17. inflammation of the cervix   _____

18. within (intra-) the cervix   _____

19. inflammation of the vagina (vagin/o)   _____

20. narrowing of the vagina (colp/o)   _____

TABLE 15-3 Roots for the Female Accessory Structures

ROOT	MEANING	EXAMPLE	DEFINITION OF EXAMPLE
vulv/o	vulva	vulvar *VUL-var*	pertaining to the vulva
episi/o	vulva	episiotomy *e-piz-ē-OT-ō-mē*	incision of the vulva
perine/o	perineum	perineal *per-i-NĒ-al*	pertaining to the perineum
clitor/o, clitorid/o	clitoris	clitorectomy *klī-tō-REK-tō-mē*	excision of the clitoris
mamm/o	breast, mammary gland	mammoplasty *mam-ō-PLAS-tē*	plastic surgery of the breast
mast/o	breast, mammary gland	amastia *a-MAS-tē-a*	absence of the breasts

Exercise 15-3

Write a word that has the same meaning as each of the following definitions:

1. any disease of the vulva (vulv/o)   _____

2. suture of the vulva (episi/o)   _____

3. pertaining to the vagina (vagin/o) and perineum   _____

4. inflammation of the clitoris   _____

5. radiograph of the breast (mamm/o)   _____

6. excision of the breast   _____

7. inflammation of the breast (mast/o)   _____

TABLE 15-4 Roots Pertaining to Pregnancy and Birth

ROOT	MEANING	EXAMPLE	DEFINITION OF EXAMPLE
amnio	amnion, amniotic sac	diamniotic _dī-am-nē-OT-ik_	developing in separate amniotic sacs
embry/o	embryo	embryonic _em-brē-ON-ik_	pertaining to the embryo
fet/o	fetus	fetoscope _FĒ-tō-skōp_	endoscope for examining the fetus
toc	labor	eutocia _ū-TŌ-sē-a_	normal labor
nat/i	birth	neonate _NĒ-ō-nāt_	newborn
lact/o	milk	lactation _lak-TĀ-shun_	secretion of milk
galact/o	milk	galactogogue _ga-LAK-tō-gog_	agent that promotes (-agogue) the flow of milk
gravida	pregnant woman	multigravida _mul-ti-GRAV-i-da_	woman who has been pregnant two or more times
para	woman who has given birth	nullipara _nul-IP-a-ra_	woman who has never (nulli-) given birth

Exercise 15-4

Define each of the following words:

1. embryology (_em-brē-OL-ō-jē_)   _____

2. postnatal (_pōst-NĀ-tal_)   _____

3. neonatal (*nē-ō-NĀ-tal*) _____

4. monoamniotic (*mon-ō-am-nē-OT-ik*) _____

5. fetometry (*fē-TOM-e-trē*) _____

6. hyperlactation (*hī-per-lak-TĀ-shun*) _____

7. agalactia (*ā-ga-LAK-shē-a*) _____

Use the appropriate roots to form a word with each of the following definitions:

8. rupture of the amniotic sac _____

9. incision of the amnion (to induce labor) _____

10. cell found in amniotic fluid _____

11. instrument for examination of the embryo _____

12. endoscopic examination of the fetus _____

13. any disease of an embryo _____

14. study of the newborn _____

15. before birth _____

16. woman who is pregnant for the first (primi-) time _____

17. woman who has never been pregnant _____

18. woman who has given birth two or more times _____

19. woman who has given birth to one (primi-) child _____

Use the suffix *-tocia*, meaning "condition of labor," to write a word that has the same meaning as each of the following definitions:

20. dry labor _____

21. slow labor _____

Use the root *galact*/o to write a word that has the same meaning as each of the following definitions:

22. cystic enlargement (-cele) of a milk duct _____

23. discharge of milk _____

Clinical Aspects of Female Reproduction

Infection

The major organisms that cause sexually transmitted diseases in both males and females are given in Table 14-1. **Pelvic inflammatory disease** (PID) is the spread of infection from the reproductive organs into the pelvic cavity. It is most often caused by the gonorrhea organism or by chlamydia, although bacteria normally living in the reproductive tract may also be responsible when conditions allow. PID is a serious disorder that may result in septicemia or shock. Inflammation of the oviducts, called **salpingitis**, may close off these tubes and cause infertility.

A fungus that infects the vulva and vagina is *Candida albicans*, causing **candidiasis**. There is **vaginitis**, a thick, white, cheesy discharge, and itching. Pregnancy, diabetes mellitus, and use of antibiotics, steroids, or birth control pills predispose to infection. If the infection is recurrent, the patient's partner should be treated to prevent reinfections. Antifungal agents (mycostatics) are used in treatment.

Endometriosis

Growth of endometrial tissue outside the uterus is termed **endometriosis**. Commonly the ovaries, oviducts, peritoneum, and other pelvic organs are involved. Stimulated by normal hormones, the endometrial tissue causes inflammation, fibrosis, and adhesions in surrounding areas. The results may be pain, **dysmenorrhea** (painful or difficult menstruation), and infertility. Laparoscopy is used to diagnose endometriosis and also to remove the abnormal tissue.

Menstrual Disorders

Menstrual abnormalities include flow that is too scanty (oligomenorrhea) or too heavy (menorrhagia), and the absence of monthly periods (amenorrhea). Dysmenorrhea, when it occurs, usually begins at the start of menstruation and lasts 1 to 2 days. Together these disorders are classified as dysfunctional uterine bleeding (DUB). These responses may be caused by hormone imbalances, systemic disorders, or uterine problems. They are most common in adolescence or near menopause. At other times they are often related to life changes and emotional upset.

Premenstrual syndrome (PMS) describes symptoms that appear during the second half of the menstrual cycle and includes emotional changes, fatigue, bloating, headaches, and appetite changes. Possible causes of PMS are under study. Symptoms may be relieved by hormone therapy, antidepressants, or antianxiety medications. Exercise, dietary control, rest, and relaxation strategies may also be helpful.

Cancer of the Female Reproductive Tract

Cancer of the endometrium is the most common cancer of the female reproductive tract. Women at risk should have biopsies taken regularly because endometrial cancer is not always detected by Pap (Papanicolaou) smear. Treatment consists of **hysterectomy** (removal of the uterus) (Fig. 15-9) and sometimes radiation therapy. A small percentage of cases occur after overgrowth (hyperplasia) of the endometrium. This tissue can be removed by **dilation and curettage** (D&C), in which the cervix is widened and the lining of the uterus is scraped with a curette.

Almost all patients with cancer of the cervix have been infected with human papilloma virus (HPV), a virus that causes genital warts. Incidence also is related to high sexual activity and other sexually transmitted viral infections, such as herpes.

In the 1940s and 1950s, the synthetic steroid DES (diethylstilbestrol) was given to prevent miscarriages. A small percentage of daughters born to women treated with this drug have shown an increased risk of developing cancer of the cervix and vagina. These women need to be examined regularly.

Cervical carcinoma is often preceded by abnormal growth (dysplasia) of the epithelial cells lining the cervix. Growth is graded as CIN I, II, or III, depending on the depth of tissue involved. CIN stands for cervical intraepithelial neoplasia. Diagnosis of cervical cancer is by a **Pap smear**, examination with a **colposcope**, and biopsy. In a **cone biopsy** (Fig. 15-10), a cone-shaped piece of tissue is removed from the lining of the cervix for study. Often in the procedure, all of the abnormal cells are removed as well.

Cancer of the ovary has a high mortality rate because it usually causes no early symptoms. Often by the time of diagnosis, the tumor has invaded the pelvis and abdomen. Removal of the ovaries (**oophorectomy**) and oviducts (**salpingectomy**) along with the uterus is required (see Fig. 15-9), in addition to chemotherapy and radiation therapy.

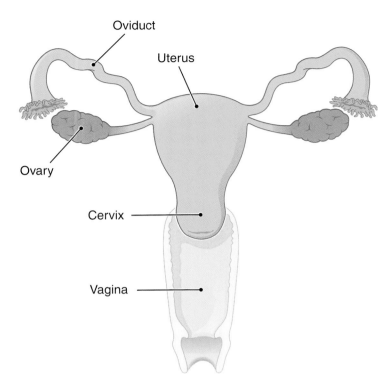

Oviduct

Uterus

Ovary

Cervix

Vagina

FIGURE 15-9. A hysterectomy is surgical removal of the uterus. Removal of the ovary (oophorectomy) and oviduct (salpingectomy) may also be required either unilaterally or bilaterally.

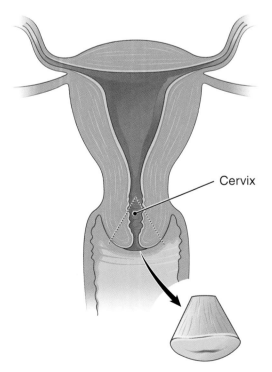

Cervix

Cone biopsy

FIGURE 15-10. Cone biopsy of the uterine cervix.

Breast Cancer

Carcinoma of the breast is second only to lung cancer in causing cancer-related deaths among women in the United States. This cancer metastasizes readily through the lymph nodes and blood to other sites such as the lung, liver, bones, and ovaries. Treatment is usually some form of **mastectomy** (removal of the breast). In a radical mastectomy, underlying muscle and axillary lymph nodes (in the armpit) also are removed; in a modified radical mastectomy, the breast and lymph nodes are removed, but muscles are left in place. Sometimes just the tumor itself is removed surgically in a segmental mastectomy or "lumpectomy." Radiation therapy, chemotherapy, and sometimes hormone therapy are also used.

Mammography is a method of diagnosing breast cancer by x-ray examination (Fig. 15-11). After the age of 45, women should be examined using this method yearly. Other diagnostic methods include palpation and cytologic study of tissue removed by aspiration or excision. Regular breast self-examination (BSE) is of utmost importance because most breast cancers are discovered by women themselves.

Clinical Aspects of Pregnancy and Birth

Pregnancy-induced hypertension (PIH), also referred to as pre-eclampsia or toxemia of pregnancy, is a state of hypertension during pregnancy in association with oliguria, proteinuria, and edema. The cause is a hormone imbalance that results in constriction of blood vessels. If untreated, PIH may lead to **eclampsia** with seizures, coma, and possible death.

Development of a fertilized egg outside of its normal position in the uterine cavity is termed an **ectopic pregnancy** (Fig. 15-12). Although it may occur elsewhere in the abdominal cavity, this abnormal development usually takes place in the oviduct, resulting in a tubal pregnancy. Salpingitis, endometriosis, and PID may lead to ectopic pregnancy by blocking passage of the egg into the uterus. Continued growth will rupture the oviduct, causing dangerous hemorrhage. Symptoms of ectopic pregnancy are pain, tenderness, swelling,

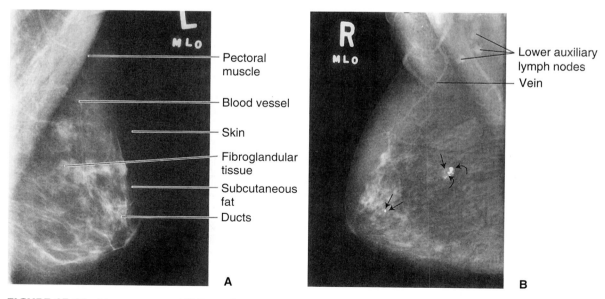

FIGURE 15-11. Mammograms. **(A)** Normal mammogram, left breast. **(B)** Mammogram of right breast showing lesions (*arrows*). (Reprinted with permission from Erkonen WE, Smith WL. Radiology 101: Basics and Fundamentals of Imaging. Philadelphia: Lippincott Williams & Wilkins, 1998.)

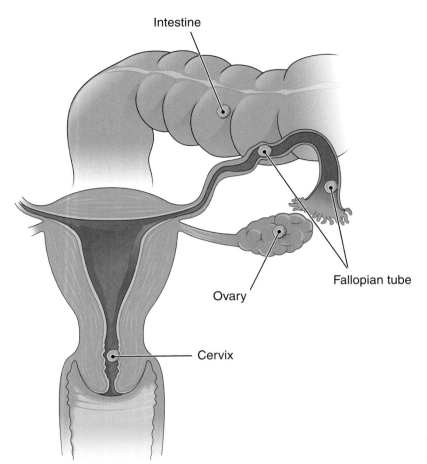

FIGURE 15-12. Sites at which an ectopic pregnancy may occur.

and shock. Diagnosis is by measurement of the hormone HCG and ultrasonography, confirmed by laparoscopic examination. Prompt surgery is required, sometimes including removal of the tube.

For a variety of reasons, a pregnancy may terminate before the fetus is capable of surviving outside the uterus. An **abortion** is loss of an embryo or fetus before the 20th week of pregnancy or before a weight of 500 g (1.1 lb). When this occurs spontaneously, it is commonly referred to as a miscarriage. Most spontaneous abortions occur within the first 3 months of pregnancy. Causes include poor maternal health, hormone imbalance, incompetence (weakness) of the cervix, immune reactions, tumors, and, most commonly, fetal abnormalities. If all gestational tissues are not eliminated, the abortion is described as incomplete and the remaining tissue must be removed.

An induced abortion is the intentional termination of a pregnancy. A common method for inducing an abortion is **dilatation and evacuation** (D&E), in which the cervix is dilated and the fetal tissue is removed by suction.

Placental Abnormalities

If the placenta attaches near or over the cervix instead of in the upper portion of the uterus, the condition is termed **placenta previa**. This disorder may cause bleeding in the later stages of pregnancy. If bleeding is heavy, it may be necessary to terminate the pregnancy.

Placental abruption (abruptio placentae) describes premature separation of the placenta from its point of attachment. The separation causes hemorrhage, which, if extensive, may result in fetal or maternal death or a need to end the pregnancy. Causative factors include injury, maternal hypertension, and advanced maternal age.

Mastitis

Inflammation of the breast, or **mastitis**, may occur at any time but usually occurs in the early weeks of breast-feeding. It is commonly caused by staphylococcus or streptococcus bacteria that enter through cracks in the nipple. The breast becomes red, swollen, and tender, and the patient may experience chills, fever, and general discomfort.

Congenital Disorders

Congenital disorders are those present at birth (birth defects). They fall into two categories: developmental disorders that occur during growth of the fetus and hereditary (familial) disorders that can be passed from parents to children through the germ cells. Genetic disorders are caused by a **mutation** (change) in the genes or chromosomes of the cells. They may involve changes in the number or structure of the chromosomes or changes in single or multiple genes. The appearance and severity of genetic disorders may also involve abnormal genes interacting with environmental factors. Examples are the diseases that "run in families," such as diabetes mellitus, heart disease, hypertension, and certain forms of cancer. Display 15-1 describes some of the most common genetic disorders.

A **carrier** of a genetic disorder is an individual who has a genetic defect that does not appear but that can be passed to offspring. Carriers of some genetic disorders can be identified using laboratory tests.

DISPLAY 15-1 Common Genetic Disorders*

DISEASE	CAUSE	DESCRIPTION
albinism	recessive gene mutation	lack of pigmentation
cystic fibrosis	recessive gene mutation	affects respiratory system, pancreas, and sweat glands; most common hereditary disease in white populations (see Chapter 11)
Down syndrome	extra chromosome 21	slanted eyes, short stature, mental retardation, and others; incidence increases with increasing maternal age
hemophilia *hē-mō-FIL-ē-a*	recessive gene mutation on the X chromosome	bleeding disease passed from mothers to sons
Huntington disease	dominant gene mutation	altered metabolism destroys specific nerve cells; appears in adulthood and is fatal within about 10 years; causes motor and mental disorders
Klinefelter syndrome	extra sex (X) chromosome	lack of sexual development, lowered intelligence
Marfan syndrome	dominant gene mutation	disease of connective tissue with weakness of the aorta
neurofibromatosis *nū-rō-fī-brō-ma-TŌ-sis*	dominant gene mutation	multiple skin tumors containing nervous tissue

DISPLAY 15-1 Common Genetic Disorders*, *continued*

DISEASE	CAUSE	DESCRIPTION
phenylketonuria (PKU) *fen-il-kē-tō-NŪ-rē-a*	recessive gene mutation	lack of enzyme to metabolize an amino acid; neurologic signs, mental retardation, lack of pigment; tested for at birth; special diet can prevent retardation
sickle cell anemia	recessive gene mutation	abnormally shaped red cells block blood vessels; mainly affects black populations
Tay-Sachs disease	recessive gene mutation	an enzyme deficiency causes lipid to accumulate in nerve cells and other tissues; causes death in early childhood; carried in Jewish populations in eastern Europe
Turner syndrome	single sex (X) chromosome	sexual immaturity, short stature, possible lowered intelligence

*A dominant gene is one for a trait that always appears if the gene is present; that is, it will affect the offspring even if inherited from only one parent. A recessive gene is one for a trait that will appear only if the gene is inherited from both parents.

Teratogens are factors that cause malformation of the developing fetus. These include infections, such as **rubella** (German measles), herpes simplex, and syphilis; alcohol; drugs; chemicals; and radiation. The fetus is most susceptible to teratogenic effects during the first 3 months of pregnancy. Examples of developmental disorders are **atresia** (absence or closure of a normal body opening), **anencephaly** (absence of a brain), **cleft lip**, **cleft palate**, and congenital heart disease. **Spina bifida** is incomplete closure of the spine, through which the spinal cord and its membranes may project (Fig. 15-13). This usually occurs in the lumbar region. If there is no herniation of tissue, the condition is spina bifida occulta. Protrusion of the meninges through the opening is a meningocele; in a myelomeningocele, both the spinal cord and membranes herniate through the defect, as seen in Figure 15-13D and Figure 15-14.

Many congenital disorders can now be detected before birth. **Ultrasonography** (Fig. 15-15), in addition to being used to monitor pregnancies and determine fetal sex, can also reveal certain fetal abnormalities. In

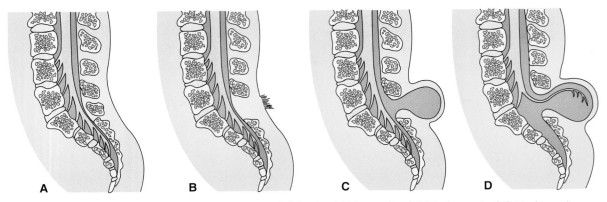

FIGURE 15-13. Spinal defects. **(A)** Normal spinal cord. **(B)** Spina bifida occulta. **(C)** Meningocele. **(D)** Myelomeningocele. (Reprinted with permission from Pillitteri A. Maternal and Child Health Nursing: Care of the Childbearing and Childrearing Family. 4th Ed. Philadelphia: Lippincott Williams & Wilkins, 2003.)

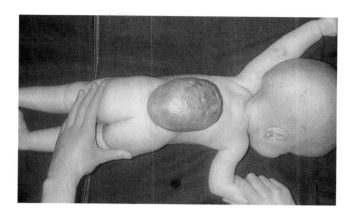

FIGURE 15-14. A myelomeningocele. (Reprinted with permission from Pillitteri A. Maternal and Child Health Nursing: Care of the Childbearing and Childrearing Family. 4th Ed. Philadelphia: Lippincott Williams & Wilkins, 2003.)

amniocentesis (Fig. 15-16), a sample is withdrawn from the amniotic cavity with a needle. The fluid obtained can be analyzed for chemical abnormalities. The cells are grown in the laboratory and tested for biochemical disorders. A **karyotype** is prepared to study the genetic material. In **chorionic villus sampling** (CVS), small amounts of the membrane around the fetus are obtained through the cervix for analysis. This can be done at 8 to 10 weeks of pregnancy, in comparison with 14 to 16 weeks for amniocentesis.

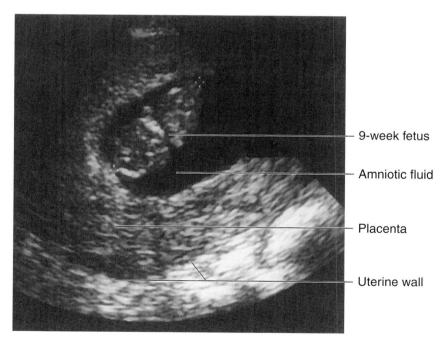

9-week fetus

Amniotic fluid

Placenta

Uterine wall

FIGURE 15-15. Transvaginal sonogram showing a 9-week-old fetus. (Reprinted with permission from Erkonen WE, Smith WL. Radiology 101: Basics and Fundamentals of Imaging. Philadelphia: Lippincott Williams & Wilkins, 1998.)

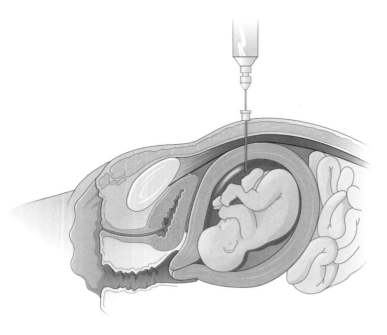

FIGURE 15-16. Amniocentesis. A sample is removed from the amniotic sac. Cells and fluid are tested for fetal abnormalities.

Key Clinical Terms

DISORDERS

Female Reproductive System

candidiasis *kan-di-DĪ-a-sis*	Infection with the fungus *Candida*, a common cause of vaginitis
dysmenorrhea *DIS-men-ō-rē-a*	Painful or difficult menstruation. A common disorder that may be caused by infection, use of an intrauterine device, endometriosis, overproduction of prostaglandins, or other factors.
endometriosis *en-dō-mē-trē-Ō-sis*	Growth of endometrial tissue outside the uterus, usually in the pelvic cavity
pelvic inflammatory disease (PID)	Condition caused by the spread of infection from the reproductive tract into the pelvic cavity. Commonly caused by sexually transmitted gonorrhea and chlamydial infections.
salpingitis *sal-pin-JĪ-tis*	Inflammation of the oviduct; typically caused by urinary tract or sexually transmitted infection. Chronic salpingitis may lead to infertility or ectopic pregnancy (development of the fertilized egg outside of the uterus).
vaginitis *vaj-i-NĪ-tis*	Inflammation of the vagina

Pregnancy and Birth

abortion *a-BOR-shun*	Termination of a pregnancy before the fetus is capable of surviving outside the uterus, usually at 20 wk or 500 g. May be spontaneous or induced. A spontaneous abortion is commonly called a miscarriage.
anencephaly *an-en-SEF-a-lē*	Congenital absence of a brain
atresia *a-TRĒ-zē-a*	Congenital absence or closure of a normal body opening
carrier	An individual who has an unexpressed genetic defect that can be passed to his or her children
cleft lip	A congenital separation of the upper lip
cleft palate	A congenital split in the roof of the mouth
congenital disorder	A disorder that is present at birth. May be developmental or hereditary.
eclampsia *e-KLAMP-sē-a*	Convulsions and coma occurring during pregnancy or after delivery and associated with the conditions of pregnancy-induced hypertension (see below) (adjective, eclamptic)
ectopic pregnancy *ek-TOP-ik*	Development of the fertilized ovum outside the body of the uterus. Usually occurs in the oviduct (tubal pregnancy) but may occur in other parts of the reproductive tract or abdominal cavity (see Fig. 15-12).
mastitis *mas-TĪ-tis*	Inflammation of the breast, usually associated with the early weeks of breastfeeding
mutation *mū-TĀ-shun*	A change in the genetic material of the cell. Most mutations are harmful. If the change appears in the sex cells, it can be passed to future generations.
placental abruption	Premature separation of the placenta; abruptio placentae
placenta previa *PRĒ-vē-a*	A placenta that is attached in the lower portion of the uterus instead of the upper portion, as is normal. May result in hemorrhage late in pregnancy.
pregnancy-induced hypertension (PIH)	A toxic condition of late pregnancy associated with hypertension, edema, and proteinuria that, if untreated, may lead to eclampsia. Also called pre-eclampsia (*prē-e-KLAMP-sē-a*) and toxemia of pregnancy.
rubella *rū-BEL-la*	German measles. The virus can cross the placenta and cause fetal abnormalities, such as eye defects, deafness, heart abnormalities, and mental retardation. The virus is most damaging during the first trimester.
spina bifida *SPĪ-na BIF-i-da*	A congenital defect in the closure of the spinal column through which the spinal cord and its membranes may project (see Figs. 15-13 and 15-14)
teratogen *ter-AT-ō-jen*	A factor that causes developmental abnormalities in the fetus (adjective, teratogenic); root terat/o means "malformed fetus"

DIAGNOSIS AND TREATMENT

Female Reproductive System

colposcope *KOL-pō-skōp*	Instrument for examining the vagina and cervix
cone biopsy	Removal of a cone of tissue from the lining of the cervix for cytologic examination; also called conization (see Fig. 15-10)
dilation and curettage (D&C)	Procedure in which the cervix is dilated (widened) and the lining of the uterus is scraped with a curette
hysterectomy *his-ter-EK-tō-mē*	Surgical removal of the uterus. Most commonly done because of tumors. Often the oviducts and ovaries are removed as well (see Fig. 15-9).
mammography *mam-OG-ra-fē*	Radiographic study of the breast for the detection of breast cancer
mastectomy *mas-TEK-tō-mē*	Excision of the breast to eliminate malignancy
oophorectomy *ō-of-ō-REK-tō-mē*	Excision of an ovary (see Fig. 15-9)
Pap smear	Study of cells collected from the cervix and vagina for early detection of cancer. Also called Papanicolaou smear or Pap test.
salpingectomy *sal-pin-JEK-tō-mē*	Surgical removal of the oviduct (see Fig. 15-9)

Pregnancy and Birth

amniocentesis *am-nē-ō-sen-TĒ-sis*	Transabdominal puncture of the amniotic sac to remove amniotic fluid for testing. Tests on the cells and fluid obtained can reveal congenital abnormalities, blood incompatibility, and sex of the fetus (see Fig. 15-16).
chorionic villus sampling (CVS)	Removal of chorionic cells through the cervix for prenatal testing. Can be done earlier in pregnancy than amniocentesis.
dilatation and evacuation (D&E)	Widening of the cervix and removal of the products of conception by suction
karyotype *KAR-ē-ō-tīp*	A picture of the chromosomes of a cell arranged in order of decreasing size; can reveal abnormalities in the chromosomes themselves or in their number or arrangement (root *kary/o* means "nucleus")
ultrasonography	The use of high-frequency sound waves to produce a photograph of an organ or tissue (see Fig. 15-15). Used in obstetrics to diagnose pregnancy, multiple births, and abnormalities and also to study and measure the fetus. The picture obtained is a sonogram or ultrasonogram.

Supplementary Terms

NORMAL STRUCTURE AND FUNCTION

Female Reproductive System

adnexa *ad-NEK-sa*	Appendages, such as the adnexa uteri—the ovaries, oviducts, and uterine ligaments
areola *a-RĒ-ō-la*	A pigmented ring, such as the dark area around the nipple of the breast
cul-de-sac *kul-di-SAK*	A blind pouch, such as the recess between the rectum and the uterus; the rectouterine pouch or pouch of Douglas
fimbriae *FIM-brē-ē*	The long fingerlike extensions of the oviduct that wave to capture the released ovum (see Fig. 15-6); singular, *fimbria*
fornix *FOR-niks*	An archlike space, such as the space between the uppermost wall of the vagina and the cervix (see Fig. 15-1)
greater vestibular gland	A small mucus-secreting gland on the side of the vestibule (see below) near the vaginal opening. Also called Bartholin (*BAR-tō-lin*) gland (see Fig. 15-6).
hymen *HĪ-men*	A fold of mucous membrane that partially covers the entrance of the vagina
menses *(MEN-sēz)*	The monthly flow of bloody discharge from the lining of the uterus
mons pubis *monz PŪ-bis*	The rounded, fleshy elevation in front of the pubic joint that is covered with hair after puberty
oocyte *Ō-ō-sīt*	An immature ovum
perimenopause *per-i-MEN-ō-pawz*	The period immediately before and after menopause
vestibule *VES-ti-būl*	The space between the labia minora that contains the openings of the urethra, vagina, and ducts of the greater vestibular glands

Pregnancy and Birth

afterbirth	The placenta and membranes delivered after birth of a child
antepartum *an-tē-PAR-tum*	Before childbirth, with reference to the mother
Braxton–Hicks contractions	Light uterine contractions that occur during pregnancy and increase in frequency and intensity during the third trimester. They strengthen the uterus for delivery.
chloasma *klō-AZ-ma*	Brownish pigmentation that appears on the face during pregnancy; melasma

Normal Structure and Function, continued

fontanel *fon-tan-EL*	A membrane-covered space between cranial bones in the fetus that later becomes ossified; a soft spot. Also spelled fontanelle.
intrapartum *in-tra-PAR-tum*	Occurring during childbirth
linea nigra *LIN-ē-a NĪ-gra*	A dark line on the abdomen from the umbilicus to the pubic region that may appear late in pregnancy
lochia *LŌ-kē-a*	The mixture of blood, mucus, and tissue discharged from the uterus after childbirth
meconium *me-KŌ-nē-um*	The first feces of the newborn
peripartum *per-i-PAR-tum*	Occurring during the end of pregnancy or the first few months after delivery, with reference to the mother
postpartum	After childbirth, with reference to the mother
premature	Describing an infant born before the organ systems are fully developed; immature
preterm	Occurring before the 37th week of gestation; describing an infant born before the 37th week of gestation
puerperium *pū-er-PĒR-ē-um*	The period of 42 days after childbirth, during which the mother's reproductive organs usually return to normal (root *puer* means "child")
striae atrophicae *STRĪ-ē a-TRŌ-fi-kē*	Pinkish or gray lines that appear where skin has been stretched, as in pregnancy; stretch marks, striae gravidarum
umbilicus *um-bi-LĪ-kus*	The scar in the middle of the abdomen that marks the point of attachment of the umbilical cord to the fetus; the navel
vernix caseosa *VER-niks kā-sē-Ō-sa*	The cheeselike deposit that covers and protects the fetus (literally "cheesy varnish")

DISORDERS

Female Reproductive System

cystocele *SIS-tō-sēl*	Herniation of the urinary bladder into the wall of the vagina (Fig. 15-17)
dyspareunia *dis-par-Ū-nē-a*	Pain during sexual intercourse
fibrocystic disease of the breast *fī-brō-SIS-tik*	A condition in which there are palpable lumps in the breasts, usually associated with pain and tenderness. These lumps or "thickenings" change with the menstrual cycle and must be distinguished from malignant tumors by palpation, mammography, and biopsy.
fibroid *FĪ-broyd*	Benign tumor of smooth muscle (see leiomyoma)

Disorders, continued

leiomyoma *lī-ō-mī-Ō-ma*	Benign tumor of smooth muscle. In the uterus, may cause bleeding and pressure on the bladder or rectum. Surgical removal or hysterectomy may be necessary. Also called fibroid or myoma.
leukorrhea *lū-kō-RĒ-a*	White or yellowish discharge from the vagina. Infection and other disorders may change the amount, color, or odor of the discharge.
prolapse of the uterus	Downward displacement of the uterus with the cervix sometimes protruding from the vagina
rectocele *REK-tō-sēl*	Herniation of the rectum into the wall of the vagina; also called proctocele (see Fig. 15-17)

Pregnancy and Birth

cephalopelvic disproportion *sef-a-lō-PEL-vik*	The condition in which the head of the fetus is larger than the pelvic outlet; also called fetopelvic disproportion
choriocarcinoma *kor-ē-ō-kar-si-NŌ-ma*	A rare malignant neoplasm composed of placental tissue
galactorrhea *ga-lak-tō-RĒ-a*	Excessive secretion of milk or continuation of milk production after breastfeeding has ceased. Often results from excess prolactin secretion and may signal a pituitary tumor.
hydatidiform mole *hī-da-TID-i-form*	A benign overgrowth of placental tissue. The placenta dilates and resembles grapelike cysts. The neoplasm may invade the wall of the uterus, causing rupture. Also called hydatid mole.
hydramnios *hī-DRAM-nē-os*	An excess of amniotic fluid; also called polyhydramnios
oligohydramnios *ol-i-gō-hī-DRAM-nē-os*	A deficiency of amniotic fluid
patent ductus arteriosus (PDA) *PĀ-tent*	Persistence of the ductus arteriosus after birth so that blood continues to shunt from the pulmonary artery to the aorta
puerperal infection *pū-ER-per-al*	Infection of the genital tract after delivery

DIAGNOSIS AND TREATMENT
Female Reproductive System

episiorrhaphy *e-pis-ē-OR-a-fē*	Suture of the vulva or suture of the perineum cut in an episiotomy
laparoscopy *lap-a-ROS-kō-pē*	Endoscopic examination of the abdomen; may include surgical procedures, such as tubal ligation (see Fig. 15-5)
sentinel nodes *SEN-ti-nel*	The first lymph nodes to receive drainage from a tumor. Biopsy of sentinel nodes is used to determine spread of cancer in planning treatment.

Diagnosis and Treatment, *continued*

speculum *SPEK-ū-lum*	An instrument used to enlarge the opening of a passage or cavity for examination

Pregnancy and Birth

alpha-fetoprotein (AFP)	A fetal protein that may be at an elevated level in amniotic fluid and maternal serum in cases of certain fetal disorders
Apgar score	A system of rating an infant's physical condition immediately after birth. Five features are rated as 0, 1, or 2 at 1 minute and 5 minutes after delivery, and sometimes thereafter. The maximum possible score at each interval is 10. Infants with low scores require medical attention.
artificial insemination (AI)	Placement of active semen into the vagina or cervix for the purpose of impregnation. The semen can be from a husband, partner, or donor.
cesarean section *se-ZAR-ē-an*	Incision of the abdominal wall and uterus for delivery of a fetus
culdocentesis *kul-dō-sen-TĒ-sis*	Puncture of the vaginal wall to sample fluid from the rectouterine space for diagnosis
extracorporeal membrane oxygenation (ECMO)	A technique for pulmonary bypass in which deoxygenated blood is removed, passed through a circuit that oxygenates the blood, and then returned. Used for selected newborn and pediatric patients in respiratory failure with an otherwise good prognosis.
in vitro fertilization (IVF)	Clinical procedure for achieving fertilization when it cannot be accomplished naturally. An oocyte (immature ovum) is removed, fertilized in the laboratory, and placed as a zygote into the uterus or fallopian tube (ZIFT, zygote intrafallopian transfer). Alternatively, an ovum can be removed and placed along with sperm cells into the fallopian tube (GIFT, gamete intrafallopian transfer).
obstetrics *ob-STET-riks*	The branch of medicine that treats women during pregnancy, childbirth, and the puerperium. Usually combined with the practice of gynecology.
pediatrics *pē-dē-AT-riks*	The branch of medicine that treats children and diseases of children (root *ped/o* means "child")
pelvimetry *pel-VIM-e-trē*	Measurement of the pelvis by manual examination or radiographic study to determine whether it will be possible to deliver a fetus through the vagina
Pitocin *pi-TŌ-sin*	Trade name for oxytocin; used to induce and hasten labor
presentation	Term describing the part of the fetus that can be felt by vaginal or rectal examination. Normally the head presents first (vertex presentation), but sometimes the buttocks (breech presentation), face, or other part presents first.

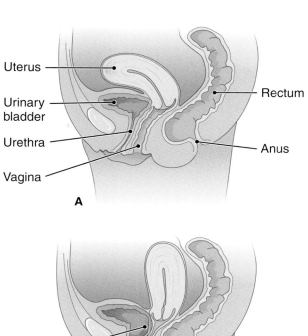

Uterus

Urinary bladder

Urethra

Vagina

Rectum

Anus

A

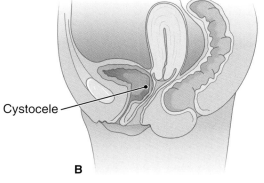

Cystocele

B

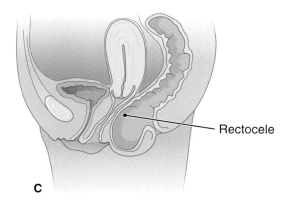

Rectocele

C

FIGURE 15-17. Herniation into the vagina.
(A) Normal. **(B)** Cystocele. **(C)** Rectocele.

ABBREVIATIONS

Female Reproductive System

BSE	Breast self-examination
BSO	Bilateral salpingo-oophorectomy
BV	Bacterial vaginosis
CIN	Cervical intraepithelial neoplasia
D&C	Dilation and curettage
DES	Diethylstilbestrol
DUB	Dysfunctional uterine bleeding
FSH	Follicle stimulating hormone
GC	Gonococcus (cause of gonorrhea)
GYN	Gynecology
HCG, hCG	Human chorionic gonadotropin
HPV	Human papilloma virus
HRT	Hormone replacement therapy
IUD	Intrauterine device
LH	Luteinizing hormone
NGU	Nongonococcal urethritis
PID	Pelvic inflammatory disease
PIH	Pregnancy-induced hypertension
PMS	Premenstrual syndrome
STD	Sexually transmitted disease
TAH	Total abdominal hysterectomy
TSS	Toxic shock syndrome
VD	Venereal disease (sexually transmitted disease)

Pregnancy and Birth

AB	Abortion
AFP	Alpha-fetoprotein
AGA	Appropriate for gestational age
AI	Artificial insemination
C section	Cesarean section
CPD	Cephalopelvic disproportion
CVS	Chorionic villus sampling
D&E	Dilatation and evacuation
ECMO	Extracorporeal membrane oxygenation
EDC	Estimated date of confinement
FHR	Fetal heart rate
FHT	Fetal heart tone
FTND	Full-term normal delivery
FTP	Full-term pregnancy
GA	Gestational age
GIFT	Gamete intrafallopian transfer
HCG	Human chorionic gonadotropin
IVF	In vitro fertilization
LMP	Last menstrual period
NB	Newborn
NICU	Neonatal intensive care unit
OB	Obstetrics
PDA	Patent ductus arteriosus
PIH	Pregnancy-induced hypertension
PKU	Phenylketonuria
SVD	Spontaneous vaginal delivery
UC	Uterine contractions
UTP	Uterine term pregnancy
VBAC	Vaginal birth after cesarean section
ZIFT	Zygote intrafallopian transfer

Labeling Exercise 15-1

Female Reproductive System

Write the name of each numbered part on the corresponding line of the answer sheet.

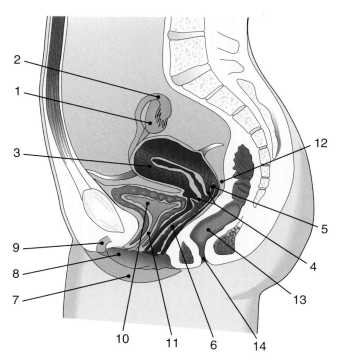

Anus
Cervix
Clitoris
Cul-de-sac
Labium majus
Labium minus
Ovary
Oviduct
Posterior fornix
Rectum
Urethra
Urinary bladder
Uterus
Vagina

1. _____	8. _____
2. _____	9. _____
3. _____	10. _____
4. _____	11. _____
5. _____	12. _____
6. _____	13. _____
7. _____	14. _____

Labeling Exercise 15-2

Female Reproductive System Showing Fertilization

Write the name of each numbered part on the corresponding line of the answer sheet.

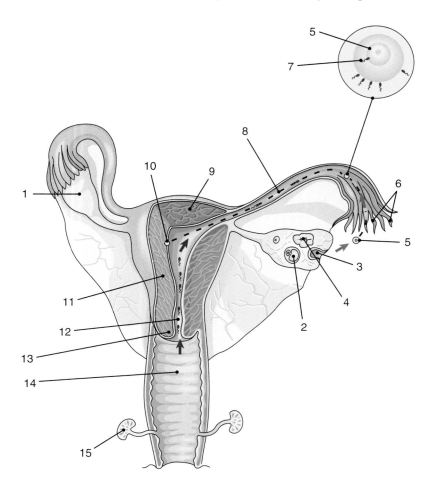

Body of uterus
Cervical canal
Cervix
Corpus luteum
Fimbriae
Fundus of uterus
Greater vestibular (Bartholin)
    gland
Implanted embryo
Maturing follicle
Ovarian follicle (ruptured)
Oviduct (fallopian tube)
Ovary
Ovum
Sperm cell
vagina

1. _____

2. _____

3. _____

4. _____

5. _____

6. _____

7. _____

8. _____

9. _____

10. _____

11. _____

12. _____

13. _____

14. _____

15. _____

Chapter Review 15-1

Match the following terms and write the appropriate letter to the left of each number:

_____ 1. clitoris

_____ 2. myometrium

_____ 3. oviduct

_____ 4. ovulation

_____ 5. vulva

a. muscle of the uterus

b. fallopian tube

c. release of an egg from the ovary

d. external female genitalia

e. female erectile tissue

_____ 6. metrorrhea

_____ 7. panhysterectomy

_____ 8. metratrophia

_____ 9. gynecogenic

_____ 10. menostasis

a. producing female characteristics

b. abnormal uterine discharge

c. wasting of uterine tissue

d. suppression of menstruation

e. removal of the entire uterus

_____ 11. chorion

_____ 12. gestation

_____ 13. zygote

_____ 14. amnion

_____ 15. parturition

a. childbirth

b. outermost layer of the embryo

c. sac that holds the fetus

d. period of development in the uterus

e. fertilized egg

_____ 16. oxytocin

_____ 17. neonate

_____ 18. dystocia

_____ 19. agalactia

_____ 20. colostrum

a. lack of milk production

b. newborn

c. first breast fluid

d. difficult labor

e. hormone that stimulates labor

_____ 21. mutation

_____ 22. karyotype

_____ 23. eclampsia

_____ 24. rubella

_____ 25. atresia

a. picture of the chromosomes used for diagnosis

b. condition associated with hypertension during pregnancy

c. congenital absence of a normal body opening

d. German measles

e. change in the genetic material

SUPPLEMENTARY TERMS

_____ 26. cul-de-sac

_____ 27. fornix

_____ 28. dyspareunia

_____ 29. fibroid

_____ 30. leukorrhea

a. leiomyoma

b. whitish vaginal discharge

c. space between the vagina and cervix

d. rectouterine pouch

e. pain during intercourse

_____ 31. hymen

_____ 32. speculum

_____ 33. vestibule

_____ 34. menarche

_____ 35. areola

a. a pigmented ring

b. membrane that covers the opening of the vagina

c. start of menstrual cycles

d. instrument used to enlarge an opening for examination

e. space between the labia

_____ 36. meconium

_____ 37. lochia

_____ 38. puerperium

_____ 39. fontanel

_____ 40. umbilicus

a. period after childbirth

b. soft spot between cranial bones

c. uterine discharge after childbirth

d. first feces of the newborn

e. navel

Fill in the blanks:

41. The female gonad is the _____.

42. The graafian follicle encloses a developing _____.

43. The inner lining of the uterus is the _____.

44. The neck of the uterus is the _____.

45. Parametritis (_par-a-mē-TRĪ-tis_) means inflammation of the tissue near the _____.

46. Polymastia (_pol-ē-MAS-tē-a_) means the presence of more than one pair of _____.

47. The stage in development between the zygote and the fetus is the _____.

48. The tissue that nourishes and maintains the developing fetus is the _____.

49. The secretion of milk from the mammary glands is called _____.

50. Loss of an embryo or fetus before 20 weeks or 500 g is termed a(n) _____.

Define each of the following terms:

51. metrorrhagia (_mē-trō-RĀ-jē-a_) _____

52. retrouterine (_re-trō-Ū-ter-in_)

53. hysteropathy (*his-te-ROP-a-thē*) _____

54. colpostenosis (*kol-pō-ste-NŌ-sis*) _____

55. pyosalpinx (*pī-ō-SAL-pinx*) _____

56. anovulatory (*an-OV-ū-la-tō-rē*) _____

57. inframammary (*in-fra-MAM-a-rē*) _____

58. congenital (*kon-JEN-i-tal*) _____

59. prenatal (*prē-NĀ-tal*) _____

60. extraembryonic (*eks-tra-em-brē-ON-ik*) _____

61. multigravida (*mul-ti-GRAV-i-da*) _____

62. tripara (*TRIP-a-ra*) _____

63. teratogenic (*TER-at-ō-jen-ik*) _____

Write a word for each of the following definitions:

64. narrowing of the uterus (metr/o) _____

65. surgical removal of the uterus (hyster/o) and oviducts _____

66. plastic repair of the vulva (episi/o-) _____

67. radiographic study of the breast (mamm/o) _____

68. hernia of an oviduct _____

69. through (-trans) the cervix _____

70. rupture of the amniotic sac _____

71. study of the embryo _____

72. direct examination of a fetus _____

73. abnormal or difficult labor _____

Write one word with the same meaning as each of the following:

74. neonate _____

75. para 1 _____

76. gravida 0 _____

Write a word that has the opposite meaning of each of the following words:

77. antepartum _____

78. postnatal _____

79. dystocia _____

80. anovulatory _____

Write the adjective form of each of the following words:

81. cervix _____

82. uterus _____

83. perineum _____

84. vagina _____

85. embryo _____

86. amnion _____

Write the plural form of each of the following words:

87. labium _____

88. cervix _____

89. fimbria _____

90. ovum _____

Write the meaning of each of the following abbreviations:

91. TAH _____

92. FSH _____

93. DUB _____

94. HRT _____

95. PDA _____

96. HCG _____

97. GA _____

98. FHR _____

99. VBAC _____

Word analysis. Define each of the following words, and give the meaning of the word parts in each. Use a dictionary if necessary.

100. gynecomastia (*jin-e-kō-MAS-tē-a*) _____
    a. gynec/o _____
    b. mast/o _____
    c. -ia _____

101. oxytocia _____
    a. oxy <u>sharp, acute</u>
    b. toc _____
    c. -ia _____

102. oligohydramnios _____
    a. oligo- _____
    b. hydr/o _____
    c. amnio(s) _____

Case Studies

Case Study 15-1: Total Abdominal Hysterectomy With Bilateral Salpingo-Oophorectomy

M.T., a 60-year-old gravida 2, para 2, had spent 3 months under the care of her gynecologist for treatment of postmenopausal bleeding and cervical dysplasia. She had had several vaginal examinations with Pap smears, a uterine ultrasound, colposcopy with endocervical biopsies, and a D&C with cone biopsy. She wanted to take hormone therapy, but her doctor thought she was at too much risk with the abnormal cells on her cervix and the excessive bleeding.

She had a TAH & BSO under general anesthesia with no complications and an uneventful recovery. Her uterus had been prolapsed on abdominal examination, but there was no sign of malignancy or PID. The pathology report revealed several leiomyomas of the uterus and stenosis of the right oviduct. She was discharged on the second postoperative day with few activity restrictions.

Case Study 15-2: In Vitro Fertilization

C.A. had worked as a technologist in the IVF lab at University Medical Center for 4 years. Her department was the Advanced Reproductive Technology Program. Although her work was primarily in the laboratory, she followed up each patient through all five phases of the IVF and embryo transfer treatment cycle: follicular development, aspiration of the preovulatory follicles, sperm preparation, IVF, and embryo transfer. Her department does both GIFT (gamete intrafallopian transfer) and ZIFT (zygote intrafallopian transfer) procedures.

While the female patient is in surgery having an ultrasound-guided transvaginal oocyte retrieval, C.A. examines the recently donated sperm for motility and quantity. She prepares to inoculate the sample into the cytoplasm of the ova as soon as she receives the cells from the OR. After inoculation, she places the sterile Petri dish with the fertilized oocytes into an incubator until they are ready to be introduced into the female patient.

Case Study 15-3: Cesarean Section Birth

A.Y., a gravida 2, para 1 at 39 weeks gestation, had been in active labor for several hours, fully effaced and dilated, yet unable to progress. She had had an uneventful pregnancy with good health, moderate weight gain, good fetal heart sounds, and no signs or symptoms of pregnancy-induced hypertension. X-ray pelvimetry revealed CPD with the fetus in right occiput posterior position. Changes in fetal heart rate indicated fetal distress. A.Y. was transported to the OR for emergency C-section under spinal anesthesia.

After being placed in the supine position, A.Y. had a urethral catheter inserted and her abdomen was prepped with antimicrobial solution. After draping, a transverse suprapubic incision was made. Dissection was continued through the muscle layers to the uterus, with care not to nick the bladder. The uterus was incised through the lower segment, 2 cm from the bladder. The fetal head was gently elevated through the incision while the assistant put gentle pressure on the fundus. The baby's mouth and nose were suctioned with a bulb syringe, and the umbilical cord was clamped and cut. The baby was handed off to an attending pediatrician and OB nurse and placed in a radiant neonate warmer bed. The Apgar score was 9/9. The placenta was gently delivered from the uterus, and the scrub nurse checked for three vessels and filled two sterile test tubes with cord blood for lab analysis. A.Y. was given an injection of Pitocin to stimulate uterine contraction. The uterus and abdomen were closed, and A.Y. was transported to the PACU (postanesthesia care unit).

Case Studies, continued

CASE STUDY QUESTIONS

Multiple choice: Select the best answer and write the letter of your choice to the left of each number.

_____ 1. M.T. is a gravida 2, para 2. This means:
   a. she has four children from two pregnancies
   b. she has had two pregnancies and two births
   c. she has had four pregnancies and two births
   d. she has had two pregnancies and two sets of twins
   e. she has one set of twins

_____ 2. An endocervical biopsy is:
   a. a tissue sample from the cul-de-sac
   b. a cone-shaped tissue sample from the uterine fundus
   c. a tissue sample from within the neck
   d. a tissue sample from the lining of the cervix
   e. a scraping of tissue cells from the vaginal wall

_____ 3. A curettage is a(n):
   a. suturing
   b. scraping
   c. cutting
   d. examination
   e. incision

_____ 4. A colposcopy is an endoscopic examination of the:
   a. vagina
   b. fundus
   c. intraperitoneal pelvic floor
   d. pouch of Douglas
   e. uterus and fallopian tubes

_____ 5. Another name for a leiomyoma is a(n):
   a. ectopic pregnancy
   b. uterine fibroid
   c. myoma
   d. a and b
   e. b and c

_____ 6. Pregnancy-induced hypertension is also called:
   a. tubal pregnancy
   b. congenital mutation
   c. ectopic pregnancy
   d. pre-eclampsia
   e. placenta previa

Case Studies, continued

_____ 7. The occiput of the fetus is the:
   a. forehead
   b. foot
   c. back of the head
   d. chin
   e. shoulder

_____ 8. Pitocin is the trade name for:
   a. progesterone
   b. estrogen
   c. chorionic gonadotropin
   d. FSH
   e. oxytocin

Write a term from the case studies with each of the following meanings:

9. displaced   _____

10. cell produced by fertilization   _____

11. measurement of the pelvis   _____

12. upper rounded portion of the uterus   _____

13. method for rating a newborn's physical condition _____

14. afterbirth   _____

Define each of the following abbreviations:

15. D&C _____

16. BSO _____

17. PID _____

18. HRT _____

19. IVF _____

20. CPD _____

21. OB _____

22. GYN _____

23. GU _____

Chapter 15 Crossword
Female Reproductive System; Pregnancy and Birth

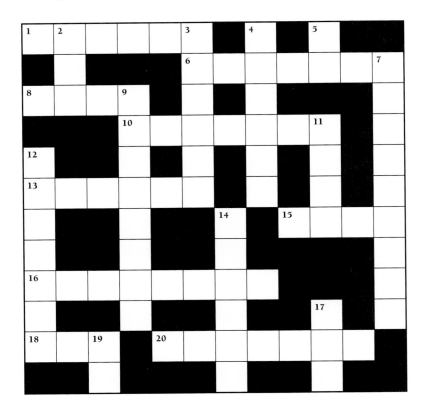

ACROSS

1. Neck of the uterus: root
6. Fallopian tube
8. Vagina: root
10. Outside the normal position
13. Tube between the uterus and the external genitalia
15. Developing infant in the uterus from the third month of gestation: combining form
16. Premature separation of the placenta: _____ placentae
18. In, within: prefix
20. The outermost layer of the embryo; forms the inner portion of the placenta

DOWN

2. Outside, away from: prefix
3. Against: prefix
4. Removal of tissue for laboratory study
5. The reproductive and urinary systems together: abbreviation
7. Substance or agent that causes birth abnormalities
9. The region between the thighs, including the genitalia
11. Hernia, localized dilation; suffix
12. To release an ovum from the ovary
14. Erectile tissue in the female: root
17. Labor: root
19. Down, without, removal: prefix

CHAPTER 15 Answer Section

Answers to Chapter Exercises

EXERCISE 15-1

1. any disease that affects women
2. between menstrual periods
3. formation of an ovum
4. pertaining to ovulation
5. rupture of an ovary
6. inflammation of an ovary
7. gynecologist (gī-ne-KOL-ō-jist)
8. anovulatory (an-OV-ū-la-tō-rē)
9. menorrhagia (men-ō-RĀ-jē-a)
10. amenorrhea (a-men-ō-RĒ-a)
11. dysmenorrhea (DIS-men-ō-rē-a)
12. oligomenorrhea (ol-i-gō-men-ō-RĒ-a)
13. ovariocele (ō-VAR-ē-ō-sēl)
14. ovariopexy (ō-var-ē-ō-PEK-sē); also oophoropexy (ō-of-ō-rō-PEK-sē)
15. ovariocentesis (ō-var-ē-ō-sen-TĒ-sis)
16. oophorectomy (ō-of-ō-REK-tō-mē)
17. oophoroma (ō-of-ō-RŌ-ma)

EXERCISE 15-2

1. plastic repair of an oviduct
2. surgical removal of the uterus
3. narrowing of the uterus
4. pertaining to the uterus and bladder
5. instrument for measuring the vagina
6. pain in the vagina
7. salpingopexy (sal-PING-gō-pek-sē)
8. salpingography (sal-ping-OG-ra-fē)
9. pyosalpinx (pi-ō-SAL-pinx)
10. hydrosalpinx (hī-drō-SAL-pinx)
11. salpingo-oophorectomy (sal-ping-gō-ō-of-ō-REK-tō-mē) also salpingo-ovariectomy (sal-ping-gō-ō-var-ē-EK-tō-me)
12. intrauterine (in-tra-Ū-ter-in)
13. hysterosalpingogram (his-ter-ō-sal-PING-gō-gram)
14. hysteropexy (his-ter-ō-PEK-sē)
15. metroptosis (mē-trō-TŌ-sis)
16. metromalacia (mē-trō-ma-LĀ-shē-a)
17. cervicitis (ser-vi-SĪ-tis)
18. intracervical (in-tra-SER-vi-kal)
19. vaginitis (vaj-i-NĪ-tis)
20. colpostenosis (kol-pō-ste-NŌ-sis)

EXERCISE 15-3

1. vulvopathy (vul-VOP-a-thē)
2. episiorrhaphy (e-piz-ē-OR-a-fē)
3. vaginoperineal (vaj-i-nō-per-i-NĒ-al)
4. clitoritis (klit-o-RĪ-tis)
5. mammogram (MAM-ō-gram)
6. mastectomy (mas-TEK-tō-mē); also mammectomy (ma-MEK-tō-mē)
7. mastitis (mas-TĪ-tis)

EXERCISE 15-4

1. study of the embryo
2. after birth
3. pertaining to the newborn
4. developing in one amniotic sac
5. measurement of the fetus
6. excess secretion of milk
7. lack of milk production
8. amniorrhexis (am-nē-ō-REK-sis)
9. amniotomy (am-nē-OT-ō-mē)
10. amniocyte (AM-nē-ō-sīt)
11. embryoscope (EM-brē-ō-skōp)
12. fetoscopy (fe-TOS-kō-pē)
13. embryopathy (em-brē-OP-a-thē)
14. neonatology (nē-ō-nā-TOL-ō-jē)
15. prenatal (prē-NĀ-tal)
16. primigravida (pri-mi-GRAV-i-da)
17. nulligravida (nul-i-GRAV-i-da)
18. multipara (mul-TIP-a-ra)
19. primipara (pri-MIP-a-ra)
20. xerotocia (zē-rō-TŌ-sē-a)
21. bradytocia (brad-ē-TŌ-sē-a)
22. galactocele (ga-LAK-to-sēl); also lactocele (LAK-tō-sēl)
23. galactorrhea (ga-lak-tō-RE-a); also lactorrhea (lak-tō-RE-a)

LABELING EXERCISE 15-1 FEMALE REPRODUCTIVE SYSTEM

1. ovary
2. oviduct (fallopian tube)
3. uterus
4. cervix
5. posterior fornix
6. vagina
7. labium majus
8. labium minus

9. clitoris
10. urinary bladder
11. urethra
12. cul-de-sac
13. rectum
14. anus

LABELING EXERCISE 15-2 FEMALE REPRODUCTIVE SYSTEM SHOWING FERTILIZATION

1. ovary
2. maturing follicle
3. ovarian follicle (ruptured)
4. corpus luteum
5. ovum
6. fimbriae
7. sperm cell
8. oviduct (fallopian tube)
9. fundus of uterus
10. implanted embryo
11. body of uterus
12. cervical canal
13. cervix
14. vagina
15. greater vestibular (Bartholin) glands

Answers to Chapter Review 15-1

1. e
2. a
3. b
4. c
5. d
6. b
7. e
8. c
9. a
10. d
11. b
12. d
13. e
14. c
15. a
16. e
17. b
18. d
19. a
20. c
21. e
22. a
23. b
24. d
25. c
26. d
27. c
28. e
29. a
30. b
31. b
32. d
33. e
34. c
35. a
36. d
37. c
38. a
39. b
40. e
41. ovary
42. ovum (egg cell)
43. endometrium
44. cervix
45. uterus
46. breasts (mammary glands)
47. embryo
48. placenta
49. lactation
50. abortion
51. abnormal uterine bleeding
52. behind the uterus
53. any disease of the uterus
54. narrowing of the vagina
55. pus in the oviduct
56. lacking ovulation
57. below the breasts
58. present at birth
59. before birth
60. outside the embryo
61. woman who has been pregnant two or more times
62. woman who had given birth three times
63. causing fetal abnormalities
64. metrostenosis
65. hysterosalpingectomy
66. episioplasty
67. mammography
68. salpingocele
69. transcervical
70. amniorrhexis
71. embryology
72. fetoscopy
73. dystocia
74. newborn
75. primipara
76. nulligravida
77. postpartum
78. prenatal
79. eutocia
80. ovulatory

81. cervical
82. uterine
83. perineal
84. vaginal
85. embryonic
86. amniotic
87. labia
88. cervices
89. fimbriae
90. ova
91. total abdominal hysterectomy
92. follicle-stimulating hormone
93. dysfunctional uterine bleeding
94. hormone replacement therapy
95. patent ductus arteriosus
96. human chorionic gonadotropin
97. gestational age
98. fetal heart rate
99. vaginal birth after cesarean section
100. excessive development of the mammary glands in the male, even to the secretion of milk
    a. woman
    b. breast
    c. condition of
101. extreme rapidity of labor
    a. sharp, acute
    b. labor
    c. condition of

102. A deficiency of amniotic fluid
    a. few, scanty
    b. fluid
    c. amnion

Answers to Case Study Questions

1. b
2. d
3. b
4. a
5. e
6. d
7. c
8. e
9. prolapsed
10. zygote
11. pelvimetry
12. fundus
13. Apgar score
14. placenta
15. dilatation and curettage
16. bilateral salpingo-oophorectomy
17. pelvic inflammatory disease
18. hormone replacement therapy
19. in vitro fertilization
20. cephalopelvic disproportion
21. obstetrics
22. gynecology
23. genitourinary

ANSWERS TO CROSSWORD PUZZLE

Female Reproductive System; Pregnancy and Birth

¹C	²E	R	V	I	³C		⁴B		⁵G		
	X			⁶O	V	I	D	U	C	⁷T	
⁸C	O	L	⁹P		N		O			E	
			¹⁰E	C	T	O	P	I	¹¹C	R	
¹²O			R		R		S		E	A	
¹³V	A	G	I	N	A		Y		L	T	
U			N			¹⁴C		¹⁵F	E	T	O
L			E			L					G
¹⁶A	B	R	U	P	T	I	O				E
T			M			T			¹⁷T		N
¹⁸E	N	¹⁹D		²⁰C	H	O	R	I	O	N	
		E				R			C		

The Endocrine System

Chapter Contents

Objectives

After study of this chapter you should be able to:

1. Define hormones.
2. Compare steroid and amino acid hormones.
3. Label a diagram of the endocrine system.
4. Name the hormones produced by the endocrine glands, and briefly describe the function of each.
5. Identify and use roots pertaining to the endocrine system.
6. Describe the main disorders of the endocrine system.
7. Interpret abbreviations used in endocrinology.
8. Analyze several case studies concerning disorders of the endocrine system.

The endocrine system consists of a widely distributed group of glands that secretes regulatory substances called **hormones**. Because these substances are released directly into the blood, the **endocrine glands** are known as the *ductless glands*. Despite the fact that hormones in the blood reach all parts of the body, only certain tissues respond. The tissue that is influenced by a specific hormone is called the **target tissue**. The cells that make up this tissue have specific **receptors** on their membranes to which the hormone attaches, enabling it to act on the cells.

Hormones

Hormones are produced in extremely small amounts and are highly potent. By means of their actions on various target tissues, they affect growth, metabolism, reproductive activity, and behavior.

Chemically, hormones fall into two categories: **steroid hormones**, made from lipids, and hormones made of amino acids, which include proteins and proteinlike compounds. Steroids are produced by the sex glands (gonads) and the outer region (cortex) of the adrenal glands. All of the remaining endocrine glands produce amino acid hormones.

The production of hormones is controlled mainly by negative feedback. That is, the hormone itself, or some product of hormone activity, acts as a control over further manufacture of the hormone—a self-regulating system. Hormone production also may be controlled by nervous stimulation or by other hormones.

The Endocrine Glands

Refer to Figure 16-1 to locate the endocrine glands described below. Display 16-1 lists the main endocrine glands and summarizes the main hormones secreted by each and their functions.

Pituitary

The **pituitary gland** (**hypophysis**) is a small gland beneath the brain. It is divided into an anterior lobe (adenohypophysis) and a posterior lobe (neurohypophysis). Both lobes are connected to and controlled by the **hypothalamus**, a part of the brain. The anterior pituitary releases six hormones. One of these is growth hormone (somatotropin), which stimulates the growth of bones and acts on other tissues as well. The remainder of the pituitary hormones regulate other glands, including the thyroid, adrenals, gonads, and mammary glands (see Display 16-1). These hormones are released in response to substances (releasing hormones) that are sent to the anterior pituitary from the hypothalamus. They can be identified by the ending *-tropin*, as in *gonadotropin*. The adjective ending is *-tropic*.

The posterior pituitary releases two hormones that are actually produced in the hypothalamus. These hormones, antidiuretic hormone and oxytocin, are stored in the posterior pituitary until nervous signals arrive from the hypothalamus to trigger their release. Antidiuretic hormone (ADH) acts on the kidneys to conserve water and also promotes constriction of blood vessels. Both of these actions serve to increase blood pressure. Oxytocin stimulates uterine contractions and promotes milk "letdown" in the breasts during lactation.

Thyroid and Parathyroids

The **thyroid gland** consists of two lobes on either side of the larynx and upper trachea (Fig. 16-2). It secretes a mixture of hormones, mainly thyroxine (T_4) and triiodothyronine (T_3). Because thyroid hormones

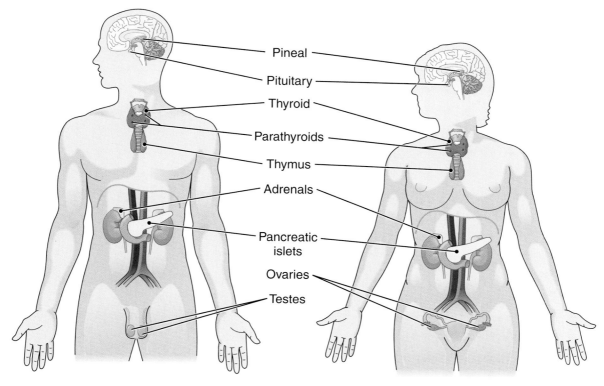

FIGURE 16-1. The endocrine glands.

contain iodine, their levels can be measured and the activity of the thyroid gland can be studied by following the uptake of iodine. Most thyroid hormone in the blood is bound to protein, mainly thyroid binding globulin (TBG).

On the posterior surface of the thyroid are four to six tiny **parathyroid glands** that affect calcium metabolism (Fig. 16-3). Parathyroid hormone increases the blood level of calcium. It works with the thyroid hormone thyrocalcitonin, which lowers blood calcium, to regulate calcium balance.

Adrenals

The **adrenal glands**, located atop each kidney, are divided into two distinct regions: an outer cortex and an inner medulla (Fig. 16-4). The hormones produced by this gland are involved in the body's response to stress. The cortex produces steroid hormones, cortisol, aldosterone, and small amounts of sex hormones. Cortisol (hydrocortisone) mobilizes reserves of fats and carbohydrates to increase the levels of these nutrients in the blood. It also acts to reduce inflammation and is used clinically for this purpose. Aldosterone acts on the kidneys to conserve sodium and water while eliminating potassium. The adrenal cortex also produces small amounts of sex hormones, mainly testosterone, but their importance is not well understood.

The medulla of the adrenal gland produces two similar hormones, epinephrine (adrenaline) and norepinephrine (noradrenaline). These are released in response to stress and work with the nervous system to help the body meet challenges.

DISPLAY 16-1 The Endocrine Glands and Their Hormones

GLAND	HORMONE	PRINCIPAL FUNCTIONS
anterior pituitary	GH (growth hormone), also called somatotropin	promotes growth of all body tissues
	TSH (thyroid-stimulating hormone)	stimulates thyroid gland to produce thyroid hormones
	ACTH (adrenocorticotropic hormone)	stimulates adrenal cortex to produce cortical hormones; aids in protecting body in stress situations (injury, pain)
	FSH (follicle-stimulating hormone)	stimulates growth and hormone activity of ovarian follicles; stimulates growth of testes; promotes development of sperm cells
	LH (luteinizing hormone); ICSH (interstitial cell-stimulating hormone)	causes development of corpus luteum at site of ruptured ovarian follicle in female; stimulates secretion of testosterone in male
	PRL (prolactin)	stimulates secretion of milk by mammary glands
posterior pituitary	ADH (antidiuretic hormone; vasopressin)	promotes reabsorption of water in kidney tubules; stimulates smooth muscle tissue of blood vessels to constrict
	oxytocin	causes contraction of uterus; causes ejection of milk from mammary glands
thyroid	thyroid hormone: thyroxine or tetraiodothyronine (T_4) and triiodothyronine (T_3)	increases metabolic rate and production of body heat, influencing both physical and mental activities; required for normal growth
	calcitonin	decreases calcium level in blood
parathyroids	parathyroid hormone	regulates exchange of calcium between blood and bones; increases calcium level in blood
adrenal medulla	epinephrine (adrenaline) and norepinephrine (noradrenaline)	active in response to stress; increases respiration, blood pressure, and heart rate
adrenal cortex	cortisol (hydrocortisone)	aids in metabolism of carbohydrates, proteins, and fats; active during stress
	aldosterone	aids in regulating electrolytes and water balance
	sex hormones	may influence secondary sexual characteristics
pancreatic islets	insulin	aids transport of glucose into cells; required for cellular metabolism of foods, especially glucose; decreases blood sugar levels
	glucagon	stimulates liver to release glucose, thereby increasing blood sugar levels
testes	testosterone	stimulates growth and development of sexual organs plus development of secondary sexual characteristics; stimulates maturation of sperm cells
ovaries	estrogens	stimulate growth of primary sexual organs and development of secondary sexual characteristics
	progesterone	stimulates development of secretory parts of mammary glands; prepares uterine lining for implantation of fertilized ovum; aids in maintaining pregnancy
thymus	thymosin	important in development of T cells needed for immunity and in early development of lymphoid tissue

BOX 16-1 Are You In a Good Humor?

In ancient times, people accepted the theory that a person's state of health depended on the balance of four body fluids. These fluids, called "humors," were yellow bile, black bile, phlegm, and blood. A predominance of any one of these humors would determine a person's mood or temperament. Yellow bile caused anger; black bile caused depression; phlegm (mucus) made a person sluggish; blood resulted in cheerfulness and optimism.

Although we no longer believe in humoralism, we still have adjectives in our vocabulary that reflect these early beliefs. Choleric describes a person under the influence of yellow bile; melancholic describes the effects of black bile (melano- means black or dark); a phlegmatic person is slow to respond; a sanguine individual "goes with the flow."

The humors persist today in the adjective "humoral," which describes substances carried in the blood or other body fluids. The term is applied to hormones and other circulating materials that influence body responses. Humoral immunity is immunity based on antibodies carried in the bloodstream.

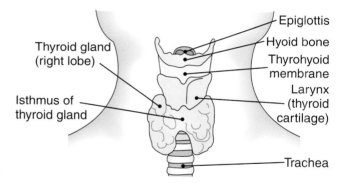

FIGURE 16-2. Thyroid gland (anterior view) in relation to the larynx and trachea. (Reprinted with permission from Cohen BJ, Wood DL. Memmler's The Human Body in Health and Disease. 9th Ed. Philadelphia: Lippincott Williams & Wilkins, 2000.)

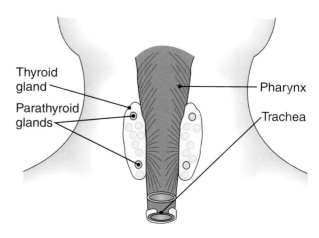

FIGURE 16-3. Posterior view of the thyroid gland showing the parathyroid glands embedded in its surface. (Reprinted with permission from Cohen BJ, Wood DL. Memmler's The Human Body in Health and Disease. 9th Ed. Philadelphia: Lippincott Williams & Wilkins, 2000.)

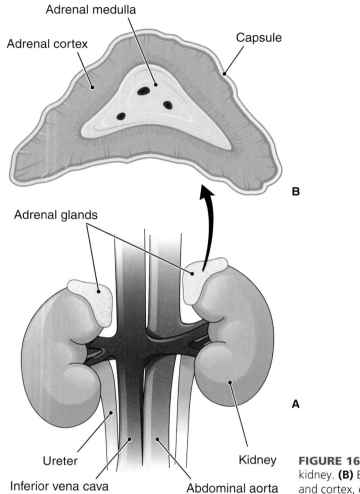

FIGURE 16-4. (A) The adrenal glands on top of each kidney. **(B)** Each adrenal gland is divided into a medulla and cortex, each secreting different hormones.

Pancreas

The endocrine portions of the pancreas are the **pancreatic islets**, small clusters of cells within the pancreatic tissue. The term *islet*, meaning "small island," is used because these cells look like little islands in the midst of the many pancreatic cells that secrete digestive juices (Fig. 16-5). The islet cells produce two hormones, insulin and glucagon, that regulate sugar metabolism. Insulin increases cellular use of glucose, thus decreasing sugar levels in the blood. Glucagon has the opposite effect of increasing blood sugar levels.

Other Endocrine Tissues

The thymus, described in Chapter 9, is considered an endocrine gland because it secretes a hormone, thymosin, which stimulates the T lymphocytes of the immune system. The gonads (Chapters 14 and 15) are also included because, in addition to producing the sex cells, they secrete hormones. Other organs, including the

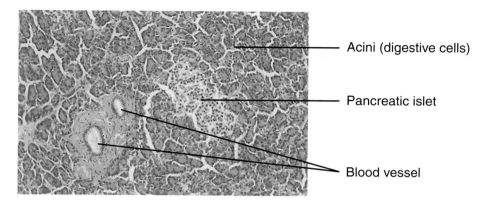

Acini (digestive cells)

Pancreatic islet

Blood vessel

FIGURE 16-5. Microscopic view of pancreatic cells. Light staining islet cells are seen among the cell clusters that produce digestive juices. (Reprinted with permission from Cohen BJ, Wood DL. Memmler's The Human Body in Health and Disease. 9th Ed. Philadelphia: Lippincott Williams & Wilkins, 2000.)

stomach, kidney, heart, and small intestine, also produce hormones. However, they have other major functions and are discussed with the systems to which they belong.

Finally, **prostaglandins** are a group of hormones produced by many cells. They have a variety of effects, including stimulation of uterine contractions, promotion of the inflammatory response, and vasomotor activities. They are called prostaglandins because they were first discovered in the prostate gland.

Key Terms

NORMAL STRUCTURE AND FUNCTION

adrenal gland a-DRĒ-nal	A gland on the upper surface of the kidney. The outer region (cortex) secretes steroid hormones; the inner region (medulla) secretes epinephrine (adrenaline) and norepinephrine (noradrenaline) (root *adren/o*)
endocrine EN-dō-krin	Pertaining to a ductless gland that secretes directly into the blood
hormone HOR-mōn	A secretion of an endocrine gland. A substance that travels in the blood and has a regulatory effect on tissues, organs, or glands.
hypophysis hī-POF-i-sis	The pituitary gland (root *hypophys*); named from *hypo* meaning "below" and *physis* meaning "growing" because the gland grows below the hypothalamus
hypothalamus hī-pō-THAL-a-mus	A portion of the brain that controls the pituitary gland and is active in maintaining homeostasis
pancreatic islets Ī-lets	Clusters of endocrine cells in the pancreas that secrete hormones that regulate sugar metabolism; also called islets of Langerhans or islet cells (root *insul/o*, meaning "island")
parathyroid glands par-a-THĪ-royd	Small glands on the back of the thyroid that act to increase blood calcium levels; there are usually four to six parathyroid glands (root *parathyr/o, parathyroid/o*); the name literally means "near the thyroid"

Normal Structure and Function, continued

pituitary gland *pi-TŪ-i-tar-ē*	A small endocrine gland at the base of the brain. The anterior lobe secretes growth hormone and hormones that stimulate other glands; the posterior lobe releases ADH and oxytocin manufactured in the hypothalamus.
prostaglandins *pros-ta-GLAN-dinz*	A group of hormones produced throughout the body that have a variety of effects, including stimulation of uterine contractions and regulation of blood pressure, blood clotting, and inflammation
receptor	A site on the cell membrane to which a substance, such as a hormone, attaches
steroid hormone *STER-oyd*	A hormone made from lipids and including the sex hormones and the hormones of the adrenal cortex
target tissue	The specific tissue on which a hormone acts; may also be referred to as the target organ
thyroid gland *THĪ-royd*	An endocrine gland on either side of the larynx and upper trachea. It secretes hormones that affect metabolism and growth and a hormone that regulates calcium balance (root *thyr/o, thyroid/o*).

Roots Pertaining to the Endocrine System

TABLE 16-1 Roots Pertaining to the Endocrine System

ROOT	MEANING	EXAMPLE	DEFINITION OF EXAMPLE
endocrin/o	endocrine glands or system	endocrinopathy *en-dō-kri-NOP-a-thē*	any disease of the endocrine glands
pituitar	pituitary gland, hypophysis	pituitarism *pi-TŪ-i-ta-rizm*	condition caused by any disorder of pituitary function
hypophys	pituitary gland, hypophysis	hypophyseal* *hī-pō-FIZ-ē-al*	pertaining to the pituitary gland
thyr/o, thyroid/o	thyroid gland	thyrotropic *thī-rō-TROP-ik*	acting on the thyroid gland
parathyr/o, parathyroid/o	parathyroid gland	parathyroidectomy *par-a-thī-royd-EK-tō-mē*	excision of a parathyroid gland
adren/o, adrenal/o	adrenal gland, epinephrine	adrenergic *ad-ren-ER-jik*	activated (erg-) by or related to epinephrine (adrenaline)
adrenocortic/o	adrenal cortex	adrenocortical *ad-rē-nō-KOR-ti-kal*	pertaining to the adrenal cortex
insul/o	pancreatic islets	insuloma *(in-sū-LŌ-ma)*	tumor of islet cells

*Note spelling.

Exercise 16-1

Define each of the following words:

1. endocrinology (*en-dō-krin-OL-ō-jē*)   _____

2. hypophysectomy (*hī-pof-i-SEK-tō-mē*)   _____

3. thyrolytic (*thī-ro-LIT-ik*)   _____

4. hyperadrenalism (*hī-per-a-drē-nal-izm*)   _____

5. insulitis (*in-sū-LĪ-tis*)   _____

Words for conditions resulting from endocrine dysfunctions are formed by adding the suffix *-ism* to the name of the gland or its root and adding the prefix *hyper-* or *hypo-* for overactivity or underactivity of the gland. Use the full name of the gland to form words with each of the following definitions:

6. condition of overactivity of the thyroid gland   _____

7. condition of underactivity of the parathyroid gland   _____

8. condition of underactivity of the adrenal gland   _____

Use the word root for the gland to form a word for each of the following definitions:

9. condition of underactivity of the adrenal cortex   _____

10. condition of overactivity of the pituitary gland (use pituitar)   _____

Word building. Write a word for each of the following definitions:

11. physician who specializes in study of the endocrine system   _____

12. incision into the thyroid gland   _____

13. any disease of the adrenal gland   _____

14. inflammation of the adrenal gland   _____

15. pertaining to (-ar) the pancreatic islets   _____

Clinical Aspects of the Endocrine System

Endocrine diseases usually result from the overproduction (hypersecretion) or underproduction (hyposecretion) of hormones. They also may result from secretion at the wrong time or from failure of the target tissue to respond. The causes of abnormal secretion may originate in the gland itself or may result from failure of the hypothalamus or the pituitary to release the proper amount of hormone stimulators. Some of the common endocrine disorders are described below. Conditions resulting from hypersecretion or hyposecretion of hormones are summarized in Display 16-2.

Pituitary

A pituitary **adenoma** (tumor) usually increases secretion of growth hormone or ACTH. Less commonly, a tumor affects the secretion of prolactin. An excess of growth hormone in children causes **gigantism**. In

DISPLAY 16-2 Disorders Associated With Endocrine Dysfunction*

HORMONE	HYPERSECRETION	HYPOSECRETION
growth hormone	gigantism (children), acromegaly (adults)	dwarfism (children)
antidiuretic hormone	syndrome of inappropriate ADH (SIADH)	diabetes insipidus
aldosterone	aldosteronism	Addison disease
cortisol	Cushing syndrome	Addison disease
thyroid hormone	Graves disease, thyrotoxicosis	congenital hypothyroidism (children), myxedema (adults)
insulin	hypoglycemia	diabetes mellitus
parathyroid hormone	bone degeneration	tetany (muscle spasms)

*Refer to key terms for pronunciations and descriptions.

adults it causes **acromegaly**, characterized by enlargement of the hands, feet, jaw, and facial features. Treatment is by surgery to remove the tumor (adenomectomy) or by drugs to reduce the level of growth hormone in the blood. Excess ACTH overstimulates the adrenal cortex, resulting in **Cushing disease**. Increased prolactin causes milk secretion, or galactorrhea, in both males and females. Radiographic studies in cases of pituitary adenoma usually show enlargement of the bony structure in the skull (sella turcica) that contains the pituitary.

Hypofunction of the pituitary, such as is caused by tumor or interruption of blood supply to the gland, may involve a single hormone but usually affects all functions and is referred to as **panhypopituitarism**. The widespread effects of this condition include dwarfism (from lack of growth hormone), lack of sexual development and sexual function, fatigue, and weakness.

A specific lack of ADH from the posterior pituitary results in **diabetes insipidus**, in which the kidneys have a decreased ability to conserve water. Symptoms are polyuria (elimination of large amounts of urine) and polydipsia (excessive thirst). Diabetes insipidus should not be confused with diabetes mellitus, a disorder of glucose metabolism described below. The two diseases share the symptoms of polyuria and polydipsia but have entirely different causes. Diabetes mellitus is the more common disorder, and when the term diabetes is used alone, it generally refers to diabetes mellitus. The word diabetes is from the Greek meaning "siphon," referring to the large urinary output in both forms of diabetes.

Thyroid

Because thyroid hormone affects the growth and function of many tissues, a deficiency of this hormone in infancy causes physical and mental retardation as well as other symptoms that together constitute **congenital hypothyroidism**, formerly called cretinism. In the adult, thyroid deficiency causes **myxedema**, in which there is weight gain, lethargy, rough, dry skin, and facial swelling. Both of these conditions are easily treated with thyroid hormone. Most U.S. states now require testing of newborns for hypothyroidism. If not diagnosed at birth, hypothyroidism will lead to mental retardation within 6 months.

The most common form of hyperthyroidism is **Graves disease**, also called diffuse toxic goiter. This is an autoimmune disorder in which antibodies stimulate an increased production of thyroid hormone. There is weight loss, irritability, hand tremor, and rapid heart rate (tachycardia). A most distinctive sign is a bulging of the eyeballs, termed **exophthalmos**, caused by swelling of the tissues behind the eyes (Fig. 16-6). Treatment for Graves disease may include antithyroid drugs, surgical removal of all or part of the thyroid, or radiation delivered in the form of radioactive iodine.

A common sign in thyroid disease is an enlarged thyroid, or **goiter**. However, a goiter is not necessarily accompanied by malfunction of the thyroid. A simple or nontoxic goiter is caused by a deficiency of iodine

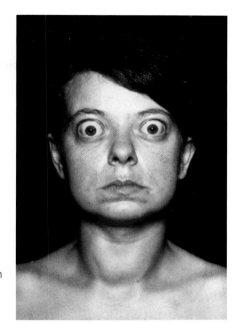

FIGURE 16-6. Graves disease. A young woman with hyperthyroidism presented with a mass in the neck and exophthalmos. (Reprinted with permission from Rubin E, Farber JL. Pathology. 3rd Ed. Philadelphia: Lippincott Williams & Wilkins, 1999.)

in the diet. With the addition of iodine to salt and other commercial foods, this form of goiter has become a thing of the past.

Thyroid function is commonly tested by measuring radioactive iodine uptake (RAIU) by the gland. Blood levels of total and free thyroxine (T_4) and triiodothyronine (T_3) are also measured, as are the levels of thyroxine-binding globulin (TBG) and thyroid-stimulating hormone (TSH) from the pituitary. Thyroid scans after the administration of radioactive iodine are also used to study the activity of this gland.

Parathyroids

Overactivity of the parathyroid glands, usually from a tumor, causes a high level of calcium in the blood. Because this calcium is obtained from the bones, there is also degeneration of the skeleton and bone pain. A common side effect is the development of kidney stones from the high levels of circulating calcium.

Damage to the parathyroids or their surgical removal, as during thyroid surgery, results in a decrease in blood calcium levels. This causes numbness and tingling in the arms and legs and around the mouth (perioral), as well as **tetany** (muscle spasms). Treatment consists of supplying calcium.

Adrenals

Hypofunction of the adrenal cortex, or **Addison disease**, is usually caused by autoimmune destruction of the gland. It may also result from a deficiency of ACTH from the pituitary. The lack of aldosterone results in water loss, low blood pressure, and electrolyte imbalance. There is also weakness, nausea, and increase of brown pigmentation. This last symptom is caused by release of a hormone from the pituitary that stimulates the pigment cells (melanocytes) in the skin. Once diagnosed, Addison disease is treated with replacement cortical hormones.

An excess of adrenal cortical hormones results in **Cushing syndrome**. Patients have a moon-shaped face, obesity localized in the torso, weakness, excess hair growth (hirsutism), and fluid retention (Fig. 16-7). The

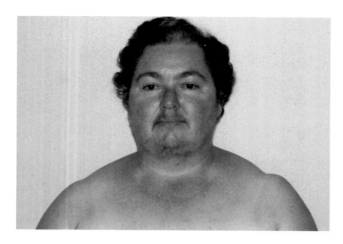

FIGURE 16-7. Cushing syndrome. The woman has a moon face, buffalo hump, increased facial hair, and thinning of the scalp hair. (Reprinted with permission from Rubin E, Farber JL. Pathology. 3rd Ed. Philadelphia: Lippincott Williams & Wilkins, 1999.)

most common cause of Cushing syndrome is the therapeutic administration of steroid hormones. It also may be caused by a tumor. If the disorder is caused by a pituitary tumor that increases production of ACTH, it is referred to as Cushing disease.

The Pancreas and Diabetes

The most common endocrine disorder, and a serious public health problem, is **diabetes mellitus**, a failure of the body cells to use glucose effectively. The excess glucose accumulates in the blood, causing **hyperglycemia**. Increased urination (polyuria) marks the effort to eliminate the excess glucose in the urine, a condition termed **glycosuria**. The result is dehydration and excessive thirst (polydipsia). There is also weakness, weight loss, and extreme hunger (polyphagia). Unable to use carbohydrates, the body burns more fat. This leads to accumulation of ketone bodies in the blood and a shift toward acidosis, a condition termed **ketoacidosis**. If untreated, diabetes will lead to starvation of the central nervous system and coma. Diabetic patients are prone to cardiovascular, neurologic, and vision problems, infections, and, sometimes, renal failure.

There are two types of diabetes mellitus. Heredity seems to be a factor in the appearance of both. Type 1, also called juvenile-onset or insulin-dependent diabetes mellitus (IDDM), usually appears in children and teenagers. It is caused by a failure of the pancreatic islets to produce insulin, resulting, perhaps, from autoimmune destruction of the cells. Because insulin levels are very low or absent, patients need careful monitoring and administration of this hormone. Blood sugar level may be tested multiple times during the day, and insulin may be given in divided doses by injection or by means of an insulin pump that delivers the hormone around the clock (continuous subcutaneous insulin infusion; CSII). Diet must be carefully regulated to keep glucose levels steady. Insulin is obtained from animals and is now also made by genetic engineering.

Type 2 diabetes mellitus, also called adult-onset or non–insulin-dependent diabetes mellitus (NIDDM), accounts for about 90% of diabetes cases. Type 2 diabetes is initiated by cellular resistance to insulin. Feedback stimulation of the pancreatic islets leads to overproduction of insulin and then to reduced insulin production by the overworked cells. **Metabolic syndrome** (also called syndrome X or insulin resistance syndrome) is the term now used to describe a state of hyperglycemia caused by insulin resistance in association with some metabolic disorders, including high levels of plasma triglycerides (fats), low levels of high-density lipoproteins (HDLs), hypertension, and coronary heart disease.

Most cases of type 2 diabetes are linked to obesity, especially upper body obesity. Although seen mostly in older people (hence the name adult-onset diabetes), the incidence of type 2 diabetes is increasing among younger generations, presumably because of increased obesity, poor diet, and sedentary habits. Exercise and weight loss for the overweight are the first approaches to treating type 2 diabetes, and these measures often lead to management of the disorder. Drugs for increasing insulin production or improving cellular responses to insulin may also be prescribed, with insulin treatment given if necessary.

Gestational diabetes mellitus (GDM) refers to glucose intolerance during pregnancy. This imbalance usually appears in women with a family history of diabetes. Women must be monitored during pregnancy for signs of diabetes mellitus, especially those with predisposing factors, because this condition can cause complications for both the mother and the fetus. Again, ensuring a proper diet is a first step to management, with insulin treatment recommended if needed.

Diabetes is diagnosed by measuring levels of glucose in blood plasma with or without fasting and by monitoring glucose levels in the blood after oral administration of glucose (oral glucose tolerance test; OGTT). Categories of impaired fasting blood glucose (IFG) and impaired glucose tolerance (IGT) are stages between a normal response to glucose and diabetes.

Excess insulin may result from a pancreatic tumor, but more often it occurs after administration of too much hormone to a diabetic patient. The resultant **hypoglycemia** leads to **insulin shock**, which is treated by administration of glucose.

Key Clinical Terms

acromegaly *ak-rō-MEG-a-lē*	Overgrowth of bone and soft tissue, especially in the hands, feet, and face, caused by an excess of growth hormone in an adult. The name comes from *acro* meaning "extremity" and *megal/o* meaning "enlargement."
Addison disease	A disease resulting from deficiency of adrenocortical hormones. It is marked by darkening of the skin, weakness, and alterations in salt and water balance.
adenoma *ad-e-NŌ-ma*	A neoplasm of a gland
congenital hypothyroidism	A condition caused by congenital lack of thyroid secretion and marked by arrested physical and mental development; formerly called cretinism (*KRĒ-tin-izm*)
Cushing disease	Overactivity of the adrenal cortex resulting from excess production of ACTH by the pituitary
Cushing syndrome	A condition resulting from an excess of hormones from the adrenal cortex. It is associated with obesity, weakness, hyperglycemia, hypertension, and hirsutism (excess hair growth).
diabetes insipidus *dī -a-BĒ-tēz in-SIP-i-dus*	A disorder caused by insufficient release of ADH from the posterior pituitary. It results in excessive thirst and production of large amounts of very dilute urine. The word *insipidus* means "tasteless," referring to the dilution of the urine.

diabetes mellitus *MEL-i-tus*	A disorder of glucose metabolism caused by deficiency of insulin production or failure of the tissues to respond to insulin. Type 1 is juvenile-onset or insulin-dependent diabetes mellitus (IDDM); type 2 is adult-onset or non–insulin-dependent diabetes mellitus (NIDDM). The word *mellitus* comes from the Latin root for honey, referring to the sugar content of the urine.
exophthalmos *ek-sof-THAL-mos*	Protrusion of the eyeballs as seen in Graves disease
gigantism *JĪ-gan-tizm*	Overgrowth caused by an excess of growth hormone from the pituitary during childhood; also called giantism
glycosuria *glī-kō-SŪ-rē-a*	Excess sugar in the urine
goiter *GOY-ter*	Enlargement of the thyroid gland. May be toxic or nontoxic. Simple (nontoxic) goiter is caused by iodine deficiency.
Graves disease	An autoimmune disease resulting in hyperthyroidism. A prominent symptom is exophthalmos (protrusion of the eyeballs). Also called exophthalmic goiter.
hyperglycemia *hī-per-glī-SĒ-mē-a*	Excess glucose in the blood
hypoglycemia *HĪ-pō-glī-SĒ-mē-a*	Abnormally low level of glucose in the blood
insulin shock	A condition resulting from an overdose of insulin, causing hypoglycemia
ketoacidosis *kē-tō-as-i-DŌ-sis*	Acidosis (increased acidity of body fluids) caused by an excess of ketone bodies, as in diabetes mellitus; diabetic acidosis
metabolic syndrome	A state of hyperglycemia caused by cellular resistance to insulin, as seen in type 2 diabetes, in association with other metabolic disorders; syndrome X or insulin resistance syndrome
myxedema *miks-e-DĒ-ma*	A condition caused by hypothyroidism in an adult. There is dry, waxy swelling most notable in the face.
panhypopituitarism *pan-hī-pō-pi-TŪ-i-ta-rism*	Underactivity of the entire pituitary gland
tetany *TET-a-nē*	Irritability and spasms of muscles; may be caused by low blood calcium and other factors

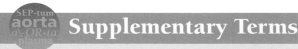

Supplementary Terms

NORMAL STRUCTURE AND FUNCTION

pineal gland *PIN-ē-al*	A small gland in the brain (see Fig. 16-1). Its function in humans is not clear, but it seems to regulate behavior and sexual development in response to environmental light.
sella turcica *SEL-a TUR-si-ka*	A saddle-shaped depression in the sphenoid bone that contains the pituitary gland (literally means "Turkish saddle")
sphenoid bone *SFĒ-noyd*	A bone at the base of the skull that houses the pituitary gland

SYMPTOMS AND CONDITIONS

adrenogenital syndrome *ad-rē-nō-JEN-i-tal*	Condition caused by overproduction of androgens from the adrenal cortex resulting in masculinization; may be congenital or acquired, usually as a result of an adrenal tumor
Conn syndrome	Hyperaldosteronism caused by an adrenal tumor
craniopharyngioma *krā-nē-ō-far-in-jē-Ō-ma*	A tumor of the pituitary gland
Hashimoto disease	A chronic thyroiditis of autoimmune origin
ketosis *kē-TŌ-sis*	Accumulation of ketone bodies, such as acetone, in the body. Usually results from deficiency or faulty metabolism of carbohydrates, as in cases of diabetes mellitus and starvation.
multiple endocrine neoplasia (MEN)	A hereditary disorder that causes tumors in several endocrine glands; classified according to the combination of glands involved
pheochromocytoma *fē-ō-krō-mō-sī-TŌ-ma*	A usually benign tumor of the adrenal medulla or other structures containing chromaffin cells (cells that stain with chromium salts). The tumor causes increased production of epinephrine and norepinephrine.
pituitary apoplexy *AP-ō-plek-sē*	Sudden massive hemorrhage and degeneration of the pituitary gland associated with a pituitary tumor. Common symptoms include severe headache, visual problems, and loss of consciousness.
Simmonds disease	Hypofunction of the anterior pituitary (panhypopituitarism), usually because of an infarction; pituitary cachexia
thyroid storm	A sudden onset of the symptoms of thyrotoxicosis occurring in patients with hyperthyroidism who are untreated or poorly treated. May be brought on by illness or trauma. Also called thyroid crisis.
thyrotoxicosis *thī-rō-tok-si-KŌ-sis*	Condition resulting from overactivity of the thyroid gland. Symptoms include anxiety, irritability, weight loss, and sweating. The main example of thyrotoxicosis is Graves disease.
von Recklinghausen disease	Degeneration of bone caused by excess production of hormone from the parathyroid glands. Also called Recklinghausen disease of bone.

DIAGNOSIS AND TREATMENT

fasting plasma glucose (FPG)	Measurement of glucose in the blood after a fast of at least 8 hours. A reading equal to or greater than 126 mg/dL indicates diabetes. Also called fasting blood glucose (FBG) or fasting blood sugar (FBS).
free thyroxine index (FTI, T_7)	Calculation based on the amount of T_4 present and T_3 uptake that is used to diagnose thyroid dysfunction
glycosylated hemoglobin (HbA_{1c}) test *glī-KŌ-si-lā-ted*	A test that measures the binding of glucose to hemoglobin during the lifespan of a red blood cell. It reflects the average blood glucose level over 2 to 3 months and is useful in evaluating long-term therapy for diabetes mellitus. Also called glycohemoglobin test.
oral glucose tolerance test (OGTT)	Measurement of glucose levels in blood plasma after administration of a challenge dose of glucose to a fasting patient. Used to measure patient's ability to metabolize glucose. A value equal to or greater than 200 mg/dL in the 2-hour sample indicates diabetes.
radioactive iodine uptake test (RAIU)	A test that measures thyroid uptake of radioactive iodine as an evaluation of thyroid function
radioimmunoassay (RIA)	A method of measuring very small amounts of a substance, especially hormones, in blood plasma using radioactively labeled hormones and specific antibodies
thyroid scan	Visualization of the thyroid gland after administration of radioactive iodine
thyroxine-binding globulin (TBG) test	Test that measures the main protein that binds T_4 in the blood
transsphenoidal adenomectomy *trans-sfē-NOY-dal* *ad-e-nō-MEK-tō-mē*	Removal of a pituitary tumor through the sphenoid sinus (space in the sphenoid bone).

Also used to diagnose endocrine disorders are imaging techniques, other measurements of hormones or their metabolites in plasma and urine, and studies involving hormone stimulation or suppression.

ABBREVIATIONS

ACTH	Adrenocorticotropic hormone	**IFG**	Impaired fasting blood glucose
ADH	Antidiuretic hormone	**IGT**	Impaired glucose tolerance
BS	Blood sugar	**MEN**	Multiple endocrine neoplasia
CSII	Continuous subcutaneous insulin infusion	**NIDDM**	Non–insulin-dependent diabetes mellitus
		NPH	Neutral protamine Hagedorn (insulin)
DM	Diabetes mellitus	**OGTT**	Oral glucose tolerance test
FBG	Fasting blood glucose	**RAIU**	Radioactive iodine uptake
FBS	Fasting blood sugar	**RIA**	Radioimmunoassay
FPG	Fasting plasma glucose	**SIADH**	Syndrome of inappropriate antidiuretic hormone (secretion)
FTI	Free thyroxine index		
GDM	Gestational diabetes mellitus	T_3	Triiodothyronine
GH	Growth hormone	T_4	Thyroxine; tetraiodothyronine
HbA$_{1c}$	Hemoglobin A_{1c}; glycohemoglobin; glycosylated hemoglobin	T_7	Free thyroxine index
		TBG	Thyroxine-binding globulin
^{131}I	Iodine 131 (radioactive iodine)	**TSH**	Thyroid-stimulating hormone
IDDM	Insulin-dependent diabetes mellitus		

Labeling Exercise 16-1

Glands of the Endocrine System

Write the name of each numbered part on the corresponding line of the answer sheet.

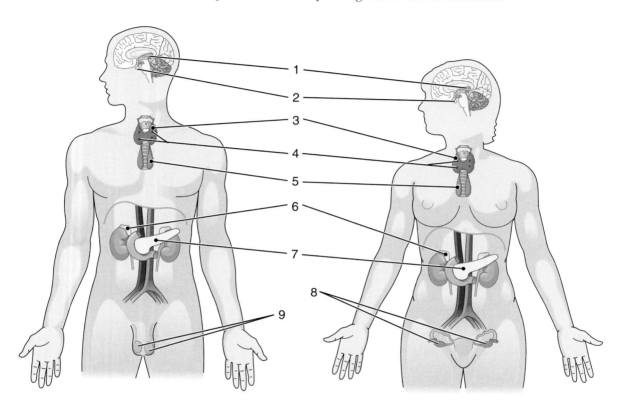

Adrenals	Parathyroids	Testes
Ovaries	Pineal	Thymus
Pancreatic islets	Pituitary (hypophysis)	Thyroid

1. _____   6. _____

2. _____   7. _____

3. _____   8. _____

4. _____   9. _____

5. _____

Chapter Review 16-1

Match the following terms and write the appropriate letter to the left of each number:

_____ 1. hypothalamus

_____ 2. cortex

_____ 3. islets

_____ 4. hypophysis

_____ 5. calcium

a. outer region of an organ

b. substance regulated by the parathyroids

c. part of the brain that controls the pituitary

d. pancreatic endocrine cells

e. pituitary

_____ 6. iodine

_____ 7. oxytocin

_____ 8. hydrocortisone

_____ 9. glucagon

_____ 10. epinephrine

a. pancreatic hormone that regulates sugar metabolism

b. hormone produced by the adrenal medulla

c. hormone that produces uterine contractions

d. ingredient in thyroid hormone

e. hormone produced by the adrenal cortex

_____ 11. OGTT

_____ 12. NPH

_____ 13. ACTH

_____ 14. ADH

_____ 15. NIDDM

a. form of diabetes mellitus

b. test of sugar metabolism

c. hormone that increases water reabsorption in the kidneys

d. a form of insulin

e. hormone that stimulates the adrenal cortex

_____ 16. Graves disease

_____ 17. myxedema

_____ 18. Cushing syndrome

_____ 19. goiter

_____ 20. Addison disease

a. enlargement of the thyroid

b. disorder caused by underactivity of the adrenal cortex

c. condition caused by hyperthyroidism

d. disorder caused by overactivity of the adrenal cortex

e. disorder caused by lack of thyroid hormone in adults

SUPPLEMENTARY TERMS

_____ 21. glycosylated hemoglobin

_____ 22. Hashimoto disease

_____ 23. pheochromocytoma

_____ 24. pineal

_____ 25. craniopharyngioma

a. tumor of the pituitary gland

b. small gland in the brain that is regulated by light

c. chronic thyroiditis

d. substance used in testing for diabetes

e. tumor of the adrenal medulla

Fill in the blanks:

26. The gland under the brain that controls other glands is the _____.

27. The gland in the neck that affects metabolic rate is the _____.

28. The endocrine glands located above the kidneys are the _____.

29. The hormone insulin is so named because it is produced by the _____.

30. The most common endocrine disorder is _____.

31. Excess sugar in the blood is called _____.

Define each of the following words:

32. hypophysitis ($h\bar{i}$-po-fi $S\bar{I}$-tis)   _____

33. hypopituitarism ($h\bar{i}$-$p\bar{o}$-pi-$T\bar{U}$-i-ta-rizm)   _____

34. adrenalectomy (ad-$r\bar{e}$-nal-EK-$t\bar{o}$-$m\bar{e}$)   _____

35. hyperthyroidism ($h\bar{i}$-per-$TH\bar{I}$-royd-ism)   _____

36. endocrinologist (en-$d\bar{o}$-kri-NOL-$\bar{o}$-jist)   _____

37. adrenocortical (ad-$r\bar{e}$-$n\bar{o}$-KOR-ti-kal)   _____

Word building. Write a word for each of the following definitions:

38. pertaining to the hypophysis   _____

39. inflammation of the pancreatic islets   _____

40. enlargement of the adrenal gland   _____

Use the full name of the gland as the root to write a word for each of the following definitions:

41. removal of one half (hemi-) of the thyroid gland   _____

42. inflammation of the thyroid gland   _____

43. surgical removal of parathyroid gland   _____

44. condition caused by underactivity of the adrenal gland   _____

Use the root *thyr/o* to write a word for each of the following definitions:

45. acting on the thyroid gland   _____

46. destructive of (-lytic) thyroid tissue   _____

47. any disease of the thyroid gland   _____

Word analysis. Define each of the following words, and give the meaning of the word parts in each. Use a dictionary if necessary.

48. euthyroidism _____
    a. eu-   _____
    b. thyroid _____
    c. -ism   _____

49. adrenocorticotropic _____
    a. adren/o _____
    b. cortic/o _____
    c. -tropic _____

50. panhypopituitarism _____
    a. pan- _____
    b. hypo- _____
    c. pituitar _____
    d. -ism _____

51. thyrotoxicosis _____
    a. thyr/o _____
    b. toxic/o _____
    c. -sis _____

Case Studies

Case Study 16-1: Acute Pancreatitis

Two weeks after his emergency cardiac bypass surgery, R.B. was admitted to the hospital with acute pancreatitis, probably triggered by the trauma of the heart surgery. As a nurse, R.B. knew that the mild form of the disease was self-limiting, whereas severe pancreatitis has a mortality rate near 50%. He was terrified, having survived heart surgery, to now have to worry about multisystem organ failure. He had once cared for a patient who died of necrotizing hemorrhagic pancreatitis.

On admission, R.B. had severe stabbing midepigastric pain that radiated to his back, nausea, vomiting, abdominal distention and rigidity, and jaundice. He also manifested a low-grade fever, hypotension, tachycardia, and decreased breath sounds over all lung fields. His cardiac enzymes were normal, but he showed an increase in serum leukocytes, amylase, and lipase. CT scan of the abdomen showed pancreatic inflammation with edema. His chest radiograph showed bilateral pleural effusion and atelectasis.

R.B.'s treatments included NPO, an NG tube, medications to decrease his pain and gastric secretions, and supplemental oxygen. He was monitored for all physiologic parameters, with close attention paid to his fluid and electrolyte balance and intravascular volume, and recovered and was discharged after 6 days.

Case Study 16-2: Hyperparathyroidism

B. E., a 58-year-old woman with a history of hypertension, had a partial nephrectomy 4 years ago for renal calculi. During a routine physical examination, her total serum calcium level was 10.8 mg/dL. Her parathyroid hormone level was WNL; she was in no apparent distress, and the remainder of her physical examination and laboratory data were noncontributory.

B.E. underwent exploratory surgery for an enlarged right superior parathyroid gland. The remaining three glands appeared normal. The enlarged gland was excised, and a biopsy was performed on the remaining glands. The pathology report showed an adenoma of the abnormal gland. On her first postoperative day, she complained of perioral numbness and tingling. She had no other symptoms, but her serum calcium was subnormal. She was given one ampule of calcium gluconate. Within 2 days, her calcium level had improved and she was discharged.

Case Studies, continued

Case Study 16-3: Diabetes Treatment With an Insulin Pump

M.G. a 32-year-old marketing executive, was diagnosed with juvenile-onset (type 1) diabetes at the age of 3 years. She vividly remembers her mother taking her to the doctor because she had an illness that caused her to feel extremely tired and very thirsty and hungry. She also had a cut on her knee that would not heal and had begun to wet her bed. Her mother had had gestational diabetes during her pregnancy with M.G.; M.G. was described as a "macrosomia" because she weighed 10 lb at birth.

M.G. has managed her disease with meticulous attention to her diet, exercise, preventative health care, regular blood glucose monitoring, and twice-daily injections of regular and NPH insulin, which she rotates among her upper arms, thighs, and abdomen. She continues in a smoking cessation program supported by weekly acupuncture treatments. She maintains good control of her disease in spite of the inconvenience and time it consumes each day. She will be married next summer and would like to start a family. M.G.'s doctor suggested she try an insulin pump to give her more freedom and enhance her quality of life. After intensive training, she has received her pump. It is about the size of a beeper with a thin catheter that she introduces through a needle into her abdominal subcutaneous tissue. She can administer her insulin in a continuous subcutaneous insulin infusion (CSII) and in calculated meal bolus doses. She still has to test her blood for hyperglycemia and hypoglycemia and her urine for ketones when her blood sugar is too high. She hopes one day to have an islet transplantation.

CASE STUDY QUESTIONS

Multiple choice: Select the best answer and write the letter of your choice to the left of each number.

_____ 1. Necrotizing hemorrhagic pancreatitis can be described as:
a. enlargement of the pancreas with anemia
b. inflammation of the pancreas with tissue death and bleeding
c. inflammation of the pancreas with overgrowth of tissue
d. marsupialization of a pancreatic pseudocyst
e. none of the above

_____ 2. R.B.'s midepigastric pain was located:
a. inferior to the sternum
b. periumbilical
c. cephalad to the clavicle
d. lateral to the anterior costal margins
e. anterolateral

_____ 3. Intravascular volume and hemodynamic stability refer to:
a. measured amount of urine in the drainage bag
b. speed with which pancreatic fluid moves
c. movement of cells through a flow cytometer
d. body fluids and blood pressure
e. blood count and clotting factors

Case Studies, continued

_____ 4. Renal calculi are:
   a. kidney stones
   b. gallstones
   c. stomach ulcers
   d. bile obstructions
   e. muscle spasms

_____ 5. B.E.'s serum calcium was 10.8 mg/dL, which is:
   a. 5.4 micrograms of calcium in her serous fluid
   b. 10.8 grams of electrolytes in parathyroid hormone
   c. 10.8 milligrams calcium in 100 cc of blood
   d. 21.6 liters of calcium in 100 grams of serum
   e. 10.8 micrograms of calcium in 100 cc of serous parathyroid fluid

_____ 6. B.E. had perioral numbness and tingling. Perioral is:
   a. peripheral to any orifice
   b. lateral to the eye
   c. within the buccal mucosa
   d. around the mouth
   e. circumferential to the perineum

_____ 7. M.G.'s diabetes is also described as:
   a. adult-onset diabetes
   b. type 2 diabetes mellitus
   c. diabetes insipidus
   d. insulin-dependent diabetes mellitus
   e. NIDDM

_____ 8. Gestational diabetes occurs:
   a. in a woman during pregnancy
   b. to any large fetus
   c. during menopause
   d. at the time of puberty
   e. at the time of delivery of a large baby with high blood sugar

_____ 9. The term _macrosomia_ describes:
   a. excessive weight gain during pregnancy
   b. a large body
   c. an excessive amount of sleep
   d. inability to sleep during pregnancy
   e. too much sugar in the amniotic fluid

_____ 10. M.G. injected the insulin into the subcutaneous tissue, which is:
   a. only present in the abdomen, thighs, and upper arms
   b. a topical application
   c. below the skin
   d. in a large artery
   e. above the pubic bone

Case Studies, continued

_____ 11. An islet transplantation refers to:
   a. transfer of parathyroid cells to the liver
   b. excision of bovine pancreatic cells
   c. surgical insertion of an insulin pump into the abdomen
   d. a total pancreas and kidney transplantation
   e. transfer of insulin-secreting cells into a pancreas

Write a term from the case studies with each of the following meanings:

12. yellowish color of the skin _____

13. enzyme that digests fats _____

14. surgical excision of a kidney _____

15. tumor of a gland _____

16. single-use glass injectable medication container _____

17. high serum glucose _____

Abbreviations. Define each of the following abbreviations:

18. NPO _____

19. NG _____

20. BUN _____

21. WNL _____

22. NPH _____

23. CSII _____

Chapter 16 Crossword
Endocrine System

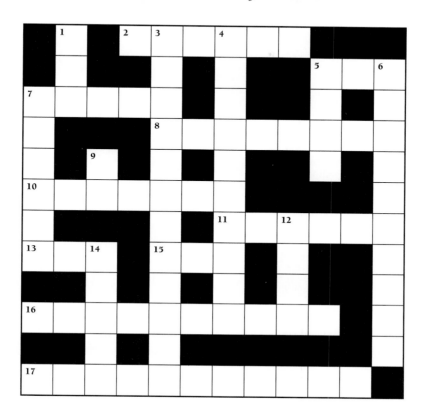

ACROSS

2. An islet is a small _____.
5. Measurement used to diagnose diabetes: abbreviation
7. Temperature: root
8. Sudden degeneration of the pituitary is pituitary _____.
10. Diabetes affects the metabolism of _____.
11. A form of hyperthyroidism is named for him.
13. Pituitary hormone that acts on the thyroid: abbreviation
15. Test for measuring hormones in the blood: abbreviation
16. Alternate name for the pituitary
17. Any disease of the adrenal gland

DOWN

1. Pituitary hormone that controls water loss: abbreviation
3. Alternate name for growth hormone
4. Disorder caused by excess growth hormone in adults
5. A form of thyroid hormones in the blood
6. Excess sugar in the urine
7. The cells or tissues a hormone acts on
9. True, normal: prefix
12. Against: prefix
14. Over, abnormally high: prefix

CHAPTER 16 Answer Section

Answers to Chapter Exercises

EXERCISE 16-1

1. study of the endocrine glands or system
2. surgical removal of the pituitary gland (hypophysis)
3. destructive to the thyroid gland
4. condition of overactivity of the adrenal gland
5. inflammation of the pancreatic islets
6. hyperthyroidism (hī-per-THĪ-royd-izm)
7. hypoparathyroidism (hī-pō-par-a-THĪ-royd-izm)
8. hypoadrenalism (hī-pō-ad-RE-nal-izm)
9. hypoadrenocorticism (hī-pō-ad-rē-nō-KOR-ti-sizm)
10. hyperpituitarism (hī-per-pi-TŪ-i-ta-rizm)
11. endocrinologist (en-dō-kri-NOL-ō-jist)
12. thyrotomy (thī-ROT-ō-mē); also thyroidotomy (thī-royd-OT-ō-mē)
13. adrenalopathy (ad-rē-nal-OP-a-thē); also adrenopathy (ad-ren-OP-a-thē)
14. adrenalitis (ad-rē-nal-Ī-tis); also adrenitis (ad-re-NĪ-tis)
15. insular (IN-sū-lar)

LABELING EXERCISE 16-1 GLANDS OF THE ENDOCRINE SYSTEM

1. pineal
2. pituitary (hypophysis)
3. thyroid
4. parathyroids
5. thymus
6. adrenals
7. pancreatic islets
8. ovaries
9. testes

Answers to Chapter Review 16-1

1. c
2. a
3. d
4. e
5. b
6. d
7. c
8. e
9. a
10. b
11. b
12. d
13. e
14. c
15. a
16. c
17. e
18. d
19. a
20. b
21. d
22. d
23. e
24. b
25. a
26. pituitary (hypophysis)
27. thyroid
28. adrenals
29. pancreatic islets
30. diabetes mellitus
31. hyperglycemia
32. inflammation of the pituitary gland (hypophysis)
33. condition caused by underactivity of the pituitary gland
34. surgical removal of the adrenal gland
35. condition caused by overactivity of the thyroid gland
36. physician who specializes in study and treatment of endocrine disorders
37. pertaining to the adrenal cortex
38. hypophyseal
39. insulitis
40. adrenomegaly
41. hemithyroidectomy
42. thyroiditis
43. parathyroidectomy
44. hypoadrenalism
45. thyrotropic
46. thyrolytic
47. thyropathy
48. normal function of the thyroid gland
    a. true, good, normal
    b. thyroid gland
    c. condition of
49. acting on the adrenal cortex
    a. adrenal gland
    b. cortex
    c. acting on
50. condition of complete underactivity of the pituitary gland
    a. all
    b. under, abnormally low
    c. pituitary gland
    d. condition of

51. a toxic condition caused by hyperactivity of the thyroid gland
    a. thyroid
    b. poisonous
    c. condition of

Answers to Case Study Questions

1. b
2. a
3. d
4. a
5. c
6. d
7. d
8. a
9. b
10. c
11. e
12. jaundice
13. lipase
14. nephrectomy
15. adenoma
16. ampule
17. hyperglycemia
18. nothing by mouth/non per os
19. nasogastric
20. blood urea nitrogen
21. within normal limits
22. neutral protamine Hagedorn
23. continuous subcutaneous insulin infusion

ANSWERS TO CROSSWORD PUZZLE

Endocrine System

The Nervous System and Behavioral Disorders

Chapter Contents

Objectives

After study of this chapter you should be able to:

1. Label a diagram showing the structural organization of the nervous system.
2. Label a diagram of a neuron.
3. Briefly describe the location and functions of the regions of the brain.
4. Describe how the central nervous system is protected.
5. Label a diagram of the spinal cord in cross section, indicating a reflex pathway.
6. Compare the sympathetic and parasympathetic systems.
7. Identify and use word parts pertaining to the nervous system.
8. Describe the major disorders of the nervous system.
9. Describe the major behavioral disorders.
10. List some common symptoms of neurologic disorders.
11. Define abbreviations used in neurology.
12. Interpret case studies involving the nervous system.

The nervous system and the endocrine system coordinate and control the body. Together they regulate our responses to the environment and maintain homeostasis. Whereas the endocrine system functions by means of hormones, the nervous system functions by means of electric impulses. For study purposes, the nervous system may be divided into the **central nervous system** (CNS), consisting of the brain and spinal cord, and the **peripheral nervous system** (PNS), consisting of all nervous tissue outside the brain and spinal cord (Fig. 17-1).

Functionally, the nervous system can be divided into the **somatic nervous system**, which controls skeletal muscles, and the visceral or **autonomic nervous system** (ANS), which controls smooth muscle, cardiac muscle, and glands. The ANS regulates responses to stress and helps to maintain homeostasis.

Two types of cells are found in the nervous system:
- **Neurons**, or nerve cells, that make up the conducting tissue of the nervous system.
- **Neuroglia**, the connective tissue cells of the nervous system that support and protect nervous tissue.

The Neuron

The neuron is the basic functional unit of the nervous system (Fig. 17-2). Each neuron has two types of fibers extending from the cell body: the **dendrite**, which carries impulses toward the cell body, and the **axon**, which carries impulses away from the cell body.

Some axons are covered with **myelin**, a whitish, fatty material that insulates and protects the axon and speeds electric conduction. Axons so covered are described as myelinated, and they make up the **white matter** of the nervous system. Unmyelinated tissue makes up the **gray matter** of the nervous system.

Each neuron is part of a relay system that carries information through the nervous system. A neuron that transmits impulses toward the CNS is a **sensory** neuron; a neuron that transmits impulses away from the CNS is a **motor** neuron. There are also connecting neurons within the CNS. The point of contact between two nerve cells is the **synapse**. At the synapse, energy is passed from one cell to another by means of a chemical **neurotransmitter**.

Nerves

Individual neuron fibers are held together in bundles like wires in a cable. If this bundle is part of the PNS, it is called a **nerve**. A collection of cell bodies along the pathway of a nerve is a **ganglion**. A few nerves (sensory nerves) contain only sensory neurons, and a few (motor nerves) contain only motor neurons, but most contain both types of fibers and are described as mixed nerves.

The Brain

The **cerebrum** is the largest part of the brain (Fig. 17-3). It is composed largely of white matter with a thin outer layer of gray matter, the **cerebral cortex**. It is within the cortex that the higher brain functions of memory, reasoning, and abstract thought occur. The cerebrum is divided into two hemispheres by a deep groove, the longitudinal fissure. Each hemisphere is further divided into lobes with specialized functions.

The **diencephalon** contains the **thalamus**, the **hypothalamus**, and the pituitary gland. The thalamus receives sensory information and directs it to the proper portion of the cortex. The hypothalamus controls the pituitary and forms a link between the endocrine and nervous systems.

The **brainstem** consists of the **midbrain**, the **pons**, and the **medulla oblongata** (see Fig. 17-3). The midbrain contains reflex centers for improved vision and hearing. The pons forms a bulge on the anterior surface

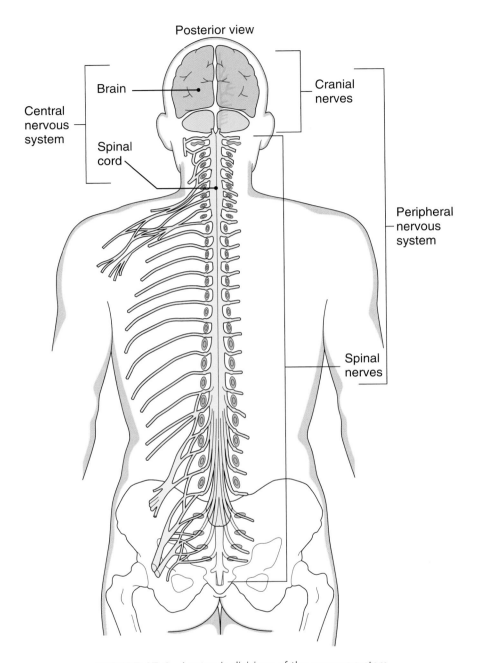

FIGURE 17-1. Anatomic divisions of the nervous system.

of the brainstem. It contains fibers that connect different regions of the brain. The medulla connects the brain with the spinal cord. All impulses passing to and from the brain travel through this region. The medulla also has vital centers for control of heart rate, respiration, and blood pressure.

The **cerebellum** is under the cerebrum and dorsal to the pons and medulla (see Fig. 17-3). Like the cerebrum, it is divided into two hemispheres. It helps to control voluntary muscle movements and to maintain posture, coordination, and balance.

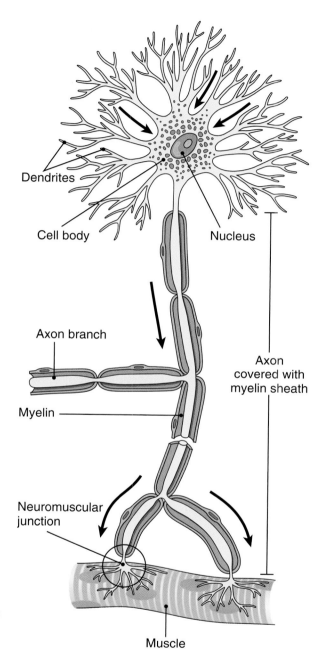

Dendrites

Cell body

Nucleus

Axon
covered with
myelin sheath

Axon branch

Myelin

Neuromuscular
junction

Muscle

FIGURE 17-2. A motor neuron. The break in the axon denotes length. The *arrows* show the direction of the nerve impulse.

Within the brain are four **ventricles** (cavities) in which **cerebrospinal fluid** (CSF) is produced. This fluid circulates around the brain and spinal cord, acting as a protective cushion for these tissues.

Covering the brain and the spinal cord are three protective layers, together called the **meninges**. The outermost and toughest of the three is the **dura mater**. The middle layer is the **arachnoid**. The thin, vascular inner layer, attached directly to the tissue of the brain and spinal cord, is the **pia mater**.

Twelve pairs of **cranial nerves** connect with the brain (see Fig. 17-1). These are identified by Roman numerals and also by name. See Display 17-1 for a summary chart of the cranial nerves.

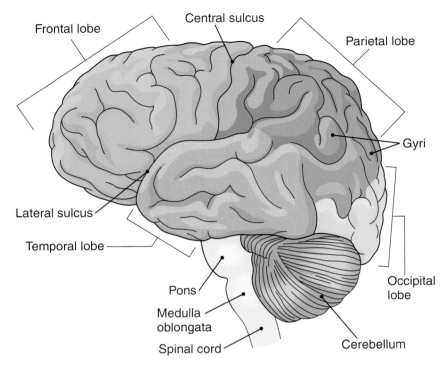

FIGURE 17-3. External surface of the brain, showing the main parts and some lobes of the cerebrum.

DISPLAY 17-1 The Cranial Nerves

NUMBER	NAME	FUNCTION
I	olfactory *ol-FAK-tō-rē*	carries impulses for the sense of smell
II	optic *OP-tik*	carries impulses for the sense of vision
III	oculomotor *ok-ū-lō-MŌ-tor*	controls movement of eye muscles
IV	trochlear *TROK-lē-ar*	controls a muscle of the eyeball
V	trigeminal *trī-JEM-i-nal*	carries sensory impulses from the face; controls chewing muscles
VI	abducens *ab-DŪ-sens*	controls a muscle of the eyeball
VII	facial *FĀ-shal*	controls muscles of facial expression, salivary glands, and tear glands; conducts some impulses for taste
VIII	vestibulocochlear *ves-tib-ū-lō-KOK-lē-ar*	conducts impulses for hearing and equilibrium; also called auditory or acoustic nerve

DISPLAY 17-1 The Cranial Nerves, *continued*

NUMBER	NAME	FUNCTION
IX	glossopharyngeal *glos-ō-fa-RIN-jē-al*	conducts sensory impulses from tongue and pharynx; stimulates parotid salivary gland and partly controls swallowing
X	vagus *VĀ-gus*	supplies most organs of thorax and abdomen; controls digestive secretions
XI	spinal accessory *ak-SES-ō-rē*	controls muscles of the neck
XII	hypoglossal *hī-pō-GLOS-al*	controls muscles of the tongue

The Spinal Cord

The **spinal cord** extends from the medulla oblongata to between the first and second lumbar vertebrae. It has a central area of gray matter surrounded by white matter. The gray matter projects toward the back and the front as the dorsal and ventral horns. The white matter contains the ascending and descending **tracts** (fiber bundles) that carry impulses to and from the brain.

Thirty-one pairs of spinal nerves connect with the spinal cord (Fig. 17-4). These nerves are grouped in the segments of the cord as follows:

- Cervical: 8
- Thoracic: 12
- Lumbar: 5
- Sacral: 5
- Coccygeal: 1

Each nerve joins the cord by two **roots** (Fig. 17-5). The dorsal, or posterior, root carries sensory impulses into the cord; the ventral, or anterior, root carries motor impulses away from the cord and out toward a muscle or gland.

A simple response that requires few neurons is a **reflex** (see Fig. 17-5). In a spinal reflex, impulses travel through the spinal cord only and do not reach the brain. An example of this type of response is the knee-jerk reflex used in physical examinations. Most neurologic responses, however, involve complex interactions among multiple neurons (interneurons) in the CNS.

The Autonomic Nervous System

The autonomic nervous system (ANS) is the division of the nervous system that controls the involuntary actions of muscles and glands (Fig. 17-6). The ANS itself has two divisions: the **sympathetic nervous system** and the **parasympathetic nervous system**. The sympathetic nervous system motivates our response to stress, the so-called "fight-or-flight" response. It increases heart rate and respiration rate, stimulates the adrenal gland, and delivers more blood to skeletal muscles. The parasympathetic system returns the body to a steady state and stimulates maintenance activities, such as digestion of food. Most organs are controlled by both systems and, in general, the two systems have opposite effects on a given organ.

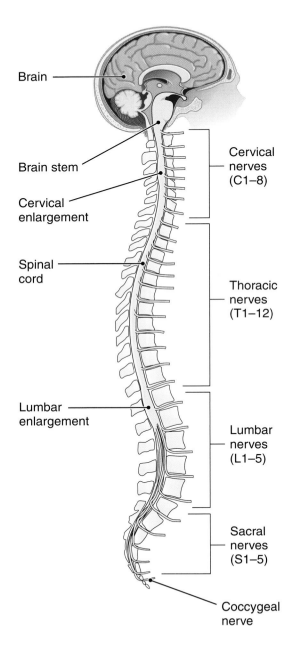

Brain

Brain stem

Cervical
enlargement

Spinal
cord

Lumbar
enlargement

Cervical
nerves
(C1–8)

Thoracic
nerves
(T1–12)

Lumbar
nerves
(L1–5)

Sacral
nerves
(S1–5)

Coccygeal
nerve

FIGURE 17-4. Spinal cord from the side, showing the divisions of the spinal nerves.

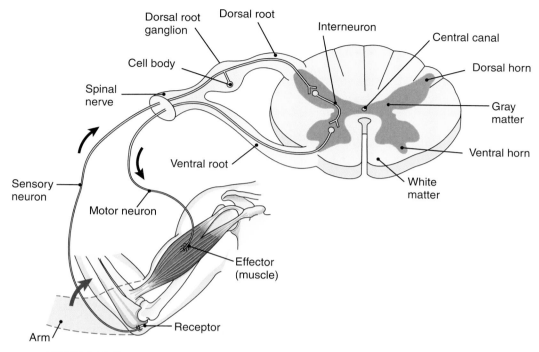

FIGURE 17-5. Cross-section of the spinal cord and pathway of impulses in a reflex arc.

Key Terms

NORMAL STRUCTURE AND FUNCTION

arachnoid *a-RAK-noyd*	The middle layer of the meninges (from the Greek word for spider, because this tissue resembles a spider web)
autonomic nervous system (ANS) *aw-tō-NOM-ik*	The division of the nervous system that regulates involuntary activities, controlling smooth muscles, cardiac muscle, and glands; the visceral nervous system
axon *AK-son*	The fiber of a neuron that conducts impulses away from the cell body
brain	The nervous tissue contained within the cranium; consists of the cerebrum, diencephalon, brainstem, and cerebellum (root *encephal/o*)
brainstem	The part of the brain that consists of the midbrain, pons, and medulla oblongata
central nervous system (CNS)	The brain and spinal cord

SYMPATHETIC SYSTEM

PARASYMPATHETIC SYSTEM

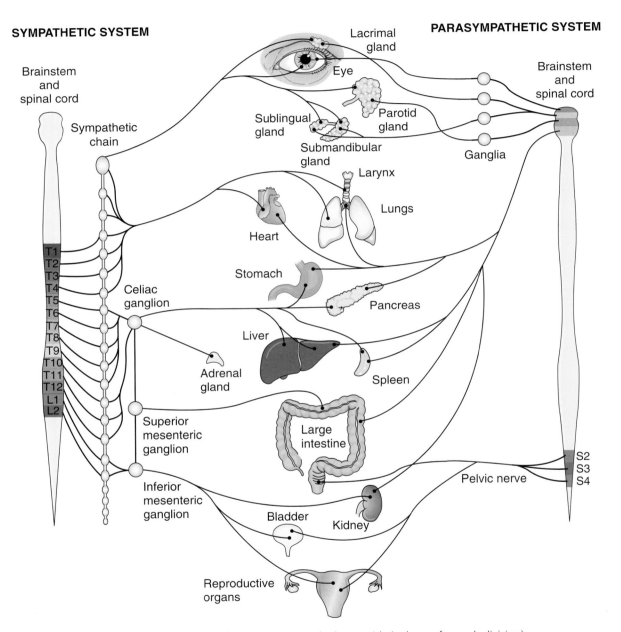

FIGURE 17-6. Autonomic nervous system (only one side is shown for each division).

Normal Structure and Function, *continued*

cerebellum ser-e-BEL-um	The posterior portion of the brain dorsal to the pons and medulla; helps to coordinate movement and to maintain balance and posture (*cerebellum* means "little brain"; root *cerebell/o*)
cerebral cortex SER-e-bral	The thin surface layer of gray matter of the cerebrum (root *cortic/o*; the cortex is the outer region of an organ)
cerebrum SER-e-brum	The large upper portion of the brain; it is divided into two hemispheres by the longitudinal fissure (root *cerebr/o*)
cerebrospinal fluid (CSF) ser-e-brō-SPĪ-nal	The watery fluid that circulates in and around the brain and spinal cord as a protection
cranial nerves	The twelve pairs of nerves that are connected to the brain
dendrite DEN-drīt	A fiber of a neuron that conducts impulses toward the cell body
diencephalon di-en-SEF-a-lon	The part of the brain that contains the thalamus, hypothalamus, and pituitary gland; located between the cerebrum and the brainstem
dura mater DŪ-ra MĀ-ter	The fibrous outermost layer of the meninges
ganglion GANG-glē-on	A collection of nerve cell bodies outside the CNS (plural, ganglia; root *gangli/o, ganglion/o*)
gray matter	Unmyelinated tissue of the nervous system
hypothalamus hī-pō-THAL-a-mus	The part of the brain that controls the pituitary gland and maintains homeostasis
medulla oblongata me-DUL-la ob-long-GA-ta	The portion of the brain that connects with the spinal cord. It has vital centers for control of respiration, heart rate, and blood pressure (root *medull/o*).
meninges men-IN-jēz	The three membranes that cover the brain and spinal cord: the dura mater, the arachnoid, and the pia mater (singular, meninx; root *mening/o, meninge/o*)
midbrain	The part of the brainstem between the diencephalon and the pons; contains centers for coordination of reflexes for vision and hearing
motor	Producing movement; describes neurons that carry impulses away from the CNS
myelin MĪ-e-lin	A whitish, fatty substance that surrounds certain axons of the nervous system
neuroglia nū-ROG-lē-a	The connective tissue cells of the nervous system; also called glial cells (from *glia* meaning "glue"; root *gli/o*)
neuron NŪ-ron	A nerve cell
neurotransmitter	A chemical that transmits energy across a synapse
nerve	A bundle of nerve cell fibers outside the CNS (root *neur/o*)

Normal Structure and Function, continued

parasympathetic nervous system	The part of the automatic nervous system that reverses the response to stress and restores homeostasis. It slows heart rate and respiration rate and stimulates activity of the digestive, urinary, and reproductive systems.
peripheral nervous system (PNS) *per-IF-er-al*	The portion of the nervous system outside the CNS
pia mater *PĒ-a MĀ-ter*	The innermost layer of the meninges
pons *ponz*	A rounded area on the ventral surface of the brainstem; contains fibers that connect regions of the brain; the adjective is pontine (*PON-tēn*)
reflex *RĒ-fleks*	A simple, rapid, and automatic response to a stimulus
root	A branch of a spinal nerve that connects with the spinal cord; the dorsal (posterior) root joins the dorsal gray horn of the spinal cord; the ventral (anterior) root joins the ventral gray horn of the spinal cord (root *radicul/o*)
sensory *SEN-so-rē*	Describing neurons that carry impulses toward the CNS
somatic nervous system	The division of the nervous system that controls skeletal (voluntary) muscles
spinal cord	The nervous tissue contained within the spinal column; extends from the medulla oblongata to the second lumbar vertebra (root *myel/o*)
spinal nerves	The 31 pairs of nerves that connect with the spinal cord
sympathetic nervous system	The part of the autonomic nervous system that mobilizes a response to stress; increases heart rate and respiration rate and delivers more blood to skeletal muscles
synapse *SIN-aps*	The junction between two neurons
thalamus *THAL-a-mus*	The part of the brain that receives all sensory impulses except those for the sense of smell and directs them to the proper portion of the cerebral cortex (root *thalam/o*)
tract *trakt*	A bundle of nerve cell fibers within the CNS
ventricle *VEN-trik-l*	A small cavity, such as one of the cavities in the brain in which CSF is produced (root *ventricul/o*)
visceral nervous system	The autonomic nervous system
white matter	Myelinated tissue of the nervous system

Word Parts Pertaining to the Nervous System

TABLE 17-1 Roots for the Nervous System and the Spinal Cord

ROOT	MEANING	EXAMPLE	DEFINITION OF EXAMPLE
neur/o, neur/i	nervous system, nervous tissue, nerve	neurotoxic *nū-rō-TOK-sik*	harmful or poisonous to a nerve or nervous tissue
gli/o	neuroglia	glioma *glī-Ō-ma*	a neuroglial tumor
gangli/o, ganglion/o	ganglion	ganglionectomy *gang-glē-o-NEK-tō-mē*	surgical removal of a ganglion
mening/o, meninge/o	meninges	meningocele *me-NING-gō-sēl*	hernia of the meninges through the skull or spinal column
myel/o	spinal cord (also bone marrow)	myelodysplasia *mī-e-lō-dis-PLĀ-sē-a*	abnormal development of the spinal cord
radicul/o	root of a spinal nerve	radiculopathy *ra-dik-ū-LOP-a-thē*	any disease of a spinal nerve root

Exercise 17-1

Define each of the following adjectives:

1. neural (*NŪ-ral*) ____pertaining to a nerve or the nervous system____

2. glial (*GLĪ-al*) _____

3. ganglionic (*gang-glē-ON-ik*) _____

4. meningeal (*me-NIN-jē-al*) _____

5. radicular (*ra-DIK-ū-lar*) _____

Fill in the blanks:

6. hematomyelia is hemorrhage into the (*hē-ma-tō-mī-E-lē-a*) _____

7. neurolysis is destruction of a(n) (*nū-ROL-i-sis*) _____

8. meningococci are bacteria that infect the (*me-ning-gō-KOK-sī*) _____

9. polyradiculitis is inflammation of many (*pol-ē-ra-dik-ū-LĪ-tis*) _____

Define each of the following terms:

10. neurology (nū-ROL-ō-jē) _____

11. myelogram (MĪ-e-lō-gram) _____

12. meningioma (combining vowel is *i*) me-nin-jē-Ō-ma _____

Write a word that has the same meaning as each of the following definitions:

13. pain in a nerve _____

14. any disease of the nervous system _____

15. inflammation of the spinal cord _____

16. tumor of a ganglion _____

17. radiographic study of the spinal cord _____

18. inflammation of the meninges _____

TABLE 17-2 Roots for the Brain

ROOT	MEANING	EXAMPLE	DEFINITION OF EXAMPLE
encephal/o	brain	encephalomalacia en-sef-a-lō-ma-LĀ-shē-a	softening of brain tissue
cerebr/o cerebr/o	cerebrum (loosely, brain)	decerebrate dē-SER-e-brāt	having no cerebral function
cortic/o	cerebral cortex, outer portion	corticospinal kor-ti-kō-SPĪ-nal	pertaining to the cerebral cortex and spinal cord
cerebell/o	cerebellum	intracerebellar in-tra-ser-e-BEL-ar	within the cerebellum
thalam/o	thalamus	thalamotomy thal-a-MOT-ō-mē	incision of the thalamus
ventricul/o	cavity, ventricle	supraventricular sū-pra-ven-TRIK-ū-lar	above a ventricle
medull/o	medulla oblongata (also spinal cord)	medullary MED-ū-lar-ē	pertaining to the medulla
psych/o	mind	psychosomatic sī-kō-sō-MAT-ik	pertaining to the mind and body (soma)
narc/o	stupor, unconsciousness	narcosis nar-KŌ-sis	state of stupor induced by drugs
somn/o, somn/i	sleep	somnolence SOM-nō-lens	sleepiness

Exercise 17-2

Fill in the blanks:

1. An electroencephalogram (EEG; $\bar{e}$-lek-tr$\bar{o}$-en-SEF-a-l$\bar{o}$-gram) is a record of the electric activity of the
   _____.

2. The term cerebrovascular (ser-e-br$\bar{o}$-VAS-k$\bar{u}$-lar) refers to the blood vessels in the
   _____.

3. The term psychogenic (s$\bar{i}$-k$\bar{o}$-JEN-ik) means originating in the _____.

4. A narcotic (nar-KOT-ik) is a drug that causes _____.

5. Somnambulism (som-NAM-b$\bar{u}$-lizm) means walking during _____.

6. Hypothalamic (h$\bar{i}$-p$\bar{o}$-tha-LAM-ik) refers to the region below the _____.

Write an adjective for each of the following definitions. Note the endings.

7. pertaining to (-al) the cerebrum   _____

8. pertaining to (-al) the cerebral cortex   _____

9. pertaining to (-ic) the thalamus   _____

10. pertaining to (-ar) the cerebellum   _____

11. pertaining to (-ar) a ventricle   _____

Define each of the following words:

12. encephalitis
    (en-sef-a-L$\bar{I}$-tis)   _____

13. extramedullary
    (eks-tra-MED-$\bar{u}$-lar-$\bar{e}$)   _____

14. psychology
    (s$\bar{i}$-KOL-$\bar{o}$-j$\bar{e}$)   _____

15. cerebrospinal
    (ser-e-br$\bar{o}$-SP$\bar{I}$-nal)   _____

16. ventriculitis
    (ven-trik-$\bar{u}$-L$\bar{I}$-tis)   _____

17. insomnia
    (in-SOM-n$\bar{e}$-a)   _____

Write a word that has the same meaning as each of the following definitions:

18. any disease of the brain   _____

19. above (supra-) the cerebellum   _____

20. pertaining to the cerebral cortex and the thalamus   _____

21. radiograph of a ventricle   _____

22. outside (extra-) the cerebrum   _____

TABLE 17-3 Suffixes for the Nervous System

SUFFIX	MEANING	EXAMPLE	DEFINITION OF EXAMPLE
-phasia	speech	heterophasia het-er-ō-FĀ-zē-a	uttering words that are different from those intended
-lalia	speech, babble	coprolalia kop-rō-LĀ-lē-a	compulsive use of obscene words (*copro-* means "feces")
-lexia	reading	dyslexia dis-LEK-sē-a	difficulty in reading
-plegia	paralysis	tetraplegia tet-ra-PLĒ-jē-a	paralysis of all four limbs
-paresis*	partial paralysis	hemiparesis hem-i-pa-RĒ-sis	partial paralysis of one side of the body
-lepsy	seizure	narcolepsy NAR-kō-lep-sē	condition marked by sudden episodes of sleep
-phobia*	persistent, irrational fear	agoraphobia ag-o-ra-FŌ-bē-a	fear of being in a public place (from Greek *agora*, meaning "marketplace")
-mania*	excited state, obsession	megalomania meg-a-lō-MĀ-nē-a	exaggerated self-importance; "delusions of grandeur"

*May be used alone as a word.

Exercise 17-3

Fill in the blanks:

1. Echolalia (*ek-ō-LĀ-lē-a*) refers to repetitive _____.

2. Epilepsy (*EP-i-lep-sē*) is a disease characterized by _____.

3. In myoparesis (*mī-ō-pa-RĒ-sis*), a muscle shows _____.

4. A person with alexia (*a-LEK-sē-a*) lacks the ability to _____.

5. Another term for quadriplegia is _____.

Define each of the following words:

6. aphasia
   (*a-FĀ-zē-a*)   _____

7. bradylexia
   (*brad-ē-LEK-sē-a*)   _____

8. pyromania
   (*pī-rō-MĀ-nē-a*)   _____

9. gynephobia
   (*jin-e-FŌ-bē-a*)   _____

Write a word that has the same meaning as each of the following definitions:

10. slowness in speech (-lalia) _____

11. paralysis of one side (hemi-) of the body _____

12. paralysis of the heart _____

13. fear of night and darkness _____

14. fear of (or abnormal sensitivity to) light _____

Clinical Aspects of the Nervous System

Vascular Disorders

The term **cerebrovascular accident** (CVA), or **stroke**, applies to any occurrence that deprives brain tissue of oxygen. These events include blockage in a vessel that supplies the brain, a ruptured blood vessel, or some other damage that leads to hemorrhage within the brain. Stroke is the third leading cause of death in developed countries, after cancer and heart attack (myocardial infarction), and is a leading cause of neurologic disability. Risk factors for a stroke include hypertension, atherosclerosis (hardening of the arteries), heart disease, diabetes mellitus, and cigarette smoking. Heredity is also a factor.

Thrombosis is the formation of a blood clot in a vessel. Often, in cases of CVA, thrombosis occurs in the carotid artery, the large vessel in the neck that supplies the brain. Sudden blockage by an obstruction traveling from another part of the body is described as an **embolism**. In cases of stroke, the embolus usually originates in the heart. These obstructions can be diagnosed by **cerebral angiography** (Fig. 17-7) with radiopaque dye, computed tomography (CT) scans, and other radiographic techniques. In cases of thrombosis, it is sometimes possible to remove the section of a vessel that is blocked and insert a graft. If the carotid artery leading to the brain is involved, a **carotid endarterectomy** may be performed to open the vessel. Drugs for dissolving ("busting") such clots are now available.

An **aneurysm** (Fig. 17-8) is a localized dilation of a vessel that may rupture and cause hemorrhage. An aneurysm may be congenital or may arise from other causes, especially atherosclerosis, which weakens the vessel wall. Hypertension then contributes to its rupture. The effects of cerebral hemorrhage vary from massive

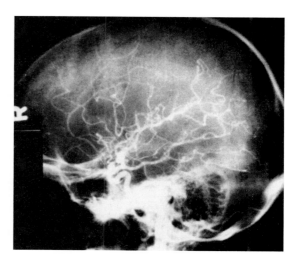

FIGURE 17-7. Cerebral angiogram showing the lateral view of filling of the left carotid and its branches. (Reprinted with permission from Sheldon H. Boyd's Introduction to the Study of Disease. 11th Ed. Philadelphia: Lea & Febiger, 1992:522.)

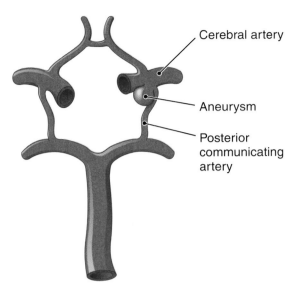

FIGURE 17-8. A cerebral aneurysm in the circle of Willis. (Reprinted with permission from Porth CM. Pathophysiology. 6th Ed. Philadelphia: Lippincott Williams & Wilkins, 2002:443.)

loss of function to mild impairment of sensory or motor activity, depending on the degree of damage. **Aphasia**, loss or impairment of speech communication, is a common aftereffect. **Hemiplegia** (paralysis of one side of the body) on the side opposite the damage is also seen. It has been found in cases of hemorrhage, as in other forms of brain injury, that immediate retraining therapy may help to restore lost function.

Trauma

A blow to the head is the usual cause of bleeding into or around the meninges, which forms a hematoma. Damage to an artery from a skull fracture, usually on the side of the head, may be the cause of an **epidural hematoma** (Fig. 17-9), which appears between the dura mater and the skull bone. The rapidly accumulating blood puts pressure on local vessels and interrupts blood flow to the brain. There may be headache, loss of consciousness, or **hemiparesis** (partial paralysis) on the side opposite the blow. Diagnosis is made by CT scan or magnetic resonance imaging (MRI). If pressure is not relieved within one or two days, death results.

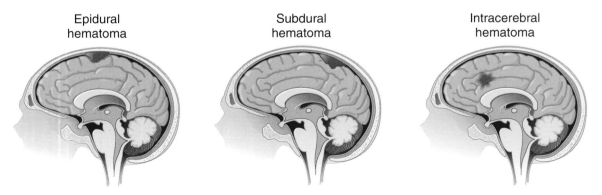

FIGURE 17-9. Location of epidural, subdural, and intracerebral hematomas.

A **subdural hematoma** (see Fig. 17-9) often results from a blow to the front or back of the head, as when the moving head hits a stationary object. The force of the blow separates the dura from the membrane below, the arachnoid. Blood from a damaged vessel, usually a vein, slowly enters this space. The gradual accumulation of blood puts pressure on the brain, causing headache, weakness, and **dementia**. If there is continued bleeding, death results. Figure 17-9 also shows a site of bleeding into the brain tissue itself, forming an intracerebral hematoma.

A cerebral **concussion** results from a blow to the head or from a fall. It may be followed by headache, dizziness, vomiting, loss of consciousness, and even paralysis, among other symptoms. Damage that occurs on the side of the brain opposite the blow as the brain is thrown against the skull is described as a **contrecoup** (*kontre-KŪ*) **injury** (from French, meaning "counterblow").

Other injuries may damage the brain directly. Injury to the base of the brain may involve vital centers in the medulla and interfere with respiration and cardiac function.

Infection

Inflammation of the meninges, or **meningitis**, is usually caused by bacteria that enter through the ear, nose, or throat or are carried by the blood. One of these organisms, the meningococcus (*Neisseria meningitidis*), is responsible for epidemics of meningitis among individuals living in close quarters. Other bacteria implicated in cases of meningitis include *Haemophilus influenzae*, *Streptococcus pneumoniae*, and *Escherichia coli*. A stiff neck is a common symptom. The presence of pus or lymphocytes in spinal fluid is also characteristic. Fluid is withdrawn for diagnosis by a **lumbar puncture** (Fig. 17-10), in which a needle is used to remove CSF from the meninges in the lumbar region of the spine. This fluid can be examined for white blood cells and bacteria in the case of meningitis, for red blood cells in the case of brain injury, or for tumor cells. The fluid also can be analyzed chemically. Normally, spinal fluid is clear, with glucose and chlorides but no protein and very few cells.

Other conditions that can cause meningitis and **encephalitis** (inflammation of the brain) include viral infections, tuberculosis, and syphilis. Viruses that can involve the central nervous system include the polio and rabies viruses; herpes virus; HIV (the cause of AIDS); tick- and mosquito-borne viruses, such as West Nile

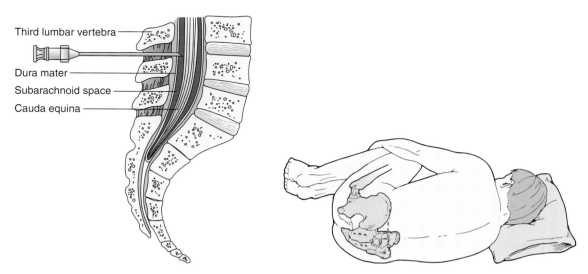

Third lumbar vertebra

Dura mater

Subarachnoid space

Cauda equina

FIGURE 17-10. Lumbar puncture. (Taylor C, Lillis CA, LeMone P: Fundamentals of Nursing. 2nd Ed. Philadelphia: JB Lippincott, 1993:543.)

Virus; and, rarely, common infections such as measles and chickenpox. Aseptic meningitis is a benign, non-bacterial form of the disease caused by a virus. Herpes zoster, the chickenpox virus, is also responsible for **shingles**, an infection that spreads along peripheral nerves, causing lesions and inflammation.

Neoplasms

Almost all tumors that originate in the nervous system are tumors of nonconducting support cells, the neuroglia. These growths are termed **gliomas** and may be named for the specific type of cell involved, such as **astrocytoma**, oligodendroglioma, or schwannoma (neurilemoma). Because they tend not to metastasize, these tumors may be described as benign. However, they do harm by compressing brain tissue. The symptoms they cause depend on their size and location. There may be **seizures**, headache, vomiting, muscle weakness, or interference with a special sense, such as vision or hearing. If present, edema and **hydrocephalus** add to the effects of the tumor. A **meningioma** is a tumor of the meninges. Because a meningioma does not spread and is localized at the surface, it can usually be removed completely by surgery.

Tumors of neural tissue generally occur in childhood, and may even originate before birth, when nervous tissue is actively multiplying. Also, cancer may metastasize to the brain from elsewhere in the body. For unknown reasons, certain forms of cancer, especially melanoma, breast cancer, and lung cancer, tend to spread to the brain.

Degenerative Diseases

Multiple sclerosis (MS) commonly attacks people in their 20s or 30s and progresses at intervals and at varying rates. It involves patchy loss of myelin with hardening (sclerosis) of tissue in the CNS. The symptoms include vision problems, tingling or numbness in the arms and legs, urinary incontinence, **tremor**, and stiff gait. MS is thought to be an autoimmune disorder, but the exact cause is not known.

Parkinson disease occurs when, for unknown reasons, certain neurons in the midbrain fail to secrete the neurotransmitter dopamine. This leads to tremors, muscle rigidity, flexion at the joints, akinesia (loss of movement), and emotional problems. Parkinson disease is treated with daily administration of the drug **L-dopa** (levodopa), a form of dopamine that can be carried by the blood into the brain.

Alzheimer disease (AD) results from unexplained degeneration of neurons and atrophy of the cerebral cortex. These changes cause progressive loss of recent memory, confusion, and mood changes. Dangers associated with AD are injury, infection, malnutrition, and aspiration of food or fluids into the lungs. Originally called presenile dementia and used only to describe cases in patients about 50 years of age, the term is now applied to these same changes when they occur in elderly patients. AD is diagnosed by CT or MRI scans and confirmed at autopsy. Histologic (tissue) studies show deposits of a substance called **amyloid** in the tissues. The disease may be hereditary. People with Down syndrome commonly develop AD after age 40, indicating that AD is associated with abnormality on chromosome 21, the same chromosome that is involved in Down syndrome.

Multi-infarct dementia (MID) resembles AD in that it is a progressive cognitive impairment associated with loss of memory, loss of judgment, aphasia, altered motor and sensory function, repetitive behavior, and loss of social skills. The disorder is caused by multiple small strokes that interrupt blood flow to brain tissue and deprive areas of oxygen.

Epilepsy

A prime characteristic of **epilepsy** is recurrent seizures brought on by abnormal electric activity of the brain. These attacks may vary from brief and mild episodes known as absence (petit mal) seizures to major tonic-clonic (grand mal) seizures with loss of consciousness, **convulsion** (intervals of violent involuntary muscle contractions), and sensory disturbances. In other cases (psychomotor seizures), there is a 1- to 2-minute period of disorientation. Epilepsy may be the result of a tumor, injury, or neurologic disease, but in most cases the cause in unknown.

Electroencephalography (EEG) studies reveal abnormalities in brain activity and can be used in diagnosis and treatment of epilepsy. The disorder is treated with antiepileptic and anticonvulsive drugs to control seizures, and sometimes surgery is of help. If seizures cannot be controlled, the individual with epilepsy may have to avoid certain activities that can lead to harm.

Sleep Disturbances

The general term dyssomnia includes a variety of possible disorders that result in excessive sleepiness or difficulty in beginning or maintaining sleep. Simple causes for such disorders include schedule changes or travel to different time zones (jet lag). **Insomnia** refers to insufficient or nonrestorative sleep despite ample opportunity to sleep. There may be physical causes for insomnia, but often it is related to emotional upset caused by stressful events. **Narcolepsy** is characterized by brief, uncontrollable attacks of sleep during the day. The disorder is treated with stimulants, regulation of sleep habits, and short daytime naps.

Sleep apnea refers to failure to breathe for brief periods during sleep. It usually results from upper airway obstruction, as is seen in obesity, alcohol consumption, or weakened throat muscles, and is usually accompanied by loud snoring with brief periods of silence. Dental appliances that move the tongue and jaw forward may help to prevent sleep apnea. Other options are surgery to correct obstruction or positive air pressure delivered through a mask.

Sleep disorders are diagnosed by physical examination, a sleep history, and a log of sleep habits, including details of the sleep environment and note of any substances consumed that may interfere with sleep. Study in a sleep laboratory with a variety of electric and other studies, composing a **polysomnography**, may also be needed.

Sleep studies characterize two components of normal sleep, each of which shows a specific EEG pattern. Non–rapid eye movement (NREM) sleep has four stages, which take a person progressively into the deepest level of sleep. If sleepwalking (somnambulism) occurs, it occurs during this stage. NREM sleep is interrupted about every 1.5 hours by episodes of rapid eye movement (REM) sleep, during which the eyes move rapidly, although they are closed. Dreaming occurs during REM sleep and muscles lose tone, while heart rate, blood pressure, and brain activity increase.

Others

Many hereditary diseases affect the nervous system. Some of these are described in Chapter 15. Hormonal imbalances that involve the nervous system are described in Chapter 16. Finally, drugs, alcohol, toxins, and nutritional deficiencies may act on the nervous system in a variety of ways.

Behavioral Disorders

Anxiety Disorders

Anxiety is a feeling of fear, worry, uneasiness, or dread. It may be associated with physical problems or drugs and is often prompted by feelings of helplessness or loss of self-esteem. Generalized anxiety disorder (GAD) is characterized by chronic excessive and uncontrollable worry about various life circumstances, often with no basis. It may be accompanied by muscle tensing, restlessness, dyspnea, palpitations, insomnia, irritability, or fatigue.

Panic disorder is a form of anxiety disorder marked by episodes of intense fear. A person with panic disorder may isolate himself or herself or avoid social situations for fear of having a panic attack or in response to attacks. A **phobia** is an extreme, persistent fear of a specific object or situation. It may center on social situations; particular objects, such as animals or blood; or activities, such as flying or driving through tunnels. **Obsessive-compulsive disorder** (OCD) is a condition marked by recurrent thoughts or images that are persistent and intrusive. To relieve anxiety about these thoughts or images, the person with OCD engages in repetitive behavior that interferes with normal daily activities, although he or she knows that such behavior is unreasonable. OCD is associated with perfectionism and rigidity in behavior.

Attention deficit–hyperactivity disorder (ADHD) is difficult to diagnose because many of its symptoms overlap or coexist with other behavioral disorders. ADHD commonly begins in childhood and is characterized by attention problems, easy boredom, impulsive behavior, and hyperactivity. ADHD has been correlated with alterations from the norm in brain structure and metabolism. It is treated with stimulant drugs, primarily methylphenidate (Ritalin).

Depression

Depression is a mental state characterized by profound feelings of sadness, emptiness, hopelessness, and lack of interest or pleasure in activities, often accompanied by suicidal tendencies. Depression frequently coexists with other physical or emotional conditions.

Dysthymia is a mild form of depression that is triggered by a serious event and lasts for several months to years. **Bipolar disorder** (formerly called manic depressive illness) is characterized by depression with episodes of **mania**, a state of elation, which may include agitation, hyperexcitability, or hyperactivity.

Most of the drugs used to treat depression affect the level of neurotransmitters in the brain. The newest of these are the selective serotonin reuptake inhibitors (SSRIs), which prolong the action of serotonin in the brain.

Psychosis

Psychosis is a mental state in which there is gross misperception of reality. This loss of touch with reality may be evidenced by **delusions** (false beliefs), including **paranoia**, delusions of persecution or threat, or **hallucinations**, imagined sensory experiences. Although the patient's condition makes it impossible for him or her to cope with the ordinary demands of life, there is lack of awareness that this behavior is inappropriate.

Schizophrenia is a form of chronic psychosis that may include bizarre behavior, paranoia, anxiety, delusions, withdrawal, and suicidal tendencies. The diagnosis of schizophrenia encompasses a broad category of

---

BOX 17-1 Phobias and Manias

Some of the terms for phobias and manias are just as strange and interesting as the behaviors themselves.

Agoraphobia is fear of being in a public place. The agora in ancient Greece was the marketplace. Xenophobia is an irrational fear of strangers, taken from the Greek root *xen/o*, which means strange or foreign. Acrophobia, a fear of heights, is taken from the root *acro-*, meaning terminal, highest, or topmost. In most medical terms, this root is used to mean extremity, as in *acrocyanosis*. Hydrophobia is a fear of or aversion to water (*hydr/o*). The term was used as an alternative name for rabies, because people infected with this paralytic disease had difficulty swallowing water and other liquids.

Trichotillomania is the odd practice of compulsively pulling out one's hair in response to stress. The word comes from the root for hair (*trich/o*) plus a Greek word that means "to pull." Kleptomania, also spelled cleptomania, is from the Greek word for thief, and describes an irresistible urge to steal in the absence of need.

disorders with many subtypes. The causes of schizophrenia are unknown, but there is evidence of hereditary factors and imbalance in brain chemistry.

Autism

Autism is a complex disorder of unknown cause that usually appears before age 3. It is marked by self-absorption and lack of response to social contact and affection. An autistic child may have low intelligence and poor language skills. He or she responds inappropriately to stimuli and may show self-destructive behavior. There may also be stereotyped (repetitive) behavior, preoccupations, and resistance to change.

Criteria for clinical diagnosis of these and other behavioral and mental disorders are set forth in the *Diagnostic and Statistical Manual of Mental Disorders* (DSM) of the American Psychiatric Association.

Drugs Used in Treatment

A **psychotropic** drug is one that acts on the mental state. This category of drugs includes antianxiety drugs or **anxiolytics**, mood stabilizers, antidepressants, and antipsychotics, also called **neuroleptics**.

Key Clinical Terms

DISORDERS

Alzheimer disease (AD) *ALTS-hī-mer*	A form of dementia caused by atrophy of the cerebral cortex; presenile dementia
amyloid *AM-i-loyd*	A starchlike substance of unknown composition that accumulates in the brain in Alzheimer and other diseases
aneurysm *AN-ū-rizm*	A localized abnormal dilation of a blood vessel that results from weakness of the vessel wall (see Fig. 17-8); an aneurysm may eventually burst
aphasia *a-FĀ-zē-a*	Specifically, loss or defect in speech communication (from Greek *phasis*, meaning "speech"). In practice, the term is applied more broadly to a range of language disorders, both spoken and written. May affect ability to understand speech (receptive aphasia) or the ability to produce speech (expressive aphasia). Both forms are combined in global aphasia.
astrocytoma *as-trō-sī-TŌ-ma*	A neuroglial tumor composed of astrocytes
cerebrovascular accident (CVA)	Sudden damage to the brain resulting from reduction of cerebral blood flow; possible causes are atherosclerosis, thrombosis, or a ruptured aneurysm; commonly called stroke
concussion *kon-KUSH-un*	Injury resulting from a violent blow or shock; a concussion of the brain usually results in loss of consciousness

Disorders, continued

contrecoup injury *kon-tre-KŪ*	Damage to the brain on the side opposite the point of a blow as a result of the brain's hitting the skull (from French, meaning "counterblow")
convulsion *kon-VUL-shun*	A series of violent, involuntary muscle contractions. A tonic convulsion involves prolonged contraction of the muscles; in a clonic convulsion there is alternation of contraction and relaxation. Both forms appear in grand mal epilepsy.
dementia *dē-MEN-shē-a*	A gradual and usually irreversible loss of intellectual function
embolism *EM-bō-lizm*	Obstruction of a blood vessel by a blood clot or other material carried in the circulation
encephalitis *en-sef-a-LĪ-tis*	Inflammation of the brain
epidural hematoma	Accumulation of blood in the epidural space (between the dura mater and the skull; see Fig. 17-9)
epilepsy *EP-i-lep-sē*	A chronic disease involving periodic sudden bursts of electric activity from the brain resulting in seizures
glioma *glī-Ō-ma*	A tumor of neuroglia cells
hemiparesis *hem-i-pa-RĒ-sis*	Partial paralysis or weakness of one side of the body
hemiplegia *hemi-i-PLĒ-jē-a*	Paralysis of one side of the body
hydrocephalus *hī-drō-SEF-a-lus*	Increased accumulation of CSF in or around the brain as a result of obstruction to flow. May be caused by tumor, inflammation, hemorrhage, or congenital abnormality.
insomnia *in-SOM-nē-a*	Insufficient or nonrestorative sleep despite ample opportunity to sleep
meningioma *men-nin-jē-Ō-ma*	Tumor of the meninges
meningitis *men-in-jĪ-tis*	Inflammation of the meninges
multi-infarct dementia	Dementia caused by chronic cerebral ischemia (lack of blood supply to the tissues) as a result of multiple small strokes. There is progressive loss of cognitive function, memory, and judgment as well as altered motor and sensory function.
multiple sclerosis	A chronic, progressive disease involving loss of myelin in the CNS
narcolepsy *NAR-kō-lep-sē*	Brief, uncontrollable episodes of sleep during the day
neurilemoma *nū-ri-lem-Ō-ma*	A tumor of the sheath (neurilemma) of a peripheral nerve; schwannoma

Disorders, continued

paralysis *pa-RAL-i-sis*	Temporary or permanent loss of function. Flaccid paralysis involves loss of muscle tone and reflexes and degeneration of muscles. Spastic paralysis involves excess muscle tone and reflexes but no degeneration.
Parkinson disease	A disorder originating in the basal ganglia and characterized by slow movements, tremor, rigidity, and masklike face. Also called Parkinsonism.
seizure *SĒ-zhur*	A sudden attack, as seen in epilepsy. The most common forms of seizure are tonic-clonic, or grand mal (gran mal; from French, meaning "great illness"); absence seizure, or petit mal (*pet-Ē mal*), meaning "small illness"; and psychomotor seizure.
shingles	An acute viral infection that follows nerve pathways causing small lesions on the skin. Also called herpes zoster (*HER-pēz ZOS-ter*), and caused by the same virus that causes chickenpox.
sleep apnea *ap-NĒ-a*	Brief periods of cessation of breathing during sleep
stroke	Sudden interference with blood flow in one or more cerebral vessels leading to oxygen deprivation and necrosis of brain tissue; caused by a blood clot in a vessel (ischemic stroke) or rupture of a vessel (hemorrhagic stroke). Cerebrovascular accident (CVA)
subdural hematoma	Accumulation of blood beneath the dura mater (see Fig. 17-9)
thrombosis *throm-BŌ-sis*	Development of a blood clot within a vessel
tremor *TREM-or*	A shaking or involuntary movement

DIAGNOSIS AND TREATMENT

carotid endarterectomy *end-ar-ter-EK-tō-mē*	Surgical removal of the lining of the carotid artery, the large artery in the neck that supplies blood to the brain
cerebral angiography	Radiographic study of the blood vessels of the brain after injection of a contrast medium (see Fig. 17-7)
electroencephalography *ē-lek-trō-en-sef-a-LOG-ra-fē*	Amplification, recording, and interpretation of the electric activity of the brain
L-dopa *DŌ-pa*	A drug used in the treatment of Parkinson disease; levodopa
lumbar puncture	Puncture of the subarachnoid space in the lumbar region of the spinal cord; spinal tap; done to remove spinal fluid for diagnosis or to inject anesthesia (see Fig. 17-10)
polysomnography *pol-ē-som-NOG-ra-fē*	Simultaneous monitoring of a variety of physiologic functions during sleep to diagnose sleep disorders

BEHAVIORAL DISORDERS

anxiety *ang-ZĪ-e-tē*	A feeling of fear, worry, uneasiness, or dread
anxiolytic *ang-zī-ō-LIT-ik*	Pertaining to relief of anxiety; a drug used to treat anxiety
attention deficit–hyperactivity disorder (ADHD)	A condition that begins in childhood and is characterized by attention problems, easy boredom, impulsive behavior, and hyperactivity
autism *AW-tizm*	A disorder of unknown cause consisting of self-absorption, lack of response to social contact and affection, preoccupations, stereotyped behavior, and resistance to change
bipolar disorder *bī-PŌ-lar*	A form of depression with episodes of mania (a state of elation); manic depressive illness
delusion *dē-LŪ-zhun*	A false belief inconsistent with knowledge and experience
depression *dē-PRESH-un*	A mental state characterized by profound feelings of sadness, emptiness, hopelessness, and lack of interest or pleasure in activities
dysthymia *dis-THĪ-mē-a*	A mild form of depression that develops in response to a serious life event
hallucination *ha-lū-si-NĀ-shun*	A false perception unrelated to reality or external stimuli
mania *MĀ-ne-a*	A state of elation, which may include agitation, hyperexcitability, or hyperactivity; adjective, manic
neuroleptic *nū-rō-LEP-tik*	Pertaining to relief of psychosis; an antipsychotic medication
obsessive-compulsive disorder (OCD)	A condition associated with recurrent and intrusive thoughts, images, and repetitive behaviors performed to relieve anxiety
panic disorder	A form of anxiety disorder marked by episodes of intense fear
paranoia *par-a-NOY-a*	A mental state characterized by jealousy, delusions of persecution, or perceptions of threat or harm
phobia *FŌ-bē-a*	An extreme, persistent fear of a specific object or situation
psychosis *sī-KŌ-sis*	A mental disorder extreme enough to cause gross misperception of reality with delusions and hallucinations
psychotropic *sī-kō-TROP-ik*	Acting on the mind, as a drug used to treat mental disorders
schizophrenia *skiz-ō-FRĒ-nē-a*	A poorly understood group of severe mental disorders with features of psychosis, delusions, hallucinations, and withdrawn or bizarre behavior (*schizo* means "split" and *phren* means "mind")

Supplementary Terms

NORMAL STRUCTURE AND FUNCTION

acetylcholine *as-ē-til-KŌ-lēn*	A neurotransmitter; activity involving acetylcholine is described as cholinergic
afferent *AF-er-ent*	Carrying toward a central point, such as the sensory neurons and nerves that transmit impulses toward the CNS
basal ganglia	Four masses of gray matter in the cerebrum and upper brainstem that are involved in movement and coordination
blood–brain barrier	A special membrane between circulating blood and the brain that prevents certain damaging substances from reaching brain tissue
Broca area *BRŌ-ka*	An area in the left frontal lobe of the cerebrum that controls speech production
circle of Willis	An interconnection (anastomosis) of several arteries supplying the brain, located at the base of the cerebrum (see Fig. 17-8)
contralateral *kon-tra-LAT-er-al*	Affecting the opposite side of the body
corpus callosum *KOR-pus ka-LŌ-sum*	A large band of connecting fibers between the cerebral hemispheres
dermatome *DER-ma-tōm*	The area of the skin supplied by a spinal nerve; term also refers to an instrument used to cut skin for grafting (see Chapter 21)
efferent *EF-er-ent*	Carrying away from a central point, such as the motor neurons and nerves that transmit impulses away from the CNS
epinephrine *ep-i-NEF-rin*	A neurotransmitter; also called adrenaline; activity involving epinephrine is described as adrenergic
gyrus *JĪ-rus*	A raised convolution of the surface of the cerebrum (see Fig. 17-3) (plural, gyri)
ipsilateral *ip-si-LAT-er-al*	On the same side; unilateral
leptomeninges *lep-to-men-IN-jēz*	The pia mater and arachnoid together
nucleus *NŪ-klē-us*	A collection of nerve cells within the central nervous system
plexus *PLEKS-us*	A network, as of nerves or blood vessels
pyramidal tracts *pi-RAM-i-dal*	A group of motor tracts involved in fine coordination. Most of the fibers in these tracts cross in the medulla to the opposite side of the spinal cord and affect the opposite side of the body. Fibers not included in the pyramidal tracts are described as extrapyramidal.

Normal Structure and Function, continued

reticular activating system (RAS) *re-TIK-ū-lar*	A widespread system in the brain that maintains wakefulness
Schwann cells *shvon*	Cells that produce the myelin sheath around peripheral axons
sulcus *SUL-kus*	A shallow furrow or groove, as on the surface of the cerebrum (see Fig. 17-3; plural, sulci)
Wernicke area *VER-ni-kē*	An area in the temporal lobe concerned with speech comprehension

SYMPTOMS AND CONDITIONS

amyotrophic lateral sclerosis (ALS) *a-mī-ō-TROF-ik*	A disorder marked by muscular weakness, spasticity, and exaggerated reflexes caused by degeneration of motor neurons; Lou Gehrig disease
amnesia *am-NĒ-zē-a*	Loss of memory
apraxia *a-PRAK-sē-a*	Inability to move with purpose or to use objects properly
ataxia *a-TAK-sē-a*	Lack of muscle coordination; dyssynergia
athetosis *ath-e-TŌ-sis*	Involuntary, slow, twisting movements in the arms, especially the hands and fingers
Bell palsy *PAWL-zē*	Paralysis of the facial nerve
berry aneurysm *AN-ū-rizm*	A small saclike aneurysm of a cerebral artery (see Fig. 17-8)
catatonia *kat-a-TŌ-nē-a*	A phase of schizophrenia in which the patient is unresponsive; there is a tendency to remain in a fixed position without moving or talking
cerebral contusion *kon-TŪ-zhun*	A bruise (ecchymosis) of brain tissue caused by a severe blow to the head
cerebral palsy *se-RĒ-bral PAWL-zē*	A nonprogressive neuromuscular disorder usually caused by damage to the CNS before, during, or shortly after birth. May include spasticity, involuntary movements, or ataxia.
chorea *KOR-ē-a*	A nervous condition marked by involuntary twitching of the limbs or facial muscles
claustrophobia *claws-trō-fō-bē-a*	Fear of being shut in or enclosed (from Latin claudere, "to shut")
coma *KŌ-ma*	A deep stupor caused by illness or injury
compulsion *kom-PUL-shun*	A repetitive, stereotyped act performed to relieve tension

Symptoms and Conditions, *continued*

Creutzfeldt-Jakob disease (CJD) *KROITS-felt YA-kob*	A slow-growing degenerative brain disease caused by a prion (*PRĪ-on*), an infectious protein agent. Related to bovine spongiform encephalopathy (BSE; "mad cow disease") in cattle.
delirium *de-LIR-ē-um*	A sudden and temporary state of confusion marked by excitement, physical restlessness, and incoherence
dysarthria *dis-AR-thrē-a*	Defect in speech articulation caused by lack of control over the required muscles
dysmetria *dis-MĒ-trē-a*	Disturbance in the path or placement of a limb during active movement. In hypometria, the limb falls short; in hypermetria, the limb extends beyond the target.
euphoria *ū-FOR-ē-a*	An exaggerated feeling of well-being; elation
glioblastoma *glī-ō-blas-TŌ-ma*	A malignant astrocytoma
Guillain-Barré syndrome *gē-YAN-bar-RĀ*	An acute polyneuritis with progressive muscular weakness that usually occurs after a viral infection; in most cases recovery is complete, but may take several months to years
hematomyelia *hē-ma-tō-mī-Ē-lē-a*	Hemorrhage of blood into the spinal cord, as from an injury
hemiballism *hem-ē-BAL-izm*	Jerking, twitching movements of one side of the body
Huntington disease	A hereditary disease of the CNS that usually appears between ages 30 and 50. The patient shows progressive dementia and chorea, and death occurs within 10 to 15 years.
hypochondriasis *hī-pō-kon-DRĪ-a-sis*	Abnormal anxiety about one's health
ictus *IK-tus*	A blow or sudden attack, such as an epileptic seizure
lethargy *LETH-ar-jē*	A state of sluggishness or stupor
migraine *MĪ-grān*	Chronic intense, throbbing headache that may result from vascular changes in cerebral arteries. Possible causes include genetic factors, stress, trauma, and hormonal fluctuations. Headache might be signaled by visual disturbances, nausea, photophobia, and tingling sensations.
neurofibromatosis *nū-rō-fī-brō-ma-TŌ-sis*	A condition involving multiple tumors of peripheral nerves
neurosis *nū-RŌ-sis*	An emotional disorder caused by unresolved conflicts, with anxiety as a main characteristic
paraplegia *par-a-PLĒ-jē-a*	Paralysis of the legs and lower part of the body

Symptoms and Conditions, continued

parasomnia *par-a-SOM-nē-a*	Condition of having undesirable phenomena, such as nightmares, occur during sleep or become worse during sleep
quadriplegia *kwod-ri-PLĒ-jē-a*	Paralysis of all four limbs; tetraplegia
Reye syndrome *rī*	A rare acute encephalopathy occurring in children after viral infections. The liver, kidney, and heart may be involved. Linked to administration of aspirin during a viral illness.
sciatica *sī-AT-i-ka*	Neuritis characterized by severe pain along the sciatic nerve and its branches
somatoform disorders *sō-MA-tō-form*	Conditions associated with symptoms of physical disease, such as pain, hypertension, or chronic fatigue, with no physical basis
somnambulism *som-NAM-bū-lizm*	Walking or performing other motor functions while asleep and out of bed; sleepwalking
stupor *STŪ-por*	A state of unconsciousness or lethargy with loss of responsiveness
syringomyelia *sir-in-gō-mī-Ē-lē-a*	A progressive disease marked by formation of fluid-filled cavities in the spinal cord
tic	Involuntary, spasmodic, recurrent, and purposeless motor movements or vocalizations
tic douloureux *tik dū-lū-RŪ*	Episodes of extreme pain in the area supplied by the trigeminal nerve; also called trigeminal neuralgia
tabes dorsalis *TĀ-bēz dor-SAL-is*	Destruction of the dorsal (posterior) portion of the spinal cord with loss of sensation and awareness of body position, as seen in advanced cases of syphilis
Tourette syndrome *tū-RET*	A tic disorder with intermittent motor and vocal manifestations that begins in childhood. There also may be obsessive and compulsive behavior, hyperactivity, and distractibility.
transient ischemic attack *(TIA)*	A sudden, brief, and temporary cerebral dysfunction usually caused by interruption of blood flow to the brain
Wallerian degeneration *wahl-LĒ-rē-an*	Degeneration of a nerve distal to an injury
whiplash	Cervical injury caused by rapid acceleration and deceleration resulting in damage to muscles, ligaments, disks, and nerves

Additional terms related to neurologic symptoms can be found in Chapters 18 (on the senses) and 20 (on the muscular system).

DIAGNOSIS AND TREATMENT

Babinski reflex	A spreading of the outer toes and extension of the big toe over the others when the sole of the foot is stroked. This response is normal in infants but indicates a lesion of specific motor tracts in adults.
evoked potentials	Record of the electric activity of the brain after sensory stimulation. Included are visual evoked potentials (VEP), brainstem auditory evoked potentials (BAEP), and somatosensory evoked potentials (SSEP), obtained by stimulating the hand or leg. These tests are used to evaluate CNS function.
Glasgow coma scale	A system for assessing level of consciousness by assigning a score to each of three responses: eye opening, motor responses, and verbal responses
Romberg sign	Inability to maintain balance when the eyes are shut and the feet are close together
sympathectomy _sim-pa-THEK-tō-mē_	Interruption of transmission by sympathetic nerves either surgically or chemically
trephination _tref-i-NĀ-shun_	Cutting a piece of bone out of the skull; the instrument used is a trepan (_tre-PAN_) or trephine (_tre-FĪN_)

ABBREVIATIONS

ACh	Acetylcholine	**ICP**	Intracranial pressure
AD	Alzheimer disease	**LMN**	Lower motor neuron
ADHD	Attention deficit–hyperactivity disorder	**LOC**	Level of consciousness
ALS	Amyotrophic lateral sclerosis	**LP**	Lumbar puncture
ANS	Autonomic nervous system	**MID**	Multi-infarct dementia
BAEP	Brainstem auditory evoked potentials	**MS**	Multiple sclerosis
CBF	Cerebral blood flow	**NICU**	Neurological intensive care unit
CJD	Creutzfeldt-Jakob disease	**NPH**	Normal-pressure hydrocephalus
CNS	Central nervous system	**NREM**	Non–rapid eye movement (sleep)
CP	Cerebral palsy	**OCD**	Obsessive-compulsive disorder
CSF	Cerebrospinal fluid	**PNS**	Peripheral nervous system
CVA	Cerebrovascular accident	**RAS**	Reticular activating system
CVD	Cerebrovascular disease	**REM**	Rapid eye movement (sleep)
DSM	_Diagnostic and Statistical Manual of Mental Disorders_	**SSEP**	Somatosensory evoked potentials
		SSRI	Selective serotonin reuptake inhibitor
DTR	Deep tendon reflexes	**TIA**	Transient ischemic attack
EEG	Electroencephalogram; electro-encephalograph	**UMN**	Upper motor neuron
		VEP	Visual evoked potentials
GAD	Generalized anxiety disorder		

Labeling Exercise 17-1

Anatomic Divisions of the Nervous System
Write the name of each numbered part on the corresponding line of the answer sheet.

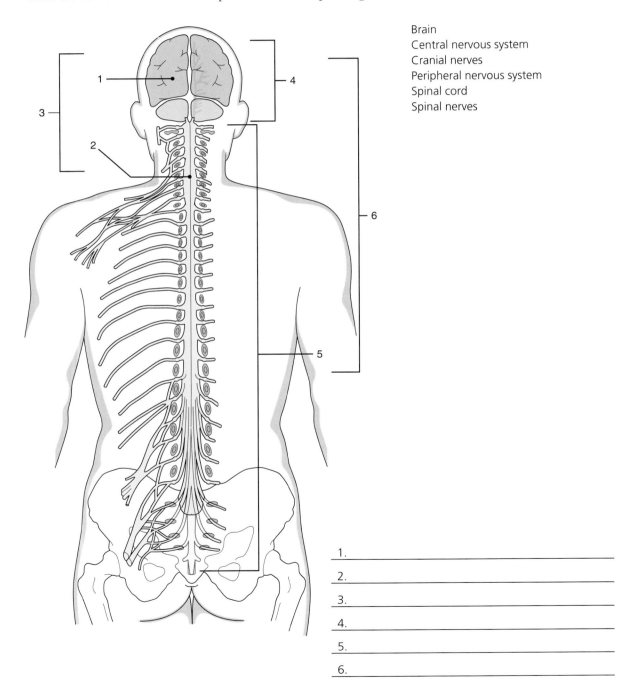

Brain
Central nervous system
Cranial nerves
Peripheral nervous system
Spinal cord
Spinal nerves

1. _____
2. _____
3. _____
4. _____
5. _____
6. _____

Labeling Exercise 17-2

Motor Neuron

Write the name of each numbered part on the corresponding line of the answer sheet.

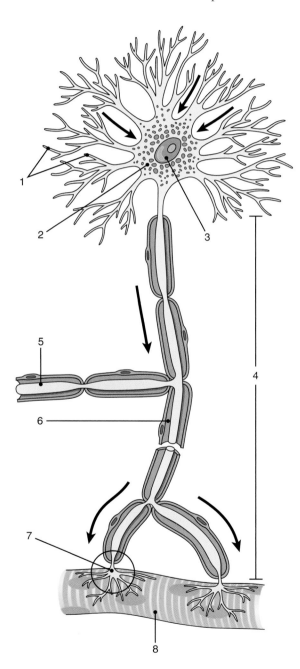

Axon
Axon branch
Cell body
Dendrites
Muscle
Myelin
Neuromuscular junction
Nucleus

1. _____

2. _____

3. _____

4. _____

5. _____

6. _____

7. _____

8. _____

Labeling Exercise 17-3

External Surface of the Brain

Write the name of each numbered part on the corresponding line of the answer sheet.

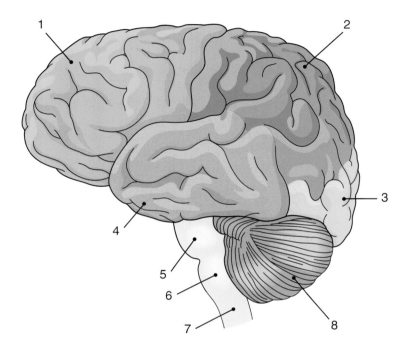

Cerebellum
Frontal lobe
Medulla oblongata
Occipital lobe
Parietal lobe
Pons
Spinal cord
Temporal lobe

1. _____

2. _____

3. _____

4. _____

5. _____

6. _____

7. _____

8. _____

Labeling Exercise 17-4

Spinal Cord and Divisions of the Spinal Nerves

Write the name of each numbered part on the corresponding line of the answer sheet.

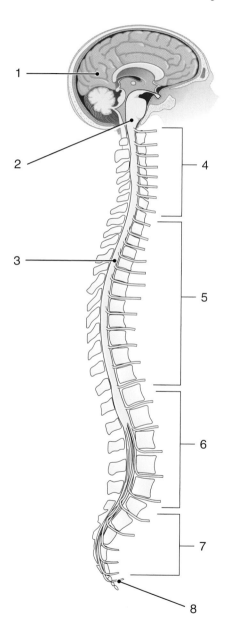

Brain
Brainstem
Cervical nerves
Coccygeal nerve
Lumbar nerves
Sacral nerves
Spinal cord
Thoracic nerves

1. _____
2. _____
3. _____
4. _____
5. _____
6. _____
7. _____
8. _____

Labeling Exercise 17-5

Cross-Section of Spinal Cord and Reflex Arc

Write the name of each numbered part on the corresponding line of the answer sheet.

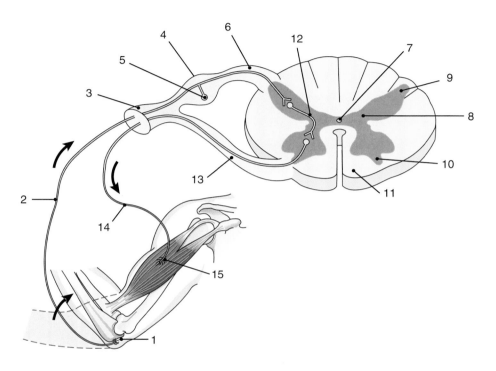

Cell body	Effector	Sensory neuron
Central canal	Gray matter	Spinal nerve
Dorsal horn	Interneuron	Ventral horn
Dorsal root	Motor neuron	Ventral root
Dorsal root ganglion	Receptor	White matter

1. _____

2. _____

3. _____

4. _____

5. _____

6. _____

7. _____

8. _____

9. _____

10. _____

11. _____

12. _____

13. _____

14. _____

15. _____

Chapter Review 17-1

Match the following terms and write the appropriate letter to the left of each number:

_____ 1. axon

_____ 2. tract

_____ 3. dendrite

_____ 4. myelin

_____ 5. ganglion

a. collection of nerve cell bodies along a nerve

b. fatty material that covers some axons

c. bundle of nerve cell fibers within the CNS

d. nerve fiber that carries impulses toward the cell body

e. nerve fiber that carries impulses away from the cell body

_____ 6. pons

_____ 7. ventricle

_____ 8. neuroglia

_____ 9. cortex

_____ 10. gray matter

a. connective tissue cells of the nervous system

b. unmyelinated tissue

c. a cavity

d. an outer region

e. rounded area on the ventral surface of the brain

_____ 11. cerebrum

_____ 12. medulla oblongata

_____ 13. gyrus

_____ 14. neurotransmitter

_____ 15. pia mater

a. chemical active at a synapse

b. region that connects the brain and spinal cord

c. innermost layer of the meninges

d. largest part of the brain

e. raised area on the surface of the brain

_____ 16. concussion

_____ 17. myeloplegia

_____ 18. paranoia

_____ 19. odynophobia

_____ 20. hydrocephalus

a. abnormal fear of pain

b. excess fluid in the brain

c. mental condition associated with delusions of persecution

d. injury caused by a violent blow

e. paralysis originating in the spinal cord

_____ 21. narcotic

_____ 22. hypersomnia

_____ 23. epidural

_____ 24. diencephalon

_____ 25. monoplegia

a. paralysis of one limb

b. above the outermost layer of the meninges

c. part of the brain between the cerebrum and brainstem

d. excessive sleepiness

e. inducing stupor

_____ 26. myelodysplasia   a. loss of speech communication

_____ 27. meningomyelocele   b. partial paralysis of a muscle

_____ 28. myoparesis   c. abnormal development of the spinal cord

_____ 29. aphasia   d. hernia of the meninges and spinal cord

_____ 30. cystoplegia   e. paralysis of the bladder

SUPPLEMENTARY TERMS

_____ 31. acetylcholine   a. network

_____ 32. Broca area   b. area of skin supplied by a spinal nerve

_____ 33. dermatome   c. shallow groove

_____ 34. plexus   d. neurotransmitter

_____ 35. sulcus   e. portion of the brain that controls speech

_____ 36. amnesia   a. sudden blow or attack

_____ 37. claustrophobia   b. abnormal anxiety about one's health

_____ 38. hypochondriasis   c. loss of memory

_____ 39. dysmetria   d. disturbance in use of a limb during movement

_____ 40. ictus   e. fear of being enclosed

_____ 41. ataxia   a. pain along the path of a nerve in the leg

_____ 42. lethargy   b. lack of muscle coordination

_____ 43. sciatica   c. sense of elation, exaggerated well-being

_____ 44. tic   d. state of sluggishness

_____ 45. euphoria   e. involuntary, spasmodic motor movement

_____ 46. CJD   a. study of brain waves

_____ 47. EEG   b. fluid in the central nervous system

_____ 48. CSF   c. stage of sleep

_____ 49. CVA   d. stroke

_____ 50. REM   e. a slow-growing brain infection

_____ 51. DSM   a. dementia caused by many small strokes

_____ 52. SSRI   b. brief loss of oxygen to part of the brain

_____ 53. TIA   c. brain and spinal cord together

_____ 54. MID
d. reference for diagnosis of mental disorders

_____ 55. CNS
e. type of psychoactive drug

Fill in the blanks:

56. The scientific name for a nerve cell is _____.

57. The junction between two nerve cells is a(n) _____.

58. A simple, rapid, automatic response to a stimulus is a(n) _____.

59. The membranes that cover the brain and spinal cord are the _____.

60. The sympathetic and parasympathetic systems make up the _____.

61. The posterior portion of the brain that coordinates muscle movement is the

_____.

Define each of the following words:

62. anencephaly (*an-en-SEF-a-lē*) _____

63. corticothalamic (*kor-ti-kō-tha-LAM-ik*) _____

64. psychotherapy (*sī-kō-THER-a-pē*) _____

65. hemiparesis (*hem-i-pa-RĒ-sis*) _____

66. dyssomnia (*dis-SOM-nē-a*) _____

67. polyneuritis (*pol-ē-nū-RĪ-tis*) _____

68. panplegia (*pan-PLĒ-jē-a*) _____

69. radicular (*ra-DIK-ū-lar*) _____

Word building. Write a word for each of the following definitions:

70. study of the nervous system _____

71. any disease of the nervous system _____

72. inflammation of the spinal cord and meninges _____

73. excision of a ganglion _____

74. incision into a brain ventricle _____

75. paralysis of one side of the body _____

76. within (intra-) the cerebellum _____

77. difficulty in reading _____

78. fear of water _____

Opposites. Write a word that has the opposite meaning of each of the following words:

79. intramedullary _____

80. ipsilateral _____

81. postganglionic _____

82. tachylalia   _____

83. sensory   _____

84. ventral   _____

85. afferent   _____

Write the adjective form of each of the following words:

86. ganglion   _____

87. cortex   _____

88. dura   _____

89. meninges   _____

90. psychosis   _____

Plurals. Write the plural form of each of the following words:

91. ganglion   _____

92. ventricle   _____

93. meninx   _____

94. sulcus   _____

Word analysis. Define each of the following words, and give the meaning of the word parts in each. Use a dictionary if necessary.

95. poliomyelitis (*pō-lē-ō-mī-e-LĪ-tis*) _____
    a. polio   ____gray____
    b. myel/o _____
    c. -itis   _____

96. polyneuroradiculitis (*pol-ē-nū-rō-ra-dik-ū-LĪ-tis*) _____
    a. poly-   _____
    b. neur/o   _____
    c. radicul/o _____
    d. -itis   _____

97. dyssynergia (*dis-sin-ER-jē-a*) _____
    a. dys-   _____
    b. syn-   _____
    c. erg   _____
    d. -ia   _____

Case Studies

Case Study 17-1: Pediatric Brain Tumor

B.C., a 6-year-old first-grade student, was referred to a pediatric neurologist by his primary pediatrician for a neuro consult. He had presented with an acute onset of headaches, vomiting on waking in the morning, and progressive ataxia. The neurologist conducted a thorough neuro exam and ordered a CT scan, MRI, and lumbar puncture (LP) to look for possible tumor cells. When the LP revealed suspicious cells and the scans showed a tissue density, he was referred to a neurosurgeon for treatment of a suspected infratentorial astrocytoma of the posterior fossa.

B.C. had a craniotomy with tumor resection 5 days later. The cerebellar tumor was found to be non-infiltrating and was enclosed within a cyst, which was totally removed. B.C. spent 2 days in the neurological intensive care unit (NICU) because he was on seizure precautions and monitoring for increased intracranial pressure (ICP). A regimen of focal radiation followed after recovery from surgery. His spine was also treated because of the potential spread of tumor cells in the CSF. B.C. did not have chemotherapy because of the danger that he might develop hydrocephalus, which generally requires a ventriculoperitoneal (VP) shunt.

B.C. was discharged 6 days after his surgery with a mild hemiparesis, which was expected to resolve within the next few weeks. He was scheduled for 6 weeks of outpatient rehabilitation, and his prognosis was good.

Case Study 17-2: Cerebrovascular Accident (CVA)

A.R., a 62-year-old man, was admitted to the ER with right hemiplegia and aphasia. He had a history of hypertension and recent transient ischemic attacks (TIAs), yet was in good health when he experienced a sudden onset of right-sided weakness. He arrived in the ER via ambulance within 15 minutes of onset and was received by a member of the hospital's stroke team. He had a rapid general assessment and neuro exam, including a Glasgow coma scale (GCS) rating, to determine his candidacy for fibrinolytic therapy.

He was sent for a noncontrast CT scan to look for evidence of hemorrhagic or ischemic stroke, post–cardiac arrest ischemia, hypertensive encephalopathy, craniocerebral or cervical trauma, meningitis, encephalitis, brain abscess, tumor, and subdural or epidural hematoma. The CT scan, read by the radiologist, did not show intracerebral or subarachnoid hemorrhage. A.R. was diagnosed with probable acute ischemic stroke within 1 hour of onset of symptoms and cleared as a candidate for immediate fibrinolytic treatment.

He was admitted to the NICU for 48-hour observation to monitor his neuro status and vital signs. He was discharged after 3 days with a prognosis of full recovery.

Case Study 17-3: Neuroleptic Malignant Syndrome

J.N., a 21-year-old woman with chronic paranoid schizophrenia, was admitted to the hospital with a diagnosis of pneumonia. She was brought to the ER by her mother, who said J.N. had been very lethargic, had a fever of 104°F, and had had muscular rigidity for 3 days. She took Haldol (haloperidol) and Cogentin (benztropine mesylate). Her mother stated that J.N.'s neuroleptic medication had been changed the week before by her psychiatrist. Her secondary diagnosis was stated as neuroleptic malignant syndrome, a rare and life-threatening disorder associated with the use of antipsychotic medications.

Case Studies, *continued*

This drug-induced condition is usually characterized by alterations in mental status, temperature regulation, and autonomic and extrapyramidal functions.

J.N. was monitored for potential hypotension, tachycardia, diaphoresis, dyspnea, dysphagia, and changes in her level of consciousness (LOC). Her medications were discontinued, she was hydrated with IV fluids, and her body temperature was monitored for fluctuations. She was treated with Bromocriptine, a dopamine antagonist, and Dantrolene, a muscle relaxant and antispasmodic.

After 5 days, J.N. was transferred to a mental health facility and restarted on low-dose neuroleptics. She was monitored to prevent a recurrence. Both J.N. and her family were educated about neuroleptic malignant syndrome in preparation for her discharge back home in 2 weeks.

CASE STUDY QUESTIONS

Multiple choice: Select the best answer and write the letter of your choice to the left of each number.

_____ 1. A neurologist is a physician who:
  a. performs brain surgery
  b. practices psychiatry
  c. practices psychology
  d. treats with natural and herbal medicine
  e. treats disorders of the nervous system

_____ 2. A diagnostic procedure in which fluid is withdrawn from the spinal subarachnoid space is a(n):
  a. thoracentesis
  b. lumbar puncture
  c. ventriculogram
  d. intracranial window
  e. trephine

_____ 3. B.C.'s tumor was in the cerebellum, which controls voluntary movement, balance, and coordination. His motor dysfunction is called:
  a. ataxia
  b. neurolepsis
  c. dysphagia
  d. dyspnea
  e. seizure

_____ 4. A VP shunt is a surgical treatment for hydrocephalus. Excess CSF is shunted (drained) from the _____ by way of tubing tunneled to the _____ cavity.
  a. vortex, ventricular
  b. ventricles, peritoneal
  c. peritoneum, ventricular
  d. ventricles, thoracic
  e. midbrain, stomach

Case Studies, continued

_____ 5. Ischemic stroke is generally caused by:
a. hemorrhage
b. hematoma
c. thrombosis
d. hemiparesis
e. hemangioma

_____ 6. Fibrinolytic therapy is directed toward the treatment of a blood clot in an artery by _____ the _____ of the clot.
a. stabilizing, blood cells
b. lysing, RBCs
c. leaking, plasma
d. dissolving, CSF
e. dissolving, fibrin matrix

_____ 7. A general term for any disorder or alteration of brain tissue is:
a. cerebrocyst
b. encephalopathy
c. neurocytoma
d. dysencephaloma
e. psychosomatic

_____ 8. J.N. had disease manifestations related to involuntary functions and to movement controlled by motor fibers outside the pyramidal tracts. These functions are:
a. antispasmodic and voluntary
b. autonomic and neuroleptic
c. autonomic and voluntary
d. extrapyramidal and pyramidal
e. autonomic and extrapyramidal

Write a term from the case studies with each of the following meanings:

9. tumor of astrocytes   _____

10. surgical opening into the skull   _____

11. sudden attack typical of epilepsy   _____

12. partial paralysis on one side   _____

13. inability to speak or understand speech   _____

14. inflammation of the meninges   _____

15. collection of blood below the dura mater   _____

16. perceived feeling of threat or harm   _____

17. drug that relieves muscle spasms   _____

Case Studies, continued

18. antipsychotic medications   _____

19. a physician who treats psychiatric disorders   _____

Define each of the following abbreviations:

20. CT   _____

21. LP   _____

22. NICU _____

23. ICP   _____

24. CSF   _____

25. CVA   _____

26. TIA   _____

27. LOC   _____

Chapter 17 Crossword
Nervous System

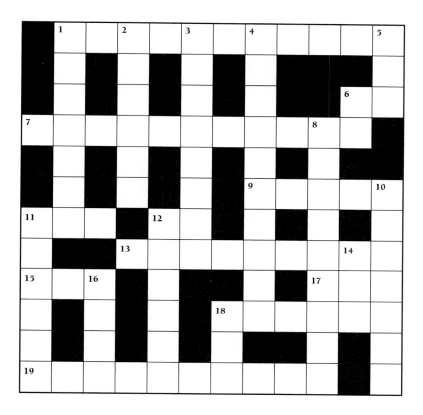

ACROSS

1. A division of the autonomic nervous system
6. Dementia caused by multiple small strokes (abbreviation): __ I __
7. Inflammation of a spinal nerve root
9. Drug used to treat Parkinson disease
11. Electric study of the brain (abbreviation)
12. Fluid around the brain and spinal cord (abbreviation): __ __ F
13. Instrument used for making computerized radiographic images
15. Order related to a patient's activity (abbreviation)
17. A sudden, brief interruption of blood flow to brain tissue (abbreviation)
18. Episodes associated with anxiety disorder
19. Mental state associated with sadness and loss of pleasure in life

DOWN

1. Junction between two neurons
2. Membranes around the brain and spinal cord: root
3. Localized dilation of a blood vessel
4. Paralysis of one side of the body
5. Slow-growing viral disease of the brain (abbreviation)
6. Disease causing progressive loss of myelin in neurons (abbreviation)
8. Feeling associated with depression and other behavioral disorders
10. Loss or defect in speech communication
11. Methods for study of the nervous system: __ __ __ __ __ __ potentials
12. Type of brain injury caused by a blow: __ __ __ __ __ coup
14. Type of catheter (abbreviation): __ __ __ C
16. Method for studying the brain involving auditory stimulation (abbreviation)
18. All of the nervous system except the brain and spinal cord (abbreviation)

CHAPTER 17 Answer Section

Answers to Chapter Exercises

EXERCISE 17-1

1. pertaining to a nerve or the nervous system
2. pertaining to neuroglia, glial cells
3. pertaining to a ganglion
4. pertaining to the meninges
5. pertaining to a spinal nerve root
6. spinal cord
7. nerve
8. meninges
9. spinal nerve roots
10. study of the nervous system
11. radiograph of the spinal cord
12. tumor of the meninges
13. neuralgia (*nū-RAL-jē-a*)
14. neuropathy (*nū-ROP-a-thē*)
15. myelitis (*mī-e-LĪ-tis*)
16. ganglioma (*gang-glē-Ō-ma*)
17. myelography (*mī-e-LOG-ra-fē*)
18. meningitis (*men-in-JĪ-tis*)

EXERCISE 17-2

1. brain
2. cerebrum, brain
3. mind
4. stupor, unconsciousness
5. sleep
6. thalamus
7. cerebral (*SER-e-bral*)
8. cortical (*KOR-ti-kal*)
9. thalamic (*tha-LAM-ik*)
10. cerebellar (*ser-e-BEL-ar*)
11. ventricular (*ven-TRIK-ū-lar*)
12. inflammation of the brain
13. outside the medulla
14. study of the mind
15. pertaining to the brain and spinal cord
16. inflammation of a ventricle
17. lack of sleep, inability to sleep
18. encephalopathy (*en-sef-a-LOP-a-thē*)
19. supracerebellar (*sū-pra-ser-e-BEL-ar*)
20. corticothalamic (*kor-ti-kō-tha-LAM-ik*)
21. ventriculogram (*ven-TRIK-ū-lō-gram*)
22. extracerebral (*eks-tra-SER-e-bral*)

EXERCISE 17-3

1. speech
2. seizures
3. partial paralysis
4. read
5. tetraplegia (*tet-ra-PLĒ-jē-a*)
6. lack of speech communication
7. slowness of reading
8. obsession with fire
9. fear of women
10. bradylalia (*brad-ē-LĀ-lē-a*)
11. hemiplegia (*hem-i-PLĒ-jē-a*)
12. cardioplegia (*kar-dē-ō-PLĒ-jē-a*)
13. noctiphobia (*nok-ti-FŌ-bē-a*); also nyctophobia (*nik-tō-FŌ-bē-a*)
14. photophobia (*fō-tō-FŌ-bē-a*)

LABELING EXERCISE 17-1 ANATOMIC DIVISIONS OF THE NERVOUS SYSTEM

1. brain
2. spinal cord
3. central nervous system
4. cranial nerves
5. spinal nerves
6. peripheral nervous system

LABELING EXERCISE 17-2 MOTOR NEURON

1. dendrites
2. cell body
3. nucleus
4. axon
5. axon branch
6. myelin
7. neuromuscular junction
8. muscle

LABELING EXERCISE 17-3 EXTERNAL SURFACE OF THE BRAIN

1. frontal lobe
2. parietal lobe
3. occipital lobe
4. temporal lobe
5. pons
6. medulla oblongata
7. spinal cord
8. cerebellum

LABELING EXERCISE 17-4 SPINAL CORD AND DIVISIONS OF THE SPINAL NERVES

1. brain
2. brainstem

3. spinal cord
4. cervical nerves
5. thoracic nerves
6. lumbar nerves
7. sacral nerves
8. coccygeal nerve

LABELING EXERCISE 17-5 CROSS-SECTION OF SPINAL CORD AND REFLEX ARC

1. receptor
2. sensory neuron
3. spinal nerve
4. dorsal root ganglion
5. cell body
6. dorsal root
7. central canal
8. gray matter
9. dorsal horn
10. ventral horn
11. white matter
12. interneuron
13. ventral root
14. motor neuron
15. effector

Answers to Chapter Review 17-1

1. e
2. c
3. d
4. b
5. a
6. e
7. c
8. a
9. d
10. b
11. d
12. b
13. e
14. a
15. c
16. d
17. e
18. c
19. a
20. b
21. e
22. d
23. b
24. c
25. a
26. c
27. d
28. b
29. a
30. e
31. d
32. e
33. b
34. a
35. c
36. c
37. e
38. b
39. d
40. a
41. b
42. d
43. a
44. e
45. c
46. e
47. a
48. b
49. d
50. c
51. d
52. e
53. b
54. a
55. c
56. neuron
57. synapse
58. reflex
59. meninges
60. autonomic nervous system
61. cerebellum
62. absence of a brain
63. pertaining to the cerebral cortex and thalamus
64. treatment of disorders of the mind
65. partial paralysis of half the body
66. sleep disorder
67. inflammation of many nerves
68. total paralysis
69. pertaining to a spinal nerve root
70. neurology
71. neuropathy
72. myelomeningitis
73. ganglionectomy; gangliectomy
74. ventriculotomy
75. hemiplegia
76. intracerebellar
77. dyslexia
78. hydrophobia
79. extramedullary
80. contralateral
81. preganglionic

82. bradylalia
83. motor
84. dorsal
85. efferent
86. ganglionic
87. cortical
88. dural
89. meningeal
90. psychotic
91. ganglia
92. ventricles
93. meninges
94. sulci
95. an acute viral disease causing inflammation of the gray matter of the spinal cord
    a. gray
    b. spinal cord
    c. inflammation
96. inflammation of many nerves and nerve roots
    a. many
    b. nerve
    c. spinal nerve root
    d. inflammation
97. disturbance of muscle coordination
    a. abnormal, difficult
    b. together
    c. work
    d. condition of

Answers to Case Study Questions

1. e
2. b
3. a
4. b
5. c
6. e
7. b
8. e
9. astrocytoma
10. craniotomy
11. seizure
12. hemiparesis
13. aphasia
14. meningitis
15. subdural hematoma
16. paranoia
17. antispasmodic
18. neuroleptics
19. psychiatrist
20. computed tomography
21. lumbar puncture
22. neurological intensive care unit (also means neonatal intensive care unit)
23. intracranial pressure
24. cerebrospinal fluid
25. cerebrovascular accident
26. transient ischemic attack
27. level of consciousness

ANSWERS TO CROSSWORD PUZZLE

Nervous System

▮	(1) S	Y	(2) M	P	(3) A	T	(4) H	E	T	I	(5) C
▮	Y	▮	E	▮	N	▮	E	▮	▮	▮	J
▮	N	▮	N	▮	E	▮	M	▮	▮	(6) M	D
(7) R	A	D	I	C	U	L	I	T	(8) I	S	▮
▮	P	▮	N	▮	R	▮	P	▮	S	▮	▮
▮	S	▮	G	▮	Y	▮	(9) L	D	O	P	(10) A
(11) E	E	G	▮	(12) C	S	▮	E	▮	L	▮	P
V	▮	▮	(13) T	O	M	O	G	R	A	(14) P	H
(15) O	O	(16) B	▮	N	▮	▮	I	▮	(17) T	I	A
K	▮	A	▮	T	▮	(18) P	A	N	I	C	S
E	▮	E	▮	R	▮	N	▮	▮	O	▮	I
(19) D	E	P	R	E	S	S	I	O	N	▮	A

The Senses

Chapter Contents

Objectives

After study of this chapter you should be able to:

1. Explain the role of the sensory system.
2. Label diagrams of the ear and the eye, and briefly describe the function of each part.
3. Describe the pathway of nerve impulses from the ear to the brain.
4. Describe the roles of the retina and the optic nerve in vision.
5. Identify and use word parts pertaining to the senses.
6. Describe the main disorders pertaining to the ear and the eye.
7. Interpret abbreviations used in the study of the ear and the eye.
8. Analyze several case studies pertaining to vision or hearing.

The sensory system is our network for detecting stimuli from the internal and external environments. It is needed to maintain homeostasis, provide us with pleasure, and protect us from harm. Pain, for example, is an important warning sign of tissue damage. The energy generated in the various **receptors** of the sensory system must be transmitted to the central nervous system for interpretation.

The Senses

The general senses are widely distributed throughout the body. These senses include pain; touch, the **tactile** sense; pressure; temperature; and **proprioception**, the awareness of body position. The special senses are localized within complex sense organs. These include the chemical senses of **gustation** (taste) and **olfaction** (smell), located in the mouth and nose, respectively; the senses of **hearing** and **equilibrium**, located in the ear; and the sense of **vision**, located in the eye. After a brief introduction, this chapter concentrates on the ear and the eye.

Key Terms: Senses

NORMAL STRUCTURE AND FUNCTION

equilibrium *ē-kwi-LIB-rē-um*	The sense of balance
gustation *gus-TĀ-shun*	The sense of taste
hearing *HĒR-ing*	The sense or perception of sound
olfaction *ol-FAK-shun*	The sense of smell
proprioception *prō-prē-ō-SEP-shun*	The awareness of posture, movement, and changes in equilibrium; receptors are located in muscles, tendons, and joints
receptor *rē-SEP-tor*	A sensory nerve ending or a specialized structure associated with a sensory nerve that responds to a stimulus
tactile *TAK-til*	Pertaining to the sense of touch
vision *VIZH-un*	The sense by which the shape, size, and color of objects are perceived by means of the light they give off

TABLE 18-1 Suffixes Pertaining to the Senses

SUFFIX	MEANING	EXAMPLE	DEFINITION OF EXAMPLE
-esthesia	sensation	cryesthesia *krī-es-THĒ-zē-a*	sensitivity to cold
-algesia	pain	hypalgesia* *hī-pal-JĒ-zē-a*	decreased sensitivity to pain
-osmia	sense of smell	parosmia *par-OS-mē-a*	abnormal (para-) sense of smell
-geusia	sense of taste	pseudogeusia *sū-dō-GŪ-zē-a*	false sense of taste

*Prefix hyp/o.

Exercise 18-1

Define each of the following words:

1. hyperesthesia (*hī-per-es-thē-zē-a*) _____

2. pseudosmia (*sū-DOZ-mē-a*) _____

3. ageusia (*a-GŪ-zē-a*) _____

Write a word that has the same meaning as each of the following definitions:

4. lack (an-) of sensation _____

5. sensitivity to temperature _____

6. excess sensitivity to pain _____

7. abnormal (dys-) sense of taste _____

8. muscular (my/o-) sensation _____

The Ear

The ear has the receptors for both hearing and equilibrium. For study purposes, it may be divided into three parts: the outer, middle, and inner ear (Fig. 18-1).

The outer ear consists of the projecting **pinna** (auricle) and the **external auditory canal** (meatus). This canal ends at the **tympanic membrane** or eardrum, which transmits sound waves to the middle ear. Glands in the external canal produce a waxy material, **cerumen**, which protects the ear and helps to prevent infection.

Spanning the middle ear cavity are three **ossicles** (small bones), each named for its shape: the **malleus** (hammer), **incus** (anvil), and **stapes** (stirrup). Sound waves traveling over the ossicles are transmitted from the footplate of the stapes to the inner ear. The **eustachian tube** connects the middle ear with the nasopharynx and serves to equalize pressure between the outer and middle ear.

The inner ear, because of its complex shape, is described as a **labyrinth** (Fig. 18-2). It consists of an outer bony framework containing a similarly shaped membranous channel. The entire labyrinth is filled with fluid.

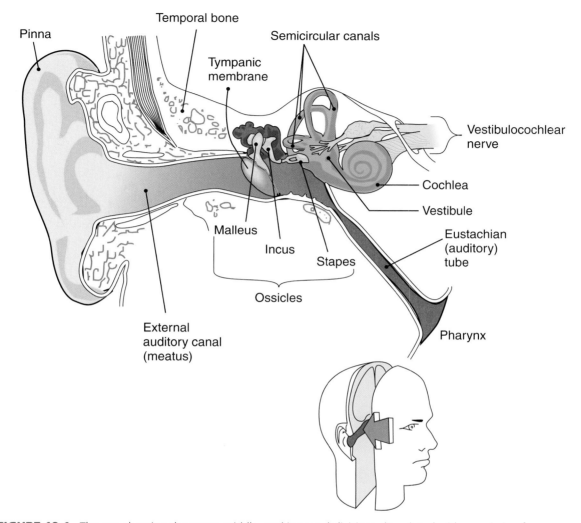

FIGURE 18-1. The ear, showing the outer, middle, and inner subdivisions. (Reprinted with permission from Cohen BJ, Wood DL. Memmler's The Human Body in Health and Disease. 9th Ed. Philadelphia: Lippincott Williams & Wilkins, 2000.)

The **cochlea**, shaped like the shell of a snail, has the specialized **organ of Corti** concerned with hearing. Cells in this receptor organ respond to sound waves traveling through the fluid-filled ducts of the cochlea. Sound waves enter the cochlea from the base of the stapes through an opening called the oval window and leave through another opening called the round window.

The sense of equilibrium is localized in the **vestibular apparatus.** This structure consists of the chamber-like **vestibule** and three projecting **semicircular canals.** Special cells within the vestibular apparatus respond to movement. (The senses of vision and proprioception are also important in maintaining balance.)

Nerve impulses are transmitted from the ear to the brain by way of the **vestibulocochlear nerve**, the eighth cranial nerve, also called the acoustic or auditory nerve. The cochlear branch of this nerve transmits impulses for hearing from the cochlea; the vestibular branch transmits impulses concerned with equilibrium from the vestibular apparatus.

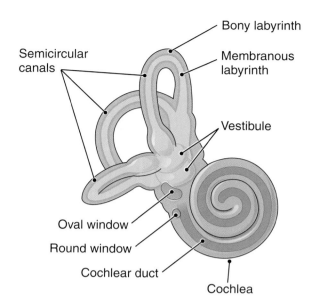

Semicircular canals

Bony labyrinth

Membranous labyrinth

Vestibule

Oval window

Round window

Cochlear duct

Cochlea

FIGURE 18-2. The inner ear. (Reprinted with permission from Smeltzer SC, Bare BG. Brunner & Suddarth's Textbook of Medical-Surgical Nursing. 9th Ed. Philadelphia: Lippincott Williams & Wilkins, 2000.)

Key Terms: The Ear

NORMAL STRUCTURE AND FUNCTION

cerumen *se-RŪ-men*	The brownish, waxlike secretion formed in the external ear canal to protect the ear and prevent infection [adjective, ceruminous (*se-RŪ-mi-nus*)]
cochlea *KOK-lē-a*	The coiled portion of the inner ear that contains the receptors for hearing (root *cochle/o*)
eustachian tube *ū-STĀ-shen*	The tube that connects the middle ear with the nasopharynx and serves to equalize pressure between the outer and middle ear (root *salping/o*)
external auditory canal	Tube that extends from the pinna of the ear to the tympanic membrane; external auditory meatus
incus *ING-kus*	The middle ossicle of the ear
labyrinth *LAB-i-rinth*	The inner ear, named for its complex structure, which resembles a maze
malleus *MAL-ē-us*	The ossicle of the middle ear that is in contact with the tympanic membrane and the incus
ossicles *OS-i-klz*	The small bones of the middle ear, the malleus, incus, and stapes
organ of Corti *KOR-tē*	The hearing receptor, which is located in the cochlea

Normal Structure and Function, *continued*

pinna *PIN-a*	The projecting part of the outer ear; auricle (*AW-ri-kl*)
semicircular canals	The three curved channels of the inner ear that hold receptors for equilibrium
stapes *STĀ-pēz*	The ossicle that is in contact with the inner ear (root *staped, stapedi/o*)
tympanic membrane *tim-PAN-ik*	The membrane between the external auditory canal and the middle ear (tympanic cavity); the eardrum. It serves to transmit sound waves to the ossicles of the middle ear (root *myring/o, tympan/o*).
vestibular apparatus *ves-TIB-ū-lar*	The portion of the inner ear that is concerned with the sense of equilibrium; consists of the vestibule and the semicircular canals (root *vestibul/o*)
vestibule *VES-ti-būl*	The chamber in the inner ear that holds some of the receptors for equilibrium
vestibulocochlear nerve *ves-tib-ū-lō-KOK-lē-ar*	The nerve that transmits impulses for hearing and equilibrium from the ear to the brain; eighth cranial nerve

TABLE 18-2 Roots Pertaining to the Ear and Hearing

ROOT	MEANING	EXAMPLE	DEFINITION OF EXAMPLE
audi/o	hearing	audition *aw-DISH-un*	act of hearing
acous, acus, cus	sound, hearing	acoustic *a-KŪ-stik*	pertaining to sound or hearing
ot/o	ear	ototoxic *ō-tō-TOKS-ik*	poisonous or harmful to the ear
myring/o	tympanic membrane	myringotome *mi-RING-gō-tōm*	knife used for surgery on the eardrum
tympan/o	tympanic cavity (middle ear), tympanic membrane	tympanometry *tim-pa-NOM-e-trē*	measurement of transmission through the tympanic membrane and middle ear
salping/o	tube, eustachian tube	salpingoscopy *sal-PING-gos-kō-pē*	examination of the eustachian tube
staped/o, stapedi/o	stapes	stapedectomy *stā-pē-DEK-tō-me*	excision of the stapes
labyrinth/o	labyrinth (inner ear)	labyrinthotomy *lab-i-rin-THOT-ō-me*	incision of the inner ear (labyrinth)
vestibul/o	vestibule, vestibular apparatus	vestibulopathy *ves-tib-ū-LOP-a-thē*	any disease of the vestibule of the inner ear
cochle/o	cochlea of inner ear	retrocochlear *ret-rō-KOK-lē-ar*	behind the cochlea

Exercise 18-2

Fill in the blanks:

1. Hyperacusis ($h\bar{\imath}$-per-a-$K\bar{U}$-sis) is abnormally high sensitivity to _____.

2. Otogenic ($\bar{o}$-$t\bar{o}$-JEN-ik) means originating in the _____.

Define each of the following adjectives:

3. cochlear (KOK-$l\bar{e}$-ar)   _____

4. vestibular (ves-TIB-$\bar{u}$-lar)   _____

5. labyrinthine (lab-i-RIN-$th\bar{e}n$)   _____

6. stapedial ($st\bar{a}$-$P\bar{E}$-$d\bar{e}$-al)   _____

7. auditory (AW-di-tor-$\bar{e}$)   _____

8. otic ($\bar{O}$-tik)   _____

Word building. Write a word for each of the following definitions:

9. an instrument for measuring hearing (audi/o-)   _____

10. pain in the ear   _____

11. plastic repair of the middle ear   _____

12. incision of the tympanic membrane   _____

13. plastic repair of the stapes   _____

14. pertaining to the vestibular apparatus and cochlea   _____

15. inflammation of the labyrinth   _____

16. instrument used to examine the eustachian tube   _____

Define each of the following words:

17. audiologist (aw-$d\bar{e}$-OL-$\bar{o}$-jist)   _____

18. otitis ($\bar{o}$-$T\bar{I}$-tis)   _____

19. myringoscope (mi-RING-$g\bar{o}$-$sk\bar{o}p$)   _____

20. salpingopharyngeal (sal-ping-$g\bar{o}$-fa-RIN-$j\bar{e}$-al)   _____

21. vestibulotomy (ves-tib-$\bar{u}$-LOT-$\bar{o}$-$m\bar{e}$)   _____

Clinical Aspects of Hearing

Hearing Loss

Hearing impairment may result from disease, injury, or developmental problems that affect the ear itself or any nervous pathways concerned with the sense of hearing. **Sensorineural hearing loss** results from damage to the eighth cranial nerve or to central auditory pathways. Heredity, toxins, exposure to loud noises, and the aging process are possible causes for this type of hearing loss. It may range from inability to hear certain frequencies of sound to a complete loss of hearing (deafness). People with extreme hearing loss that originates in the inner ear may benefit from a cochlear implant. This prosthesis stimulates the cochlear nerve directly, bypassing the receptor cells of the inner ear, and may allow the recipient to hear medium to loud sounds.

Conductive hearing loss results from blockage in sound transmission to the inner ear. Causes include obstruction, severe infection, or fixation of the middle ear ossicles. Often the conditions that cause conductive hearing loss can be treated successfully.

Otitis

Otitis is any inflammation of the ear. **Otitis media** refers to an infection that leads to the accumulation of fluid in the middle ear cavity. One cause is malfunction or obstruction of the eustachian tube, such as by allergy, enlarged adenoids, injury, or congenital abnormalities. Another cause is infection that spreads to the middle ear, most commonly from the upper respiratory tract. Continued infection may lead to accumulation of pus and perforation of the eardrum. Otitis media usually affects children under 5 years of age and may result in hearing loss. If untreated, the infection may spread to other regions of the ear and head. Treatment is with antibiotics. A tube also may be placed in the tympanic membrane to ventilate the middle ear cavity, a procedure called a **myringotomy**.

Otitis externa is inflammation of the external auditory canal. Infections in this region may be caused by a fungus or bacterium and are most common among those living in hot climates and among swimmers, leading to the alternate name, "swimmer's ear."

Otosclerosis

In **otosclerosis**, the bony structure of the inner ear deteriorates and then reforms into spongy bone tissue that may eventually harden. Most commonly, the stapes becomes fixed against the inner ear and is unable to vibrate, resulting in conductive hearing loss. The cause is unknown, but some cases are hereditary. The damaged bone can usually be removed surgically. In a **stapedectomy**, the stapes is removed and a prosthetic bone is inserted.

Ménière Disease

Ménière disease is a disorder that affects the inner ear. It seems to involve the production and circulation of the fluid that fills the inner ear, but the cause is unknown. The symptoms are **vertigo** (dizziness), hearing loss, pronounced **tinnitus** (ringing in the ears), and feeling of pressure in the ear. The course of the disease is uneven, and symptoms may become less severe with time. Ménière disease is treated with drugs to control nausea and dizziness, such as those used to treat motion sickness. In severe cases, the inner ear or part of the eighth cranial nerve may be destroyed surgically.

Acoustic Neuroma

An **acoustic neuroma** (also called a schwannoma or neurilemoma) is a tumor that arises from the neurilemma (sheath) of the eighth cranial nerve. As the tumor enlarges, it presses on surrounding nerves and interferes with blood supply. This leads to tinnitus, dizziness, and progressive hearing loss. Other symptoms develop as the tumor presses on the brainstem and other cranial nerves. Usually it is necessary to remove the tumor surgically.

Key Clinical Terms: The Ear

DISORDERS

acoustic neuroma *a-KŪ-stik*	A tumor of the eighth cranial nerve sheath; although benign, it can press on surrounding tissue and produce symptoms; also called a schwannoma or neurilemoma
conductive hearing loss	Hearing impairment that results from blockage of sound transmission to the inner ear
Ménière disease *men-ē-ĀR*	A disease associated with increased fluid pressure in the inner ear and characterized by hearing loss, vertigo, and tinnitus
otitis externa *ō-TĪ-tis ex-TER-na*	Inflammation of the external auditory canal; swimmer's ear
otitis media *ō-TĪ-tis MĒ-dē-a*	Inflammation of the middle ear with accumulation of watery (serous) or mucoid fluid
otosclerosis *ō-tō-skle-RŌ-sis*	Formation of abnormal and sometimes hardened bony tissue in the ear. It usually occurs around the oval window and the footplate (base) of the stapes, causing immobilization of the stapes and progressive loss of hearing.
sensorineural hearing loss *sen-sō-rē-NŪ-ral*	Hearing impairment that results from damage to the eighth cranial nerve or to auditory pathways in the brain
tinnitus *tin-Ī-tus*	A sensation of noises, such as ringing or tinkling, in the ear
vertigo *VER-ti-gō*	An illusion of movement, as of the body moving in space or the environment moving about the body; usually caused by disturbances in the vestibular apparatus; loosely used to mean dizziness or lightheadedness

TREATMENT

myringotomy *mir-in-GOT-ō-mē*	Surgical incision of the tympanic membrane; performed to drain the middle ear cavity or to insert a tube into the tympanic membrane for drainage
otorhinolaryngology (ORL) *ō-tō-rī-nō-lar-in-GOL-ō-jē*	The branch of medicine that deals with diseases of the ear(s), nose, and throat (ENT); also called otolaryngology (OL)
stapedectomy *stā-pē-DEK-tō-mē*	Surgical removal of the stapes; it may be combined with insertion of a prosthesis to correct otosclerosis

Supplementary Terms

NORMAL STRUCTURE AND FUNCTION

aural *AW-ral*	Pertaining to or perceived by the ear
decibel (dB) *DES-i-bel*	A unit for measuring the relative intensity of sound
hertz (Hz)	A unit for measuring the frequency (pitch) of sound
mastoid process	A small projection of the temporal bone behind the external auditory canal; it consists of loosely arranged bony material and small, air-filled cavities
oval window	An oval opening in the inner ear that is in contact with the footplate of the stapes
stapedius *stā-PĒ-dē-us*	A small muscle attached to the stapes. It contracts in the presence of a loud sound, producing the acoustic reflex.

SYMPTOMS AND CONDITIONS

cholesteatoma *kō-lē-stē-a-TŌ-ma*	A cystlike mass containing cholesterol that is most common in the middle ear and mastoid region; a possible complication of chronic middle ear infection
labyrinthitis *lab-i-rin-THĪ-tis*	Inflammation of the labyrinth of the ear (inner ear); otitis interna
mastoiditis *mas-toyd-Ī-tis*	Inflammation of the air cells of the mastoid process
presbyacusis *prez-bē-a-KŪ-sis*	Loss of hearing caused by aging; also presbyacusia, presbycusis

DIAGNOSIS AND TREATMENT

audiometry *aw-de-OM-e-trē*	Measurement of hearing
electronystagmography (ENG) *ē-lek-trō-nis-tag-MOG-ra-fē*	A method for recording eye movements by means of electrical responses; such movements may reflect vestibular dysfunction
otoscope *Ō-tō-skōp*	Instrument for examining the ear (see Fig. 7-2)
Rinne test	Test that measures hearing by comparing results of bone conduction and air conduction (Fig. 18-3)
spondee *spon-dē*	A two-syllable word with equal stress on each syllable; used in hearing tests; examples are toothbrush, baseball, cowboy, pancake
Weber test	Test for hearing loss that uses a vibrating tuning fork placed at the center of the head (Fig. 18-4)

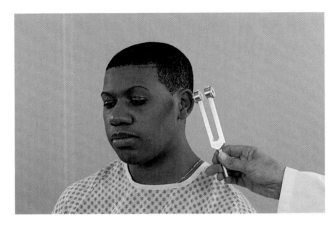

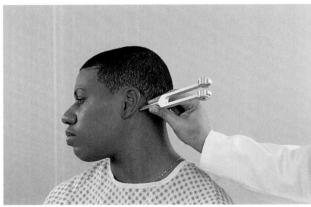

FIGURE 18-3. The Rinne test assesses both air and bone conduction of sound. (Reprinted with permission from Smeltzer SC, Bare BG. Brunner & Suddarth's Textbook of Medical-Surgical Nursing. 9th Ed. Philadelphia: Lippincott Williams & Wilkins, 2000.)

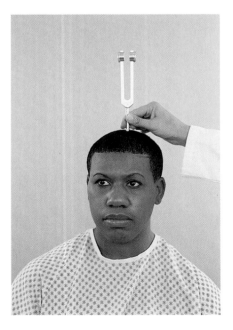

FIGURE 18-4. The Weber test assesses bone conduction of sound. (Reprinted with permission from Smeltzer SC, Bare BG. Brunner & Suddarth's Textbook of Medical-Surgical Nursing. 9th Ed. Philadelphia: Lippincott Williams & Wilkins, 2000.)

ABBREVIATIONS

ABR	Auditory brainstem response	**HL**	Hearing level
AC	Air conduction	**Hz**	Hertz
AD	Right ear (Latin, *Auris dexter*)	**OL**	Otolaryngology
AS	Left ear (Latin, *Auris sinistra*)	**OM**	Otitis media
BAEP	Brainstem auditory evoked potentials	**ORL**	Otorhinolaryngology
BC	Bone conduction	**ST**	Speech threshold
dB	Decibel	**TM**	Tympanic membrane
ENG	Electronystagmography	**TTS**	Temporary threshold shift
ENT	Ear(s), nose, and throat		

The Eye and Vision

The wall of the **eye** is composed of three layers (Fig. 18-5). The outermost is a tough protective layer, the **sclera**, commonly called the *white of the eye*. This layer extends over the front of the eye as the transparent **cornea**. The middle layer is a vascular layer, the **uvea**, which consists of the **choroid**, the **ciliary body**, and the **iris**. The iris, by which we assign the color of the eye, is a muscular ring that controls the size of the **pupil**,

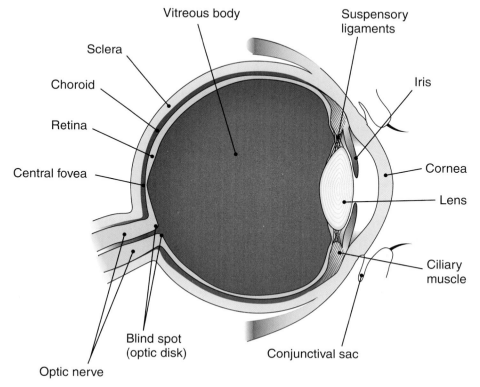

FIGURE 18-5. The eye. (Reprinted with permission from Cohen BJ, Wood DL. Memmler's The Human Body in Health and Disease. 9th Ed. Philadelphia: Lippincott Williams & Wilkins, 2000.)

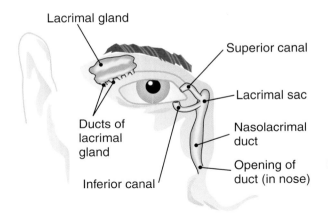

FIGURE 18-6. Lacrimal apparatus. (Reprinted with permission from Cohen BJ, Wood DL. Memmler's The Human Body in Health and Disease. 9th Ed. Philadelphia: Lippincott Williams & Wilkins, 2000.)

thus regulating the amount of light that enters the eye. The ciliary body contains a muscle that controls the shape of the **lens** to allow for near and far vision, a process known as **accommodation**.

The **retina** is the innermost layer and the actual visual receptor. It consists of specialized cells, **rods** and **cones**, which respond to light. The rods function in dim light, have low visual acuity, and do not respond to color. The cones are active in bright light, have high visual acuity, and respond to color. Proper vision requires the **refraction** (bending) of light rays as they pass through the structures of the eye to focus on a specific point on the retina. The energy generated within the rods and cones is transmitted to the brain by way of the optic nerve (second cranial nerve). Where the optic nerve connects to the retina, there are no rods or cones. This point, at which there is no visual perception, is called the **optic disk**, or blind spot. In the retina, near the optic nerve, is the **fovea**, a tiny depression that has a high concentration of cone cells and is the point of greatest **visual acuity** (sharpness). The fovea is surrounded by a yellowish spot called the **macula**.

The eye is protected by its position within a bony socket or **orbit**. It is also protected by the **eyelids**, eyebrows, eyelashes, and tears. The **lacrimal** (tear) **glands** (Fig. 18-6) constantly bathe the eyes with a lubricating fluid that drains into the nose. There is also a protective **conjunctiva**, a thin membrane that lines the eyelids and covers the anterior portion of the eye.

The eyeball is filled with a jellylike **vitreous body** (see Fig. 18-5).

Six muscles attached to the outside of each eye coordinate eye movements to achieve **convergence**, that is, coordinated movement of the eyes so that they both are fixed on the same point.

Key Terms: The Eye

NORMAL STRUCTURE AND FUNCTION

accommodation *a-kom-ō-DĀ-shun*	Adjustment of the curvature of the lens to allow for vision at various distances
conjunctiva *kon-junk-TĪ-va*	The mucous membrane that lines the eyelids and covers the anterior portion of the eyeball
choroid *KOR-oyd*	The dark, vascular, middle layer of the eye; part of the uvea (see below; root *chori/o, choroid/o*)

Normal Structure and Function, continued

ciliary body *SIL-ē-ar-ē*	The muscular portion of the uvea that surrounds the lens and adjusts its shape for near and far vision (root *cycl/o*)
cone	A specialized cell in the retina of the eye that responds to light; cones have high visual acuity, function in bright light, and can discriminate colors
convergence *kon-VER-jens*	Coordinated movement of the eyes toward fixation on the same point
cornea *KOR-nē-a*	The clear, anterior portion of the sclera (root *corne/o, kerat/o*)
eye	The organ of vision (root *opt/o, ocul/o, ophthalm/o*)
eyelid	A protective fold (upper and lower) that closes over the anterior surface of the eye (root *palpebr/o, blephar/o*)
fovea *FŌ-vē-a*	The tiny depression in the retina that is the point of sharpest vision; fovea centralis, central fovea
iris *Ī-ris*	The muscular colored ring between the lens and the cornea; regulates the amount of light that enters the eye by altering the size of the pupil at its center (plural, irides) (roots *ir, irid/o, irit/o*)
lacrimal glands *LAK-ri-mal*	Pertaining to tears (roots *lacrim/o, dacry/o*)
lens *lenz*	The transparent, biconvex structure in the anterior portion of the eye that refracts light and functions in accommodation (roots *lent/i, phak/o*)
macula *MAK-ū-la*	A small spot or colored area; used alone to mean the yellowish spot in the retina that contains the fovea
optic disk	The point where the optic nerve joins the retina; at this point there are no rods or cones; also called the blind spot or optic papilla
orbit *OR-bit*	The bony cavity that contains the eyeball
pupil *PŪ-pil*	The opening at the center of the iris (*pupill/o*)
refraction *rē-FRAK-shun*	The bending of light rays as they pass through the eye to focus on a specific point on the retina; also the determination and correction of ocular refractive errors
retina *RET-i-na*	The innermost, light-sensitive layer of the eye; contains the rods and cones, the specialized receptor cells for vision (root *retin/o*)
rod	A specialized cell in the retina of the eye that responds to light; rods have low visual acuity, function in dim light, and do not discriminate color
sclera *SKLĒR-a*	The tough, white, fibrous outermost layer of the eye; the white of the eye (root *scler/o*)

Normal Structure and Function, continued	
uvea *Ū-vē-a*	The middle, vascular layer of the eye; consists of the choroid, ciliary body, and iris (root *uve/o*)
visual acuity *a-KŪ-i-tē*	Sharpness of vision; commonly measured with the Snellen eye chart
vitreous body *VIT-rē-us*	The transparent jellylike mass that fills the main cavity of the eyeball; also called vitreous humor

Word Parts Pertaining to the Eye and Vision

TABLE 18-3 Roots for External Eye Structures

ROOT	MEANING	EXAMPLE	DEFINITION OF EXAMPLE
palpebr/o	eyelid	palpebral *PAL-pe-bral*	pertaining to an eyelid
blephar/o	eyelid	symblepharon *sim-BLEF-a-ron*	adhesion of the eyelid to the eyeball
lacrim/o	tear, lacrimal apparatus	lacrimation *lak-ri-MA-shun*	secretion of tears
dacry/o	tear, lacrimal apparatus	dacryolith *DAK-rē-ō-lith*	stone in the lacrimal apparatus
dacryocyst/o	lacrimal sac	dacryocystocele *dak-rē-ō-SIS-tō-sēl*	hernia of the lacrimal sac

Exercise 18-3

Define each of the following words:

1. interpalpebral (*in-ter-PAL-pe-bral*) _____

2. blepharoplegia (*BLEF-a-rō-plē-jē-a*) _____

3. nasolacrimal (*nā-zō-LAK-ri-mal*) _____

4. dacryocystectomy (*dak-rē-ō-sis-TEK-tō-mē*) _____

Word building. Use the roots indicated to write a word with each of the following meanings:

5. spasm of the eyelid (blephar/o) _____

6. discharge from the lacrimal apparatus (dacry/o) _____

7. inflammation of a lacrimal sac _____

BOX 18-1 The Greek Influence

Some of our most beautiful (and difficult to spell and pronounce) words come from Greek. Esthesi/o means sensation. It appears in the word *anesthesia*, a state in which there is lack of sensation, particularly pain. It is found in the word *esthetics* (also spelled aesthetics), which pertains to beauty, artistry, and appearance. The prefix *presby*, in the terms *presbyacusis* and *presbyopia*, means "old," and these conditions appear with aging. The root *cyclo*, pertaining to the ringlike ciliary body of the eye, is from the Greek word for circle or wheel. The same root appears in the words *bicycle* and *tricycle*. Also pertaining to the eye, the term *iris* means "rainbow" in Greek, and the iris is the colored part of the eye.

The root *-sthen/o* means "strength," and occurs in the words *asthenia*, meaning lack of strength or weakness, and *neurasthenia*, an old term for vague "nervous exhaustion," now applied to conditions involving chronic symptoms of generalized fatigue, anxiety, and pain. The root also appears in the word *calisthenics* in combination with the root *cali-*, meaning "beauty." So the rhythmic strengthening and conditioning exercises that are done in calisthenics literally give us beauty through strength.

The Greek root *steth/o* means "chest," although a stethoscope is used to listen to sounds in other parts of the body as well as the chest. *Asphyxia* is from a Greek word meaning "stoppage of the pulse," which is exactly what happens when one suffocates.

A sphygmomanometer, used to measure blood pressure, also contains the Greek root for pulse. One look at the word and one attempt to pronounce it make clear why most people call the apparatus a blood pressure cuff.

TABLE 18-4 Roots for the Eye and Vision

ROOT	MEANING	EXAMPLE	DEFINITION OF EXAMPLE
opt/o	eye, vision	optometer *op-TOM-e-ter*	instrument for measuring the refractive power of the eye
ocul/o	eye	dextrocular *deks-TROK-ū-lar*	pertaining to the right eye
ophthalm/o	eye	exophthalmos *eks-of-THAL-mos*	protrusion of the eyeball
scler/o	sclera	subscleral *sub-SKLĒR-al*	below the sclera
corne/o	cornea	circumcorneal *sir-kum-KOR-nē-al*	around the cornea
kerat/o	cornea	keratoplasty *KER-a-tō-plas-tē*	plastic repair of the cornea; corneal transplant
lent/i	lens	lenticular *len-TIK-ū-lar*	pertaining to the lens
phak/o, phac/o	lens	aphakia *a-FĀ-kē-a*	absence of a lens
uve/o	uvea	uveitis *ū-vē-Ī-tis*	inflammation of the uvea

TABLE 18-4 Roots for the Eye and Vision, *continued*

ROOT	MEANING	EXAMPLE	DEFINITION OF EXAMPLE
chori/o, choroid/o	choroid	choroidal *kor-OYD-al*	pertaining to the choroid
cycl/o	ciliary body, ciliary muscle	cycloplegic *sī-klō-PLĒ-jik*	pertaining to or causing paralysis of the ciliary muscle
ir, irit/o, irid/o	iris	iridotomy *ir-i-DOT-ō-mē*	incision of the iris
pupill/o	pupil	iridopupillary *ir-i-dō-PŪ-pi-ler-ē*	pertaining to the iris and the pupil
retin/o	retina	retinoschisis *ret-i-NOS-ki-sis*	splitting of the retina

Exercise 18-4

Fill in the blanks:

1. The science of orthoptics (*or-THOP-tiks*) deals with correcting defects in

   _____.

2. The oculomotor (*ok-ū-lō-MŌ-tor*) nerve controls movements of the

   _____.

3. A keratometer (*ker-a-TOM-e-ter*) is an instrument for measuring the curves of the

   _____.

4. The term phacolysis (*fa-KOL-i-sis*) means destruction of the _____.

5. Lenticonus is conical protrusion of the _____.

Identify and define the roots pertaining to the eye in the following words:

	Root	Meaning of Root
6. microphthalmos (*mī-krof-THAL-mus*)	_____	_____
7. interpupillary (*in-ter-PŪ-pi-ler-ē*)	_____	_____
8. lentiform (*LEN-ti-form*)	_____	_____
9. uveal (*Ū-vē-al*)	_____	_____
10. phacotoxic (*fak-ō-TOK-sik*)	_____	_____
11. iridodilator (*ir-id-ō-DĪ-lā-tor*)	_____	_____
12. retinoscopy (*ret-in-OS-kō-pē*)	_____	_____
13. optometrist (*op-TOM-e-trist*)	_____	_____

Write a word that has the same meaning as each of the following definitions:

14. inflammation of the uvea and sclera _____

15. softening of the lens (use phac/o) _____

16. pertaining to the pupil _____

17. inflammation of the ciliary body _____

18. any disease of the retina _____

Use the root *ophthalm/o* to write a word that has the same meaning as each of the following definitions:

19. an instrument used to examine the eye _____

20. the medical specialty that deals with the eye and diseases of the eye _____

Use the root *irid/o* to write a word that has the same meaning as each of the following definitions:

21. surgical removal of (part of) the iris _____

22. paralysis of the iris _____

Define each of the following words:

23. optical (*OP-ti-kal*) _____

24. intraocular (*in-tra-OK-ū-lar*) _____

25. iridoschisis (*ir-i-DOS-ki-sis*) _____

26. sclerotome (*SKLĒR-ō-tōm*) _____

27. keratitis (*ker-a-TĪ-tis*) _____

28. retrolental (*ret-rō-LEN-tal*) _____

29. cyclotomy (*sī-KLOT-ō-mē*) _____

30. chorioretinal (*kor-ē-ō-RET-i-nal*) _____

31. iridocyclitis (*ir-i-dō-sī-KLĪ-tis*) _____

Table 18-5 Suffixes for the Eye and Vision*

SUFFIX	MEANING	EXAMPLE	DEFINITION OF EXAMPLE
-opsia	vision	heteropsia het-er-OP-sē-a	unequal vision in the two eyes
-opia	eye, vision	hemianopia hem-ē-an-Ō-pe-a	blindness in half the visual field

*Compounds of *-ops* (eye) + *-ia*.

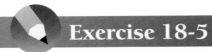

Exercise 18-5

Use the suffix *-opsia* to write a word that has the same meaning as each of the following definitions:

1. a visual defect in which objects seem larger (macr/o) than they are

   _____

2. lack of (a-) color (chromat/o) vision (complete color blindness) _____

Use the suffix *-opia* to write a word that has the same meaning as each of the following definitions:

3. double vision _____

4. changes in vision due to old age (use the prefix *presby-* meaning "old")

   _____

The suffix *-opia* is added to the root *metr/o* (measure) to form words pertaining to the refractive power of the eye. Add a prefix to *-metropia* to form a word that has the same meaning as each of the following definitions:

5. a lack of perfect refractive power in the eye _____

6. unequal refractive powers in the two eyes _____

Clinical Aspects of Vision

Errors of Refraction

If the eyeball is too long, images will form in front of the retina. To focus clearly, an object must be brought closer to the eye. This condition of nearsightedness is technically called **myopia** (Fig. 18-7). The opposite condition is **hyperopia**, or farsightedness, in which the eyeball is too short and images form behind the retina. Objects must be moved away from the eye for the focus to be clear. The same effect is produced by **presbyopia**, which accompanies aging. The lens loses elasticity and can no longer accommodate for near vision. The person becomes increasingly farsighted. An **astigmatism** is an irregularity in the curve of the cornea or lens that distorts light entering the eye and blurs vision. Glasses can compensate for most of these impairments.

Infection

Several microorganisms can cause **conjunctivitis** (inflammation of the conjunctiva). This is a highly infectious disease commonly called pinkeye.

The bacterium *Chlamydia trachomatis* causes **trachoma**, inflammation of the cornea and conjunctiva that results in scarring. This disease is rare in the United States but is a common cause of blindness in underdeveloped countries, although it is easily cured with sulfa drugs and antibiotics.

Gonorrhea is the usual cause of an acute conjunctivitis in newborns called **ophthalmia neonatorum**. An antibiotic ointment is routinely used to prevent such eye infections in newborns.

Disorders of the Retina

Retinal detachment, separation of the retina from the underlying layer of the eye (the choroid), may be caused by a tumor, hemorrhage, or injury to the eye (Fig. 18-8). This condition interferes with vision and is commonly repaired with laser surgery.

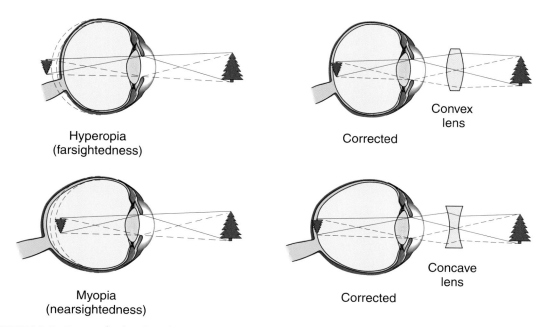

Hyperopia
(farsightedness)

Corrected

Convex
lens

Myopia
(nearsightedness)

Corrected

Concave
lens

FIGURE 18-7. Errors of refraction. (Reprinted with permission from Cohen BJ, Wood DL. Memmler's The Human Body in Health and Disease. 9th Ed. Philadelphia: Lippincott Williams & Wilkins, 2000.)

Degeneration of the macula, the point of sharpest vision, is a common cause of visual problems in the elderly. When associated with aging, this deterioration is described as **age-related macular degeneration** (AMD). Macular degeneration typically affects central vision but not peripheral vision (Fig. 18-9). Other causes of macular degeneration are drug toxicity and hereditary diseases.

Circulatory problems associated with diabetes mellitus eventually cause changes in the retina referred to as **diabetic retinopathy**. In addition to vascular damage, there is a yellowish, waxy exudate high in lipopro-

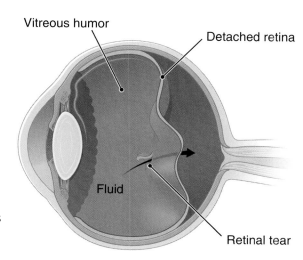

Vitreous humor

Detached retina

Fluid

Retinal tear

FIGURE 18-8. Retinal detachment. (Reprinted with permission from Smeltzer SC, Bare BG. Brunner & Suddarth's Textbook of Medical-Surgical Nursing. 9th Ed. Philadelphia: Lippincott Williams & Wilkins, 2000.)

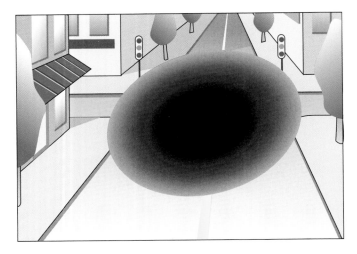

FIGURE 18-9. Visual loss associated with macular degeneration. (Reprinted with permission from Smeltzer SC, Bare BG. Brunner & Suddarth's Textbook of Medical-Surgical Nursing. 9th Ed. Philadelphia: Lippincott Williams & Wilkins, 2000.)

teins. With time, new blood vessels form and penetrate the vitreous humor, causing hemorrhage, detachment of the retina, and blindness.

Cataract

A **cataract** is an opacity (cloudiness) of the lens. Causes of cataract include disease, injury, chemicals, and exposure to physical forces, especially the ultraviolet radiation in sunlight. The cataracts that frequently appear with age may result from exposure to environmental factors in combination with degeneration attributable to aging. To prevent blindness, the cloudy lens must be removed surgically. Commonly, the anterior capsule of the lens is removed along with the cataract, leaving the posterior capsule in place (Fig. 18-10). In

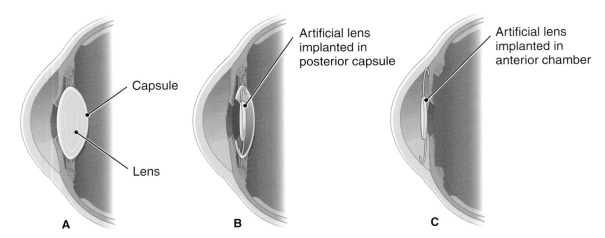

FIGURE 18-10. Cataract extraction surgeries. **(A)** Cross-section of normal eye anatomy. **(B)** Extracapsular lens extraction involves removing the lens but leaving the posterior capsule intact to receive a synthetic intraocular lens. **(C)** Intracapsular lens extraction involves removing the lens and lens capsule and implanting a synthetic intraocular lens in the anterior chamber.

phacoemulsification, the lens is fragmented with high-frequency ultrasound and extracted through a small incision. Often, after cataract removal, an artificial intraocular lens (IOL) is implanted to compensate for the missing lens. Alternatively, the person can wear a contact lens or special glasses.

Glaucoma

Glaucoma is an abnormal increase in pressure within the eyeball. It occurs when more aqueous humor is produced than can be drained away from the eye. There is pressure on blood vessels in the eye and on the optic nerve, leading to blindness. There are many causes of glaucoma, and screening for glaucoma should be a part of every routine eye examination. Fetal infection with German measles (rubella) early in pregnancy can cause glaucoma, as well as cataracts and hearing impairment. Glaucoma is usually treated with medication to reduce pressure in the eye and occasionally is treated with surgery.

Key Clinical Terms: The Eye

astigmatism *a-STIG-ma-tizm*	An error of refraction caused by irregularity in the curvature of the cornea or lens
cataract *KAT-a-rakt*	Opacity of the lens of the eye
conjunctivitis *kon-junk-ti-VĪ-tis*	Inflammation of the conjunctiva; pinkeye
diabetic retinopathy *ret-i-NOP-a-thē*	Degenerative changes in the retina associated with diabetes mellitus
glaucoma *glaw-KŌ-ma*	A disease of the eye caused by increased intraocular pressure that damages the optic disk and causes loss of vision. Usually results from faulty drainage of fluids from the anterior portion of the eye.
hyperopia *hī-per-Ō-pē-a*	An error of refraction in which light rays focus behind the retina and objects can be seen clearly only when far from the eye; farsightedness; also called hypermetropia
myopia *mī-Ō-pē-a*	An error of refraction in which light rays focus in front of the retina and objects can be seen clearly only when very close to the eye; nearsightedness
ophthalmia neonatorum *of-THAL-mē-a* *nē-ō-nā-TOR-um*	Severe conjunctivitis usually caused by infection with gonococcus during birth
phacoemulsification *fak-ō-ē-MUL-si-fi-kā-shun*	Removal of a cataract by ultrasonic destruction and extraction of the lens
presbyopia *prez-bē-Ō-pē-a*	Changes in the eye that occur with age; the lens loses elasticity and the ability to accommodate for near vision
retinal detachment	Separation of the retina from the underlying layer of the eye

senile macular degeneration (SMD)	Deterioration of the macula associated with aging; impairs central vision
trachoma *tra-KŌ-ma*	An infection caused by *Chlamydia trachomatis* leading to inflammation and scarring of the cornea and conjunctiva; a common cause of blindness in underdeveloped countries

Supplementary Terms: The Eye

NORMAL STRUCTURE AND FUNCTION

canthus *KAN-thus*	The angle at either end of the slit between the eyelids
diopter *DĪ-op-ter*	A unit of measurement for the refractive power of a lens
emmetropia *em-e-TRŌ-pē-a*	The normal condition of the eye in refraction, in which parallel light rays focus exactly on the retina
fundus *FUN-dus*	A bottom or base; the region farthest from the opening of a structure. The fundus of the eye is the back portion of the inside of the eyeball as seen with an ophthalmoscope.
meibomian gland *mī-BŌ-mē-an*	A sebaceous gland in the eyelid
tarsus *TAR-sus*	The framework of dense connective tissue that gives shape to the eyelid; tarsal plate
zonule *ZON-ūl*	A system of fibers that holds the lens in place; also called suspensory ligaments

SYMPTOMS AND CONDITIONS

amblyopia *am-blē-Ō-pē-a*	A condition that occurs when visual acuity is not the same in the two eyes in children. (Prefix *ambly* means "dim.") Disuse of the poorer eye will result in blindness if not corrected. Also called "lazy eye."
blepharoptosis *blef-a-rop-TŌ-sis*	Drooping of the eyelid
chalazion *ka-LĀ-zē-on*	A small mass on the eyelid resulting from inflammation and blockage of a meibomian gland
druzen *DRŪ-zen*	Small growths that appear as tiny yellowish spots beneath the retina of the eye; typically occur with age but also occur in certain abnormal conditions
hordeolum *hor-DĒ-ō-lum*	Inflammation of a sebaceous gland of the eyelid; a sty

Symptoms and Conditions, continued

keratoconus *ker-a-tō-KŌ-nus*	Conical protrusion of the center of the cornea
miosis *mī-Ō-sis*	Abnormal contraction of the pupils (from Greek, meaning "diminution")
mydriasis *mi-DRĪ-a-sis*	Pronounced or abnormal dilation of the pupil
night blindness	Difficulty in seeing at night because of lack of vitamin A, which is used to make the pigment needed for vision in dim light
nyctalopia *nik-ta-LŌ-pē-a*	Inability to see well in dim light or at night; night blindness (root *nyct/o* means "night")
nystagmus *nis-TAG-mus*	Rapid, involuntary, rhythmic movements of the eyeball; may occur in neurologic diseases or disorders of the vestibular apparatus of the inner ear
papilledema *pap-il-e-DĒ-ma*	Swelling of the optic disk (papilla); choked disk
phlyctenule *FLIK-ten-ūl*	A small blister or nodule on the cornea or conjunctiva
pseudophakia *sū-dō-FĀ-kē-a*	A condition in which a cataractous lens has been removed and replaced with a plastic lens implant
retinitis *ret-in-Ī-tis*	Inflammation of the retina; causes include systemic disease, infection, hemorrhage, exposure to light
retinitis pigmentosa *ret-in-Ī-tis pig-men-TŌ-sa*	A hereditary chronic degenerative disease of the retina that begins in early childhood. There is atrophy of the optic nerve and clumping of pigment in the retina.
retinoblastoma *ret-in-ō-blas-TŌ-ma*	A malignant glioma of the retina; usually appears in early childhood and is sometimes hereditary; fatal if untreated, but current cure rates are high
scotoma *skō-TŌ-ma*	An area of diminished vision within the visual field
strabismus *stra-BIZ-mus*	A deviation of the eye in which the visual lines of each eye are not directed to the same object at the same time. Also called heterotropia or squint. The various forms are referred to as *-tropias*, with the direction of turning indicated by a prefix, such as esotropia (inward), exotropia (outward), hypertropia (upward), and hypotropia (downward). The suffix *-phoria* is also used, as in esophoria.
synechia *sin-EK-ē-a*	Adhesion of parts, especially adhesion of the iris to the lens and cornea (plural, synechiae)
xanthoma *zan-THŌ-ma*	A soft, slightly raised, yellowish patch or nodule usually on the eyelids; occurs in the elderly; also called xanthelasma

DIAGNOSIS AND TREATMENT

canthotomy *kan-THOT-ō-mē*	Surgical division of a canthus
cystitome *SIS-ti-tōm*	Instrument for incising the capsule of the lens
electroretinography (ERG) *ē-lek-trō-ret-i-NOG-ra-fē*	Study of the electrical response of the retina to light stimulation
enucleation *ē-nū-klē-Ā-shun*	Surgical removal of the eyeball
gonioscopy *gō-nē-OS-kō-pē*	Examination of the angle between the cornea and the iris (anterior chamber angle) where fluids drain out of the eye (root *goni/o* means "angle")
keratometer *ker-a-TOM-e-ter*	An instrument for measuring the curvature of the cornea
mydriatic *mid-rē-AT-ik*	A drug that causes dilation of the pupil
phorometer *fo-ROM-e-ter*	An instrument for determining the degree and kind of strabismus
retinoscope *RET-in-ō-skōp*	An instrument used to determine refractive errors of the eye; also called a skiascope (*SKĪ-a-skōp*)
slit lamp biomicroscope	An instrument for examining the eye under magnification
tarsorrhaphy *tar-SOR-a-fē*	Suturing together of all or part of the upper and lower eyelids
tonometer *tō-NOM-e-ter*	An instrument used to measure the pressure of fluids in the eye

ABBREVIATIONS

A, Acc	Accommodation		**IOP**	Intraocular pressure
AMD	Age-related macular degeneration		**NRC**	Normal retinal correspondence
ARC	Abnormal retinal correspondence		**NV**	Near vision
As, AST	Astigmatism		**OD**	Right eye (Latin, *oculus dexter*)
cc	With correction		**ORL**	Otorhinolaryngology
Em	Emmetropia		**OS**	Left eye (Latin, *oculus sinister*)
EOM	Extraocular movement, muscles		**OU**	Both eyes (Latin, *oculi unitas*); also each eye (Latin, *oculus uterque*)
ERG	Electroretinography			
ET	Esotropia		**sc**	Without correction
FC	Finger counting		**VA**	Visual acuity
HM	Hand movements		**VF**	Visual field
IOL	Intraocular lens		**XT**	Exotropia

Labeling Exercise 18-1

The Ear

Write the name of each numbered part on the corresponding line of the answer sheet.

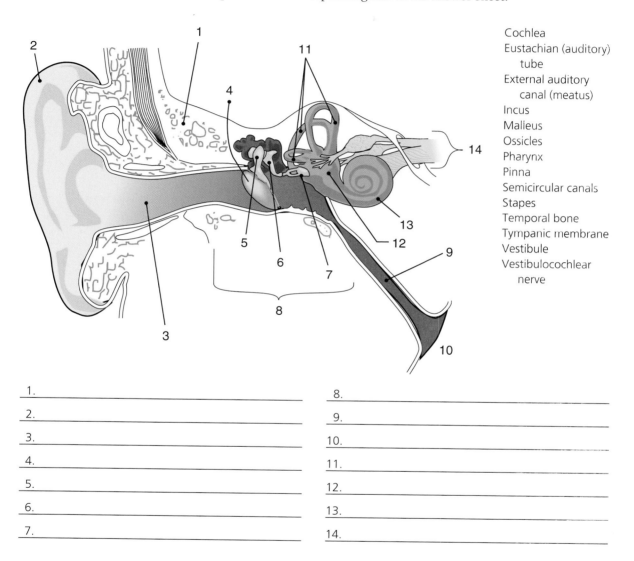

Cochlea
Eustachian (auditory)
    tube
External auditory
    canal (meatus)
Incus
Malleus
Ossicles
Pharynx
Pinna
Semicircular canals
Stapes
Temporal bone
Tympanic membrane
Vestibule
Vestibulocochlear
    nerve

1. _____
2. _____
3. _____
4. _____
5. _____
6. _____
7. _____

8. _____
9. _____
10. _____
11. _____
12. _____
13. _____
14. _____

Labeling Exercise 18-2

The Eye

Write the name of each numbered part on the corresponding line of the answer sheet.

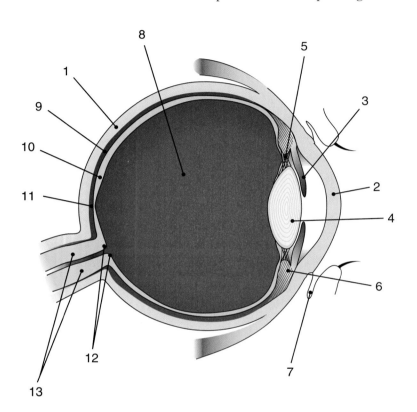

Blind spot (optic disk)
Choroid
Ciliary muscle
Conjunctival sac
Cornea
Fovea centralis
Iris
Lens
Optic nerve
Retina
Sclera
Suspensory ligaments
Vitreous body

1. _____   8. _____
2. _____   9. _____
3. _____   10. _____
4. _____   11. _____
5. _____   12. _____
6. _____   13. _____
7. _____

Chapter Review 18-1

Match the following terms and write the appropriate letter to the left of each number:

_____ 1. myesthesia

_____ 2. parosmia

_____ 3. nyctalopia

_____ 4. hypergeusia

_____ 5. hemianopia

a. night blindness

b. abnormal increase in the sense of taste

c. muscular sensation

d. abnormal smell perception

e. blindness in half the visual field

_____ 6. proprioception

_____ 7. tactile

_____ 8. vitreous body

_____ 9. olfaction

_____ 10. gustation

a. sense of smell

b. sense of taste

c. pertaining to touch

d. awareness of body position

e. material that fills the eyeball

_____ 11. lens

_____ 12. sclera

_____ 13. conjunctiva

_____ 14. vestibular apparatus

_____ 15. eustachian tube

a. membrane that lines the eyelid

b. structure that changes shape for near and far vision

c. passage that connects the middle ear and pharynx

d. part of the ear that contains the receptors for equilibrium

e. outermost layer of the eye

_____ 16. fovea

_____ 17. labyrinth

_____ 18. rods and cones

_____ 19. ossicles

_____ 20. iris

a. inner ear

b. point of sharpest vision

c. small bones of the middle ear

d. receptors for vision

e. muscular ring that regulates light entering the eye

_____ 21. anacusis

_____ 22. tinnitus

_____ 23. achromatopsia

_____ 24. cataract

_____ 25. myopia

a. complete color blindness

b. opacity of the lens

c. nearsightedness

d. sensation of noises in the ear

e. total loss of hearing

_____ 26. hemotympanum

a. corneal transplant

_____ 27. phacosclerosis

b. blood in the middle ear

_____ 28. blepharedema

c. excessive flow of tears

_____ 29. keratoplasty

d. swelling of the eyelid

_____ 30. dacryorrhea

e. hardening of the lens

SUPPLEMENTARY TERMS

_____ 31. aural

a. loss of hearing due to age

_____ 32. mastoid process

b. unit for measuring the frequency of sound

_____ 33. stapedius

c. bony projection of the temporal bone

_____ 34. presbycusis

d. small muscle attached to an ear ossicle

_____ 35. hertz

e. pertaining to the ear

_____ 36. fundus

a. abnormal contraction of the pupil

_____ 37. diopter

b. deviation of the eye

_____ 38. miosis

c. back portion of the eye

_____ 39. strabismus

d. rapid, involuntary eye movements

_____ 40. nystagmus

e. unit for measuring the refractive power of the lens

_____ 41. xanthoma

a. surgical removal of the eye

_____ 42. emmetropia

b. a raised, yellowish patch on the eyelid

_____ 43. tonometer

c. night blindness

_____ 44. enucleation

d. instrument used to measure pressure in the eye

_____ 45. nyctalopia

e. normal refraction of the eye

_____ 46. As

a. unit for measuring the intensity of sound

_____ 47. VA

b. study of the ears, nose, and throat

_____ 48. dB

c. sharpness of vision

_____ 49. OU

d. both eyes

_____ 50. ORL

e. irregularity in the curve of the eye

Fill in the blanks:

51. The coiled portion of the inner ear that contains the receptor for hearing is the

_____.

52. The waxy material secreted into the external ear canal is _____.

53. The ossicle that is in contact with the inner ear is the _____.

54. The innermost layer of the eye that contains the receptors for vision is the

_____.

55. The bending of light rays as they pass through the eye is _____.

56. The transparent extension of the sclera that covers the front of the eye is the

_____.

57. The scientific name for the eardrum is _____.

58. The muscular ring that adjusts the size of the pupil is the _____.

Define each of the following words:

59. audiology _____

60. aphakia _____

61. hyposcleral _____

62. ophthalmometer _____

63. keratoiritis _____

64. iridotomy _____

65. circumlental _____

66. chorioretinal _____

67. myringitis _____

Word building. Write a word for each of the following definitions:

68. absence of pain _____

69. drooping of the eyelid _____

70. surgical removal of the stapes _____

71. plastic repair of the ear _____

72. measurement of the pupil _____

73. any disease of the retina _____

74. pertaining to tears _____

75. surgical incision of the tympanic membrane _____

76. instrument for examination of the eustachian tube _____

77. pertaining to the vestibular apparatus and cochlea _____

78. excision of (part of) the ciliary body _____

Adjectives. Write the adjective form of each of the following words:

79. cochlea _____

80. uvea _____

81. vestibule _____

82. sclera   _____

83. pupil   _____

84. cornea   _____

Opposites. Write a word that has the opposite meaning of each of the following words:

85. miosis   _____

86. esotropia   _____

87. cc   _____

88. myopia   _____

89. hypoesthesia   _____

90. AD   _____

Word analysis. Define each of the following words, and give the meaning of the word parts in each. Use a dictionary if necessary.

91. anisometropia (*an-Ī-sō-me-TRŌ-pē-a*) _____
    a. an-   _____
    b. iso-   _____
    c. metr/o _____
    d. -opia   _____

92. paresthesia (*par-es-THĒ-zē-a*) _____
    a. par/a   ___abnormal___
    b. esthesi/o _____
    c. -ia   _____

93. hemianopia (*hem-ē-an-Ō-pē-a*) _____
    a. hemi- _____
    b. an-   _____
    c. -opia _____

94. hyperchromatopsia (*hī-per-krō-ma-TOP-sē-a*) _____
    a. hyper-   _____
    b. chromat/o _____
    c. -opsia   _____

Case Studies

Case Study 18-1: Medical Records

An electrical fire in the physicians' dictation room left a charred mass of burned and water-damaged medical records. Discharge charts had been stacked awaiting physician sign-off before they could be returned to Medical Records for storage. Several medical transcriptionists spent 3 days sorting through the remains to reassemble the charts, all of which were from the patients of the large otorhinolaryngology practice. In addition to patient identification information, the transcriptionists matched word cues to create piles of similar documents. Middle ear and inner ear patients were identified with words such as stapedectomy, tympanoplasty, myringotomy, cochlear, cholesteatoma, otosclerosis, labyrinth, otitis media, and acoustic neuroma. External ear patients were grouped using terms such as otoplasty, pinna, postauricular, and otitis externa. Mastoid, laryngeal, and nasal surgery patients were grouped separately. Restoring the charts was an impossible task, and the records were determined to be either incomplete or a total loss. The only document to survive the fire was an audiology report.

Case Study 18-2: Audiology Report

S.R., a 55-year-old man, was seen with the complaint of decreased hearing sensitivity in his left ear for the past 3 years. In addition to hearing loss, he was experiencing tinnitus and aural fullness. Pure tone test results revealed normal hearing sensitivity for the right ear and a moderate sensorineural hearing loss in the left ear. Speech thresholds were appropriate for the degree of hearing loss noted. Word recognition was excellent for the right ear and poor for the left ear when the signal was present at a suprathreshold level. Tympanograms were characterized by normal shape, amplitude, and peak pressure points bilaterally. The contralateral acoustic reflex was normal for the right ear but absent for the left ear at the frequencies tested (500 to 4000 Hz). The ipsilateral acoustic reflex was present with the probe in the right ear and absent with the probe in the left ear. Brainstem auditory evoked potentials (BAEP) were within normal range for the right ear. No repeatable response was observed from the left ear. A subsequent MRI showed a 1-cm acoustic neuroma.

Case Study 18-3: Phacoemulsification With Intraocular Lens Implant

W.S., a 68-year-old woman, was scheduled for surgery for a cataract and relief from "floaters," which she had noticed in her visual field since her surgery for a retinal detachment last year. She reported to the ambulatory surgery center an hour before her scheduled procedure. Before transfer to the operating room, she spoke with her ophthalmologist and reviewed the surgical plan. Her right eye was identified as the operative eye and it was marked with a "yes" and the surgeon's initials on the lid. She was given anesthetic drops in the right eye and an intravenous bolus of 2.0 mg of midazolam (Versed).

In the OR, W.S. and her operative eye were again identified by the surgeon, anesthetist, and nurses. After anesthesia and akinesia were achieved, the eye area was prepped and draped in sterile sheets. An operating microscope with video system was positioned over her eye. A 5-0 silk suture was placed through the superior rectus muscle to retract the eye. A lid speculum was placed to open the eye. A minimal conjunctival peritotomy was performed, and hemostasis was achieved with wet-field cautery. The anterior chamber was entered at the 10:30 o'clock position. A capsulotomy was performed after Healon was placed in the anterior chamber. Phacoemulsification was carried out without difficulty. The remaining cortex was removed by irrigation and aspiration.

Case Studies, continued

An intraocular lens (IOL) was placed into the posterior chamber. Miochol was injected to achieve papillary miosis, and the wound was closed with one 10-0 suture. Subconjunctival Celestone and Garamycin were injected. The lid speculum and retraction suture were removed. After application of Eserine and Bacitracin ointments, the eye was patched and a shield was applied. W.S. left the OR in good condition and was discharged to home 4 hours later.

CASE STUDY QUESTIONS

Multiple choice: Select the best answer and write the letter of your choice to the left of each number.

_____ 1. The medical specialty of otorhinolaryngology is most often referred to as:
   a. ENT or ear, nose, and throat
   b. optometry
   c. PERLA
   d. oral surgery
   e. EENT/dental

_____ 2. The surgery to remove one of the microscopic bones of the middle ear is a(n):
   a. stapedectomy
   b. mastoidectomy
   c. myringotomy
   d. tympanoplasty
   e. otoplasty

_____ 3. The procedure in question 2 may require construction of a new ear drum, a procedure called a(n):
   a. otoplasty
   b. myringotomy
   c. stapes transfer
   d. tympanoplasty
   e. otoscope

_____ 4. Mastoid surgery incisions are made postauricular, which is:
   a. anterior to the ear drum
   b. over the left ear
   c. behind the ear
   d. inferior to the tympanic membrane
   e. between the ears

_____ 5. The study of hearing is termed:
   a. acousticology
   b. radio frequency
   c. light spectrum
   d. otology
   e. audiology

Case Studies, continued

_____ 6. Sensorineural hearing loss results from:
   a. damage to the second cranial nerve
   b. otitis media
   c. otosclerosis
   d. damage to the eighth cranial nerve
   e. stapedectomy

_____ 7. Ultrasound destruction and aspiration of the lens is called:
   a. catarectomy
   b. phacoemulsification
   c. stapedectomy
   d. radial keratotomy
   e. refraction

_____ 8. The term *akinesia* means:
   a. movement
   b. lack of sensation
   c. washing
   d. lack of movement
   e. incision

_____ 9. The term that means "on the same side" is:
   a. contralateral
   b. bilateral
   c. distal
   d. ventral
   e. ipsilateral

_____ 10. Another name for an acoustic neuroma is:
   a. macular degeneration
   b. neurilemoma
   c. otosclerosis
   d. labyrinthitis
   e. glaucoma

Write a term from the case studies with each of the following meanings:

11. record obtained by tympanometry _____

12. pertaining to or perceived by the ear _____

13. inflammation of the middle ear _____

14. inflammation of the external ear _____

15. physician who specializes in conditions of the eye _____

16. within the eye _____

17. abnormal contraction of the pupil _____

18. generic drug name for Versed _____

Case Studies, continued

Abbreviations. Define the following abbreviations:

19. Hz _____

20. BAEP _____

21. OD _____

22. IOL _____

Chapter 18 Crossword
The Senses

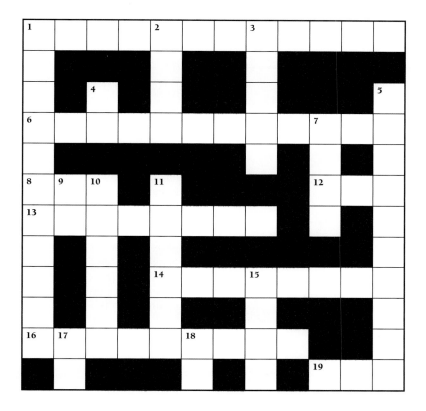

ACROSS

1. Membranes that line the eyelids and cover the fronts of the eyes
6. Sharpness of vision
8. A light-sensitive cell of the retina
12. Lens implant: abbreviation
13. Eye disorder caused by increased pressure
14. Pertaining to tears
16. Inward deviation of the eye
19. Three: prefix

DOWN

1. Coordinated movement of the eyes toward fixation on the same point
2. The middle layer of the eye
3. The tactile sense
4. Left ear: abbreviation
5. Paralysis of the ciliary body:

   _ _ _ _ _ _ _ _ _ _ a
7. Iris: root
9. Medical specialty treating the ear and throat: abbreviation
10. Tear, lacrimal apparatus: combining form
11. Pertaining to the eye
15. Nose: root
17. Without correction: abbreviation
18. Right eye: abbreviation

CHAPTER 18 Answer Section

Answers to Chapter Exercises

EXERCISE 18-1

1. excess sensitivity to stimuli
2. false sense of smell
3. lack of taste sensation
4. anesthesia (*an-es-THE-ze-a*)
5. thermesthesia (*ther-mes-THE-ze-a*)
6. hyperalgesia (*hi-per-al-JE-ze-a*)
7. dysgeusia (*dis-GU-ze-a*)
8. myesthesia (*MI-es-the-se-a*)

EXERCISE 18-2

1. sound
2. ear
3. pertaining to the cochlea
4. pertaining to the vestibule or vestibular apparatus
5. pertaining to the labyrinth (inner ear)
6. pertaining to the stapes
7. pertaining to hearing
8. pertaining to the ear
9. audiometer (*aw-de-OM-e-ter*)
10. otalgia (*o-TAL-je-a*)
11. tympanoplasty (*tim-PAN-o-plas-te*)
12. myringotomy (*mir-in-GOT-o-me*); also tympanotomy (*tim-pan-OT-o-me*)
13. stapedoplasty (*sta-pe-do-PLAS-te*)
14. vestibulocochlear (*ves-tib-u-lo-KOK-le-ar*)
15. labyrinthitis (*lab-i-rin-THI-tis*)
16. salpingoscope (*sal-PING-go-skop*)
17. a specialist in the diagnosis and treatment of hearing disorders
18. inflammation of the ear
19. instrument used to examine the eardrum
20. pertaining to the eustachian tube and pharynx
21. surgical incision of the vestibule or vestibular apparatus

EXERCISE 18-3

1. between the eyelids
2. paralysis of the eyelid
3. pertaining to the nose and lacrimal apparatus
4. excision of a lacrimal sac
5. blepharospasm (*BLEF-a-ro-spasm*)
6. dacryorrhea (*dak-re-o-RE-a*)
7. dacryocystitis (*dak-re-o-sis-TI-tis*)

EXERCISE 18-4

1. vision
2. eye
3. cornea
4. lens of the eye
5. lens
6. ophthalm/o; eye
7. pupill/o; pupil
8. lent/i; lens
9. uve/o; uvea
10. phak/o; lens
11. irid/o; iris
12. retin/o; retina
13. opt/o; eye, vision
14. uveoscleritis (*u-ve-o-skle-RI-tis*)
15. phacomalacia (*fak-o-ma-LA-she-a*)
16. pupillary (*PU-pi-ler-e*)
17. cyclitis (*si-KLI-tis*)
18. retinopathy (*ret-i-NOP-a-the*)
19. ophthalmoscope (*of-THAL-mo-skop*)
20. ophthalmology (*of-thal-MOL-o-je*)
21. iridectomy (*ir-i-DEK-to-me*)
22. iridoplegia (*ir-id-o-PLE-je-a*)
23. pertaining to the eye or vision
24. within the eye
25. splitting of the iris
26. instrument used to incise the sclera
27. inflammation of the cornea
28. behind the lens
29. incision of the ciliary muscle
30. pertaining to the choroid and retina
31. inflammation of the iris and ciliary body

EXERCISE 18-5

1. macropsia (*mak-ROP-se-a*)
2. achromatopsia (*a-kro-ma-TOP-se-a*)
3. diplopia (*dip-LO-pe-a*)
4. presbyopia (*pres-be-O-pe-a*)
5. ametropia (*am-e-TRO-pe-a*)
6. heterometropia (*het-er-o-me-TRO-pe-a*)

LABELING EXERCISE 18-1 THE EAR

1. temporal bone
2. pinna
3. external auditory canal (meatus)
4. tympanic membrane

5. malleus
6. incus
7. stapes
8. ossicles
9. eustachian (auditory) tube
10. pharynx
11. semicircular canals
12. vestibule
13. cochlea
14. vestibulocochlear nerve

LABELING EXERCISE 18-2 THE EYE

1. sclera
2. cornea
3. iris
4. lens
5. suspensory ligaments
6. ciliary muscle
7. conjunctival sac
8. vitreous body
9. choroid
10. retina
11. central fovea
12. blind spot (optic disk)
13. optic nerve

Answers to Chapter Review 18-1

1. c
2. d
3. a
4. b
5. e
6. d
7. c
8. e
9. a
10. b
11. b
12. e
13. a
14. d
15. c
16. b
17. a
18. d
19. c
20. e
21. e
22. d
23. a
24. b
25. c

26. b
27. e
28. d
29. a
30. c
31. e
32. c
33. d
34. a
35. b
36. c
37. e
38. a
39. b
40. d
41. b
42. e
43. d
44. a
45. c
46. e
47. c
48. a
49. d
50. b
51. cochlea
52. cerumen
53. stapes
54. retina
55. refraction
56. cornea
57. tympanic membrane
58. iris
59. study and treatment of hearing disorders
60. absence of a lens
61. beneath the sclera
62. instrument used to measure the eye
63. inflammation of the cornea and iris
64. incision of the iris
65. around the lens
66. pertaining to the choroid and retina
67. inflammation of the tympanic membrane
68. analgesia (an-al-JĒ-zē-a)
69. blepharoptosis
70. stapedectomy
71. otoplasty
72. pupillometry
73. retinopathy
74. lacrimal
75. myringotomy, tympanotomy
76. salpingoscope
77. vestibulocochlear
78. cyclectomy
79. cochlear

80. uveal
81. vestibular
82. scleral
83. pupillary
84. corneal
85. mydriasis
86. exotropia
87. sc
88. hyperopia
89. hyperesthesia
90. AS
91. unequal refractive powers in the two eyes
    a. not, without
    b. equal
    c. measure
    d. vision
92. abnormal sensation
    a. abnormal
    b. sensation
    c. condition of
93. blindness in one half of the visual field
    a. half
    b. without, lack of
    c. vision
94. defect of vision in which all objects appear colored
    a. excess
    b. color
    c. vision

Answers to Case Study Questions

1. a
2. a
3. d
4. c
5. e
6. d
7. b
8. b
9. e
10. b
11. tympanogram
12. aural
13. otitis media
14. otitis externa
15. ophthalmologist
16. intraocular
17. miosis
18. midazolam
19. hertz
20. brainstem auditory evoked potentials
21. right eye
22. intraocular lens

ANSWERS TO CROSSWORD PUZZLE

The Senses

¹C	O	N	J	²U	N	C	³T	I	V	A	E	
O				V			O					
N		⁴A		E			U				⁵C	
⁶V	I	S	U	A	L	A	C	U	⁷I	T	Y	
E							H		R		C	
⁸R	⁹O	¹⁰D		¹¹O				¹²I	O	L		
¹³G	L	A	U	C	O	M	A	D		O		
E		C		U						P		
N		R		¹⁴L	A	C	¹⁵R	I	M	A	L	
C		Y		A			H			E		
¹⁶E	¹⁷S	O	T	R	¹⁸O	P	I	A		G		
	C				D		N	¹⁹T	R	I		

The Skeleton

Chapter Contents

Objectives

After study of this chapter you should be able to:

1. Compare the axial skeleton and the appendicular skeleton.
2. Briefly describe formation of bone tissue.
3. Describe the structure of a long bone.
4. Compare a suture, a symphysis, and a synovial joint.
5. Identify and use roots pertaining to the skeleton.
6. Describe the main disorders that affect the skeleton and joints.
7. Describe the common methods used to diagnose and treat disorders of the skeleton.
8. Interpret abbreviations used in relation to the skeleton.
9. Label diagrams of the skeleton.
10. Analyze several case studies pertaining to bones and joints.

Divisions of the Skeleton

The **skeleton** forms the framework of the body, protects vital organs, and works with the muscular system to produce movement. The human adult skeleton is composed of 206 **bones**. It is divided for study into the axial skeleton and the appendicular skeleton (Fig. 19-1).

    The axial skeleton consists of the skull, the spinal column, the ribs, and the sternum. The skull consists of eight cranial bones and the 14 bones of the face (Fig. 19-2). Skull bones are joined by nonmoveable joints (sutures), except for the joint between the lower jaw (mandible) and the temporal bone of the cranium, the temporomandibular joint (TMJ). As shown in Figure 19-3, the 26 vertebrae of the spinal column are divided into five regions: cervical (7); thoracic (12); lumbar (5); the sacrum (5 fused); and the coccyx (4 to 5 fused). Between the vertebrae are disks of cartilage that add strength and flexibility to the spine.

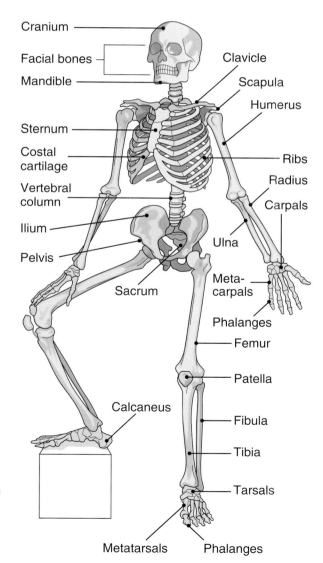

FIGURE 19-1. The skeleton. The axial skeleton is shown in yellow; the appendicular skeleton is shown in blue. (Reprinted with permission from Cohen BJ, Wood DL. Memmler's The Human Body in Health and Disease. 9th Ed. Philadelphia: Lippincott Williams & Wilkins, 2000.)

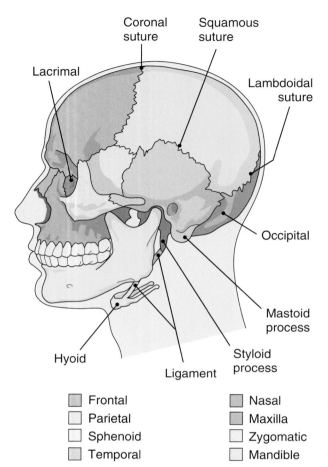

FIGURE 19-2. The skull from the left. An additional cranial bone, the ethmoid, is visible mainly from the interior of the skull. (Reprinted with permission from Cohen BJ, Wood DL. Memmler's The Human Body in Health and Disease. 9th Ed. Philadelphia: Lippincott Williams & Wilkins, 2000.)

- Frontal
- Parietal
- Sphenoid
- Temporal
- Nasal
- Maxilla
- Zygomatic
- Mandible

The appendicular skeleton consists of the bones of the arms and legs, the shoulder girdle, and the pelvis. Each of the two pelvic bones is formed of three fused bones (Fig. 19-4). The large, flared, upper bone is the **ilium.**

Bone Formation

Bone is formed by the gradual addition of calcium and phosphorus salts to **cartilage,** a type of dense connective tissue. This process of **ossification** begins before birth and continues to adulthood. Although bone appears to be inert, it is actually living tissue that is constantly being replaced and remodeled throughout life. Three types of bone cells are involved in these changes: **osteoblasts** are the cells that produce bone; **osteocytes** are mature bone cells; and **osteoclasts** are involved in the breakdown of bone tissue to release needed minerals or to allow for reshaping and repair. The process of destroying bone so that its components can be taken into the circulation is called **resorption.** This process occurs normally throughout life; in disease states, resorption may occur more rapidly or more slowly than bone production.

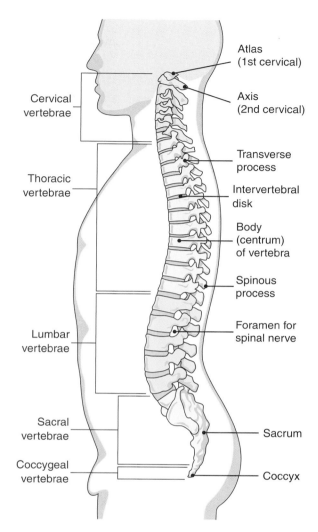

FIGURE 19-3. Vertebral column from the side. (Reprinted with permission from Cohen BJ, Wood DL. Memmler's The Human Body in Health and Disease. 9th Ed. Philadelphia: Lippincott Williams & Wilkins, 2000.)

Structure of a Long Bone

A typical long bone (Fig. 19-5) has a shaft or **diaphysis** composed of compact bone tissue. Within the shaft is a medullary cavity containing the yellow form of **bone marrow**, which is high in fat. The irregular **epiphysis** at either end is made of a less dense, spongy bone tissue containing the blood-forming red bone marrow. A thin layer of cartilage covers the epiphysis and protects the bone surface. Between the diaphysis and the epiphysis at each end of the bone, in a region called the **metaphysis**, is the growth region or **epiphyseal plate**. When the bone stops growing in length, this area becomes fully calcified but remains visible as the epiphyseal line. The thin layer of fibrous tissue that covers the outside of the bone, the **periosteum**, nourishes and protects the bone and also generates new bone cells for growth and repair.

Long bones are found in the arms, legs, hands, and feet. Other types of bones are described as flat (i.e., cranial bones), short (i.e., wrist and ankle bones), or irregular (i.e., facial bones and vertebrae).

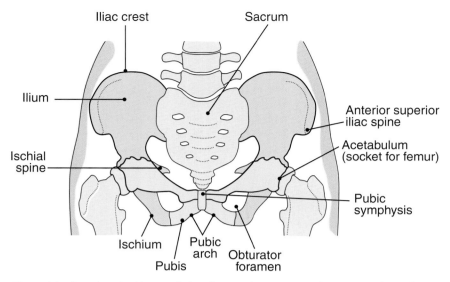

FIGURE 19-4. The pelvis. (Reprinted with permission from Cohen BJ, Wood DL. Memmler's The Human Body in Health and Disease. 9th Ed. Philadelphia: Lippincott Williams & Wilkins, 2000.)

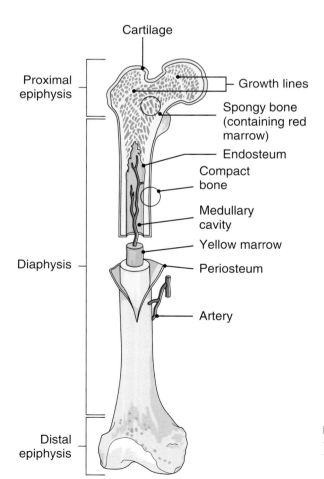

FIGURE 19-5. Structure of a long bone. (Reprinted with permission from Cohen BJ, Wood DL. Memmler's The Human Body in Health and Disease. 9th Ed. Philadelphia: Lippincott Williams & Wilkins, 2000.)

Joints

The joints or **articulations** are classified according to the degree of movement they allow. A **suture** is an immovable joint held together by fibrous connective tissue, as is found between the bones of the skull (see Fig. 19-2). A **symphysis** is a slightly movable joint connected by fibrous cartilage. Examples are the joints between the bodies of the vertebrae (see Fig. 19-3) and the joint between the pubic bones (see Fig. 19-4). A freely movable joint is called a **synovial joint** or **diarthrosis**. Such joints allow for a wide range of movements, as described in Chapter 20. **Tendons** attach muscles to bones to produce movement at the joints.

Freely moveable joints are subject to wear and tear, and they therefore have some protective features. The cavity of a diarthrotic joint contains **synovial fluid**, which cushions and lubricates the joint. This fluid is produced by the synovial membrane that lines the joint cavity. The ends of the articulating bones are cushioned and protected by cartilage. Synovial joints are stabilized and strengthened by **ligaments**, which connect the articulating bones. **A bursa** is a small sac of synovial fluid that cushions the area around a joint. Bursae are found at stress points between tendons, ligaments, and bones.

Key Terms

NORMAL STRUCTURE AND FUNCTION

articulation *ar-tik-ū-LĀ-shun*	A joint; adjective, articular
bone	A calcified form of dense connective tissue; osseous tissue; also an individual unit of the skeleton made of such tissue (root *oste/o*)
bone marrow	The soft material that fills the cavities of a bone. Yellow marrow fills the central cavity of the long bones; blood cells are formed in red bone marrow, which is located in spongy bone tissue (root *myel/o*).
bursa *BUR-sa*	A fluid-filled sac that reduces friction near a joint (root *burs/o*)
cartilage *KAR-ti-lij*	A type of dense connective tissue that is found in the skeleton, larynx, trachea, and bronchi. It is the precursor to most bone tissue (root *chondr/o*).
diarthrosis *di-ar-THRŌ-sis*	A freely movable joint; also called a synovial joint (adjective, diarthrotic)
diaphysis *dī-AF-i-sis*	The shaft of a long bone
epiphysis *e-PIF-i-sis*	The irregularly shaped end of a long bone
epiphyseal plate *ep-i-FIZ-ē-al*	The growth region of a long bone; located in the metaphysis, between the diaphysis and epiphysis. When bone growth ceases, this area appears as the epiphyseal line.
ilium *IL-ē-um*	The large, flared, upper portion of the pelvic bone; adjective, iliac (root *ili/o*)

Normal Structure and Function, *continued*

joint	The junction between two bones; articulation (root *arthr/o*)
ligament *LIG-a-ment*	A strong band of connective tissue that joins one bone to another
metaphysis *me-TAF-i-sis*	The region of a long bone between the diaphysis (shaft) and epiphysis (end); during development, the growing region of a long bone
ossification *os-i-fi-KĀ-shun*	The formation of bone tissue (from Latin *os*, meaning "bone")
osteoblast *OS-tē-ō-blast*	A cell that produces bone tissue
osteoclast *OS-tē-ō-clast*	A cell that destroys bone tissue
osteocyte *OS-tē-ō-sīt*	A mature bone cell that nourishes and maintains bone tissue
periosteum *per-ē-OS-tē-um*	The fibrous membrane that covers the surface of a bone
resorption *rē-SORP-shun*	Removal of bone by breakdown and absorption into the circulation
skeleton *SKEL-e-ton*	The bony framework of the body, consisting of 206 bones. The axial portion (80 bones) is composed of the skull, spinal column, ribs, and sternum. The appendicular skeleton (126 bones) contains the bones of the arms and legs, shoulder girdle, and pelvis.
suture *SŪ-chur*	An immovable joint, such as the joints between the bones of the skull
symphysis *SIM-fi-sis*	A slightly movable joint
synovial fluid *sin-O-vē-al*	The fluid contained in a freely movable (diarthrotic) joint; synovia (root *synov/i*)
synovial joint	A freely movable joint; has a joint cavity containing synovial fluid; a diarthrosis
tendon *TEN-don*	A fibrous band of connective tissue that attaches a muscle to a bone

Roots Pertaining to the Skeleton, Bones, and Joints

TABLE 19-1 Roots for Bones and Joints

ROOT	MEANING	EXAMPLE	DEFINITION OF EXAMPLE
oste/o	bone	osteolytic *os-tē-ō-LIT-ik*	destroying or dissolving bone
myel/o	bone marrow; also, spinal cord	myeloblast *MĪ-e-lō-blast*	immature bone marrow cell
chondr/o	cartilage	chondromalacia *kon-drō-ma-LĀ-shē-a*	softening of cartilage
arthr/o	joint	arthrosis *ar-THRŌ-sis*	joint; condition affecting a joint
synov/i	synovial fluid, joint, or membrane	asynovia *a-sin-Ō-vē-a*	lack of synovial fluid
burs/o	bursa	bursotomy *bur-SOT-ō-mē*	incision into a bursa

Exercise 19-1

Fill in the blanks:

1. The term osteoid (*os-tē-oyd*) means resembling _____.

2. Arthrodesis (*ar-thrō-DĒ-sis*) is fusion of a(n) _____.

3. A chondrocyte (*KON-drō-sīt*) is a cell found in _____.

4. A bursolith (*BUR-sō-lith*) is a stone in a(n) _____.

Define each of the following words:

5. osteogenesis (*os-tē-ō-JEN-e-sis*) _____

6. chondroma (*kon-DRŌ-ma*) _____

7. arthroplasty (*AR-thrō-plas-tē*) _____

8. peribursal (*per-i-BER-sal*) _____

9. myeloid (*MĪ-e-loyd*) _____

Word building. Write a word for each of the following definitions:

10. deficiency (-penia) of bone tissue _____

11. inflammation of bone and bone marrow _____

12. any disease of a joint _____

13. tumor of bone marrow _____

14. pertaining to or resembling cartilage _____

15. instrument for examining the interior of a joint _____

16. narrowing (-stenosis) of a joint _____

17. inflammation of a synovial membrane _____

The word *ostosis* means "bone growth." Use this as a suffix for the following two words:

18. excess growth of bone _____

19. abnormal growth of bone _____

TABLE 19-2 Roots for the Skeleton

ROOT	MEANING	EXAMPLE	DEFINITION OF EXAMPLE
crani/o	skull, cranium	craniostosis *krā-nē-os-TŌ-sis*	ossification of the cranial sutures
spondyl/o	vertebra	spondylolysis *spon-di-LOL-i-sis*	destruction and separation of a vertebra
vertebr/o	vertebra, spinal column	paravertebral *pa-ra-VER-te-bral*	before or in front of the spinal column
rachi/o	spine	rachischisis *rā-KIS-ki-sis*	fissure of the spine; spina bifida
cost/o	rib	costochondral *kos-tō-KON-dral*	pertaining to a rib and its cartilage
sacr/o	sacrum	presacral *prē-SĀ-kral*	in front of the sacrum
coccy, coccyg/o	coccyx	coccygeal* *kok-SIJ-ē-al*	pertaining to the coccyx
pelvi/o	pelvis	pelvimetry *pel-VIM-e-trē*	measurement of the pelvis
ili/o	ilium	iliopelvic *il-ē-ō-PEL-vik*	pertaining to the ilium and pelvis

*Note spelling.

Exercise 19-2

Write the adjective that fits each of the following definitions:

1. pertaining to (-al) the skull _____

2. pertaining to (-al) a rib _____

3. pertaining to (-ic) the pelvis _____

4. pertaining to (-ac) the ilium _____

5. pertaining to (-al) the spinal column _____

6. pertaining to (-al) the sacrum _____

Define each of the following terms:

7. craniometry (*krā-nē-OM-e-trē*) _____

8. endocranial (*en-dō-KRĀ-nē-al*) _____

9. spondylodynia (*spon-di-lō-DIN-ē-a*) _____

10. prevertebral (*prē-VER-te-bral*) _____

11. suprapelvic (*sū-pra-PEL-vik*) _____

Word building. Write a word for each of the following definitions:

12. fissure of the skull _____

13. incision of the cranium _____

14. inflammation of the vertebrae (use spondyl/o) _____

15. surgical puncture of the spine; spinal tap _____

16. surgical excision of a rib _____

17. pertaining to the sacrum and ilium _____

18. pertaining to the cranium and sacrum _____

19. near the sacrum _____

20. excision of the coccyx _____

21. pertaining to the ilium and coccyx _____

22. below (infra-) the ribs _____

Clinical Aspects of the Skeleton

Disorders of the skeleton often involve surrounding tissues—ligaments, tendons, and muscles—and may be studied together as diseases of the musculoskeletal system. (The muscular system is described in Chapter 20.) The medical specialty that concentrates on diseases of the skeletal and muscular systems is **orthopedics**. Physical therapists and occupational therapists must also understand these systems.

Most abnormalities of the bones and joints appear on simple radiographs (see Fig. 19-6 for a radiograph of a normal joint). Radioactive bone scans, computed tomography (CT), and magnetic resonance imaging (MRI) scans are used as well. Also indicative of disorders are changes in blood levels of calcium and **alkaline phosphatase**, an enzyme needed for calcification of bone.

Infection

Osteomyelitis is an inflammation of bone caused by pus-forming bacteria that enter through a wound or are carried by the blood. Often the blood-rich ends of the long bones are invaded, and the infection then spreads to other regions, such as the bone marrow and even the joints. The use of antibiotics has greatly reduced the threat of osteomyelitis.

Tuberculosis may spread to bone, especially the long bones of the arms and legs and the bones of the wrist and ankle. Tuberculosis of the spine is **Pott disease**. Infected vertebrae are weakened and may collapse, causing pain, deformity, and pressure on the spinal cord. Antibiotics can be used to control tuberculosis as long as the strains are not resistant to these drugs and the host is not weakened by other diseases.

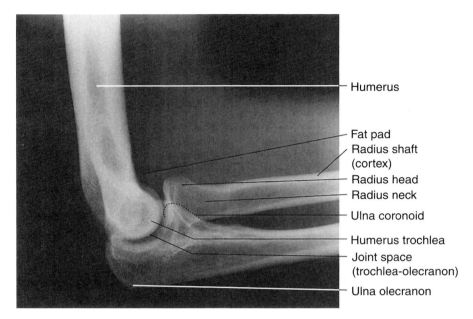

FIGURE 19-6. Radiograph of left elbow. Lateral view. Normal. (Reprinted with permission from Erkonen WE, Smith WL. Radiology 101: Basics and Fundamentals of Imaging. Philadelphia: Lippincott Williams & Wilkins, 1998.)

Fractures

A **fracture** is a break in a bone, usually caused by trauma. The effects of a fracture depend on the location and severity of the break; the amount of associated injury; possible complications, such as infections; and success of healing, which may take months. In a closed or simple fracture, the skin is not broken. If the fracture is accompanied by a wound in the skin, it is described as an open fracture. Various types of fractures are listed in Display 19-1 and illustrated in Figure 19-7.

DISPLAY 19-1 Types of Fractures

FRACTURE	DESCRIPTION
closed	a simple fracture with no open wound
Colles *KOL-ēz*	fracture of the distal end of the radius with backward displacement of the hand
comminuted *COM-i-nū-ted*	fracture in which the bone is splintered or crushed
compression	fracture caused by force from both ends, as to a vertebra
greenstick	one side of the bone is broken and the other side is bent
impacted	one fragment is driven into the other
oblique	break occurs at an angle across the bone; usually one fragment slips by the other
open	fracture is associated with an open wound, or broken bone protrudes through the skin
Pott	fracture of the distal end of the fibula with injury to the tibial joint
spiral	fracture is in a spiral or S shape; usually caused by twisting injuries
transverse	a break at right angles to the long axis of a bone

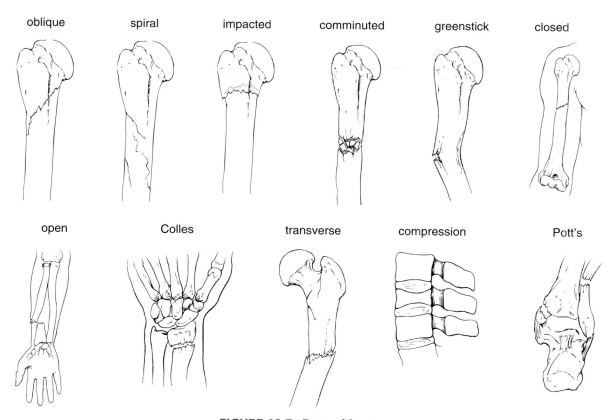

FIGURE 19-7. Types of fractures.

Reduction of a fracture refers to realignment of the broken bone. If no surgery is required, the reduction is described as closed; an open reduction is one that requires surgery to place the bone in proper position. Rods, plates, or screws might be needed to ensure proper healing. A splint or cast is often needed during the healing phase to immobilize the bone. **Traction** refers to using pulleys and weights to maintain alignment of a fractured bone during healing. A traction device may be attached to the skin or attached to the bone itself by means of a pin or wire.

Metabolic Bone Diseases

Osteoporosis is a loss of bone mass that results in weakening of the bones (Fig. 19-8). A decrease in estrogens after menopause makes women over age 50 most susceptible to the effects of this disorder. Efforts to prevent osteoporosis include adequate intake of calcium and engaging in weight-bearing exercise. Because of safety concerns, hormone replacement therapy (HRT) is currently being re-evaluated for use in prevention of osteoporosis. Some drugs are available for reducing bone resorption and increasing bone density. Osteoporosis can be diagnosed and monitored using a DEXA (dual-energy x-ray absorptiometry) scan, an imaging technique that measures bone mineral density (BMD).

Other conditions that can lead to osteoporosis include nutritional deficiencies; disuse, as in paralysis or immobilization in a cast; and excess steroids from the adrenal cortex. Overactivity of the parathyroid glands also leads to osteoporosis because parathyroid hormone releases calcium from bones to raise blood calcium levels. Certain drugs, smoking, lack of exercise, and high intake of alcohol, caffeine, and proteins may also contribute to the development of osteoporosis.

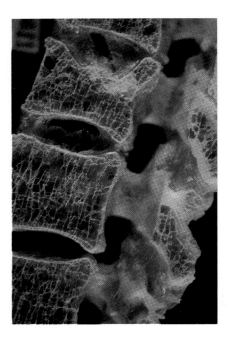

FIGURE 19-8. Osteoporosis. A section of the vertebral column showing a loss of bone tissue and a compression fracture of a vertebra (*top*). (Reprinted with permission from Rubin E, Farber JL. Pathology. 3rd Ed. Philadelphia: Lippincott Williams & Wilkins, 1999.)

In **osteomalacia** there is a softening of bone tissue because of lack of formation of calcium salts. Possible causes include deficiency of vitamin D, needed to absorb calcium and phosphorus from the intestine; renal disorders; liver disease; and certain intestinal disorders. When osteomalacia occurs in children, the disease is called **rickets** (Fig. 19-9). Rickets is usually caused by a deficiency of vitamin D.

Paget disease (osteitis deformans) is a disorder of aging in which bones become overgrown and thicker, but deformed. The disease results in bowing of the long bones and distortion of the flat bones, such as those of the skull. Paget disease usually involves the bones of the axial skeleton, causing pain, fractures, and hearing loss. With time, there may be neurologic signs, heart failure, and predisposition to cancer of the bones.

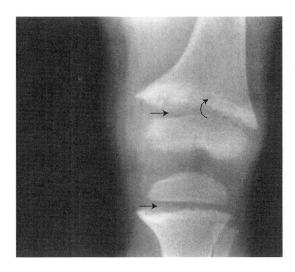

FIGURE 19-9. Rickets. Radiograph of the left knee joint showing widening of the growth regions of the bones (*arrows*). (Reprinted with permission from Erkonen WE, Smith WL. Radiology 101: Basics and Fundamentals of Imaging. Philadelphia: Lippincott Williams & Wilkins, 1998.)

Neoplasms

Osteogenic sarcoma (osteosarcoma) most commonly occurs in the growing region of a bone, especially around the knee. This is a highly malignant tumor that often requires amputation. It most commonly metastasizes to the lungs.

Chondrosarcoma usually appears in midlife. As the name implies, this tumor arises in cartilage. It may require amputation and most frequently metastasizes to the lungs.

In cases of malignant bone tumors, early surgical removal is important for prevention of metastasis. Signs of bone tumors are pain, easy fracture, and increases in serum calcium and alkaline phosphatase levels. Aside from primary tumors, neoplasms at other sites often metastasize to bone, most commonly to the spine.

Arthritis

In general, **arthritis** means inflammation of a joint. The most common form is **osteoarthritis** or **degenerative joint disease** (DJD) (Fig. 19-10). This is a gradual degeneration of articular (joint) cartilage caused by wear and tear. It usually appears at midlife and beyond and involves the weight-bearing joints and joints of the fingers. Radiographs show a narrowing of the joint cavity and thickening of the bone. The cartilage may crack and break loose, causing inflammation in the joint and exposing the underlying bone. Osteoarthritis is treated with analgesics to relieve pain, **anti-inflammatory agents**, such as corticosteroids and **nonsteroidal anti-inflammatory drugs** (NSAIDs), and physical therapy. Predisposing factors are age, heredity, injury, congenital skeletal abnormalities, and endocrine disorders.

Rheumatoid arthritis is a systemic inflammatory disease of the joints that commonly appears in young adult women. Its exact causes are unknown, but it may involve immunologic reactions. A group of antibodies called **rheumatoid factor** often appears in the blood, but is not always specific for rheumatoid arthritis because it may occur in other systemic diseases as well. There is an overgrowth of the synovial membrane that lines the joint cavity. As this membrane covers and destroys the joint cartilage, synovial fluid accumulates, causing swelling of the joint (Fig. 19-11). There is degeneration of the underlying bone eventually causing fusion of the bones, or **ankylosis**. Treatment includes rest, physical therapy, analgesics, and anti-inflammatory drugs.

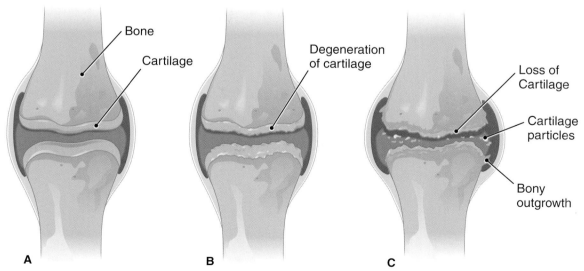

FIGURE 19-10. Osteoarthritis. **(A)** Normal joint. **(B)** Early stage of osteoarthritis. **(C)** Late stage of disease.

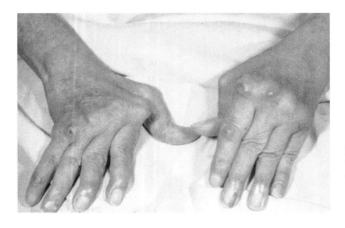

FIGURE 19-11. Advanced rheumatoid arthritis. The hands show swelling of the joints and deviation of the fingers. (Reprinted with permission from Rubin E, Farber JL. Pathology. 3rd Ed. Philadelphia: Lippincott Williams & Wilkins, 1999.)

Gout is caused by an increased level of uric acid in the blood, salts of which are deposited in the joints. It mostly occurs in middle-aged men and almost always involves pain at the base of the great toe. Gout may result from a primary metabolic disturbance or may be a secondary effect of another disease, as of the kidneys. Gout is treated with drugs to suppress formation of uric acid or to increase elimination of uric acid (uricosuric agent).

Disorders of the Spine

Ankylosing spondylitis is a disease of the spine that appears mainly in males. Joint cartilage is destroyed; eventually the disks between the vertebrae calcify and there is fusion of the bones (ankylosis) (Fig. 19-12). Changes begin low in the spine and progress upward, limiting mobility.

In cases of a **herniated disk** (Fig. 19-13), the central mass (nucleus pulposus) of an intervertebral disk protrudes through the weakened outer ring (anulus fibrosus) of the disk into the spinal canal. This commonly occurs in the lumbosacral or cervical regions of the spine as a result of injury or heavy lifting. The herniated or "slipped" disk puts pressure on the spinal cord or spinal nerves, often causing pain along the sciatic nerve (**sciatica**). There may be spasms of the back muscles, leading to disability.

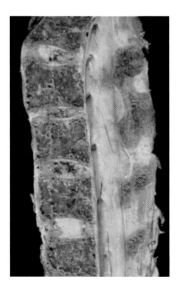

FIGURE 19-12. Ankylosing spondylitis. Bone bridges fuse one vertebra to the next across the intervertebral discs and fuse the posterior portions of the vertebrae. There is osteoporosis from disuse. (Reprinted with permission from Rubin E, Farber JL. Pathology. 3rd Ed. Philadelphia: Lippincott Williams & Wilkins, 1999.)

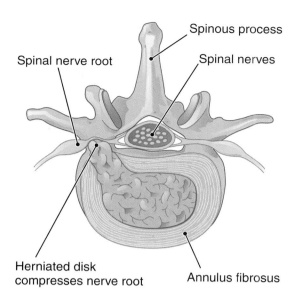

Spinous process

Spinal nerve root

Spinal nerves

Herniated disk
compresses nerve root

Annulus fibrosus

FIGURE 19-13. Herniated disk.

A herniated disk is diagnosed by myelography, CT scan, MRI, and neuromuscular tests. Treatment is bed rest; drugs to reduce pain, muscle spasms, and inflammation; followed by an exercise program to strengthen muscles. In severe cases, it may be necessary to remove the disk surgically in a **discectomy**, sometimes followed by fusion of the vertebrae with a bone graft to stabilize the spine. Using techniques of microsurgery, surgery done through a small incision under magnification, it is now possible to remove an exact amount of extruded disk tissue instead of the entire disk.

BOX 19-1 Names That Are Like Pictures

Some conditions are named by terms that are very descriptive. In orthopedics, several names for types of bursitis are based on the repetitive stress that leads to the irritation. For example, "tailor's bottom" involves the ischial ("sit") bones of the pelvis, as might be irritated by sitting tailor-fashion to sew. "Housemaid's knee" comes from the days of scrubbing floors on hands and knees, and "tennis elbow" is named for the sport that is its most common cause. "Student's elbow" results from leaning to pore over books while studying, although today a student is more likely to have neck and wrist problems from sitting at a computer.

The term knock-knee describes genu valgum, in which the knees are abnormally close and the space between the ankles is wide. The opposite is genu varum, in which the knees are far apart and the bottom of the legs are close together, giving rise to the term bowleg. A dowager's hump appears dorsally between the shoulders as a result of osteoporosis and is most commonly seen in elderly women.

Injury to the roots of nerves that supply the arm may cause the arm to abduct slightly and rotate medially with the wrist flexed and the fingers pointing backward, a condition colorfully named "waiter's tip position." "Popeye's shoulder" is sign of a separation or tear at the head of the biceps tendon. The affected arm, when abducted with the elbow flexed, reveals a bulge on the upper arm—just like Popeye's!

Key Clinical Terms

DISORDERS

ankylosing spondylitis *ang-ki-LŌ-sing* *spon-di-LĪ-tis*	A chronic, progressive inflammatory disease involving the joints of the spine and surrounding soft tissue, most common in young males; also called rheumatoid spondylitis
ankylosis *ang-ki-LŌ-sis*	Immobility and fixation of a joint
arthritis *ar-THRĪ-tis*	Inflammation of a joint
chondrosarcoma *kon-drō-sar-KŌ-ma*	A malignant tumor of cartilage
degenerative joint disease (DJD)	Osteoarthritis (see below)
fracture	A break in a bone. In a closed or simple fracture, the broken bone does not penetrate the skin; in an open fracture, there is an accompanying wound in the skin.
gout *gowt*	A form of acute arthritis, usually beginning in the knee or foot, caused by deposit of uric acid salts in the joints
herniated disk	Protrusion of the center (nucleus pulposus) of an intervertebral disk into the spinal canal; ruptured or "slipped" disk
osteoarthritis (OA) *os-tē-ō-ar-THRĪ-tis*	Progressive deterioration of joint cartilage with growth of new bone and soft tissue in and around the joint; the most common form of arthritis; results from wear and tear, injury, or disease; also called degenerative joint disease (DJD)
osteogenic sarcoma *os-tē-ō-JEN-ik*	A malignant bone tumor; osteosarcoma
osteomalacia *os-tē-ō-ma-LĀ-shē-a*	A softening and weakening of the bones due to vitamin D deficiency or other disease
osteomyelitis *os-tē-ō-mī-e-LĪ-tis*	Inflammation of bone and bone marrow caused by infection, usually bacterial
osteoporosis *os-tē-ō-po-RŌ-sis*	A condition characterized by reduction in bone density, most common in white women past menopause; causative factors include, diet, activity, and estrogen levels
Paget disease *PAJ-et*	Skeletal disease of the elderly characterized by thickening and distortion of bones with bowing of long bones; osteitis deformans
Pott disease	Inflammation of the vertebrae, usually caused by tuberculosis
rheumatoid arthritis *RŪ-ma-toyd*	A chronic autoimmune disease of unknown origin resulting in inflammation of peripheral joints and related structures; more common in women than in men

Disorders, *continued*

rheumatoid factor	A group of antibodies found in the blood in cases of rheumatoid arthritis and other systemic diseases
rickets *RIK-ets*	Faulty bone formation in children usually caused by a deficiency of vitamin D
sciatica *sī-AT-i-ka*	Severe pain in the leg along the course of the sciatic nerve, usually related to irritation of a spinal nerve root

TREATMENT

alkaline phosphatase *AL-ka-lin FOS-fa-tās*	An enzyme needed in the formation of bone; serum activity of this enzyme is useful in diagnosis
anti-inflammatory agent	Drug that reduces inflammation; includes steroids, such as cortisone, and nonsteroidal anti-inflammatory drugs (NSAIDs)
discectomy *dis-KEK-tō-mē*	Surgical removal of a herniated intervertebral disk
nonsteroidal anti-inflammatory drug (NSAID)	Drug that reduces inflammation but is not a steroid; examples include aspirin and ibuprofen and other inhibitors of prostaglandins, naturally produced substances that promote inflammation
orthopedics *or-thō-PĒ-diks*	The study and treatment of disorders of the skeleton, muscles, and associated structures; literally "straight" (ortho) "child" (ped); also spelled orthopaedics
reduction of a fracture	Return of a fractured bone to a normal position; may be closed (not requiring surgery) or open (requiring surgery)
traction *TRAK-shun*	The process of drawing or pulling, such as traction of the head in the treatment of injuries to the cervical vertebrae

Supplementary Terms

NORMAL STRUCTURE AND FUNCTION*

acetabulum *as-e-TAB-ū-lum*	The bony socket in the hip bone that holds the head of the femur
annulus fibrosus *AN-ū-lus fī-BRŌ-sus*	The outer ringlike portion of an intervertebral disk
atlas *AT-las*	The first cervical vertebra (see Fig. 19-3; root *atlant/o*)
axis	The second cervical vertebra (see Fig. 19-3)
calvaria *kal-VAR-ē-a*	The domelike upper portion of the skull

Normal Structure and Function, continued

coxa *KOK-sa*	Hip
cruciate ligaments *KRŪ-shē-āt*	Ligaments that cross in the knee joint to connect the tibia and fibula. They are the anterior cruciate ligament (ACL) and the posterior cruciate ligament (PCL). *Cruciate* means "shaped like a cross."
genu *JE-nu*	The knee
glenoid cavity *GLEN-oyd*	The bony socket in the scapula that articulates with the head of the humerus
hallux *HAL-uks*	The great toe
ischium *IS-kē-um*	The lower portion of the pelvic bone (see Fig. 19-4)
malleolus *ma-LĒ-ō-lus*	The projection of the tibia or fibula on either side of the ankle
meniscus *me-NIS-kus*	Crescent-shaped disc of cartilage found in certain joints, such as the knee joint. In the knee, the medial meniscus and the lateral meniscus separate the tibia and femur. Plural, menisci (*me-NIS-kī*); meniscus means "crescent."
olecranon *ō-LEK-ra-non*	The process of the ulna that forms the elbow
os	Bone; plural, ossa
osseous *OS-ē-us*	Pertaining to bone
patella *pa-TEL-la*	The kneecap
pubis *PŪ-bis*	The anterior part of the pelvic bone. The two pubic bones join anteriorly at the pubic symphysis (see Fig. 19-4).
symphysis pubis *SIM-fi-sis*	The anterior joint of the pelvis, formed by the union of the two pubic bones (see Fig. 19-4); also called pubic symphysis

*See Display 19-2 for a list of bone markings.

SYMPTOMS AND CONDITIONS

achondroplasia *a-kon-drō-PLĀ-zha*	Decreased growth of cartilage in the growth plate of long bones resulting in dwarfism; a genetic disorder
bunion *BUN-yun*	Inflammation and enlargement of the metatarsal joint of the great toe, usually with displacement of the great toe toward the other toes
bursitis *bur-SĪ-tis*	Inflammation of a bursa, a small fluid-filled sac near a joint; causes include injury, irritation, and joint disease; the shoulder, hip, elbow, and knee are common sites

Symptoms and Conditions, continued

carpal tunnel syndrome	Numbness and weakness of the hand caused by pressure on the median nerve as it passes through a tunnel formed by carpal bones
chondroma *kon-DRŌ-ma*	A benign tumor of cartilage
curvature of the spine	An exaggerated curve of the spine; includes scoliosis (sideways curve in any region), lordosis (lumbar curve), and kyphosis (thoracic curve; Fig. 19-14)
Ewing tumor	A bone tumor that usually appears in children 5 to 15 years of age. It begins in the shaft of a bone and spreads readily to other bones. It may respond to radiation therapy, but then returns. Also called Ewing sarcoma.
exostosis *eks-os-TŌ-sis*	A bony outgrowth from the surface of a bone
giant cell tumor	A bone tumor that usually appears in children and young adults. The ends of the bones are destroyed, commonly at the knee, by a large mass that does not metastasize.
hammertoe *HAM-er-tō*	Change in position of the toe joints so that the toe takes on a clawlike appearance and the first joint protrudes upward, causing irritation and pain on walking.
hallux valgus	Painful condition involving lateral displacement of the great toe at the metatarsal joint. There is also enlargement of the metatarsal head and bunion formation.
Heberden nodes *HĒ-ber-den*	Small, hard nodules formed in the cartilage of the distal joints of the fingers in osteoarthritis
hemarthrosis *hē-mar-THRŌ-sis*	Bleeding into a joint cavity
kyphosis *kī-FŌ-sis*	An exaggerated curve of the spine in the thoracic region; hunchback, humpback (see Fig. 19-14)
Legg-Calvé-Perthes disease *leg-kahl-vā-PER-tez*	Degeneration (osteochondrosis) of the proximal growth center of the femur. The bone is eventually restored, but there may be deformity and weakness. Most common in young boys. Also called coxa plana.
lordosis *lor-DŌ-sis*	An exaggerated curve of the spine in the lumbar region; swayback (see Fig. 19-14)
multiple myeloma *mī-e-LŌ-ma*	A cancer of blood-forming cells in bone marrow (see Chapter 10)
neurogenic arthropathy *nū-rō-JEN-ik ar-THROP-a thē*	Degenerative disease of joints caused by impaired nervous stimulation; most common cause is diabetes mellitus; Charcot arthropathy
Osgood-Schlatter disease *oz-good-SHLAHT-er*	Degeneration (osteochondrosis) of the proximal growth center of the tibia causing pain and tendinitis at the knee

Symptoms and Conditions, *continued*

osteochondroma *os-tē-ō-kon-DRŌ-ma*	A benign tumor consisting of cartilage and bone
osteochondrosis *os-tē-ō-kon-DRŌ-sis*	Disease of the growth center of a bone in children; degeneration of the tissue is followed by recalcification
osteodystrophy *os-tē-ō-DIS-trō-fē*	Abnormal bone development
osteogenesis imperfecta (OI) *os-tē-ō-JEN-e-sis* *im-per-FEK-ta*	A hereditary disease resulting in the formation of brittle bones that fracture easily. There is faulty synthesis of collagen, the main structural protein in connective tissue.
osteoma	A benign bone tumor that usually remains small and localized
osteopenia *os-tē-ō-PĒ-nē-a*	Lack of bone tissue; decrease of bone density as seen in osteoporosis
Reiter syndrome *RĪ-ter*	Chronic polyarthritis that usually affects young men; occurs after a bacterial infection and is common in those infected with HIV; may also involve the eyes and genitourinary tract
scoliosis *skō-lē-Ō-sis*	A sideways curvature of the spine in any region (see Fig. 19-14)
spondylolisthesis *spon-di-lō-LIS-the-sis*	A forward displacement of one vertebra over another (-*listhesis*) means "a slipping")
spondylosis *spon-di-LŌ-sis*	Degeneration and ankylosis of the vertebrae resulting in pressure on the spinal cord and nerve roots
sprain	Trauma to a joint involving the ligaments
subluxation *sub-luk-SĀ-shun*	A partial dislocation
talipes *TAL-i-pēz*	A deformity of the foot, especially one occurring congenitally; clubfoot
valgus *VAL-gus*	Bent outward
varus *VAR-us*	Bent inward
von Recklinghausen disease	Loss of bone tissue caused by increased parathyroid hormone; bones become decalcified, deformed, and fracture easily

DIAGNOSIS AND TREATMENT

allograft *AL-ō-graft*	Graft of tissue between individuals of the same species but different genetic makeup; homograft, allogenic graft (see autograft)
arthrocentesis *ar-thrō-sen-TĒ-sis*	Puncture and removal of fluid (aspiration) of a joint
arthroclasia *ar-thrō-KLĀ-zha*	Surgical breaking of an ankylosed joint to provide movement

Diagnosis and Treatment, *continued*

arthroplasty *AR-thrō-plas-tē*	Partial or total replacement of a joint with a prosthesis
arthroscope	An endoscope for examining the interior of a joint (Fig. 19-15); may also be used to perform surgery on the joint, for example, to remove damaged cartilage
arthroscopy *ar-THROS-kō-pē*	Use of an arthroscope to examine the interior of a joint or to perform surgery on the joint (see Fig. 19-15)
aspiration *as-pi-RĀ-shun*	Removal by suction, as removal of fluid from a body cavity; also inhalation, such as accidental inhalation of material into the respiratory tract
autograft *AW-tō-graft*	Graft of tissue taken from a site on or in the body of the person receiving the graft; autologous graft (see allograft)
biphosphonate *bī-FOS-fō-nāt*	A drug that inhibits resorption (loss) of bone tissue in the treatment of osteoporosis and other disorders that weaken the bones (an example is Fosamax)
calcitonin *kal-si-TŌ-nin*	A hormone from the thyroid gland that decreases resorption (loss) of bone tissue; used in the treatment of Paget disease and osteoporosis; also called thyrocalcitonin
chondroitin *kon-DRŌ-i-tin*	A complex polysaccharide found in connective tissue; used as a dietary supplement, usually with glucosamine, for treatment of joint pain
glucosamine	A dietary supplement used in the treatment of joint pain
goniometer *gō-nē-OM-e-ter*	A device used to measure joint angles and movements (root *goni/o* means "angle")
laminectomy *lam-i-NEK-tō-mē*	Excision of the posterior arch (lamina) of a vertebra
meniscectomy *men-i-SEK-tō-mē*	Removal of the crescent-shaped cartilage (meniscus) of the knee joint
myelogram *MĪ-e-lō-gram*	Radiograph of the spinal canal after injection of a radiopaque dye; used to evaluate a herniated disk
osteoplasty *OS-tē-ō-plas-tē*	Scraping and removal of damaged bone from a joint
prosthesis *PROS-thē-sis*	An artificial organ or part, such as an artificial limb
selective estrogen receptor modulator (SERM)	A drug that decreases resorption (loss) of bone tissue in the treatment of osteoporosis; it binds to certain estrogen receptors, activating some estrogenic pathways and inhibiting others [an example is raloxifene (Evista)]

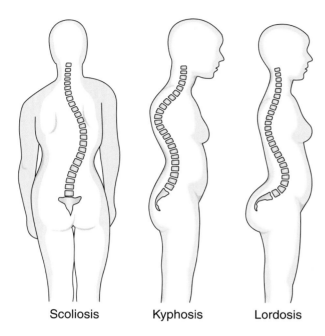

Scoliosis   Kyphosis   Lordosis

FIGURE 19-14. Abnormalities of the spinal curves. (Reprinted with permission from Cohen BJ, Wood DL. Memmler's The Human Body in Health and Disease. 9th Ed. Philadelphia: Lippincott Williams & Wilkins, 2000.)

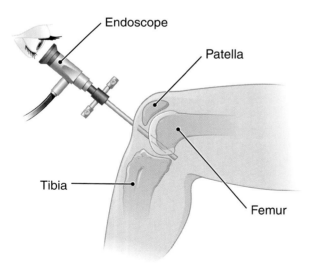

FIGURE 19-15. Arthroscopic examination of the knee. Endoscope is inserted between projections at the end of the femur to view the posterior of the knee.

DISPLAY 19-2 Bone Markings

MARKING	DESCRIPTION
condyle *KON-dīl*	smooth, rounded protuberance at a joint
crest	raised, narrow ridge (see iliac crest in Fig. 19-4)
epicondyle *ep-i-KON-dīl*	projection above a condyle
facet *FAS-et*	small, flattened surface
foramen *for-Ā-men*	rounded opening (see foramen for spinal nerve in Fig. 19-3)
fossa *FOS-a*	hollow cavity
meatus *mē-Ā-tus*	long channel within a bone
process	projection (see mastoid process and styloid process in Fig. 19-2)
sinus *SĪ-nus*	air-filled space or channel
spine	sharp projection (see ischial spine in Fig. 19-4)
trochanter *trō-KAN-ter*	large, blunt projection as at the top of the femur
tubercle *TŪ-ber-kl*	small, rounded projection
tuberosity *tū-ber-OS-i-tē*	large, rounded projection

ABBREVIATIONS

AE	Above the elbow	NSAID(s)	Nonsteroidal anti-inflammatory drug(s)
AK	Above the knee	OA	Osteoarthritis
ASF	Anterior spinal fusion	OI	Osteogenesis imperfecta
BE	Below the elbow	ORIF	Open reduction internal fixation
BK	Below the knee	ortho, ORTH	Orthopedics
BMD	Bone mineral density		
C	Cervical vertebra; numbered C1–C7	PIP	Proximal interphalangeal (joint)
Co	Coccyx; coccygeal	PSF	Posterior spinal fusion
DEXA	Dual-energy x-ray absorptiometry (scan)	RA	Rheumatoid arthritis
DIP	Distal interphalangeal (joint)	S	Sacrum; sacral
DJD	Degenerative joint disease	SERM	Selective estrogen receptor modulator
Fx	Fracture	T	Thoracic vertebra; numbered T1–T12
HNP	Herniated nucleus pulposus	THA	Total hip arthroplasty
IM	Intramedullary	TKA	Total knee arthroplasty
L	Lumbar vertebra; numbered L1–L5	TMJ	Temporomandibular joint
MCP	Metacarpophalangeal (joint)	Tx	Traction
MTP	Metatarsophalangeal (joint)		

Labeling Exercise 19-1

The Skeleton

Write the name of each numbered part on the corresponding line of the answer sheet.

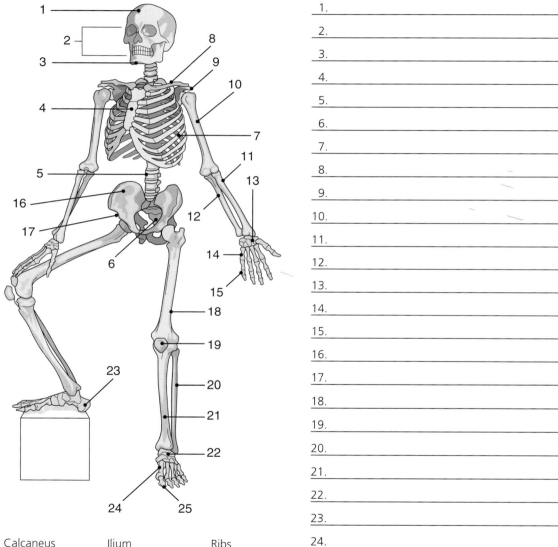

1. _____
2. _____
3. _____
4. _____
5. _____
6. _____
7. _____
8. _____
9. _____
10. _____
11. _____
12. _____
13. _____
14. _____
15. _____
16. _____
17. _____
18. _____
19. _____
20. _____
21. _____
22. _____
23. _____
24. _____
25. _____

Calcaneus   Ilium   Ribs
Carpals   Mandible   Sacrum
Clavicle   Metacarpals   Scapula
Cranium   Metatarsals   Sternum
Facial bones   Patella   Tarsals
Femur   Pelvis   Tibia
Fibula   Phalanges   Ulna
Humerus   Radius   Vertebral column

Labeling Exercise 19-2

Skull From the Left

Write the name of each numbered part on the corresponding line of the answer sheet.

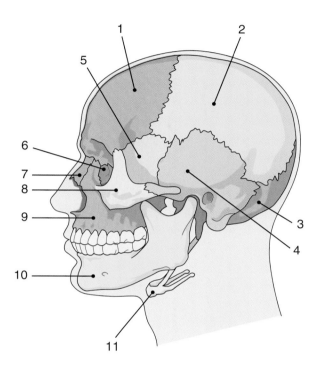

Frontal
Hyoid
Lacrimal
Mandible
Maxilla
Nasal
Occipital
Parietal
Sphenoid
Temporal
Zygomatic

1. _____

2. _____

3. _____

4. _____

5. _____

6. _____

7. _____

8. _____

9. _____

10. _____

11. _____

Labeling Exercise 19-3

Vertebral Column From the Side

Write the name of each numbered part on the corresponding line of the answer sheet.

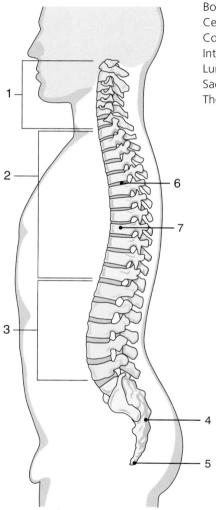

Body (centrum) of vertebra
Cervical vertebrae
Coccyx
Intervertebral disc
Lumbar vertebrae
Sacrum
Thoracic vertebrae

1. _____
2. _____
3. _____
4. _____

5. _____
6. _____
7. _____

Labeling Exercise 19-4

The Pelvis

Write the name of each numbered part on the corresponding line of the answer sheet.

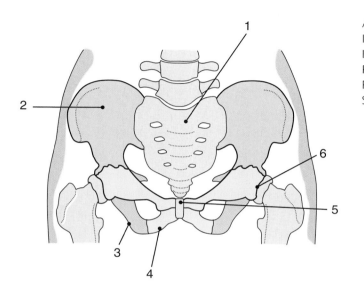

Acetabulum
Ilium
Ischium
Pubic symphysis
Pubis
Sacrum

1. _____
2. _____
3. _____
4. _____
5. _____
6. _____

Labeling Exercise 19-5

Structure of a Long Bone

Write the name of each numbered part on the corresponding line of the answer sheet.

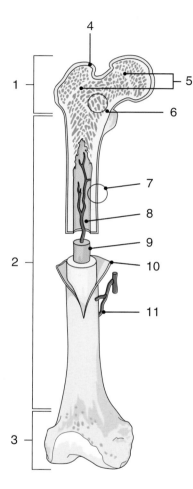

Artery
Cartilage
Compact bone
Diaphysis
Distal epiphysis
Growth lines
Medullary cavity
Periosteum
Proximal epiphysis
Spongy bone
Yellow marrow

1. _____
2. _____
3. _____
4. _____
5. _____
6. _____
7. _____
8. _____
9. _____
10. _____
11. _____

Chapter Review 19-1

Multiple choice: Select the best answer and write the letter of your choice to the left of each number.

_____ 1. bursa
_____ 2. periosteum
_____ 3. phalanges
_____ 4. ilium
_____ 5. zygomatic

a. upper portion of the pelvic bone
b. fluid-filled sac near a joint
c. bones of the fingers and toes
d. facial bone
e. membrane that covers a bone

_____ 6. patella
_____ 7. symphysis
_____ 8. osteoclasts
_____ 9. metaphysis
_____ 10. resorption

a. growth region of a long bone
b. kneecap
c. breakdown and removal of bone tissue
d. slightly movable joint
e. cells that break down bone

_____ 11. polyarticular
_____ 12. hemarthrosis
_____ 13. ankylosis
_____ 14. myelopoiesis
_____ 15. osteoporosis

a. formation of bone marrow
b. immobility of a joint
c. loss of bone mass
d. bleeding into a joint cavity
e. pertaining to many joints

_____ 16. rachiocentesis
_____ 17. spondylolisthesis
_____ 18. osteitis
_____ 19. comminuted
_____ 20. gout

a. inflammation of bone
b. spinal tap
c. metabolic disorder that affects joints
d. displacement of a vertebra
e. fracture in which bone is splintered or crushed

SUPPLEMENTARY TERMS

_____ 21. coxalgia
_____ 22. scoliosis
_____ 23. intraosseous
_____ 24. lordosis
_____ 25. achondroplasia

a. exaggerated lumbar curve of the spine
b. pain in the hip
c. abnormal growth of cartilage
d. within bone
e. sideways curvature of the spine

_____ 26. calvaria   a. knee

_____ 27. subluxation   b. partial dislocation

_____ 28. genu   c. upper portion of the skull

_____ 29. olecranon   d. like or resembling a cross

_____ 30. cruciate   e. part of the ulna that forms the elbow

_____ 31. atlas   a. lower part of the pelvic bone

_____ 32. foramen   b. first cervical vertebra

_____ 33. exostosis   c. a rounded hole

_____ 34. ischium   d. great toe

_____ 35. hallux   e. outgrowth of bone

_____ 36. laminectomy   a. artificial part

_____ 37. goniometer   b. removal of knee cartilage

_____ 38. prosthesis   c. excision of part of a vertebra

_____ 39. arthroclasis   d. device used to measure joint angles

_____ 40. meniscectomy   e. surgical breaking of a fused joint

True-False. Examine each of the following statements. If the statement is true, write T in the first blank. If the statement is false, write F in the first blank and correct the statement by replacing the underlined word in the second blank.

41. The end of a long bone is the epiphysis.   _____ _____

42. The carpal bones are found in the ankle.   _____ _____

43. An immovable joint is a suture.   _____ _____

44. The radius is part of the axial skeleton.   _____ _____

45. The cervical vertebrae are located in the neck.   _____ _____

46. The cells that produce bone tissue are osteoblasts.   _____ _____

47. Blood cells are formed in yellow bone marrow.   _____ _____

48. A sideways curvature of the spine is called kyphosis.   _____ _____

49. The term valgus means bent outward.   _____ _____

Fill in the blanks:

50. The type of tissue that covers the ends of the bones at the joints is _____.

51. The fluid that fills a freely movable joint is _____.

52. A band of connective tissue that connects a bone to another bone is a(n) _____.

53. The part of the vertebral column that articulates with the ilium is the _____.

54. The thigh bone is the _____.

55. The study and treatment of disorders of the skeleton, muscles, and associated structures is

_____.

56. The term costochondral refers to a rib and its _____.

57. Spondylarthritis (*spon-dil-ar-THRĪ-tis*) is arthritis of the _____.

58. Rachischisis (*rā-KIS-ki-sis*) is fissure of the _____.

Define each of the following words:

59. chondrogenesis (*kon-drō-JEN-i-sis*)   _____

60. osteoplasty (*OS-tē-ō-plas-tē*)   _____

61. arthrotome (*AR-thrō-tōm*)   _____

62. synovectomy (*sin-ō-VEK-tō-mē*)   _____

63. peribursal (*per-i-BER-sal*)   _____

64. craniotomy (*krā-nē-OT-ō-mē*)   _____

65. spondylodynia (*spon-di-lō-DIN-ē-a*)   _____

66. subcostal (*sub-KOS-tal*)   _____

67. iliopelvic (*il-ē-ō-PEL-vic*)   _____

68. coccygeal (*kok-SIJ-ē-al*)   _____

Word building. Write a word for each of the following definitions:

69. within the cranium   _____

70. death (-necrosis) of bone tissue   _____

71. inflammation of bone marrow   _____

72. tumor of bone and cartilage   _____

73. surgical excision of cartilage   _____

74. fusion (-desis) of a joint   _____

75. narrowing of a joint   _____

76. instrument for examining the inside of a joint   _____

77. radiographic image of a joint   _____

78. stone in a bursa   _____

79. measurement of the pelvis   _____

80. pertaining to the sacrum and ilium   _____

81. pertaining to a vertebra (use vertebr/o) and a rib   _____

82. surgical excision of the coccyx   _____

83. near the sacrum   _____

84. inflammation of a joint   _____

Adjectives. Write the adjective form of each of the following words:

85. cranium   _____

86. ilium   _____

87. coccyx   _____

88. pelvis   _____

89. vertebra   _____

Word analysis. Define each of the following words, and give the meaning of the word parts in each. Use a dictionary if necessary.

90. achondroplasia (*a-kon-drō-PLĀ-zha*) _____
    a. a-   _____
    b. chondr/o   _____
    c. -plasia   _____

91. chondroblastoma (*kon-drō-blas-TŌ-ma*) _____
    a. chondr/o   _____
    b. blast   _____
    c. -oma   _____

92. spondylosyndesis (*spon-di-lō-SIN-de-sis*) _____
    a. spondyl/o   _____
    b. syn-   _____
    c. -desis   _____

Case Studies

Case Study 19-1: Arthroplasty of the Right TMJ

S.A., a 38-year-old teacher, was admitted for surgery for degenerative joint disease (DJD) of her right temporomandibular joint (TMJ). She has experienced chronic pain in her right jaw, neck, and ear since her automobile accident the previous year. S.A.'s diagnosis was confirmed by CT scan and was followed up with conservative therapy, which included a bite plate, NSAIDs, and steroid injections. She had also tried hypnosis in an attempt to manage her pain but was not able to gain relief. Her doctor referred her to an oral surgeon who specializes in TMJ disorders. S.A. was scheduled for an arthroplasty of the right TMJ to remove diseased bone on the articular surface of the right mandibular condyle.

On the following day, she was transported to the OR for surgery. She was given general endotracheal anesthesia, and a vertical incision was made from the superior aspect of the right ear down to the base of the attachment of the right earlobe. After appropriate dissection and retraction, the posterior-superior aspect of the right zygomatic arch was bluntly dissected anteroposteriorly. With a nerve stimulator, the zygomatic branch of the facial nerve was identified and retracted from the surgical field with a vessel loop. The periosteum was then incised along the superior aspect of the arch. An inferior dissection was then made along the capsular ligament and retracted posteriorly. With a Freer elevator, the meniscus was freed, and a horizontal incision was made to the condyle. With a Hall drill and saline coolant, a high condylectomy of approximately 3 mm of bone was removed while conserving function of the external pterygoid muscle. The stump of the condyle was filed smooth and irrigated copiously with NSS. The lateral capsule, periosteum, subcutaneous tissue, and skin were then closed with sutures. The facial nerve was tested before closing and confirmed to be intact. A pressure pack and Barton bandage were applied. The sponge, needle, and instrument counts were correct. Estimated blood loss (EBL) was approximately 50 mL.

S.A. was discharged on the second postoperative day with instructions for soft diet; daily mouth opening exercises; an antibiotic (Keflex 500 mg po q6h); Tylenol no. 3 po q4h prn for pain; and four weekly postoperative appointments.

Case Study 19-2: Osteogenesis Imperfecta

M.H., a 3-year-old boy with osteogenesis imperfecta (OI) type III, was admitted to the pediatric orthopedic hospital for treatment of yet another fracture. Since he was born he has had 15 fractures of his arms and legs. His congenital disease is manifested by a defect in the creation of bone matrix, which gives normal bone its strength. His bones are very brittle and break with little pressure or trauma. This latest fracture occurred when he twisted at the hip while standing in his wheeled walker. He has been in a research study and receives a bisphosphonates infusion every 2 months. He is short in stature with short limbs for his age, and has bowing of both legs. He also has a pectus cavernosus of his chest, an inversion or concavity of the sternum.

M.H. was transferred to the OR and carefully lifted to the OR table by the staff. After he was anesthetized, he was positioned with gentle manipulation, and his left hip was elevated on a small gel pillow. After skin preparation and sterile draping, a stainless steel rod was inserted into the medullary canal of his left femur to reduce and stabilize the femoral fracture. The muscle, fascia, subcutaneous tissue, and skin were sutured closed. Three nurses gently held M.H. in position on a pediatric spica box while the surgeon applied a hip spica (body cast) to stabilize the fixation, protect the leg, and maintain abduction. M.H. was transferred to the PACU for recovery. The surgeon dictated the procedure as an open reduction internal fixation (ORIF) of the left femur with intramedullary rodding (IM) and application of spica cast.

Case Studies, continued

Case Study 19-3: Idiopathic Adolescent Scoliosis

Four years ago, L.R., who is now 15, had a posterior spinal fusion (PSF) for correction of idiopathic adolescent scoliosis in a pediatric orthopedic hospital in another state. Her spinal curvature had been surgically corrected with the insertion of bilateral laminar and pedicle hooks and two $\frac{3}{16}$-inch rods. A bone autograft was taken from her right posterior superior ilium and applied along the lateral processes of T4 to L2 to complete the fusion.

During a follow-up visit, she presented with a significant prominence of the right scapula and back pain in the mid and lower back. She denied numbness or tingling of the lower extremities, bowel or bladder problems, chest pain, and shortness of breath. A CT scan of the upper thoracic spine showed a prominent rotatory scoliosis deformity of the right posterior thorax with acute angulation of the ribs. Her deformity is a common consequence of overcorrection of prior spinal fusion surgery, called crank shaft phenomenon.

L.R. was referred to the chief spinal surgeon of a local pediatric orthopedic hospital for removal of the spinal instrumentation, posterior spinal osteotomies from T4 to L2, insertion of replacement hooks and rods, bilateral rib resections, autograft bone from the resected ribs, partial scapulectomy, and possible allograft bone and bilateral chest tube placement. The surgical plan was explained to her and her mother and consent was obtained and signed. The surgical procedure as well as the potential benefits versus risks were discussed. L.R. and her mother stated that they fully understood and provided consent to proceed with the plan for surgery.

CASE STUDY QUESTIONS

Multiple choice: Select the best answer and write the letter of your choice to the left of each number.

_____ 1. A condylectomy is:
   a. removal of a joint capsule
   b. plastic repair of a vertebra
   c. removal of a rounded bone protuberance
   d. enlargement of a cavity
   e. removal of a tumor

_____ 2. The articulating surface of a bone is located:
   a. under the epiphysis
   b. in a joint
   c. around the bone marrow
   d. at a muscle attachment
   e. at a tendon attachment

_____ 3. The dissection of the zygomatic arch was directed anteroposteriorly, which describes:
   a. posterior-superior
   b. circumferential
   c. front to back
   d. top to bottom
   e. perpendicular to the mandible

Case Studies, continued

_____ 4. Another term for bow-legged is:
   a. internal rotation
   b. knock-kneed
   c. adduction
   d. varus
   e. valgus

_____ 5. An IM rod is placed:
   a. inferior to the femoral condyle
   b. into the acetabulum
   c. within the medullary canal
   d. on top of the periosteum
   e. lateral to the epiphyseal growth plates

_____ 6. The anatomic area described as thoracic or the thorax is the:
   a. chest
   b. lower pelvis
   c. between sternum and umbilicus
   d. shoulders
   e. posterior abdomen

_____ 7. L.R.'s spinal fusion will immobilize the spinal levels of T4 to L2. These segments describe the _____ and _____ vertebrae.
   a. cervical and lumbar
   b. sacral and cranial
   c. lamina and disks
   d. thoracic and lumbar
   e. lumbar and thoracic

_____ 8. The grafted bone for L.R.'s fusion came from her own right ilium. The proper name for this is a(n):

   a. allograft
   b. autograft
   c. heterograft
   d. iliograft
   e. homograft

Write a term from the case studies with each of the following meanings:

 9. pertaining to the cheekbone _____

10. the membrane around the bone _____

11. a crescent-shaped cartilage in a joint _____

12. on both sides _____

13. breastbone _____

Case Studies, continued

14. plastic repair of a joint   _____

15. term for a disease of unknown origin   _____

16. removal of the shoulder blade   _____

17. a break in the integrity of a bone   _____

18. surgical openings into bones   _____

Abbreviations. Define the following abbreviations:

19. DJD   _____

20. MRI   _____

21. NSAIDs   _____

22. CT   _____

23. NSS   _____

24. TMJ   _____

25. OI   _____

26. ORIF   _____

27. PSF   _____

28. EBL   _____

Chapter 19 Crossword
The Skeleton

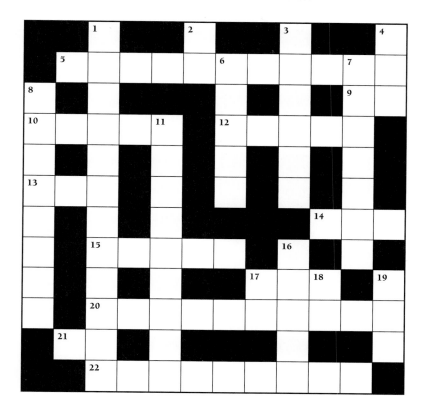

ACROSS

5. Study and treatment of the skeleton, muscles, and associated structures
9. Abbreviation used in taking medical histories
10. Deficiency of: suffix
12. Instrument for measuring joint angles: _ _ _ _ _ meter
13. New: prefix
14. Cold: root
15. First cervical vertebra
17. Twice per day: abbreviation
20. Breakdown and removal of bone
21. Type of arthritis: abbreviation
22. Slipping of a vertebra: spondylo _ _ _ _ _ _ _ _ _

DOWN

1. Pertaining to the cranium and sacrum
2. Last portion of the spinal column: abbreviation
3. Pain: suffix
4. Same, equal: prefix
6. A bone disease is named for him
7. Cartilage: combining form
8. Vertebra: combining form
11. Immobility of a joint
16. Stones: suffix
17. Blood pressure: abbreviation
18. Two, twice: prefix
19. Meaning of the prefix tel/o

CHAPTER 19 Answer Section

Answers to Chapter Exercises

EXERCISE 19-1

1. bone, bone tissue
2. joint
3. cartilage
4. bursa
5. formation of bone
6. tumor of cartilage
7. plastic repair of a joint
8. around a bursa
9. pertaining to or resembling bone marrow
10. osteopenia (os-tē-ō-Pē-nē-a)
11. osteomyelitis (os-tē-ō-mī-e-Lī-tis)
12. arthropathy (ar-THROP-a-thē)
13. myeloma (mī-e-LŌ-ma)
14. chondroid (KON-droyd)
15. arthroscope (AR-thrō-skōp)
16. arthrostenosis (ar-thrō-ste-NŌ-sis)
17. synovitis (si-nō-Vī-tis)
18. hyperostosis (hī-per-os-TŌ-sis)
19. dysostosis (dis-os-TŌ-sis)

EXERCISE 19-2

1. cranial
2. costal
3. pelvic
4. iliac
5. vertebral
6. sacral
7. measurement of the skull (cranium)
8. within the skull
9. pain in a vertebra
10. in front of a vertebra or the spinal column
11. above the pelvis
12. cranioschisis (krā-nē-OS-ki-sis)
13. craniotomy (krā-nē-OT-ō-mē)
14. spondylitis (spon-di-Lī-tis)
15. rachiocentesis (rā-kē-ō-sen-TĒ-sis); also rachicentesis (rā-kē-sen-TĒ-sis)
16. costectomy (kos-TEK-tō-mē)
17. sacroiliac (sā-krō-IL-ē-ak)
18. craniosacral (krā-nē-ō-SĀ-kral)
19. parasacral (par-a-SĀ-kral)
20. coccygectomy (kok-si-JEK-tō-mē)
21. iliococcygeal (il-ē-ō-kok-SIJ-ē-al)
22. infracostal (in-fra-KOS-tal)

LABELING EXERCISE 19-1 THE SKELETON

1. cranium
2. facial bones
3. mandible
4. sternum
5. vertebral column
6. sacrum
7. ribs
8. clavicle
9. scapula (SKAP-ū-la)
10. humerus (HŪ-mer-us)
11. radius (RĀ-dē-us)
12. ulna (UL-na)
13. carpals (KAR-pals)
14. metacarpals (met-a-KAR-pals)
15. phalanges (fa-LAN-jēz)
16. ilium (IL-ē-um)
17. pelvis (PEL-vis)
18. femur (FĒ-mur)
19. patella (pa-TEL-a)
20. fibula (FIB-ū-la)
21. tibia (TIB-ē-a)
22. tarsals (TAR-sals)
23. calcaneus (kal-KĀ-nē-us)
24. metatarsals (met-a-TAR-sals)
25. phalanges

LABELING EXERCISE 19-2
SKULL FROM THE LEFT

1. frontal (FRON-tal)
2. parietal (pa-Rī-e-tal)
3. occipital (ok-SIP-i-tal)
4. temporal (TEM-por-al)
5. sphenoid (SFĒ-noyd)
6. lacrimal (LAK-ri-mal)
7. nasal (NĀ-zal)
8. zygomatic (zī-gō-MAT-ik)
9. maxilla (mak-SIL-a)
10. mandible (MAN-di-bl)
11. hyoid (Hī-oyd)

LABELING EXERCISE 19-3
VERTEBRAL COLUMN FROM THE SIDE

1. cervical vertebrae
2. thoracic vertebrae
3. lumbar vertebrae
4. sacrum

5. coccyx
6. intervertebral disk
7. body (centrum) of vertebra

LABELING EXERCISE 19-4 THE PELVIS

1. sacrum (SĀ-krum)
2. ilium (IL-ē-um)
3. ischium (IS-kē-um)
4. pubis
5. pubic symphysis
6. acetabulum (as-e-TAB-ū-lum)

LABELING EXERCISE 19-5
STRUCTURE OF A LONG BONE

1. proximal epiphysis (e-PIF-i-sis)
2. diaphysis (dī-AF-i-sis)
3. distal epiphysis
4. cartilage
5. growth lines
6. spongy bone
7. compact bone
8. medullary cavity
9. yellow marrow
10. periosteum (per-ē-OS-tē-um)
11. artery

Answers to Chapter Review 19-1

1. b
2. e
3. c
4. a
5. d
6. b
7. d
8. e
9. a
10. c
11. e
12. d
13. b
14. a
15. c
16. b
17. d
18. a
19. e
20. c
21. b
22. e
23. d
24. a
25. c
26. c
27. b
28. a
29. e
30. d
31. b
32. c
33. e
34. a
35. d
36. c
37. d
38. a
39. e
40. b
41. T
42. F wrist
43. T
44. F appendicular
45. T
46. T
47. F red
48. F scoliosis
49. T
50. cartilage
51. synovial fluid; synovia
52. ligament
53. sacrum
54. femur
55. orthopedics
56. cartilage
57. vertebrae
58. spine
59. formation of cartilage
60. plastic repair of bone
61. instrument for incising a joint
62. excision of synovial membrane
63. around a bursa
64. incision into the cranium (skull)
65. pain in a vertebra
66. below a rib or the ribs
67. pertaining to the ilium and pelvis
68. pertaining to the coccyx
69. endocranial
70. osteonecrosis
71. myelitis
72. osteochondroma
73. chondrectomy
74. arthrodesis
75. arthrostenosis
76. arthroscope
77. arthrogram
78. bursolith
79. pelvimetry

80. sacroiliac
81. vertebrocostal
82. coccygectomy
83. parasacral
84. arthritis
85. cranial
86. iliac
87. coccygeal
88. pelvic
89. vertebral
90. decreased growth of cartilage in the growth plate of long bones resulting in dwarfism
    a. lack of
    b. cartilage
    c. formation, molding
91. benign tumor of cartilage-forming cells
    a. cartilage
    b. immature, productive cell
    c. tumor
92. surgical fusion (ankylosis) between vertebrae
    a. vertebra
    b. together
    c. fusion, binding

Answers to Case Study Questions
1. c
2. b
3. c
4. e
5. c
6. a
7. d
8. b
9. zygomatic
10. periosteum
11. meniscus
12. bilateral
13. sternum
14. arthroplasty
15. idiopathic
16. scapulectomy
17. fracture
18. osteotomies
19. degenerative joint disease
20. magnetic resonance imaging
21. nonsteroidal anti-inflammatory drugs
22. computed tomography
23. normal saline solution
24. temporomandibular joint
25. osteogenesis imperfecta
26. open reduction internal fixation
27. posterior spinal fusion
28. estimated blood loss

ANSWERS TO CROSSWORD PUZZLE

The Skeleton

The Muscular System

Chapter Contents

Objectives

After study of this chapter you should be able to:

1. Compare the location and function of smooth, cardiac, and skeletal muscle.
2. Briefly describe the mechanism of muscle contraction.
3. Explain how muscles work together to produce movement.
4. Describe the main types of movements produced by muscles.
5. List some of the criteria for naming muscles.
6. Briefly describe the structure of a muscle.
7. Identify and use the roots pertaining to the muscular system.
8. Describe the main disorders that affect muscles.
9. Label diagrams of the superficial anterior and posterior muscles.
10. Interpret abbreviations pertaining to muscles.
11. Analyze several case studies involving muscles.

The main characteristic of muscle tissue is its ability to contract. When stimulated, muscles shorten to produce movement of the skeleton, vessels, or internal organs. Muscles also may remain partially contracted to maintain posture. In addition, the heat generated by muscle contraction is the main source of body heat.

Types of Muscle

There are three types of muscle tissue in the body:
- **Smooth (visceral) muscle.** This makes up the walls of the hollow organs and the walls of ducts, such as the blood vessels and bronchioles. This muscle operates involuntarily and is responsible for peristalsis, the wavelike movements that propel materials through the systems.
- **Cardiac muscle.** This makes up the myocardium of the heart wall. It functions involuntarily and is responsible for the pumping of the heart.
- **Skeletal muscle.** This is attached to the bones of the skeleton and is responsible for voluntary movement. It also maintains posture and generates a large proportion of body heat. All of these voluntary muscles together make up the muscular system.

The discussion that follows describes the characteristics of skeletal muscle, which has been the most extensively studied of the three types of muscle tissue.

Muscle Contraction

Skeletal muscles are stimulated to contract by motor neurons of the nervous system. At the **neuromuscular junction (NMJ)**, the point where a branch of a neuron meets a muscle cell, the neurotransmitter **acetylcholine** is released, prompting contraction of the cell (Fig. 20-1). Two special proteins in the cell, **actin** and **myosin**, interact to produce the contraction. ATP (the cell's energy compound) and calcium are needed for this response.

Most skeletal muscles contract rapidly to produce movement and then relax rapidly unless stimulation continues. Sometimes muscles are kept in a steady partially contracted state, to maintain posture, for example. This state of firmness is called **tonus**, or muscle tone.

Muscle Action

Muscles work in pairs to produce movement at the joints (see Display 20-1 for a description of various types of movement). As one muscle, the **prime mover**, contracts, an opposing muscle, the **antagonist**, must relax. For example, when the biceps brachii on the anterior surface of the upper arm contracts to flex the arm, the triceps brachii on the posterior surface must relax (Fig. 20-2). When the arm is extended, these actions are reversed. In a given movement, the point where the muscle is attached to a stable part of the skeleton is the **origin**; the point where a muscle is attached to a moving part of the skeleton is the **insertion**.

Naming of Muscles

A muscle can be named by its location (near a bone, for example), by the direction of its fibers, or by its size, its shape, or its number of attachment points (heads), as indicated by the suffix *-ceps*. It may also be

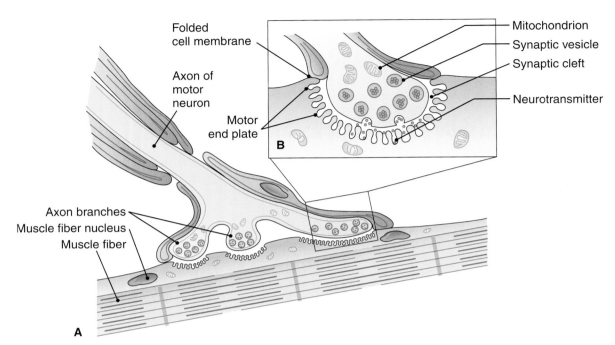

FIGURE 20-1. Neuromuscular junction. **(A)** The branched end of a motor neuron makes contact with the membrane of a muscle fiber (cell). **(B)** Enlarged view. (Reprinted with permission from Cohen BJ, Wood DL. Memmler's The Human Body in Health and Disease. 9th Ed. Philadelphia: Lippincott Williams & Wilkins, 2000.)

DISPLAY 20-1 Types of Movement Produced by Muscles

MOVEMENT	DEFINITION	EXAMPLE
flexion *FLEK-shun*	closing the angle at a joint	bending at the knee or elbow
extension *eks-TEN-shun*	opening the angle at a joint	straightening at the knee or elbow
abduction *ab-DUK-shun*	movement away from the midline of the body	outward movement of the arms at the shoulders
adduction *a-DUK-shun*	movement toward the midline of the body	return of lifted arms to the body
rotation *rō-TĀ-shun*	turning of a body part on its own axis	turning of the forearm from the elbow
circumduction *ser-kum-DUK-shun*	circular movement from a central point	describing a circle with an outstretched arm
pronation *prō-NĀ-shun*	turning downward	turning the palm of the hand downward

DISPLAY 20-1 Types of Movement Produced by Muscles, *continued*

MOVEMENT	DEFINITION	EXAMPLE
supination *sū-pin-Ā-shun*	turning upward	turning the palm of the hand upward
eversion *ē-VER-zhun*	turning outward	turning the sole of the foot outward
inversion *in-VER-zhun*	turning inward	turning the sole of the foot inward
dorsiflexion *dor-si-FLEK-shun*	bending backward	moving the foot so that the toes point upward, away from the sole of the foot
plantar flexion	bending the sole of the foot	pointing the toes downward

named for its action, adding the suffix *-or* to the root for the action. For example, a muscle that produces flexion at a joint is a flexor. Examine the muscle diagrams in Figures 20-3 and 20-4. See how many of these criteria you can find in the names of the muscles. Note that sometimes more than one criterion is used in the name.

Muscle Structure

Muscles are composed of individual cells, often referred to as fibers because they are so long and thread-like. These cells are held together in bundles by connective tissue (Fig. 20-5). Covering each muscle is a sheath of connective tissue or **fascia.** These supporting tissues merge to form the **tendon** that attaches the muscle to a bone.

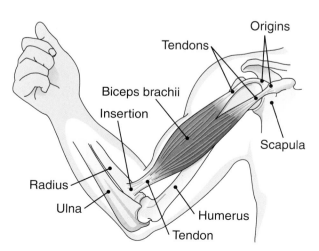

FIGURE 20-2. Diagram of a muscle showing three attachments to bones—two origins and one insertion. (Reprinted with permission from Cohen BJ, Wood DL. Memmler's The Human Body in Health and Disease. 9th Ed. Philadelphia: Lippincott Williams & Wilkins, 2000.)

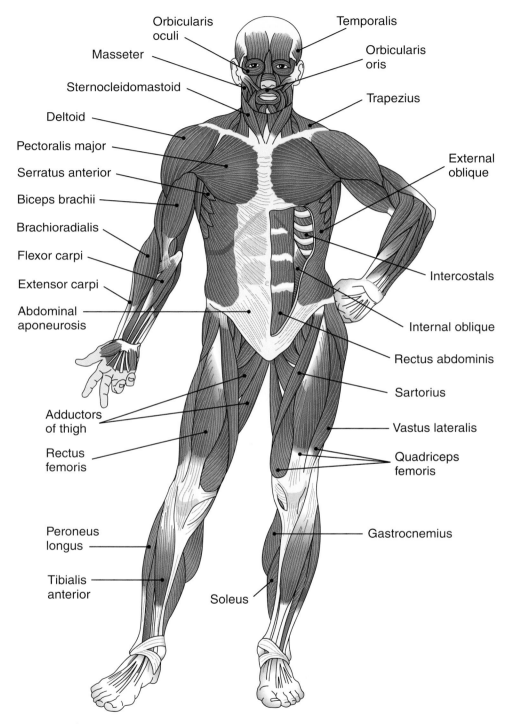

Orbicularis oculi

Masseter

Sternocleidomastoid

Deltoid

Pectoralis major

Serratus anterior

Biceps brachii

Brachioradialis

Flexor carpi

Extensor carpi

Abdominal aponeurosis

Adductors of thigh

Rectus femoris

Peroneus longus

Tibialis anterior

Temporalis

Orbicularis oris

Trapezius

External oblique

Intercostals

Internal oblique

Rectus abdominis

Sartorius

Vastus lateralis

Quadriceps femoris

Gastrocnemius

Soleus

FIGURE 20-3. Superficial muscles, anterior view. (Reprinted with permission from Cohen BJ, Wood DL. Memmler's The Human Body in Health and Disease. 9th Ed. Philadelphia: Lippincott Williams & Wilkins, 2000.)

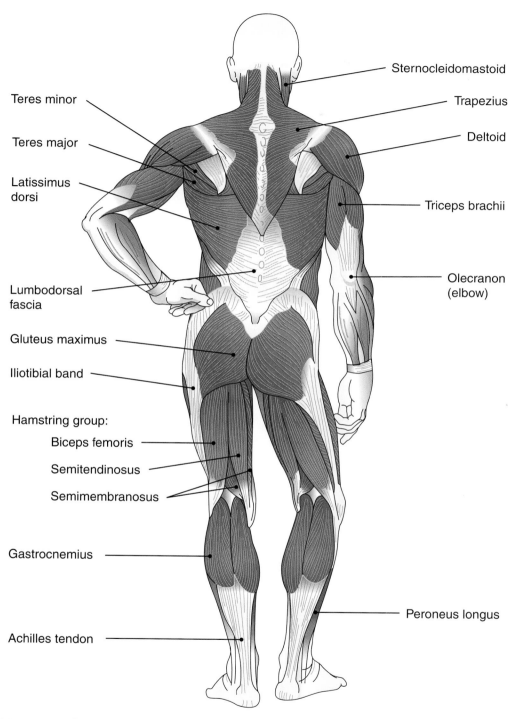

Teres minor

Teres major

Latissimus
dorsi

Lumbodorsal
fascia

Gluteus maximus

Iliotibial band

Hamstring group:

Biceps femoris

Semitendinosus

Semimembranosus

Gastrocnemius

Achilles tendon

Sternocleidomastoid

Trapezius

Deltoid

Triceps brachii

Olecranon
(elbow)

Peroneus longus

FIGURE 20-4. Superficial muscles, posterior view. (Reprinted with permission from Cohen BJ, Wood DL. Memmler's The Human Body in Health and Disease. 9th Ed. Philadelphia: Lippincott Williams & Wilkins, 2000.)

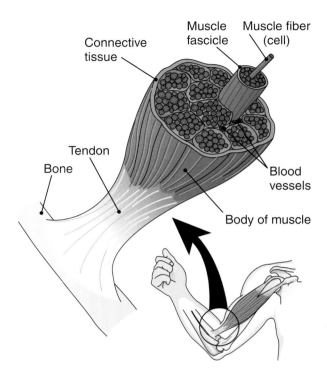

Connective
tissue

Muscle
fascicle

Muscle fiber
(cell)

Tendon

Bone

Blood
vessels

Body of muscle

FIGURE 20-5. Structure of a skeletal muscle showing connective tissue coverings. (Reprinted with permission from Cohen BJ, Wood DL. Memmler's The Human Body in Health and Disease. 9th Ed. Philadelphia: Lippincott Williams & Wilkins, 2000.)

Key Terms

NORMAL STRUCTURE AND FUNCTION

acetylcholine *as-e-til-KŌ-lēn*	A neurotransmitter that stimulates contraction of skeletal muscles
actin *AK-tin*	One of the two contractile proteins in muscle cells; the other is myosin
antagonist *an-TAG-ō-nist*	The muscle that opposes a prime mover; it must relax when the prime mover contracts
cardiac muscle *KAR-dē-ak*	Involuntary muscle that makes up the wall of the heart
fascia *FASH-ē-a*	The fibrous sheath of connective tissue that covers a muscle; called *deep fascia* to differentiate it from the superficial fascia that underlies the skin (plural, fasciae; root *fasci/o*)
insertion *in-SER-shun*	In a given movement, the point where a muscle is attached to a moving part of the skeleton
muscle *MUS-el*	An organ that produces movement by contracting; also the tissue that composes such organs (root *my/o, muscul/o*)

Normal Structure and Function, *continued*

myosin MĪ-ŏ-sin	One of the two contractile proteins in muscle cells; the other is actin
neuromuscular junction (NMJ) nū-rō-MUS-kū-lar JUNK-shun	The point of contact between a branch of a motor neuron and a muscle cell
origin OR-i-jin	In a given movement, the point where a muscle is attached to a stable part of the skeleton
prime mover PRĪM	The muscle that carries out a given movement; agonist
skeletal muscle SKEL-e-tal	Voluntary muscle that moves the skeleton and maintains posture
smooth muscle	Involuntary muscle that makes up the wall of the hollow organs, vessels, and ducts; visceral muscle
tendon TEN-dun	A fibrous band of connective tissue that attaches a muscle to a bone (root *ten/o*, *tendin/o*)
tonus TŌ-nus	A state of steady, partial contraction of muscle that maintains firmness; muscle tone (root *ton/o*)

Roots Pertaining to Muscles

TABLE 20-1 Roots Pertaining to Muscles

ROOT	MEANING	EXAMPLE	DEFINITION OF EXAMPLE
my/o	muscle	myositis* mī-ŏ-SĪ-tis	inflammation of muscle
muscul/o	muscle	musculoskeletal mus-kū-lō-SKEL-e-tal	pertaining to muscle and skeleton
in/o	fiber	inotropic in-ō-TROP-ik	acting on muscle fibers
fasci/o	fascia	fasciodesis fash-ē-OD-e-sis	suturing of a fascia to a tendon or other fascia
ten/o, tendin/o	tendon	tenorrhaphy ten-OR-a-fē	suture of a tendon
ton/o	tone	cardiotonic kar-dē-ō-TON-ik	having a strengthening action on the heart
kine, kinesi/o kinet/o	movement	dyskinesia dis-kī-NĒ-zē-a	abnormality of movement

*Note addition of *s* to this root before the suffix *–itis*.

Exercise 20-1

Define each of the following adjectives:

1. muscular   _____

2. fascial   _____

3. tendinous   _____

4. kinetic   _____

Fill in the blanks:

5. Myoedema (*mī-ō-e-DĒ-ma*) is accumulation of fluid in a(n) _____.

6. Dystonia (*dis-TŌ-nē-a*) is abnormal muscle _____.

7. Tenostosis (*ten-os-TŌ-sis*) is ossification of a(n) _____.

8. Kinesitherapy (*ki-nē-si-THER-a-pē*) is treatment by means of _____.

9. Fasciitis (*fash-ē-Ī-tis*) is inflammation of _____.

10. Inosclerosis (*in-ō-skle-RŌ-sis*) is hardening of tissue because of an increase in
 _____.

11. Myofibrils (*mī-ō-FĪ-brils*) are small fibers found in _____.

Define each of the following terms:

12. atony (*AT-ō-nē*)   _____

13. myalgia (*mī-AL-jē-a*)   _____

14. musculotendinous (*mus-kū-lō-TEN-di-nus*)   _____

15. tendinitis (*ten-di-NI-tis*) or tenositis (*ten-ō-SĪ-tis*)
 (note spelling)   _____

16. hypermyotonia (*hī-per-mī-ō-TŌ-nē-a*)   _____

17. kinesiology (*ki-nē-sē-OL-ō-jē*)   _____

18. fasciorrhaphy (*fash-ē-OR-a-fē*)   _____

19. myofascial (*mī-ō-FASH-ē-al*)   _____

20. tenomyoplasty (*ten-ō-MĪ-ō-plas-tē*)   _____

Write a word that has the same meaning as each of the following definitions:

21. inflammation of many (poly-) muscles   _____

22. any disease of muscle   _____

23. excision of fascia   _____

24. incision of a tendon (use ten/o)   _____

25. inflammation of a muscle and its tendon (use ten/o)   _____

Clinical Aspects of the Muscular System

Muscle function may be affected by disorders elsewhere, particularly in the nervous system and connective tissue. The conditions described below affect the muscular system directly or involve the muscles and have not been described in other chapters. Any disorder of muscles is described as a myopathy.

Techniques for diagnosing muscle disorders include electrical studies of muscle in action, **electromyography** (EMG), and serum assay of enzymes released in increased amounts from damaged muscles, mainly **creatine kinase** (CK).

Muscular Dystrophy

Muscular dystrophy refers to a group of hereditary diseases involving progressive, noninflammatory degeneration of muscles. There is weakness and wasting of muscle tissue with gradual replacement by connective tissue and fat. There also may be cardiomyopathy (disease of cardiac muscle) and mental impairment.

The most common form is Duchenne muscular dystrophy, a sex-linked disease passed from mother to son. This appears at age 3 to 4, and patients are incapacitated by age 10 to 15. Death is commonly caused by respiratory failure or infection.

Multiple System Disorders Involving Muscles

Polymyositis

Polymyositis is inflammation of skeletal muscle leading to weakness, frequently associated with dysphagia (difficulty in swallowing) or cardiac problems. The cause is unknown and may be related to viral infection or autoimmunity. Often the disorder is associated with some other systemic disease such as rheumatoid arthritis or lupus erythematosus.

When the skin is involved, the condition is termed **dermatomyositis**. In this case, there is erythema (redness of the skin), dermatitis (inflammation of the skin), and a typical lilac-colored rash, predominantly on the face. In addition to enzyme studies and EMG, muscle biopsy is used in diagnosis.

Fibromyalgia Syndrome

Fibromyalgia syndrome (FMS) is a difficult-to-diagnose condition involving the muscles. It is associated with widespread muscle aches, tenderness, and stiffness along with fatigue and sleep disorders in the absence of neurologic abnormalities or any other known cause. The disorder may coexist with other chronic diseases, may follow a viral infection, and may involve immune system dysfunction. Treatments for FMS may include a carefully planned exercise program and medication with pain relievers, muscle relaxants, or antidepressants.

Chronic Fatigue Syndrome

Chronic fatigue syndrome (CFS) involves persistent fatigue of no known cause that may be associated with impaired memory, sore throat, painful lymph nodes, muscle and joint pain, headaches, sleep problems, and immune disorders. The condition often occurs after a viral infection. Epstein-Barr virus (the agent that causes mononucleosis), herpesvirus, and other viruses have been suggested as possible causes of CFS. No traditional or alternative therapies have been consistently successful in treating CFS.

Myasthenia Gravis

Myasthenia gravis is an acquired autoimmune disease in which antibodies interfere with muscle stimulation at the neuromuscular junction. There is a progressive loss of muscle power, especially in the external eye muscles and other muscles of the face.

Key Clinical Terms

DISORDERS

chronic fatigue syndrome (CFS)	A disease of unknown cause that involves persistent fatigue along with muscle and joint pain and other symptoms; may be virally induced
dermatomyositis *der-ma-tō-mī-ō-SĪ-tis*	A disease of unknown origin involving inflammation of muscles as well as dermatitis and skin rashes
fibromyalgia syndrome (FMS) *fī-brō-mī-AL-jē-a*	A disorder associated with widespread muscular aches and stiffness and having no known cause
muscular dystrophy *DIS-trō-fē*	A group of hereditary muscular disorders marked by progressive weakness and atrophy of muscles
myasthenia gravis (MG) *mī-as-THĒ-nē-a GRA-vis*	A disease characterized by progressive muscular weakness; an autoimmune disease affecting the neuromuscular junction
polymyositis *pol-ē-mī-ō-SĪ-tis*	A disease of unknown cause involving muscle inflammation and weakness

DIAGNOSIS

creatine kinase (CK) *KRĒ-a-tin KĪ-nās*	An enzyme found in muscle tissue; the serum level of CK increases in cases of muscle damage; creatine phosphokinase (CPK)
electromyography (EMG) *ē-lek-trō-mī-OG-ra-fē*	Study of the electrical activity of muscles during contraction

BOX 20-1 Origins of Some Common Terms

Some common terms for musculoskeletal disorders have interesting origins. A charley horse describes muscular strain and soreness, especially in the legs. The term comes from common use of the name Charley for old lame horses that were kept around for family use when they could no longer be used for hard work. Wryneck, technically torticollis, uses the word *wry* meaning twisted or turned, as in the word awry (*a-RĪ*), meaning amiss or out of position.

A bunion, technically called hallux valgus, is an enlargement of the first joint of the great toe with bursitis at the joint. It probably comes from the word bony, changed to bunny, and used to mean a bump on the head and then a swelling on a joint. A clavus is commonly called a corn because it is a hardened or horny thickening of the skin in an area of friction or pressure.

Supplementary Terms

NORMAL STRUCTURE AND FUNCTION

Achilles tendon a-KIL-ēz	The strong cordlike tendon that attaches the calf muscles to the heel (see Fig. 20-4)
aponeurosis ap-ō-nū-RŌ-sis	A flat, white, sheetlike tendon that connects a muscle with the part that it moves (see abdominal aponeurosis, Fig. 20-3)
creatine KRĒ-a-tin	A substance in muscle cells that stores energy for contraction
glycogen GLĪ-kō-jen	A complex sugar that is stored for energy in muscles and in the liver
hamstring muscles	Three muscles of the posterior thigh: the biceps femoris, semitendinosus, and semimembranosus. They flex the leg and adduct and extend the thigh (see Fig. 20-4).
isometric ī-sō-MET-rik	Pertaining to a muscle action in which the muscle tenses but does not shorten
isotonic ī-sō-TON-ik	Pertaining to a muscle action in which the muscle shortens to accomplish movement
kinesthesia kin-es-THĒ-zē-a	Awareness of movement; perception of the weight, direction, and degree of movement (-*esthesia* means "sensation")
lactic acid LAK-tik	An acid that accumulates in muscle cells functioning without enough oxygen (anaerobically), as in times of great physical exertion. The lactic acid leads to muscle fatigue, after which it is gradually removed from the tissues.
motor unit	A single motor neuron and all of the muscle cells that its branches stimulate
myoglobin mī-ō-GLŌ-bin	A pigment similar to hemoglobin that stores oxygen in muscle cells
oxygen debt	The period during which muscles are functioning without enough oxygen. Lactic acid accumulates and leads to fatigue.
quadriceps muscle KWOD-ri-seps	A four-part muscle at the front and sides of the thigh; includes the rectus femoris, vastus intermedius, vastus lateralis, and vastus medialis; inserts at the patella and flexes the leg (see Fig. 20-3)
rotator cuff rō-TĀ-tor	A group of muscles and tendons around the capsule of the shoulder joint that provides mobility and strength to the joint

SYMPTOMS AND CONDITIONS

amyotrophic lateral sclerosis (ALS) a-mī-ō-TROF-ik	A condition caused by degeneration of motor neurons; marked by muscular weakness and atrophy with spasticity and hyperreflexia; Lou Gehrig disease
asterixis as-ter-IK-sis	Rapid, jerky movements, especially in the hands, caused by intermittent loss of muscle tone

Symptoms and Conditions, *continued*

asthenia *as-THĒ-nē-a*	Weakness (prefix *a-* meaning "without" with root *-sthen/o* meaning "strength)"
ataxia *a-TAK-sē-a*	Lack of muscle coordination (from root *tax/o* meaning "order, arrangement"; adjective, ataxic)
athetosis *ath-e-TŌ-sis*	A condition marked by slow, irregular, twisting movements, especially in the hands and fingers (adjective, athetotic)
atrophy *AT-rō-fē*	A wasting away; a decrease in the size of a tissue or organ, such as the wasting of muscle from disuse
avulsion *a-VUL-shun*	Forcible tearing away of a part
clonus *KLŌ-nus*	Alternating spasmodic contraction and relaxation in a muscle (adjective, clonic)
contracture *kon-TRAK-chur*	Permanent contraction of a muscle
fibromyositis *fī-brō-mī-ō-SĪ-tis*	A nonspecific term for pain, tenderness, and stiffness in muscles and joints
fibrositis *fī-brō-SĪ-tis*	Inflammation of fibrous connective tissue, especially the muscle fasciae; marked by pain and stiffness
rhabdomyolysis *rab-dō-mī-OL-i-sis*	An acute disease involving diffuse destruction of skeletal muscle cells (root *rhabd/o* means "rod," referring to the long, rodlike muscle cells)
rhabdomyoma *rab-dō-mī-Ō-ma*	A benign tumor of skeletal muscle
rhabdomyosarcoma *rab-dō-mī-ō-sar-KŌ-ma*	A highly malignant tumor of skeletal muscle
rheumatism *rū-ma-tizm*	A general term for inflammation, soreness, and stiffness of muscles associated with pain in joints (adjective, rheumatic, rheumatoid)
spasm	A sudden, involuntary muscle contraction; may be clonic (contraction alternating with relaxation) or tonic (sustained); a strong and painful spasm may be called a cramp (adjectives, spastic, spasmodic)
spasticity *spas-TIS-i-tē*	Increased tone or contractions of muscles causing stiff and awkward movements
strain	Trauma to a muscle because of overuse or excessive stretch; if severe, may involve tearing of muscle, bleeding, or separation of muscle from its tendon or separation of a tendon from bone
tendinitis *ten-di-NĪ-tis*	Inflammation of a tendon, usually caused by injury or overuse; the shoulder, elbow, and hip are common sites
tenosynovitis *ten-ō-sin-ō-VĪ-tis*	Inflammation of a tendon sheath

Symptoms and Conditions, continued

tetanus *TET-a-nus*	An acute infectious disease caused by the anaerobic bacillus *Clostridium tetani*. It is marked by persistent painful spasms of voluntary muscles; lockjaw.
tetany *TET-a-nē*	A condition marked by spasms, cramps, and muscle twitching caused by a metabolic imbalance, such as low blood calcium caused by underactivity of the parathyroid glands
torticollis *tor-ti-KOL-is*	Spasmodic contraction of the neck muscles causing stiffness and twisting of the neck; wryneck

DIAGNOSIS AND TREATMENT

anti-inflammatory agent	Drug that reduces inflammation; includes steroids, such as cortisone, and nonsteroidal anti-inflammatory drugs
Chvostek sign *VOS-tek*	Spasm of facial muscles after a tap over the facial nerve; evidence of tetany
muscle relaxant *rē-LAX-ant*	A drug that reduces muscle tension; different forms may be used to relax muscles during surgery, to control spasticity, or to relieve pain of musculoskeletal disorders
nonsteroidal anti-inflammatory drug (NSAID)	Drug that reduces inflammation but is not a steroid; examples include aspirin and ibuprofen and other inhibitors of prostaglandins, naturally produced substances that promote inflammation
occupational therapy	Health profession concerned with increasing function and preventing disability through work and play activities. The goal of occupational therapy is to increase the patient's independence and quality of daily life.
physical therapy	Health profession concerned with physical rehabilitation and prevention of disability. Exercise, massage, and other therapeutic methods are used to restore proper movement.
rheumatology *rū-ma-TOL-ō-jē*	The study and treatment of rheumatic diseases
Trousseau sign *tru-SŌ*	Spasmodic contractions caused by pressing the nerve supplying a muscle; seen in tetany

ABBREVIATIONS

Ach	Acetylcholine	**MG**	Myasthenia gravis
ALS	Amyotrophic lateral sclerosis	**NMJ**	Neuromuscular junction
CFS	Chronic fatigue syndrome	**OT**	Occupational therapy, therapist
C(P)K	Creatine (phospho)kinase	**PT**	Physical therapy, therapist
EMG	Electromyography, electromyogram	**ROM**	Range of motion
FMS	Fibromyalgia syndrome		

Labeling Exercise 20-1

Superficial Muscles, Anterior View

Write the name of each numbered part on the corresponding line of the answer sheet.

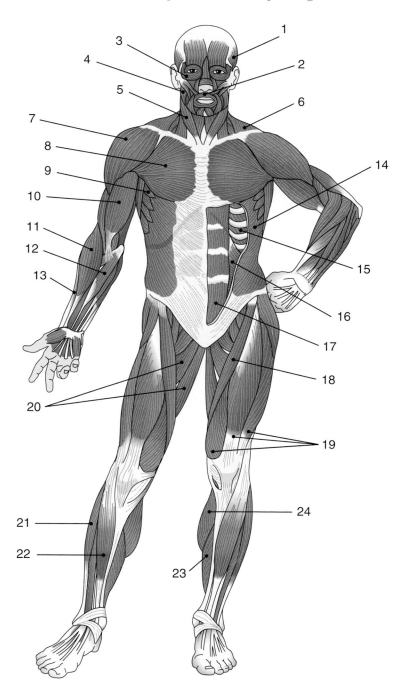

Adductors of thigh
Biceps brachii
Brachioradialis
Deltoid
Extensor carpi
External oblique
Flexor carpi
Gastrocnemius
Intercostals
Internal oblique
Masseter
Orbicularis oculi
Orbicularis oris
Pectoralis major
Peroneus longus
Quadriceps femoris
Rectus abdominis
Sartorius
Serratus anterior
Soleus
Sternocleidomastoid
Temporalis
Tibialis anterior
Trapezius

1. _____

2. _____

3. _____

4. _____

5. _____

6. _____

7. _____

8. _____

9. _____

10. _____

11. _____

12. _____

13. _____

14. _____

15. _____

16. _____

17. _____

18. _____

19. _____

20. _____

21. _____

22. _____

23. _____

24. _____

Labeling Exercise 20-2

Superficial Muscles, Posterior View

Write the name of each numbered part on the corresponding line of the answer sheet.

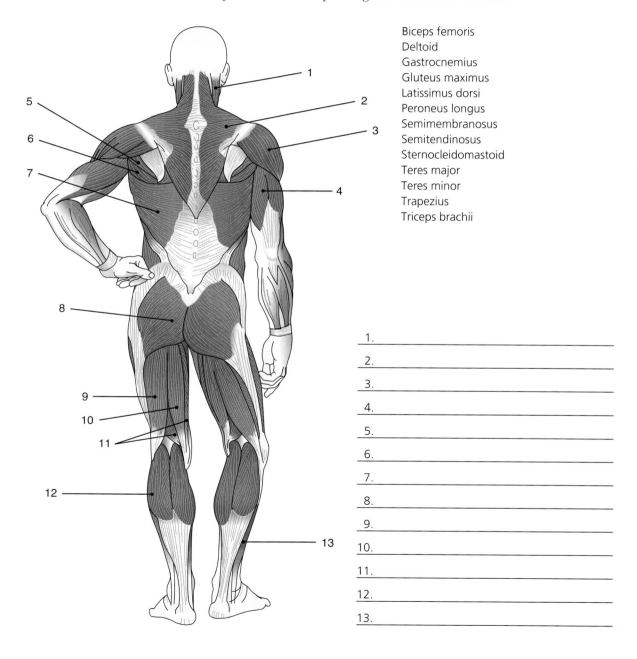

Biceps femoris
Deltoid
Gastrocnemius
Gluteus maximus
Latissimus dorsi
Peroneus longus
Semimembranosus
Semitendinosus
Sternocleidomastoid
Teres major
Teres minor
Trapezius
Triceps brachii

1. _____
2. _____
3. _____
4. _____
5. _____
6. _____
7. _____
8. _____
9. _____
10. _____
11. _____
12. _____
13. _____

Chapter Review 20-1

Match the following terms and write the appropriate letter to the left of each number:

_____ 1. biceps brachii

_____ 2. deltoid

_____ 3. semitendinosus

_____ 4. gastrocnemius

_____ 5. quadriceps femoris

a. main muscle of the calf

b. triangular muscle that covers the shoulder

c. one of the hamstring muscles

d. anterior muscle of the upper arm that flexes the forearm

e. large muscle group of the anterior thigh

_____ 6. pectoralis major

_____ 7. rectus abdominis

_____ 8. intercostal

_____ 9. latissimus dorsi

_____ 10. gluteus maximus

a. muscle that runs vertically at the center of the anterior trunk

b. main muscle of the buttocks

c. muscle between the ribs

d. large muscle of the upper chest

e. large muscle across the back below the trapezius

_____ 11. bradykinesia

_____ 12. inotropic

_____ 13. dystonia

_____ 14. actin

_____ 15. inosemia

a. abnormal muscle tone

b. excess fibrin in the blood

c. a contractile protein in muscle cells

d. slowness of movement

e. acting on muscle fibers

SUPPLEMENTARY TERMS

_____ 16. aponeurosis

_____ 17. rotator cuff

_____ 18. isometric

_____ 19. creatine

_____ 20. lactic acid

a. substance that stores energy in muscle cells

b. flat, white, sheetlike tendon

c. substance that accumulates in muscles working anaerobically

d. group of muscles around the shoulder joint

e. a type of muscle contraction

_____ 21. tetany

_____ 22. ataxia

_____ 23. rhabdomyolysis

_____ 24. asthenia

_____ 25. atrophy

a. weakness

b. lack of muscle coordination

c. muscular spasms and cramps

d. wasting or decrease in size of tissue

e. disease involving destruction of muscle cells

_____ 26. avulsion

_____ 27. torticollis

_____ 28. athetosis

_____ 29. kinesthesia

_____ 30. myoglobin

a. pigment that stores oxygen in muscle cells

b. awareness of movement

c. wryneck

d. forcible tearing away of a part

e. condition marked by slow, twisting movements

Fill in the blanks:

31. The neurotransmitter released at the neuromuscular junction is _____.

32. A muscle that produces flexion at a joint is called a(n) _____.

33. The number of origins (heads) in the biceps brachii muscle is _____.

34. The sheath of connective tissue that covers a muscle is called _____.

35. A band of connective tissue that attaches a muscle to a bone is a(n) _____.

36. The strong, cordlike tendon that attaches the calf muscle to the heel is the
_____.

37. Movement toward the midline of the body is termed _____.

Define each of the following words:

38. myofascial (mī-ō-FASH-ē-al) _____

39. myonecrosis (mī-ō-ne-KRO-sis) _____

40. inositis (in-ō-SĪ-tis) _____

41. tenorrhaphy (ten-OR-a-fē) _____

42. hypotonia (hī-pō-TŌ-nē-a) _____

43. hyperkinesia (hī-per-ki-NE-sē-a) _____

Word building. Write a word for each of the following definitions:

44. study of muscles (use my/o-) _____

45. pain in a muscle (use my/o-) _____

46. incision of fascia _____

47. inflammation of fascia _____

48. study of movement _____

49. plastic repair of a tendon (use ten/o-) _____

50. pertaining to a tendon _____

Opposites. Write a word that has the opposite meaning of each of the following terms as they pertain to muscles:

51. antagonist _____

52. insertion _____

53. adduction _____

54. pronation   _____

55. extension   _____

Supplementary terms. Write the adjective form of each of the following words:

56. ataxia   _____

57. athetosis   _____

58. spasm   _____

59. clonus   _____

Abbreviations. Write the meaning of each of the following:

60. EMG   _____

61. Ach   _____

62. OT   _____

63. ROM   _____

64. FMS   _____

Word analysis. Define each of the following words, and give the meaning of the word parts in each. Use a dictionary if necessary.

65. isometric _____
    a. iso- _____
    b. metr/o _____
    c. -ic _____

66. amyotrophic _____
    a. a- _____
    b. my/o _____
    c. troph/o _____
    d. -ic _____

67. myasthenia _____
    a. my/o _____
    b. a- _____
    c. sthen/o _____
    d. -ia _____

Case Studies

Case Study 20-1: Rotator Cuff Tear

M.L., a 56-year-old business executive and former college football player, was referred to an orthopedic surgeon for recurrent shoulder pain. M.L. was unable to abduct his right arm without pain even after 6 months of physical therapy and NSAIDs. In addition, he had taken supplements of glucosamine, chondroitin, and S-adenosylmethionine for several months in an effort to protect the flexibility of his shoulder joint. M.L. recalled a shoulder dislocation resulting from a football injury 35 years earlier. The surgeon recommended the Bankart procedure for M.L.'s complete tear to restore his joint stability, alleviate his pain, and permit him to return to his former normal activities, including golf.

After anesthesia induction and positioning in a semisitting (beach chair) position, the surgeon made an anterosuperior deltoid incision (the standard deltopectoral approach) and divided the coracoacromial ligament at the acromial attachment. The rotator cuff was identified after the deltoid was retracted and the clavipectoral fascia was incised. The subscapularis tendon was incised proximal to its insertion. After incision of the capsule, inspection showed a large pouch inferiorly in the capsule, consistent with laxity (instability). The torn edges of the capsule were anchored to the rim of the glenoid fossa with heavy nonabsorbable sutures. A flap from the subscapularis tendon was transposed and sutured to the supraspinatus and infraspinatus muscles to bridge the gap. An intraoperative ROM examination showed that the external rotation could be performed past neutral and that the shoulder did not dislocate. The wound was closed, and a shoulder immobilizer sling was applied. M.L. was referred to PT to begin therapy in 3 weeks and was assured he would be able to play golf in 6 months.

Case Study 20-2: Brachial Plexus Injury

T.D., a 16-year-old high school student, had a severe football accident 3 months before his admission. He sustained a right brachial plexus injury, resulting in a flail arm. He had no recovery and was on medication for neurologic pain. He reported that he had no feeling or motion in his right shoulder or arm. He had atrophy over the supraspinatus and infraspinatus muscles and also subluxation of his shoulder and atrophy of the deltoid. He had no active motion of the right upper extremity and no sensation. The rest of his orthopedic exam showed full ROM of his hips, knees, and ankles with intact sensation and palpable distal pulses as well as normal motor function. He was diagnosed with a possible middle trunk brachial plexus injury from C7. He was scheduled for an EMG, nerve conduction studies, and somatosensory evoked potentials (SSEPs). His diaphragm was examined under fluoroscopy to R/O phrenic nerve injury.

With middle trunk brachial plexus injury, damage to the subscapular nerve will interrupt conduction to the subscapularis and teres major muscles. Damage to the long thoracic nerve prevents conduction to the serratus anterior muscles. Injury to the pectoral nerves affects the pectoralis major and minor muscles.

T.D. was scheduled for a brachial plexus exploration with possible nerve graft, nerve transfer, bilateral sural (calf) nerve harvest, or gracilis muscle graft from his right thigh.

Case Study 20-3: "Wake Up" Test During Spinal Fusion Surgery

L.N.'s somatosensory evoked potentials (SSEPs) were monitored throughout her spinal fusion surgery to provide continuous information on the functional state of her sensory pathways from the median and posterior tibial nerves through the dorsal column to the primary somatosensory cortex. Before surgery, needle electrodes were inserted into L.N.'s right and left quadriceps muscles to determine nerve conduction through L2 to L4, into the anterior tibialis muscles to measure passage through L5, and into the gastrocnemius muscles to measure S1 to S2. Electrodes were placed in her rectus abdominus to monitor S1 to S2. All electrodes were taped in place, and the wires were plugged into a transformer box with feed-

Case Studies, continued

back to a computer. A neuromonitoring technologist placed the electrodes and attended the computer monitor throughout the case. During the procedure, selected muscle groups were stimulated with 15 to 40 milliamps (mA) of current to test the nerves and muscles. Feedback data into the computer confirmed the neuromuscular integrity and status of the spinal fixation of the instrumentation and implants.

After the pedicle screws, hooks, and wires were in place and the spinal rods were cinched down to straighten the spine, L.N. was permitted to emerge temporarily from anesthesia and muscle paralysis medication to a lightly sedated but pain-free state. She was given commands to move her feet, straighten her legs, and wiggle her toes to test all neuromuscular groups that could be affected by misplaced or compressed spinal fixation devices. Her feet were watched, and movement was announced to the team. Dorsiflexion cleared the tibialis anterior muscles; plantar flexion cleared the gastrocnemius muscles. Knee flexion cleared the hamstring muscle group, and knee extension determined function of the quadriceps group. L.N. had a successful "wake-up" test. She was put back into deep anesthesia, and her incision was closed. A postoperative "wake-up" test was repeated after she was moved to her bed. The surgical instruments and tables were kept sterile until after all of the monitored muscle groups were tested and showed voluntary movement. The electrodes were removed, and she was taken to PACU for recovery.

CASE STUDY QUESTIONS

Multiple choice: Select the best answer and write the letter of your choice to the left of each number.

_____ 1. The insertion of the muscle is:
   a. the thick middle portion
   b. the point of attachment to the moving bone
   c. the point of attachment to the stable bone
   d. the fibrous sheath
   e. the connective tissue

_____ 2. M.L. was unable to abduct his affected arm. This motion is:
   a. toward the midline
   b. circumferential
   c. in the same direction as the muscle fibers
   d. away from the midline
   e. a position with the palm facing upward

_____ 3. An anterosuperior deltoid incision would be made:
   a. perpendicular to the muscle fibers
   b. below the fascia sheath
   c. behind the glenoid fossa
   d. in the best area
   e. at the top and to the front of the deltoid muscle

_____ 4. The subscapularis tendon arises from the subscapularis:
   a. fascia
   b. nerve
   c. bone
   d. extensor
   e. flexor

Case Studies, continued

5. The intraoperative ROM examination was performed:
   a. in the OR corridor
   b. during surgery
   c. before surgery
   d. after surgery
   e. in the interventional radiology suite

6. M.L.'s arm and shoulder were immobilized after surgery to:
   a. encourage movement beyond the point of pain
   b. minimize rapid ROM
   c. maintain adduction and external rotation
   d. prevent movement
   e. stop bleeding

7. T.D. had atrophy of the supraspinatus and infraspinatus muscles. The term atrophy here refers to:
   a. hypercontraction
   b. intermittent contraction and relaxation
   c. muscle tissue wasting
   d. paralysis
   e. painful discoloration

8. Another term for subluxation is:
   a. dislocation
   b. hyperextension
   c. turning inside out
   d. overlapping
   e. stretched beyond original shape

9. A palpable distal pulse means that the pulse can be:
   a. heard at the foot
   b. felt at the top of the thigh
   c. felt at the foot
   d. obliterated with light
   e. undetectable

10. The pectoralis major and pectoralis minor muscles are located:
    a. below the knees
    b. behind the thighs
    c. in the lower back
    d. in the upper chest
    e. on the lateral side of the arms

11. The quadriceps muscle group is made up of:
    a. smooth and cardiac muscle fibers
    b. four muscles in the thigh
    c. three muscles in the leg and one in the anterior chest
    d. fascia and tendon sheaths
    e. tendons and fascia around the shoulder

Case Studies, continued

_____ 12. The nerve supply for the rectus abdominus muscle runs through S1-S2. This anatomic region is:
   a. the first and second sural sheath
   b. subluxation and suppuration
   c. sacral disk space 1 and 2
   d. sacral disk space 3
   e. somatosensory electrodes 1 and 2

_____ 13. The joint motion characterized by elevating the toes toward the anterior ankle is:
   a. supination
   b. pronation
   c. dorsiflexion
   d. plantar flexion
   e. external rotation

_____ 14. Knee extension results in:
   a. a bent knee
   b. a ballet position with the toes turned out
   c. bilateral abduction
   d. inversion
   e. a straight leg

Write a term from the case studies with each of the following meanings:

15. pertaining to the arm   _____

16. pertaining to treatment of skeletal and muscular   _____
    disorders

17. bending at a joint   _____

18. to point the toes downward   _____

Abbreviations. Define the following abbreviations:

19. PT   _____

20. ROM   _____

21. R/O   _____

22. EMG   _____

23. SSEP   _____

24. PACU   _____

Chapter 20 Crossword
Muscular System

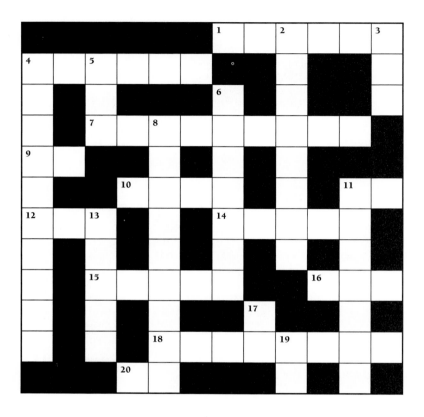

ACROSS

1. Around: prefix
4. Rod, such as a muscle cell: combining form
7. Muscle group at the back of the thigh
9. Not: prefix
10. Muscle tone: combining form
11. Down, without, removal: prefix
12. Disease caused by degeneration of motor neurons, with weakness, atrophy, and spasticity: abbreviation
14. Muscle that carries out a given movement, _ _ _ _ _ mover
15. Lack of muscle tone
16. Referring to a joint in the foot: abbreviation
18. Adjective for a type of muscle contraction
20. Fiber: root

DOWN

2. Muscle of the forearm, brachio _ _ _ _ _ _ _ _
3. Muscle: combining form
4. Referring to rheumatism
5. Neurotransmitter active in the muscular system: abbreviation
6. Wasting of tissue
8. Substance that stores oxygen in muscles
11. Muscle that covers the shoulder
13. Sudden involuntary muscle contraction
17. Health profession concerned with physical rehabilitation and prevention of disability: abbreviation
19. Health profession concerned with working to increase function and independence in daily life: abbreviation

CHAPTER 20 Answer Section

Answers to Chapter Exercises

EXERCISE 20-1

1. pertaining to muscle
2. pertaining to fascia
3. pertaining to a tendon
4. pertaining to movement
5. muscle
6. tone
7. tendon
8. movement
9. fascia
10. fibers
11. muscle
12. lack of muscle tone
13. pain in a muscle
14. pertaining to muscle and tendon
15. inflammation of a tendon
16. excess muscle tone
17. study of movement
18. suture of fascia
19. pertaining to muscle and fascia
20. plastic repair of tendon and muscle
21. polymyositis (*pol-ē-mi-ō-SĪ-tis*)
22. myopathy (*mī-OP-a-thē*)
23. fasciectomy (*fash-ē-EK-tō-mē*)
24. tenotomy (*ten-OT-ō-mē*)
25. myotenositis (*mī-ō-ten-ō-SĪ-tis*)

LABELING EXERCISE 20-1
SUPERFICIAL MUSCLES, ANTERIOR VIEW

1. temporalis (*tem-pō-RĀ-lis*)
2. orbicularis oris (*OR-is*)
3. orbicularis oculi (*or-bik-ū-LĀ-ris OK-ū-li*)
4. masseter (*MAS-e-ter*)
5. sternocleidomastoid (*ster-nō-klī-dō-MAS-toyd*)
6. trapezius (*tra-PĒ-zē-us*)
7. deltoid (*DEL-toyd*)
8. pectoralis (*pek-tō-RĀ-lis*) major
9. serratus (*ser-Ā-tus*) anterior
10. biceps brachii (*BĪ-seps BRĀ-kē-Ī*)
11. brachioradialis (*brā-kē-ō-rā-dē-AL-is*)
12. flexor carpi (*KAR-pī*)
13. extensor carpi
14. external oblique (*ō-BLĒK*)
15. internal oblique
16. rectus abdominis

17. adductor longus
18. sartorius (*sar-TŌ-rē-us*)
19. quadriceps femoris (*KWOD-ri-seps FEM-or-is*)
20. adductors of thigh
21. peroneus longus (*per-ō-NĒ-us LONG-us*)
22. tibialis (*tib-ē-Ā-lis*) anterior
23. soleus (*SŌ-lē-us*)
24. gastrocnemius (*gas-trok-NĒ-mē-us*)

LABELING EXERCISE 20-2 SUPERFICIAL MUSCLES, POSTERIOR VIEW

1. sternocleidomastoid
2. trapezius (*tra-PĒ-zē-us*)
3. deltoid
4. triceps brachii (*BRĀ kē-ī*)
5. teres (*TĒ-rez*) minor
6. teres major
7. latissimus dorsi (*la-TIS-i-mus DOR-sī*)
8. gluteus (*GLŪ-tē-us*) maximus
9. biceps femoris
10. semitendinosus (*sem-ē-ten-di-NŌ-sus*)
11. semimembranosus (*sem-ē-mem-bra-NŌ-sus*)
12. gastrocnemius
13. peroneus longus

Answers to Chapter Review 20-1

1. d
2. b
3. c
4. a
5. e
6. d
7. a
8. c
9. e
10. b
11. d
12. e
13. a
14. c
15. b
16. b
17. d
18. e
19. a
20. c
21. c
22. b

23. e
24. a
25. d
26. d
27. c
28. e
29. b
30. a
31. acetylcholine
32. flexor
33. two
34. fascia
35. tendon
36. Achilles tendon
37. adduction
38. pertaining to muscle and fascia
39. death of muscle tissue
40. inflammation of fibers (fibrous tissue)
41. suture of a tendon
42. decreased muscle tone
43. abnormally increased movement
44. myology
45. myalgia
46. fasciotomy
47. fasciitis, also fascitis
48. kinesiology
49. tenoplasty
50. tendinous
51. prime mover; agonist
52. origin
53. abduction
54. supination
55. flexion
56. ataxic
57. athetotic
58. spastic, spasmodic
59. clonic
60. electromyography, electromyogram
61. acetylcholine
62. occupational therapy
63. range of motion
64. fibromyalgia syndrome
65. pertaining to muscle action in which the muscle tenses but does not shorten
    a. the same, equal
    b. measure
    c. pertaining to
66. pertaining to muscle wasting, atrophy
    a. lack of
    b. muscle
    c. nourishment
    d. pertaining to
67. muscular weakness
    a. muscle
    b. lack of
    c. strength
    d. condition of

Answers to Case Study Questions

1. b
2. d
3. e
4. a
5. b
6. d
7. c
8. a
9. c
10. d
11. b
12. c
13. c
14. e
15. brachial
16. orthopedic
17. flexion
18. plantar flexion
19. physical therapy
20. range of motion
21. rule out
22. electromyogram
23. somatosensory evoked potentials
24. postanesthetic care unit

ANSWERS TO CROSSWORD PUZZLE

Muscular System

					1.C	I	R	2.C	U	3.M	
4.R	H	5.A	B	D	O			A		Y	
H		C			6.A			D		O	
E		7.H	8.A	M	S	T	R	I	N	G	
9.U	N			Y		R		A			
M			10.T	O	N	O		L	11.D	E	
12.A	L	13.S		G		14.P	R	I	M	E	
T		P		L	H		S		L		
I		15.A	T	O	N	Y		16.M	T	P	
I		S		B		17.P			O		
D		M		18.I	S	O	T	19.O	N	I	C
			20.I	N			T		D		

The Skin

Chapter Contents

Objectives

After study of this chapter you should be able to:

1. Compare the epidermis, dermis, and subcutaneous tissue.
2. Describe the roles of keratin and melanin in the skin.
3. Name and describe the glands in the skin.
4. Describe the structure of hair and of nails.
5. Identify and use roots pertaining to the skin.
6. Describe the main disorders that affect the skin.
7. Label a diagram of the skin.
8. Analyze several case studies involving the skin.

L ike the eyes, the **skin** is a readily visible reflection of one's health. Its color, texture, and resilience reveal much, as does the condition of the **hair** and **nails**. The skin and its associated structures make up the **integumentary system**. This body-covering system protects against infection, dehydration, ultraviolet radiation, and injury. Extensive damage to the skin, such as by burns, can result in a host of dangerous complications. The skin also serves in temperature regulation and sensory perception. The adjective **cutaneous** refers to the skin.

Anatomy of the Skin

The outermost portion of the skin is the **epidermis**, consisting of 4 to 5 layers (strata) of epithelial cells (Fig. 21-1). The deepest layer, the stratum basale, or basal layer, produces new cells. As these cells gradually rise toward the surface, they die and become filled with **keratin**, a protein that thickens and toughens the skin. The outermost (horny) layer of the epidermis, the stratum corneum, is composed of flat, dead, protective cells that are constantly being shed and replaced. Some of the cells in the epidermis produce **melanin**, a pigment that gives color to the skin and protects against sunlight.

The **dermis** is beneath the epidermis. It is composed of connective tissue, nerves, blood vessels, and lymphatics. This layer supplies support and nourishment for the skin. The **subcutaneous tissue** beneath the dermis is composed mainly of connective tissue and fat.

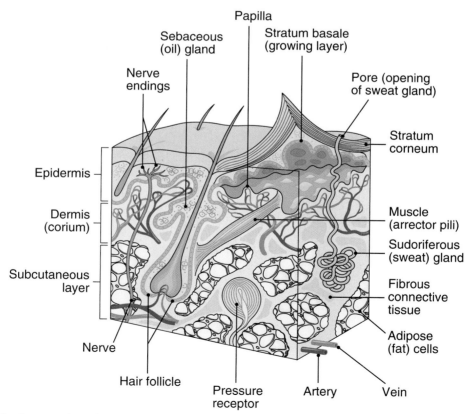

FIGURE 21-1. Cross-section of the skin. (Reprinted with permission from Cohen BJ, Wood DL. Memmler's The Human Body in Health and Disease. 9th Ed. Philadelphia: Lippincott Williams & Wilkins, 2000.)

Associated Skin Structures

The **sudoriferous** (sweat) **glands** act mainly in temperature regulation by releasing a watery fluid that evaporates to cool the body.

The **sebaceous glands** release an oily fluid, **sebum,** that lubricates the hair and skin and prevents drying.

Hair is widely distributed over the body. Each hair develops within a sheath or **hair follicle** and grows from its base within the deep layers of the skin. Both hair and nails function in protection. Each nail develops from a growing region at its proximal end. Hair and nails are composed of nonliving material consisting mainly of keratin.

Key Terms

NORMAL STRUCTURE AND FUNCTION

cutaneous kū-TĀ-nē-us	Pertaining to the skin (from Latin *cutis,* meaning "skin")
dermis DER-mis	The layer of the skin between the epidermis and the subcutaneous tissue; the true skin or corium
epidermis ep-i-DER-mis	The outermost layer of the skin (from *epi-,* meaning "upon or over" and *derm,* meaning "skin")
hair	A threadlike keratinized outgrowth from the skin (root *trich/o*)
hair follicle FOL-i-kl	The sheath in which a hair develops
integumentary system in-teg-ū-MEN-ta-rē	The skin and its associated glands, hair, and nails
keratin KER-a-tin	A protein that thickens and toughens the skin and makes up hair and nails (root *kerat/o*)
melanin MEL-a-nin	A dark pigment that gives color to the hair and skin and protects the skin against the sun's radiation (root *melan/o*)
nail	A platelike keratinized outgrowth of the skin that covers the dorsal surface of the terminal phalanges (root *onych/o*)
sebaceous gland se-BA-shus	A gland that produces sebum; usually associated with a hair follicle (root *seb/o*)
sebum SE-bum	A fatty secretion of the sebaceous glands that lubricates the hair and skin (root *seb/o*)
skin	The tissue that covers the body; the integument (root *derm/o, dermat/o*)
subcutaneous tissue sub-kū-TĀ-nē-us	The layer of tissue beneath the skin; also called the hypodermis
sudoriferous gland sū-dor-IF-er-us	A sweat gland (root *hidr/o, idr/o*)

Roots Pertaining to the Skin

TABLE 21-1 Roots Pertaining to the Skin			
ROOT	**MEANING**	**EXAMPLE**	**DEFINITION OF EXAMPLE**
derm/o, dermat/o	skin	dermabrasion *derm-a-BRĀ-zhun*	surgical procedure used to resurface the skin and remove imperfections
kerat/o	keratin, horny layer of the skin	keratosis *ker-a-TŌ-sis*	horny growth of the skin
melan/o	dark, black, melanin	melanosome *MEL-a-nō-sōm*	a small body in the cell that produces melanin
hidr/o, idr/o	sweat, perspiration	hyperhidrosis *hī-per-hī-DRŌ-sis*	abnormally high production of sweat
seb/o	sebum, sebaceous gland	seborrhea *seb-or-Ē-a*	excess flow of sebum
trich/o	hair	trichomycosis *trik-ō-mī-KŌ-sis*	fungal infection of the hair
onych/o	nail	onychia *ō-NIK-ē-a*	inflammation of the nail and nail bed (not an *-itis* ending)

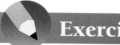

Exercise 21-1

Identify and define the roots in each of the following words:

	Root	Meaning of Root
1. hypodermis (*hī-pō-DĒR-mis*)	_____	_____
2. hypomelanosis (*hī-pō-mel-a-NŌ-sis*)	_____	_____
3. seborrheic (*seb-ō-RĒ-ik*)	_____	_____
4. keratogenous (*ker-a-TOJ-e-nus*)	_____	_____
5. anidrosis (*an-Ī-DRŌ-sis*)	_____	_____
6. hyponychium (*hī-pō-NIK-ē-um*)	_____	_____
7. hypertrichosis (*hī-per-tri-KŌ-sis*)	_____	_____

Fill in the blanks:

8. Dermatopathology (*der-ma-tō-pa-THOL-ō-jē*) refers to any disease of the

_____.

9. Dyskeratosis (*dis-ker-a-TŌ-sis*) is an abnormality in the skin's formation of

_____.

10. A melanocyte (*MEL-a-nō-sīt*) is a cell that produces _____.

11. Hidradenitis (*hī-drad-i-NĪ-tis*) is inflammation of a gland that produces

    _____.

12. Trichoid (*TRIK-oyd*) means resembling a(n) _____.

13. Onychomycosis (*on-i-kō-mī-KŌ-sis*) is a fungal infection of a(n) _____.

14. A hypodermic (*hī-pō-DER-mik*) injection is given under the _____.

Word building. Write a word for each of the following definitions:

15. study of the skin and skin diseases   _____

16. inflammation of the skin   _____

17. formation (-genesis) of keratin   _____

18. a tumor containing melanin   _____

19. abnormally low production of sweat   _____

20. study of the hair   _____

21. softening of a nail   _____

22. instrument for cutting the skin   _____

Use the suffix *-derma* meaning "condition of the skin" to write a word with each of the following meanings:

23. hardening of the skin   _____

24. presence of pus in the skin   _____

Clinical Aspects of the Skin

Many diseases are manifested by changes in the quality of the skin or by specific lesions. Some types of skin lesions are described and illustrated in Display 21-1. The study of the skin and diseases of the skin is **dermatology**, but careful observation of the skin, hair, and nails should be part of every physical examination. The skin should be examined for color, unusual pigmentation, and lesions. It should be palpated to evaluate its texture, temperature, moisture, firmness, and any tenderness.

Wounds

Wounds are caused by trauma, such as in cases of accidents or attacks, or by surgery and other therapeutic or diagnostic procedures. Wounds may affect not only the injured area but also other body systems. Infection and hemorrhage may complicate wounds, as do **dehiscence**, disruption of the wound layers, and **evisceration**, protrusion of internal organs through the lesion.

As a wound heals, fluid and cells drain from the damaged tissue. This drainage, called **exudate**, may be clear, bloody (sanguinous), or pus-containing (purulent). Tubes may be used to remove exudate from the site of a wound.

Proper wound healing depends on cleanliness and care of the lesion and also on proper circulation, good general health, and good nutrition. Various types of dressings are used to protect wounded areas and promote healing. Vacuum-assisted closure (VAC) uses negative pressure to close the tissues and begin the healing process. Healing may be promoted by **débridement**, the removal of dead or damaged tissue from

DISPLAY 21-1   Types of Skin Lesions

LESION	DESCRIPTION
bulla *BUL-a*	raised, fluid-filled lesion larger than a vesicle (plural, bullae)
fissure *FISH-ur*	crack or break in the skin
macule *MAK-ūl*	flat, colored spot
nodule *NOD-ūl*	solid, raised lesion larger than a papule; often indicative of systemic disease
papule *PAP-ūl*	small, circular, raised lesion at the surface of the skin
plaque *plak*	patch
pustule *PUS-tūl*	raised lesion containing pus; often in a hair follicle or sweat pore
ulcer *UL-ser*	lesion resulting from destruction of the skin and perhaps subcutaneous tissue
vesicle *VES-i-kl*	small, fluid-filled, raised lesion; a blister or bleb
wheal *wēl*	smooth, rounded, slightly raised area often associated with itching; seen in urticaria (hives) such as resulting from allergy

Bulla

Fissure

Macule

Nodule

Papule

Plaque

Pustule

Ulcer

Vesicle

Wheal

a wound. This may be accomplished by cutting or scrubbing away the dead tissue or by means of enzymes. A thick, dark crust or scab (eschar) may be removed in an **escharotomy**. Deep wounds may require skin grafting for proper healing. Grafts may be a full-thickness skin graft (FTSG), which consists of the epidermis and dermis, or a split-thickness skin graft (STSG), consisting of the epidermis only. Skin is cut for grafting with a **dermatome**.

BOX 21-1 The French Connection

Many scientific and medical terms are adapted from foreign languages. Most of the roots come from Latin and Greek; others are derived from German or French. Sometimes a foreign word is used "as is." Débridement, removal of dead or damaged tissue from a wound, comes from the French, meaning removal of a restraint, such as the bridle of a harness. Also from French, a contrecoup injury occurs when the head is thrown forward and back, as in a car accident, and the brain is injured by hitting the skull on the side opposite the blow. Contrecoup in French means "counter blow." Tic douloureux, a disorder causing pain along the path of the trigeminal nerve in the face, translates literally as "painful spasm."

A sound heard while listening to the body with a stethoscope is a bruit, a word in French that literally means "noise." Lavage, which refers to irrigation of a cavity, is a French word meaning "washing."

BURNS

Most burns are caused by hot objects, explosions, or scalding. They may also be caused by electrical malfunctions, contact with harmful chemicals, or abrasion. Burns are assessed in terms of the depth of damage and the percentage of body surface area (BSA) involved. Depth of tissue destruction is categorized as follows:

- Superficial partial-thickness, which involves the epidermis and perhaps a portion of the dermis. The tissue is reddened and may blister, as in cases of sunburn.
- Deep partial-thickness, which involves the epidermis and portions of the dermis. The tissue is blistered and broken and has a weeping surface. Causes include scalding and flash flame.
- Full-thickness, which involves the full skin and sometimes subcutaneous tissue and underlying tissues as well. The tissue is broken and is dry and pale or charred. These injuries may result in loss of digits or limbs and require skin grafting.

The above classification replaces an older system of ranking burns as first-, second-, and third-degree according to the depth of tissue damage.

The amount of BSA involved in a burn may be estimated by using the **rule of nines**, in which areas of body surface are assigned percentages in multiples of nine (Fig. 21-2). The more accurate Lund and Browder method divides the body into small areas and estimates the proportion of BSA that each contributes.

Infection is a common complication of burns because a major defense against invasion of microorganisms is damaged. Respiratory complications and shock may also occur.

Treatment of burns includes respiratory care, administration of fluids, wound care, and pain control. Monitoring for cardiovascular complications, infections, and signs of posttraumatic stress are also important.

PRESSURE ULCERS

Pressure ulcers are necrotic skin lesions that appear where the body rests on skin that covers bony projections, such as the sacrum, heel, elbow, ischial bone of the pelvis, or greater trochanter of the femur. The pressure interrupts circulation, leading to thrombosis, ulceration, and death of tissue. Poor general health, malnutrition, age, obesity, and infection contribute to the development of pressure ulcers.

Lesions first appear as redness of the skin. If ignored, they may penetrate the skin and underlying muscle, extending even to bone, and may require months to heal.

Pads or mattresses to relieve pressure, regular cleansing and drying of the skin, frequent change in position, and good nutrition help to prevent pressure ulcers. Other terms for pressure ulcers are *decubitus ulcer* and *bedsore*. Both of these terms refer to lying down in bed, although pressure ulcers may appear in anyone with limited movement, not only those who are confined to bed.

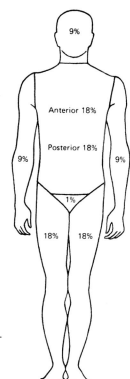

FIGURE 21-2. The rule of nines. Percentage of body surface area (BSA) in the adult is esti-mated by sectioning the body surface into areas with numerical values related to nine. (Reprinted with permission from Smeltzer SC, Bare BG. Brunner & Suddarth's Textbook of Medical-Surgical Nursing. 9th Ed. Philadelphia: Lippincott Williams & Wilkins, 2000.)

Dermatitis

Dermatitis is inflammation of the skin, which may be acute or chronic. A chronic allergic form of this disorder that appears early in childhood is called **eczema** or **atopic dermatitis.** Although its exact cause is unknown, atopic dermatitis is made worse by allergies, infection, temperature extremes, and skin irritants.

Other forms of dermatitis include contact dermatitis, caused by chemical irritants; seborrheic dermatitis, which involves areas with large numbers of sebaceous glands such as the scalp and face; and stasis dermati-tis, caused by poor circulation.

Psoriasis

Psoriasis is a chronic overgrowth (hyperplasia) of the epidermis, producing large, erythematous (red) plaques with silvery scales (Fig. 21-3). The cause is unknown but there is sometimes a hereditary pattern, and autoimmunity may be involved. Psoriasis is treated with topical corticosteroids and with exposure to ultraviolet (UV) light. Severe cases have been treated with a combination of a drug, psoralen (P), to increase sensitivity to light, followed by exposure to a form of UV light (UV-A).

Autoimmune Disorders

The diseases discussed below are caused, at least in part, by autoimmune reactions. They are diagnosed by biopsy of lesions and by antibody studies.

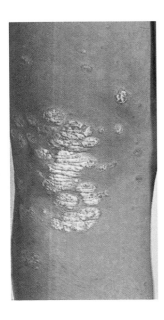

FIGURE 21-3. Psoriasis. Plaques with scales seen at the front of the knee. (Reprinted with permission from Bickley LS. Bate's Guide to Physical Examination and History Taking. 8th Ed. Philadelphia: Lippincott Williams & Wilkins, 2003.)

Pemphigus is characterized by the formation of blisters (bullae) in the skin and mucous membranes caused by a separation of epidermal cells from underlying layers (Fig. 21-4). Rupture of these lesions leaves deeper areas of the skin unprotected from infection and fluid loss, much as in cases of burns. The cause is an autoimmune reaction to epithelial cells. Pemphigus is fatal unless treated by suppressing the immune system.

Lupus erythematosus (LE) is a chronic inflammatory autoimmune disease of connective tissue. The more widespread form of the disease, systemic lupus erythematosus (SLE), involves the skin and other organs. The discoid form (DLE) involves only the skin. It is seen as rough, raised, violet-tinted papules, usually limited to the face and scalp. There may also be a butterfly-shaped rash across the nose and cheeks that is typical of this disease.

The skin lesions of lupus are worsened by exposure to the ultraviolet radiation in sunlight. SLE is more prevalent in women than in men and has a higher incidence among Asians and blacks than in other populations.

Scleroderma is a disease of unknown cause that involves thickening and tightening of the skin. There is gradual fibrosis of the dermis because of overproduction of collagen. Sweat glands and hair follicles are also involved. A very early sign of scleroderma is Raynaud disease, in which blood vessels in the fingers and toes constrict in the cold, causing numbness, pain, coldness, and tingling. Skin symptoms first appear on the fore-

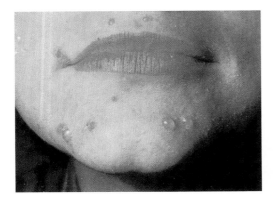

FIGURE 21-4. Pemphigus, showing vesicles on the chin. (Reprinted with permission from Bickley LS. Bate's Guide to Physical Examination and History Taking. 8th Ed. Philadelphia: Lippincott Williams & Wilkins, 2003.)

arms and around the mouth. Internal organs become involved in a diffuse form of scleroderma called progressive systemic sclerosis (PSS).

Skin Cancer

Skin cancer is the most common type of human cancer. Its rate has been increasing in recent years, mainly because of the mutation-causing effects of the ultraviolet rays in sunlight.

Malignant melanoma results from an overgrowth of melanocytes, the pigment-producing cells in the epidermis. It is the most dangerous form of skin cancer because of its tendency to metastasize. This cancer appears as a lesion that is variable in color with an irregular border (Fig. 21-5). It may spread superficially for up to 1 or 2 years before it begins to invade the deeper tissues of the skin and to metastasize through blood and lymph. The prognosis for cure is good if the lesion is recognized and removed surgically before it enters this invasive stage.

Squamous cell carcinoma and **basal cell carcinoma** are both cancers of epithelial cells. Both appear in areas exposed to sunlight, such as the face. Squamous cell carcinoma appears as a painless, firm, red nodule or plaque that may develop surface scales, ulceration, or crusting (Fig. 21-6). This cancer may invade underlying tissue but tends not to metastasize. It is treated by surgical removal and sometimes with x-irradiation or chemotherapy.

Basal cell carcinoma constitutes more than 75% of all skin cancers. It usually appears as a smooth, pearly papule (Fig. 21-7). Because these cancers are easily seen and do not metastasize, the cure rate after excision is greater than 95%.

Kaposi sarcoma, once considered rare, is now seen frequently in association with AIDS. It usually appears as distinct brownish areas on the legs. These plaques become raised and firm as the tumor progresses. In those with weakened immune systems, such as AIDS patients, the cancer can metastasize.

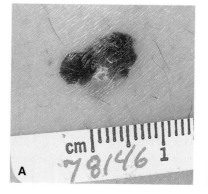
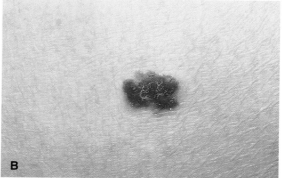
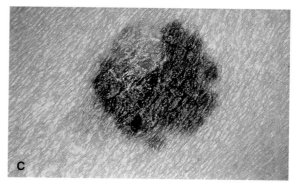

FIGURE 21-5. Characteristics of malignant melanoma. **(A)** Shows asymmetry. **(B)** Shows irregular borders. **(C)** Shows variation in color, a diameter greater than 6 mm, and elevation. (Courtesy of The American Cancer Society; American Academy of Dermatology.)

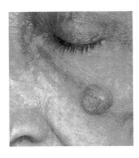 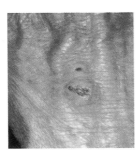

FIGURE 21-6. Squamous cell carcinoma shown on the face and the back of the hand, sun-exposed areas that are commonly affected. (Reprinted with permission from Bickley LS. Bate's Guide to Physical Examination and History Taking. 8th Ed. Philadelphia: Lippincott Williams & Wilkins, 2003.)

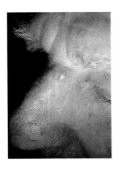

FIGURE 21-7. Basal cell carcinoma. An initial translucent nodule spreads, leaving a depressed center and a firm, elevated border. (Reprinted with permission from Bickley LS. Bate's Guide to Physical Examination and History Taking. 8th Ed. Philadelphia: Lippincott Williams & Wilkins, 2003.)

Key Clinical Terms

atopic dermatitis *a-TOP-ik der-ma-TĪ-tis*	Hereditary, allergic, chronic inflammation of the skin with pruritus; eczema
basal cell carcinoma	An epithelial tumor that rarely metastasizes and has a high cure rate with surgical removal
débridement *da-brē-DMON*	Removal of dead or damaged tissue, as from a wound
dehiscence *dē-HIS-ens*	Splitting or bursting, as when the layers of a wound separate
dermatitis *der-ma-TĪ-tis*	Inflammation of the skin, often associated with redness and itching; may be caused by allergy, irritants (contact dermatitis), or a variety of diseases
dermatology *der-ma-TOL-ō-jē*	Study of the skin and diseases of the skin
dermatome *DER-ma-tōm*	Instrument for cutting thin sections of skin for skin grafting
eczema *EK-zē-ma*	A general term for an inflammation of the skin with redness, lesions, and itching; atopic dermatitis

escharotomy *es-kar-OT-ō-mē*	Removal of scab tissue (eschar) resulting from burns or other skin injuries
evisceration *ē-vis-er-Ā-shun*	Protrusion of internal organs (viscera) through an opening, as through a wound
exudate *EKS-ū-dāt*	Material, which may include fluid, cells, pus, or blood, that escapes from damaged tissue
Kaposi sarcoma *KAP-ō-sē*	Cancerous lesion of the skin and other tissues seen most often in patients with AIDS
lupus erythematosus (LE) *LŪ-pus er-i-thē-ma-TŌ-sis*	A chronic, inflammatory, autoimmune disease of connective tissue that often involves the skin; types include the more widespread systemic lupus erythematosus (SLE) and a discoid form (DLE) that involves only the skin
malignant melanoma	A metastasizing pigmented tumor of the skin
pemphigus *PEM-fi-gus*	An autoimmune disease of the skin characterized by sudden, intermittent formation of bullae (blisters); may be fatal if untreated
pressure ulcer	An ulcer caused by pressure to an area of the body, as from a bed or chair; decubitus (*dē-KŪ-bi-tus*) ulcer, bedsore, pressure sore
psoriasis *so-RĪ-a-sis*	A chronic hereditary dermatitis with red lesions covered by silvery scales
rule of nines	A method for estimating the extent of body surface area involved in a burn by assigning percentages in multiples of nine to various regions of the body
scleroderma *sklē r-ō-DER-ma*	A chronic disease that is characterized by thickening and tightening of the skin and that often involves internal organs in a form called progressive systemic sclerosis (PSS)
squamous cell carcinoma	An epidermal cancer that may invade deeper tissues but tends not to metastasize

Supplementary Terms

SEP-tum
aorta
a-OR-ta
plasma

SYMPTOMS AND CONDITIONS

acne *AK-nē*	An inflammatory disease of the sebaceous glands and hair follicles usually associated with excess secretion of sebum; acne vulgaris
actinic *ak-TIN-ik*	Pertaining to the effects of radiant energy, such as sunlight, ultraviolet light, and x-rays
albinism *AL-bin-izm*	A hereditary lack of pigment in the skin, hair, and eyes

Symptoms and Conditions, continued

alopecia *al-ō-PĒ-shē-a*	Absence or loss of hair; baldness
Beau lines *bō*	White lines across the fingernails; usually a sign of systemic disease or injury (Fig. 21-8)
bromhidrosis *brō-mi-DRŌ-sis*	Sweat that has a foul odor because of bacterial decomposition; also called bromidrosis
carbuncle *CAR-bung-kl*	A localized infection of the skin and subcutaneous tissue, usually caused by staphylococcus, and associated with pain and discharge of pus
cicatrix *SIK-a-triks*	A scar; scar formation is called cicatrization
comedo *KOM-e-dō*	A plug of sebum, often containing bacteria, in a hair follicle; a blackhead (plural, comedones)
dermatophytosis *der-ma-tō-fī-TŌ-sis*	Fungal infection of the skin, especially between the toes; athlete's foot (root *phyt/o* means "plant")
diaphoresis *dī-a-fō-RĒ-sis*	Profuse sweating
dyskeratosis *dis-ker-a-TŌ-sis*	Any abnormality in keratin formation in epithelial cells
ecchymosis *ek-i-MŌ-sis*	A collection of blood under the skin caused by leakage from small vessels
erysipelas *er-i-SIP-e-las*	An acute infectious disease of the skin with localized redness and swelling and systemic symptoms
erythema *er-i-THĒ-ma*	Diffuse redness of the skin
erythema nodosum *nō-DŌ-sum*	Inflammation of subcutaneous tissues resulting in tender, erythematous nodules; may be an abnormal immune response to a systemic disease, an infection, or a drug
exanthem *eks-AN-them*	Any eruption of the skin that accompanies a disease, such as measles; a rash
excoriation *eks-kō-rē-Ā-shun*	Lesion caused by scratching or abrasion (Fig. 21-9)
folliculitis *fō-lik-ū-LĪ-tis*	Inflammation of a hair follicle
furuncle *FŪ-rung-kl*	A painful skin nodule caused by staphylococci that enter through a hair follicle; a boil
hemangioma *hē-man-jē-Ō-ma*	A benign tumor of blood vessels; in the skin, called birthmarks or port wine stains

Symptoms and Conditions, continued

herpes simplex *HER-pēz SIM-pleks*	A group of acute infections caused by herpes simplex virus. Type I herpes simplex virus produces fluid-filled vesicles, usually on the lips, after fever, exposure to the sun, injury, or stress; cold sore, fever blister. Type II infections usually involve the genital organs.
hirsutism *HIR-sū-tizm*	Excessive growth of hair
ichthyosis *ik-thē-ō-sis*	A dry, scaly condition of the skin (from the root *ichthy/o*, meaning "fish")
impetigo *im-pe-TĪ-gō*	A bacterial skin infection with pustules that rupture and form crusts; most commonly seen in children, usually on the face
keloid *KĒ-loyd*	A raised, thickened scar caused by overgrowth of tissue during scar formation
keratosis *ker-a-TŌ-sis*	Any skin condition marked by thickened or horny growth. Seborrheic keratosis is a benign tumor, yellow or light brown in color, that appears in the elderly. Actinic keratosis is caused by exposure to sunlight and may lead to squamous cell carcinoma.
lichenification *lī-ken-i-fi-KĀ-shun*	Thickened marks caused by chronic rubbing, as seen in atopic dermatitis (a lichen is a flat, branching type of plant that grows on rocks and bark; see Fig. 21-9)
mycosis fungoides *mī-KŌ-sis fun-GOY-dēz*	A rare malignant disease that originates in the skin and involves the internal organs and lymph nodes. There are large, painful, ulcerating tumors.
nevus *NĒ-vus*	A defined discoloration of the skin; a congenital vascular tumor of the skin; a mole, birthmark
paronychia *par-ō-NIK-ē-a*	Infection around a nail
pediculosis *pe-dik-ū-LŌ-sis*	Infestation with lice
petechiae *pē-TĒ-kē-ē*	Flat, pinpoint, purplish-red spots caused by bleeding within the skin or mucous membrane (singular, petechia)
pruritus *prū-RĪ-tus*	Severe itching
purpura *PUR-pū-ra*	A condition characterized by hemorrhages into the skin and other tissues
rosacea *rō-ZĀ-shē-a*	A condition of unknown cause involving redness of the skin, pustules, and overactivity of sebaceous glands, mainly on the face
scabies *SKĀ-bēz*	A highly contagious skin disease caused by a mite

Symptoms and Conditions, continued

senile lentigines *len-TIJ-i-nēz*	Brown macules that appear on sun-exposed skin in adults; liver spots
shingles	An acute eruption of vesicles along the path of a nerve; herpes zoster (*HER-pēz ZOS-ter*); caused by the same virus that causes chicken pox
tinea *TIN-ē-a*	A fungal infection of the skin; ringworm
tinea versicolor *VER-si-kol-or*	Superficial chronic fungal infection that causes varied pigmentation of the skin
urticaria *ur-ti-KĀ-rē-a*	A skin reaction marked by temporary, smooth, raised areas (wheals) associated with itching; hives
venous stasis ulcer	Ulcer caused by venous insufficiency and stasis of venous blood; usually forms near the ankle
verruca *ver-RŪ-ka*	An epidermal tumor; a wart
vitiligo *vit-i-LĪ-gō*	Patchy disappearance of pigment in the skin; leukoderma (Fig. 21-10)
xeroderma pigmentosum *zē-rō-DER-ma* *pig-men-TŌ-sum*	A fatal hereditary disease that begins in childhood with discolorations and ulcers of the skin and muscle atrophy. There is increased sensitivity to the sun and increased susceptibility to cancer.

DIAGNOSIS AND TREATMENT

aloe *A-lō*	A plant (Aloe vera), the leaves of which contain a gel that is used in treatment of burns and minor skin irritations
antipruritic *an-ti-prū-RIT-ik*	Agent that prevents or relieves itching
cautery *KAW-ter-ē*	Destruction of tissue by physical or chemical means; cauterization; also the instrument or chemical used for this purpose
dermabrasion *DERM-a-brā-zhun*	A plastic surgical procedure for removing scars or birthmarks by chemical or mechanical destruction of epidermal tissue
dermatoplasty *DER-ma-tō-plas-tē*	Transplantation of human skin; skin grafting
diascopy *dī-AS-kō-pē*	Examination of skin lesions by pressing a glass plate against the skin
fulguration *ful-gū-RĀ-shun*	Destruction of tissue by high-frequency electric sparks
skin turgor *TUR-gor*	Resistance of the skin to deformation. Evidenced by the ability of the skin to return to position when pinched. Skin turgor is a measure of the skin's elasticity and state of hydration. It typically declines with age and may also be a sign of poor nutrition.
Wood lamp	An ultraviolet light used to diagnose fungal infections

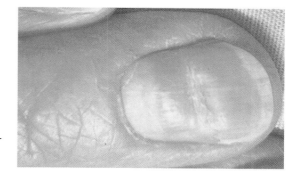

FIGURE 21-8. Beau lines, transverse depressions in the nails associated with acute severe illness. (Reprinted with permission from Bickley LS. Bate's Guide to Physical Examination and History Taking. 8th Ed. Philadelphia: Lippincott Williams & Wilkins, 2003.)

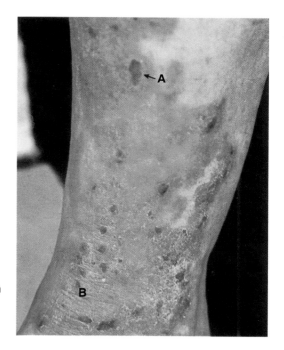

FIGURE 21-9. **(A)** Excoriation and **(B)** lichenification seen on the leg. (Reprinted with permission from Bickley LS. Bate's Guide to Physical Examination and History Taking. 8th Ed. Philadelphia: Lippincott Williams & Wilkins, 2003.)

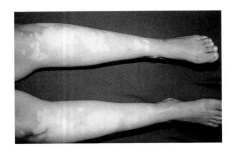

FIGURE 21-10. Vitiligo. Depigmented macules appear on the skin and may merge into large areas that lack melanin. The brown pigment seen in the illustration is the person's normal skin color; the pale areas are caused by vitiligo. (Reprinted with permission from Bickley LS. Bate's Guide to Physical Examination and History Taking. 8th Ed. Philadelphia: Lippincott Williams & Wilkins, 2003.)

ABBREVIATIONS

BSA	Body surface area	**SLE**	Systemic lupus erythematosus
DLE	Discoid lupus erythematosus	**SPF**	Sun protection factor
FTSG	Full-thickness skin graft	**STSG**	Split-thickness skin graft
LE	Lupus erythematosus	**UV**	Ultraviolet
PSS	Progressive systemic sclerosis	**VAC**	Vacuum-assisted closure
PUVA	Psoralen UV-A		
SCLE	Subacute cutaneous lupus erythematosus		

Labeling Exercise 21-1

Cross-Section of the Skin

Write the name of each numbered part on the corresponding line of the answer sheet.

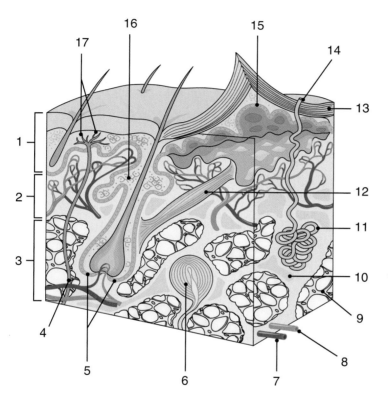

Adipose (fat) cells
Artery
Dermis
Epidermis
Fibrous connective tissue
Hair follicle
Muscle (arrector pili)
Nerve
Nerve endings
Pore
Pressure receptor
Sebaceous gland
Stratum basale
Stratum corneum
Subcutaneous layer
Sudoriferous (sweat) gland
Vein

1. _____   10. _____

2. _____   11. _____

3. _____   12. _____

4. _____   13. _____

5. _____   14. _____

6. _____   15. _____

7. _____   16. _____

8. _____   17. _____

9. _____

Chapter Review 21-1

Multiple choice: Select the best answer and write the letter of your choice to the left of each number.

_____ 1. cutaneous   a. oily secretion of the skin

_____ 2. follicle   b. growing layer of the epidermis

_____ 3. stratum basale   c. sheath that contains a hair

_____ 4. stratum corneum   d. referring to the skin

_____ 5. sebum   e. uppermost, thickened layer of the epidermis

_____ 6. macule   a. crack or break in the skin

_____ 7. vesicle   b. solid, raised lesion

_____ 8. nodule   c. flat, colored spot

_____ 9. fissure   d. blister

_____ 10. wheal   e. smooth, raised area with itching

_____ 11. débridement   a. autoimmune disorder that involves the skin

_____ 12. pressure ulcer   b. removal of dead tissue from a wound

_____ 13. psoriasis   c. chronic dermatitis with silvery scales

_____ 14. lupus erythematosus   d. cancerous skin lesion seen in debilitated people

_____ 15. Kaposi sarcoma   e. bedsore

SUPPLEMENTARY TERMS

_____ 16. alopecia   a. severe itching

_____ 17. diaphoresis   b. redness of the skin

_____ 18. erythema   c. baldness

_____ 19. keloid   d. profuse sweating

_____ 20. pruritus   e. thickened scar

_____ 21. urticaria   a. hemorrhages into the skin

_____ 22. furuncle   b. hives

_____ 23. nevus   c. viral infection of the skin

_____ 24. purpura   d. mole or birthmark

_____ 25. herpes simplex   e. painful infectious nodule; boil

_____ 26. bromhidrosis   a. scar

_____ 27. comedo   b. fungal infection

_____ 28. actinic   c. blackhead

_____ 29. cicatrix   d. referring to radiation

_____ 30. tinea   e. sweat with a foul odor

_____ 31. fulguration   a. condition causing redness and pustules, mainly on the face

_____ 32. petechiae   b. pinpoint red spots caused by bleeding into the skin

_____ 33. impetigo   c. bacterial skin infection

_____ 34. paronychia   d. destruction of tissue by electric spark

_____ 35. rosacea   e. infection around a nail

Fill in the blanks:

36. The skin and its associated structures make up the _____ system.

37. A sudoriferous gland produces _____.

38. The layer of the skin under the epidermis is the _____.

39. The main pigment in skin is _____.

40. The oil-producing glands of the skin are the _____.

41. The protein that thickens the skin and makes up hair and nails is _____.

Define each of the following words:

42. percutaneous (_per-kū-TĀ-nē-us_)   _____

43. keratogenic (_ker-a-tō-JEN-ik_)   _____

44. melanocyte (_MEL-an-ō-sīt_)   _____

45. xeroderma (_zē-rō-DER-ma_)   _____

46. pachyderma (_pak-ē-DER-ma_)   _____

47. hypertrichosis (_hī-per-tri-KŌ-sis_)   _____

48. onychomycosis (_on-i-kō-mī-KŌ-sis_)   _____

Word building. Write a word for each of the following definitions:

49. any disease of the skin   _____

50. insufficient production of melanin   _____

51. hardening of the skin   _____

52. tumor containing melanin   _____

53. discharge of sebum   _____

54. instrument for cutting the skin   _____

55. loosening or separation (-lysis) of a nail   _____

56. study of hair   _____

Use the word *hidrosis* (sweating) or the ending *-idrosis* as an ending to make a word with each of the following meanings:

57. absence (an-) of sweating   _____

58. excess sweating   _____

59. excretion of colored (chrom/o) sweat   _____

Word analysis. Define each of the following words, and give the meaning of the word parts in each. Use a dictionary if necessary.

60. onychocryptosis (*on-i-kō-krip-TŌ-sis*) _____
    a. onych/o _____
    b. crypt/o _____
    c. -sis _____

61. achromotrichia (*a-krō-mō-TRIK-ē-a*) _____
    a. a- _____
    b. chrom/o _____
    c. trich/o _____
    d. -ia _____

62. hidradenoma (*hī-drad-e-NŌ-ma*) _____
    a. hidr/o _____
    b. aden/o _____
    c. -oma _____

Case Studies

Case Study 21-1: Basal Cell Carcinoma (BSC)

K.B., a 32-year-old fitness instructor, had noticed a "tiny hard lump" at the base of her left nostril while cleansing her face. The lesion had been present for about 2 months when she consulted a dermatologist. She had recently moved north from Florida, where she had worked as a lifeguard. She thought the lump might have been triggered by the regular tanning salon sessions she had used to retain her tan because it did not resemble the acne pustules, blackheads, or resulting scars of her adolescent years. Although dermabrasion had removed the obvious acne scars and left several areas of dense skin, this lump was brown-pigmented and different. K.B. was afraid it might be a malignant melanoma. On examination, the dermatologist noted a small pearly-white nodule at the lower portion of the left ala (outer flared portion of the nostril). There were no other lesions on her face or neck.

A plastic surgeon excised the lesion and was able to re-approximate the wound edges without a full-thickness skin graft. The pathology report identified the lesion as a basal cell carcinoma with clean margins of normal skin and subcutaneous tissue and stated that the entire lesion had been excised. K.B. was advised to wear SPF 30 sun protection on her face at all times and to avoid excessive sun exposure and tanning salons.

Case Study 21-2: Cutaneous Lymphoma

L.C., a 52-year-old female research chemist, has had a history of T-cell lymphoma for 8 years. She was initially treated with systemic chemotherapy with methotrexate until she contracted stomatitis. Continued therapy with topical chemotherapeutic agents brought some measurable improvement. She also had a history of hidradenitis.

A recent physical examination showed diffuse erythroderma with scaling and hyperkeratosis, plus alopecia. She had painful leukoplakia and ulcerations of the mouth and tongue. L.C. was hospitalized and given two courses of topical chemotherapy. She was referred to Dental Medicine for treatment of the oral lesions and discharged in stable condition with an appointment for follow-up in 4 weeks. Her discharge medications included hydrocortisone ointment 2% to affected lesions q hs, Keralyt gel bid for the hyperkeratosis, and Dyclone and Benadryl for her mouth ulcers prn.

Case Study 21-3: Pressure Ulcer

L.N., an elderly woman in failing health, had recently moved in with her daughter after her hospitalization for a stroke. The daughter reported to the home care nurse that her mother had minimal appetite, was confused and disoriented, and had developed a blister on her lower back since she had been confined to bed. The nurse noted that L.N. had lost weight since her last visit and that her skin was dry with poor skin turgor. She was wearing an "adult diaper," which was wet. After examining L.N.'s sacrum, the nurse noted a nickel-sized open area, 2 cm in diameter and 1 cm in depth (stage II pressure ulcer), with a 0.5-cm reddened surrounding area with no drainage. L.N. moaned when the nurse palpated the lesion. The nurse also noted reddened areas on L.N.'s elbows and heels.

The nurse provided L.N.'s daughter with instructions for proper skin care, incontinence management, enhanced nutrition, and frequent repositioning to prevent pressure ischemia to the prominent body areas. However, 6 months later L.N.'s pressure ulcer had deteriorated to a class III. She was hospitalized under the care of a plastic surgeon and wound-ostomy care nurse. Surgery was scheduled to débride the sacral wound and close it with a full-thickness skin graft taken from her thigh. L.N. was

Case Studies, continued

discharged 8 days later to a long-term care facility with orders for an alternating pressure mattress, position change every 2 hours, supplemental nutrition, and meticulous wound care.

CASE STUDY QUESTIONS

Multiple choice: Select the best answer and write the letter of your choice to the left of each number.

_____ 1. K.B.'s basal cell carcinoma may have been caused by chronic exposure to the sun and ultraviolet tanning bed use. The scientific explanation for this is the:
a. autoimmune response
b. actinic effect
c. allergic reaction
d. sun block tanning lotion theory
e. dermatophytosis

_____ 2. The characteristic pimples of adolescent acne are whiteheads and blackheads. The medical terms for these lesions are:
a. vesicles and lymphotomes
b. pustules and blisters
c. pustules and comedones
d. vitiligo and macules
e. furuncle and sebaceous cyst

_____ 3. Which skin cancer is an overgrowth of pigment-producing epidermal cells:
a. basal cell carcinoma
b. Kaposi sarcoma
c. cutaneous lymphoma
d. melanoma
e. erythema nodosum

_____ 4. Basal cell carcinoma involves:
a. subcutaneous tissue
b. hair follicles
c. connective tissue
d. adipose tissue
e. epithelial cells

_____ 5. Hydradenitis is inflammation of a:
a. sweat gland
b. salivary gland
c. sebaceous gland
d. ceruminous gland
e. meibomian gland

_____ 6. Leukoplakia is:
a. baldness
b. ulceration
c. formation of white patches in the mouth

Case Studies, continued

d. formation of yellow patches on the skin

e. formation of scales on the skin

_____ 7. Hydrocortisone is a(n):

a. vitamin

b. steroid

c. analgesic

d. lubricant

e. diuretic

_____ 8. An example of a topical drug is a:

a. systemic chemotherapeutic agent

b. drug derived from rain forest plants

c. subdermal allergy test antigens

d. skin ointment

e. Benadryl capsule 25 mg

_____ 9. Stomatitis, a common side effect of systemic chemotherapy, is an inflammatory condition of the:

a. mouth

b. colostomy

c. stomach

d. teeth and hair

e. nails

_____ 10. Skin turgor is an indicator of:

a. elasticity

b. hydration

c. aging

d. nutrition

e. all of the above

_____ 11. Another name for a pressure ulcer is a:

a. shearing force

b. bedsore

c. decubitus ulcer

d. a and b

e. b and c

_____ 12. A FTSG is usually harvested (taken) from another body area with a scalpel, whereas a STSG is harvested with an instrument called a(n) _____, which can cut a thinner graft.

a. tissue slicer

b. Keralyt

c. erythroderm

d. dermatome

e. débridement

Case Studies, continued

Write a term from the case studies with each of the following meanings:

13. skin sanding procedure _____

14. a solid raised lesion larger than a papule _____

15. physician who cares for patients with skin diseases _____

16. connective tissue and fat layer beneath the dermis _____

17. diffuse redness of the skin _____

18. increased production of keratin in the skin _____

19. removal of dead or damaged skin _____

20. reduced blood flow to the tissue _____

Abbreviations. Define the following abbreviations:

21. FTSG _____

22. STSG _____

23. SPF _____

24. hs _____

25. bid _____

Chapter 21 Crossword
The Skin

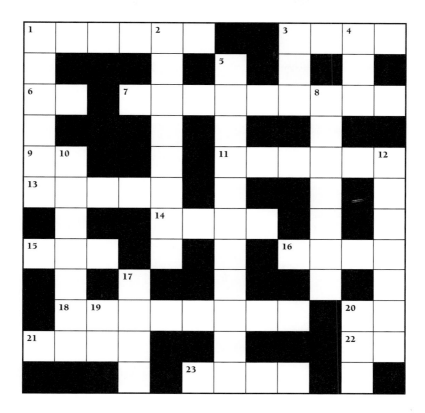

ACROSS

1. Horny layer of the skin: combining form
3. Inflammation of a sweat gland: __ __ __ __ adenitis
6. Autoimmune disease that affects the skin: abbreviation
7. Excess growth of hair
9. Within the skin: abbreviation
11. Viral disease that affects the skin
13. Skin: combining form
14. Sweat: combining form
15. Three: prefix
16. Scar: __ __ __ __trix
18. Examination by pressing a glass plate against the skin
20. True, good, easy: prefix
21. Half: prefix
22. Part of a medical history: __ __ H: abbreviation
23. Under, below, decreased: prefix

DOWN

1. Raised, thickened scar
2. Pertaining to a hair
3. Measurement of packed red cells: abbreviation
4. Abnormal, painful: prefix
5. Removal of scab tissue
8. Bacterial skin infection common in children: __ __ __ __ __ __ __ o
10. Remove dead tissue, as from a wound
12. A layer, as of the skin
17. Meaning of the root onych/o
19. A route of injection: abbreviation
20. On, over: prefix

CHAPTER 21 Answer Section

Answers to Chapter Exercises

EXERCISE 21-1

1. derm/o; skin
2. melan/o; melanin
3. seb/o; sebum
4. kerat/o; keratin, horny layer of the skin
5. idr/o; sweat
6. onych/o; nail
7. trich/o; hair
8. skin
9. keratin
10. melanin
11. sweat, perspiration
12. hair
13. nail
14. skin
15. dermatology (*der-ma-TOL-ō-jē*)
16. dermatitis (*der-ma-TĪ-tis*)
17. keratogenesis (*ker-a-tō-JEN-e-sis*)
18. melanoma (*mel-a-NŌ-ma*)
19. hypohidrosis (*hī-pō-hī-DRŌ-sis*)
20. trichology (*trik-OL-ō-jē*)
21. onychomalacia (*on-i-kō-ma-LĀ-shē-a*)
22. dermatome (*DER-ma-tōm*)
23. scleroderma (*sklēr-ō-DER-ma*)
24. pyoderma (*pī-ō-DER-ma*)

LABELING EXERCISE 21-1
CROSS-SECTION OF THE SKIN

1. epidermis
2. dermis (corium)
3. subcutaneous tissue
4. nerve
5. hair follicle
6. pressure receptor
7. artery
8. vein
9. adipose (fat) cells
10. fibrous connective tissue
11. sudoriferous (sweat) gland
12. muscle (arrector pili)
13. stratum corneum
14. pore (opening of sweat gland)
15. stratum basale (growing layer)
16. sebaceous (oil) gland
17. nerve endings

Answers to Chapter Review 21-1

1. d
2. c
3. b
4. e
5. a
6. c
7. d
8. b
9. a
10. e
11. b
12. e
13. c
14. a
15. d
16. c
17. d
18. b
19. e
20. a
21. b
22. e
23. d
24. a
25. c
26. e
27. c
28. d
29. a
30. b
31. d
32. b
33. c
34. e
35. a
36. integumentary
37. sweat
38. dermis
39. melanin
40. sebaceous glands
41. keratin
42. through the skin
43. producing keratin
44. cell that produces melanin
45. dryness of the skin
46. thickening of the skin
47. condition of having excess hair

48. fungal infection of a nail
49. dermatopathy, dermopathy
50. hypomelanosis
51. scleroderma, dermatosclerosis
52. melanoma
53. seborrhea
54. dermatome
55. onycholysis
56. trichology
57. anhidrosis, anidrosis
58. hyperhidrosis, hyperidrosis
59. chromhidrosis, chromidrosis
60. ingrown toenail
    a. nail
    b. hidden
    c. condition of
61. lack of color or graying of the hair
    a. lack of
    b. color
    c. hair
    d. condition of
62. benign tumor of a sweat gland
    a. sweat
    b. gland
    c. tumor

Answers to Case Study Questions

1. b
2. c
3. d
4. e
5. a
6. c
7. b
8. d
9. a
10. e
11. e
12. d
13. dermabrasion
14. nodule
15. dermatologist
16. subcutaneous tissue
17. erythema/erythroderma
18. hyperkeratosis
19. débridement
20. ischemia
21. full-thickness skin graft
22. split-thickness skin graft
23. sun protection factor
24. at bedtime
25. twice per day

ANSWERS TO CROSSWORD PUZZLE

The Skin

Commonly Used Symbols

SYMBOL	MEANING	CHAPTER
1°	primary	7
2°	secondary (to)	7
Δ	change (Greek delta)	7
Ⓛ	left	7
Ⓡ	right	7
↑	increase(s)	7
↓	decrease(s)	7
♂	male	7
♀	female	7
°	degree	7
>	greater than	7
<	less than	7
#	number, pound	7
×	times	7

Abbreviations and Their Meanings

ABBREVIATIONS	MEANING	CHAPTER
$\overline{a}$	before	7
A, Acc	accommodation	18
$\overline{a}\,\overline{a}$	of each	7
Ab	antibody	10
AB	abortion	15
ABC	aspiration biopsy cytology	7
ABG(s)	arterial blood gas(es)	11
ABR	auditory brainstem response	18
ac	before meals	8
AC	air conduction	18
ACE	angiotensin-converting enzyme	9
ACh	acetylcholine	17, 20
ACL	anterior cruciate ligament	19
ACTH	adrenocorticotropic hormone	16
ad lib	as desired	7
AD	Alzheimer disease, right ear	17, 18
ADH	antidiuretic hormone	13
ADHD	attention deficit hyperactivity disorder	17
ADL	activities of daily living	7
AE	above the elbow	19
AF	atrial fibrillation	9
AFB	acid-fast bacillus	11
AFP	alpha-fetoprotein	7, 15
Ag	antigen	9
AGA	appropriate for gestational age	15
AI	artificial insemination	15
AIDS	acquired immunodeficiency syndrome	10
AK	above the knee	19
ALL	acute lymphoblastic (lymphocytic) leukemia	10
ALS	amyotrophic lateral sclerosis	17, 20
AMA	against medical advice	7
AMB	ambulatory	7
AMD	age-related macular degeneration	18
AMI	acute myocardial infarction	9
AML	acute myeloblastic (myelogenous) leukemia	10
ANS	autonomic nervous system	17
AP	anteroposterior	7

ABBREVIATIONS	MEANING	CHAPTER
APAP	acetaminophen	8
APC	atrial premature complex	9
APPT	activated partial thromboplastin time	10
aq	water, aqueous	7
AR	aortic regurgitation	9
ARC	abnormal retinal correspondence	18
ARDS	acute respiratory distress syndrome	11
ARF	acute respiratory failure	11
ARF	acute renal failure	13
ASA	acetylsalicylic acid (aspirin)	8
As, Ast	astigmatism	18
AS	atrial stenosis; arteriosclerosis	9
AS	left ear	18
ASCVD	arteriosclerotic cardiovascular disease	9
ASD	atrial septal defect	9
ASF	anterior spinal fusion	19
ASHD	arteriosclerotic heart disease	9
AST	aspartate aminotransferase (SGOT)	9
AT	atrial tachycardia	9
ATN	acute tubular necrosis	13
AV	atrioventricular	9
BAEP	brainstem auditory evoked potentials	17
BBB	bundle branch block	9
BC	bone conduction	17
BE	barium enema	12
BE	below the elbow	19
bid	twice per day	7
BK	below the knee	19
BM	bowel movement	12
BMD	bone mineral density	19
BNO	bladder neck obstruction	14
BP	blood pressure	7
BPH	benign prostatic hyperplasia (hypertrophy)	14
BPM	beats per minute	7, 9
BRP	bathroom privileges	7
BS	bowel sounds, blood sugar	7, 16
BSA	body surface area	21
BSE	breast self-examination	15
BSO	bilateral salpingo-oophorectomy	15
BT	bleeding time	10
BUN	blood urea nitrogen	13
BV	bacterial vaginosis	15
bx	biopsy	7
$\bar{c}$	with	7
C	Celsius (centigrade)	7
C	compliance	11

ABBREVIATIONS	MEANING	CHAPTER
C	cervical vertebra	19
C section	cesarean section	15
CA	cancer	6
CABG	coronary artery bypass graft	9
CAD	coronary artery disease	9
CAM	complementary and alternative medicine	7
cap	capsule	7, 8
CAPD	continuous ambulatory peritoneal dialysis	13
CBC	complete blood count	10
CBD	common bile duct	12
CBF	cerebral blood flow	17
CBR	complete bed rest	7
cc	cubic centimeter, with correction	8, appendix 5, 18
CC	chief complaint	7
CCPD	continuous cyclic peritoneal dialysis	13
CCU	coronary care unit, cardiac care unit	9
CD	cardiovascular disease	9
CF	cystic fibrosis	11
CFS	chronic fatigue syndrome	20
CHD	coronary heart disease	9
CHF	congestive heart failure	9
Ci	Curie	7
CIN	cervical intraepithelial neoplasia	13
CIS	carcinoma in situ	6
CJD	Creutzfeldt-Jakob disease	17
CLL	chronic lymphocytic leukemia	10
cm	centimeter	appendix 5
CMG	cystometrography, cystometrogram	13
CML	chronic myelogenous leukemia	10
CNS	central nervous system	17
c/o	complains of	7
Co	coccyx; coccygeal	19
CO_2	carbon dioxide	11
COLD	chronic obstructive lung disease	11
COPD	chronic obstructive pulmonary disease	11
CP	cerebral palsy	17
CPAP	continuous positive airway pressure	11
CPD	cephalopelvic disproportion	15
C(P)K	creatine (phospho)kinase	9, 20
CPR	cardiopulmonary resuscitation	9
CRF	chronic renal failure	13
crit	hematocrit	10
C&S	culture and sensitivity	7
CSF	cerebrospinal fluid	17
CSII	continuous subcutaneous insulin infusion	16
CT	computed tomography	7
CVA	cerebrovascular accident	9, 17

ABBREVIATIONS	MEANING	CHAPTER
CVD	cerebrovascular disease	17
CVI	chronic venous insufficiency	9
CVP	central venous pressure	9
CVS	chorionic villus sampling	15
CXR	chest x-ray	11
D&C	dilatation and curettage	15
dB	decibel	18
dc, DC	discontinue, discharge	7
D/C	discharge	7
D&E	dilatation and evacuation	15
DES	diethylstilbestrol	15
DEXA	dual-energy x-ray absorptiometry (scan)	19
DIC	disseminated intravascular coagulation	10
DIFF	differential count	10
DIP	distal interphalangeal	19
DJD	degenerative joint disease	19
dL	deciliter	appendix 5
DLE	discoid lupus erythematosus	21
DM	diabetes mellitus	16
DNR	do not resuscitate	7
DOE	dyspnea on exertion	9
DRE	digital rectal examination	14
DS	double strength	8
DSM	Diagnostic and Statistical Manual of Mental Disorders	17
DTR	deep tendon reflex(es)	17
DUB	dysfunctional uterine bleeding	15
DVT	deep vein thrombosis	9
Dx	diagnosis	7
EBL	estimated blood loss	7
EBV	Epstein-Barr virus	10
EDC	estimated date of confinement	15
EEG	electroencephalogram; electroencephalograph	17
ECG (EKG)	electrocardiogram	9
ELISA	enzyme-linked immunosorbent assay	10
elix	elixir	8
EM	emmetropia	18
EMG	electromyography, electromyogram	20
ENG	electronystagmography	18
ENT	ear(s), nose, and throat	18
EOM	extraocular movement, muscles	18
EOMI	extraocular muscles intact	7
EPO	erythropoietin	10, 13
ERCP	endoscopic retrograde cholangiopancreatography	12
ERV	expiratory reserve volume	11
ESR	erythrocyte sedimentation rate	10

ABBREVIATIONS	MEANING	CHAPTER
ESRD	end-stage renal disease	13
ESWL	extracorporeal shock wave lithotripsy	13
ET	esotropia	18
ETOH	alcohol, ethyl alcohol	7
F	Fahrenheit	7
FAP	familial adenomatous polyposis	12
FBG	fasting blood glucose	16
FBS	fasting blood sugar	16
FC	finger counting	18
FDA	Food and Drug Administration	8
FEV	forced expiratory volume	11
FFP	fresh frozen plasma	10
FHR	fetal heart rate	15
FHT	fetal heart tone	15
FM	fibromyalgia syndrome	20
FPG	fasting plasma glucose	16
FRC	functional residual capacity	11
FSH	follicle-stimulating hormone	14, 15
FTI	free thyroxine index	16
FTND	full-term normal delivery	15
FTP	full-term pregnancy	15
FTSG	full-thickness skin graft	21
FUO	fever of unknown origin	6
FVC	forced vital capacity	11
Fx	fracture	19
g	gram	appendix 5
GA	gestational age	15
GAD	generalized anxiety disorder	17
GC	gonococcus	14, 15
GDM	gestational diabetes mellitus	16
GERD	gastroesophageal reflux disease	12
GFR	glomerular filtration rate	13
GH	growth hormone	16
GI	gastrointestinal	12
GIFT	gamete intrafallopian transfer	15
GTT	glucose tolerance test	16
gt(t)	drop(s)	7
GU	genitourinary	13
GYN	gynecology	15
H&P	history and physical examination	7
HAV	hepatitis A virus	12
Hb, Hgb	hemoglobin	10
HBA$_{1c}$	hemoglobin A$_{1c}$; glycohemoglobin; glycosylated hemoglobin	16
HBV	hepatitis B virus	12

ABBREVIATIONS	MEANING	CHAPTER
HCG, hCG	human chorionic gonadotropin	15
HCl	hydrochloric acid	12
Hct, Ht	hematocrit	10
HCV	hepatitis C virus	12
HDL	high-density lipoprotein	9
HDN	hemolytic disease of the newborn	10
HEENT	head, eyes, ears, nose, and throat	7
HIV	human immunodeficiency virus	10
HL	hearing level	18
HM	hand movements	18
HNP	herniated nucleus pulposus	19
h/o	history of	7
HPI	history of present illness	7
HPV	human papilloma virus	15
HRT	hormone replacement therapy	15
hs	at bedtime	7
HTN	hypertension	9
Hx	history	7
Hz	Hertz	18
^{131}I	iodine 131	16
I&D	incision and drainage	7
I&O	intake and output	7
IABP	intra-aortic balloon pump	9
IBD	inflammatory bowel disease	12
IBS	irritable bowel syndrome	12
IC	inspiratory capacity	11
ICD	implantable cardioverter defibrillator	9
ICP	intracranial pressure	17
ICSH	interstitial cell-stimulating hormone	14
ICU	intensive care unit	7
ID	intradermal	8
IDDM	insulin-dependent diabetes mellitus	16
IF	intrinsic factor	10
IFG	impaired fasting blood glucose	16
Ig	immunoglobulin	10
IGT	impaired glucose tolerance	16
IM	intramuscular(ly), intramedullary	7, 19
INH	isoniazid	8, 11
IOL	intraocular lens	18
IOP	intraocular pressure	18
IPPA	inspection, palpation, percussion, auscultation	7
IPPB	intermittent positive pressure breathing	11
IPPV	intermittent positive pressure ventilation	11
IRV	inspiratory reserve volume	11
ITP	idiopathic thrombocytopenic purpura	10
IU	international unit	7

ABBREVIATIONS	MEANING	CHAPTER
IUD	intrauterine device	15
IV	intravenous(ly)	7, 8
IVC	intravenous cholangiogram	12
IVCD	intraventricular conduction delay	9
IVDA	intravenous drug abuse	7
IVF	in vitro fertilization	15
IVP	intravenous pyelography	13
IVPB	intravenous piggyback	7
IVU	intravenous urography	13
JVP	jugular venous pulse	9
K	potassium	13
kg	kilogram	appendix 5
km	kilometer	appendix 5
KUB	kidney-ureter-bladder	13
KVO	keep vein open	7
L	lumbar vertebra	19
L	liter	appendix 5
LA	long-acting	8
LAD	left anterior descending (coronary artery)	9
LAHB	left anterior hemiblock	9
LDH	lactic dehydrogenase	9
LDL	low-density lipoprotein	9
LE	lupus erythematosus	21
LH	luteinizing hormone	14, 15
LL	left lateral	7
LLL	left lower lobe (of lung)	11
LLQ	left lower quadrant	5
LMN	lower motor neuron	17
LMP	last menstrual period	15
LOC	level of consciousness	17
LP	lumbar puncture	17
LUL	left upper lobe (of lung)	11
LUQ	left upper quadrant	5
LV	left ventricle	9
LVAD	left ventricular assist device	9
LVEDP	left ventricular end-diastolic pressure	9
LVH	left ventricular hypertrophy	9
lytes	electrolytes	10
μg, mcg	microgram	appendix 5
μL	microliter	appendix 5
μm	micrometer	appendix 5
m	meter	appendix 5
mcg	microgram	appendix 5

ABBREVIATIONS	MEANING	CHAPTER
MCH	mean corpuscular hemoglobin	10
MCHC	mean corpuscular hemoglobin concentration	10
MCP	metacarpophalangeal	19
MCV	mean corpuscular volume	9
MED(s)	medicine(s), medication(s)	8
MEFR	maximal expiratory flow rate	11
MEN	multiple endocrine neoplasia	16
mEq	milliequivalent	10
MET	metastasis	7
mg	milligram	appendix 5
MG	myasthenia gravis	20
MI	myocardial infarction	9
MID	multi-infarct dementia	17
mL	milliliter	appendix 5
mm	millimeter	appendix 5
MMFR	maximum midexpiratory flow rate	11
mm Hg	millimeters of mercury	9
MN	myoneural	20
MR	mitral regurgitation, reflux	9
MRI	magnetic resonance imaging	7
MRSA	methicillin-resistant *Staphylococcus aureus*	6
MS	mitral stenosis	9
MS	multiple sclerosis	17
MTP	metatarsophalangeal	19
MUGA	multigated acquisition (scan)	9
MVP	mitral valve prolapse	9
MVR	mitral valve replacement	9
Na	sodium	13
NAD	no apparent distress	7
n&v	nausea and vomiting	12
NB	newborn	15
NCCAM	National Center for Complementary and Alternative Medicine	7
NG	nasogastric	12
NGU	nongonococcal urethritis	14, 15
NHL	non-Hodgkin lymphoma	10
NICU	neonatal intensive care unit, neurologic intensive care unit	15, 17
NIDDM	non–insulin-dependent diabetes mellitus	16
NKDA	no known drug allergies	7
NMJ	neuromuscular junction	20
NPH	neutral protamine Hagedorn (insulin)	16
NPH	normal pressure hydrocephalus	17
NPO	nothing by mouth	7
NRC	normal retinal correspondence	18
NREM	non–rapid eye movement (sleep)	17
NSAID(s)	nonsteroidal anti-inflammatory drug(s)	8, 19
NSR	normal sinus rhythm	9

ABBREVIATIONS	MEANING	CHAPTER
NSS	normal sterile saline	7
NV	near vision	18
N/V, N&V	nausea and vomiting	12
N/V/D	nausea, vomiting, diarrhea	12
O_2	oxygen	11
OA	osteoarthritis	19
OB	obstetrics	15
OCD	obsessive-compulsive disorder	17
OD	right eye	18
ODA	Office of Dietary Supplements	8
OGTT	oral glucose tolerance test	16
OJ	osteogenesis imperfecta	19
OOB	out of bed	7
OM	otitis media	18
ORIF	open reduction internal fixation	19
ORL	otorhinolaryngology	18
ortho, ORTH	orthopedics	19
OS	left eye	18
OT	occupational therapy	20
OTC	over-the-counter	8
OU	both eyes; each eye	18
$\bar{p}$	after, post	7
P	pulse	7
PA	posteroanterior; physician assistant	7
PAC	premature atrial contraction	9
$Paco_2$	arterial partial pressure of carbon dioxide	11
PACU	postanesthetic care unit	7
Pao_2	arterial partial pressure of oxygen	11
PAP	pulmonary arterial pressure	9
pc	after meals	7
PCA	patient-controlled analgesia	7
PCL	posterior cruciate ligament	20
PCP	*Pneumocystis carinii* pneumonia; pneumocystic pneumonia	10
PCV	packed cell volume	10
PDA	patent ductus arteriosus	15
PDR	*Physicians' Desk Reference*	8
PE	physical examination	7
PEG	percutaneous endoscopic gastrostomy (tube)	12
PEP	protein electrophoresis	13
PE(R)RLA	pupils equal, (regular) react to light and accommodation	7
PEEP	positive end-expiratory pressure	11
PEFR	peak expiratory flow rate	11
PET	positron emission tomography	7
PFT	pulmonary function test(s)	11
pH	scale for measuring hydrogen ion concentration (acidity)	10

ABBREVIATIONS	MEANING	CHAPTER
Ph	Philadelphia chromosome	10
PICC	peripherally inserted central catheter	7
PID	pelvic inflammatory disease	14
PIH	pregnancy-induced hypertension	15
PIP	peak inspiratory pressure	11
PIP	proximal interphalangeal	19
PKU	phenylketonuria	15
PMH	past medical history	7
PMI	point of maximal impulse	9
PMN	polymorphonuclear (neutrophil)	10
PMS	premenstrual syndrome	15
PND	paroxysmal nocturnal dyspnea	11
poly, polymorph	neutrophil	10
PONV	postoperative nausea and vomiting	12
PNS	peripheral nervous system	17
po	by mouth, orally	7, 8
post op	postoperative	7
pp	postprandial (after a meal)	7
PPD	purified protein derivative (tuberculin)	11
pre op	preoperative	7
prn	as needed	7
PSA	prostate-specific antigen	14
PSF	posterior spinal fusion	19
PSS	physiologic saline solution, progressive systemic sclerosis	7, 21
PSVT	paroxysmal supraventricular tachycardia	9
pt	patient	7
PT	physical therapy, therapist	20
PT, ProTime	prothrombin time	10
PTCA	percutaneous transluminal coronary angioplasty	9
PTT	partial thromboplastin time	10
PUVA	psoralen UV-A	21
PVC	premature ventricular contraction	9
PVD	peripheral vascular disease	9
PWP	pulmonary (artery) wedge pressure	9
PYP	pyrophosphate	9
qam	every morning	7
qd	every day	7
qh	every hour	7
q __ h	every __ hours	7
qid	four times per day	7
QNS	quantity not sufficient	7
qod	every other day	7
QS	quantity sufficient	7
R	respiration	7
RA	rheumatoid arthritis	19

ABBREVIATIONS	MEANING	CHAPTER
RAIU	radioactive iodine uptake	16
RAS	reticular activating system	17
RATx	radiation therapy	7
RBC	red blood cell; red blood (cell) count	10
RDS	respiratory distress syndrome	11
REM	rapid eye movement (sleep)	17
RIA	radioimmunoassay	16
RL	right lateral	7
RLL	right lower lobe (of lung)	11
RLQ	right lower quadrant	5
RML	right middle lobe (of lung)	11
R/O	rule out	7
ROM	range of motion	20
ROS	review of systems	7
RSV	respiratory syncytial virus	11
RUL	right upper lobe (of lung)	11
RUQ	right upper quadrant	5
RV	residual volume	11
Rx	drug, prescription, therapy	7, 8
$\overline{s}$	without	7
S	sacrum; sacral	19
S_1	the first heart sound	9
S_2	the second heart sound	9
SA	sustained action, sinoatrial	8, 9
Sao_2	oxygen percent saturation (arterial)	11
SBE	subacute bacterial endocarditis	9
sc	without correction	18
SC, SQ, subcu.	subcutaneous(ly)	7, 8
seg	neutrophil	10
SERM	selective estrogen receptor modulator	19
SG	specific gravity	13
SGOT	serum glutamic oxaloacetic transaminase (AST)	9
SIADH	syndrome of inappropriate antidiuretic hormone	16
SIDS	sudden infant death syndrome	11
SK	streptokinase	9
SL	sublingual	8
SLE	systemic lupus erythematosus	10, 21
SPECT	single photon emission computed tomography	7
SPF	skin protection factor	21
SR	sustained release	8
$\overline{ss}$	half	7
SSEP	somatosensory evoked potentials	17
SSRI	selective serotonin reuptake inhibitor	17
ST	speech threshold	18
staph	staphylococcus	6
STAT	immediately	7

ABBREVIATIONS	MEANING	CHAPTER
STD	sexually transmitted disease	14, 15
strep	streptococcus	6
STSG	split-thickness skin graft	21
supp	suppository	7, 8
susp	suspension	7, 8
SVD	spontaneous vaginal delivery	15
SVT	supraventricular tachycardia	9
T	thoracic vertebra	19
T	temperature	7
T_3	tri-iodothyronine	16
T_4	thyroxine	16
T_7	free thyroxine index	16
T&A	tonsils and adenoids, tonsillectomy and adenoidectomy	11
tab	tablet	8
TAH	total abdominal hysterectomy	15
TB	tuberculosis	11
TBG	thyroxine binding globulin	16
^{99m}Tc	technetium-99m	9
TEE	transesophageal echocardiography	9
TGV	thoracic gas volume	11
THA	total hip arthroplasty	19
TIA	transient ischemic attack	17
tid	three times per day	7
tinct	tincture	7, 8
TKA	total knee arthroplasty	19
TKO	to keep open	7
TLC	total lung capacity	11
Tm	maximal transport capacity; tubular maximum	13
TM	tympanic membrane	18
TNM	(primary) tumor, (regional lymph) nodes, (distant) metastases	7
TMJ	temporomandibular joint	19
tPA	tissue plasminogen activator	9
TPN	total parenteral nutrition	12
TPR	temperature, pulse, respiration	7
TPUR	transperineal urethral resection	14
TSE	testicular self-examination	14
TSH	thyroid-stimulating hormone	16
TSS	toxic shock syndrome	15
T(C)T	thrombin (clotting) time	10
TTP	thrombotic thrombocytopenic purpura	10
TTS	temporary threshold shift	18
TUIP	transurethral incision of prostate	14
TURP	transurethral resection of prostate	14
TV	tidal volume	11
Tx	traction	19

ABBREVIATIONS	MEANING	CHAPTER
U	units	7
UA	urinalysis	13
UC	uterine contractions	15
UGI	upper gastrointestinal	12
UMN	upper motor neuron	17
ung	ointment	7, 8
URI	upper respiratory infection	11
USP	*United States Pharmacopeia*	8
UTI	urinary tract infection	13
UTP	uterine term pregnancy	15
UV	ultraviolet	7, 21
VA	visual acuity	18
VAC	vacuum-assisted closure	21
VAD	ventricular assist device	9
VBAC	vaginal birth after cesarean section	15
VC	vital capacity	11
VD	venereal disease	14, 15
VDRL	Venereal Disease Research Laboratory	14
VEP	visual evoked potentials	17
VF	ventricular fibrillation, visual field	9, 18
VPC	ventricular premature complex	9
VRSA	vancomycin-resistant *Staphylococcus aureus*	6
VS	vital signs	7
VSD	ventricular septal defect	9
VT	ventricular tachycardia	9
VTE	venous thromboembolism	9
VTG	thoracic gas volume	11
vWF	von Willebrand factor	10
WBC	white blood cell; white blood (cell) count	10
WD	well developed	7
WNL	within normal limits	7
w/o	without	7
WPW	Wolff-Parkinson-White syndrome	9
XT	exotropia	18
ZIFT	zygote intrafallopian transfer	15

Word Parts and Their Meanings

WORD PART	MEANING	REFERENCE PAGE
a-	not, without, lack of, absence	31
ab-	away from	33
abdomin/o	abdomen	72
-ac	pertaining to	19
acous, acus	sound, hearing	505
acro-	extremity, end	73
ad-	toward, near	33
aden/o	gland	51
adip/o	fat	54
adren/o	adrenal gland, epinephrine	432
adrenal/o	adrenal gland	432
adrenocortic/o	adrenal cortex	432
aer/o	air, gas	124
-al	pertaining to	19
alg/o, algi/o, algesi/o	pain	98, 144
-algesia	pain	100, 502
-algia	pain	100
ambly-	dim	522
amnio	amnion	393
amyl/o	starch	54
an-	not, without, lack of	31
andr/o	male	358
angi/o	vessel	179
an/o	anus	290
ante-	before	36
anti-	against	31, 143
aort/o	aorta	179
-ar	pertaining to	19
arter/o, arteri/o	artery	179
arteriol/o	arteriole	179
arthr/o	joint	547
-ary	pertaining to	19
-ase	enzyme	54
atel/o	incomplete	263
atri/o	atrium	178
audi/o	hearing	505

WORD PART	MEANING	REFERENCE PAGE
auto-	self	229
azot/o	nitrogen compounds	224
bacill/i, bacill/o	bacillus	103
bacteri/o	bacterium	103
bar/o	pressure	124
bi-	two, twice	29
bili	bile	291
blast/o, -blast	immature cell, productive cell, embryonic cell	53
blephar/o	eyelid	515
brachi/o	arm	73
brady-	slow	99
bronch/i, bronch/o	bronchus	255
bronchiol	bronchiole	255
bucc/o	cheek	288
burs/o	bursa	547
calc/i	calcium	224
cali, calic	calyx	327
-capnia	carbon dioxide (level of)	254
carcin/o	cancer, carcinoma	98
cardi/o	heart	178
cec/o	cecum	289
-cele	hernia, localized dilation	100
celi/o	abdomen	72
centesis	puncture, tap	126
cephal/o	head	72
cerebell/o	cerebellum	464
cerebr/o	cerebrum	464
cervic/o	neck, cervix	72, 391
chem/o	chemical	144
cholangi/o	bile duct	291
chol/e, chol/o	bile, gall	291
cholecyst/o	gallbladder	291
choledoch/o	common bile duct	291
chondr/o	cartilage	547
chori/o, choroid/o	choroid	516
chrom/o, chromat/o	color, stain	124
chron/o	time	124
circum-	around	74
clasis, -clasia	breaking	100
clitor/o, clitorid/o	clitoris	392
coccy, coccyg/o	coccyx	548
cochle/o	cochlea (of inner ear)	505
col/o, colon/o	colon	289
colp/o	vagina	391
contra-	against, opposite	31, 144

WORD PART	MEANING	REFERENCE PAGE
corne/o	cornea	515
cortic/o	outer portion, cerebral cortex	464
cost/o	rib	548
counter	opposite, against	144
crani/o	skull, cranium	548
cry/o	cold	124
crypt/o	hidden	364
cus	sound, hearing	505
cyan/o-	blue	30
cycl/o	ciliary body, ciliary muscle (of eye)	516
cyst/o, cyst/i	filled sac or pouch, cyst, bladder, urinary bladder	98, 328
-cyte, cyt/o	cell	50
dacry/o	tear, lacrimal apparatus	514
dacryocyst/o	lacrimal sac	514
dactyl/o	finger, toe	73
de-	down, without, removal, loss	31
dent/o, dent/i	tooth, teeth	288
derm/o, dermat/o	skin	613
-desis	binding, fusion	126
dextr/o-	right	37
di-	two, twice	29
dia-	through	33
dilation, dilatation	expansion, widening	101
dipl/o-	double	29
dis-	absence, removal, separation	31
duoden/o	duodenum	289
dys-	abnormal, painful, difficult	99
ec-	out, outside	37
ectasia, ectasis	dilation, dilatation	101
ecto-	out, outside	37
-ectomy	excision, surgical removal	126
edema	accumulation of fluid, swelling	101
electr/o	electricity	124
embryo/o	embryo	393
emesis	vomiting	298
-emia	condition of blood	221
encephal/o	brain	464
end/o-	in, within	37
endocrin/o	endocrine	432
enter/o	intestine	289
epi-	on, over	74
epididym/o	epididymis	360
episi/o	vulva	392
equi-	equal, same	34
erg/o	work	124
erythr/o-	red, red blood cell	30, 222

WORD PART	MEANING	REFERENCE PAGE
erythrocyt/o	red blood cell	222
esophag/o	esophagus	289
-esthesia, -esthesi/o	sensation	502, 593
eu-	true, good, easy, normal	34
ex/o	away from, outside	37
extra-	outside	74
fasci/o	fascia	589
ferr/i, ferr/o	iron	224
fet/o	fetus	393
fibr/o	fiber	50
-form	like, resembling	19
galact/o	milk	393
gangli/o, ganglion/o	ganglion	463
gastr/o	stomach	289
gen, genesis	origin, formation	53
ger/e, ger/o	old age	32
-geusia	sense of taste	502
gingiv/o	gum	288
gli/o	neuroglia	463
glomerul/o	glomerulus	327
gloss/o	tongue	288
gluc/o	glucose	54
glyc/o	sugar, glucose	54
gnath/o	jaw	288
-gram	record of data	125
-graph	instrument for recording data	125
-graphy	act of recording data	125
gravida	pregnant woman	393
gyn/o, gynec/o	woman	390
hem/o, hemat/o	blood	222
hemi-	half, one side	29
-hemia	condition of blood	221
hepat/o	liver	291
hetero-	other, different, unequal	34
hidr/o	sweat, perspiration	613
hist/o, histi/o	tissue	50
homo-, homeo-	same, unchanging	34
hydr/o	water, fluid	54
hyper-	over, excess, increased, abnormally high	34
hypn/o	sleep	144
hypo-	under, below, decreased, abnormally low	34
hypophys	pituitary, hypophysis	432
hyster/o	uterus	391

WORD PART	MEANING	REFERENCE PAGE
-ia	condition of	15
-ian	specialist	17
-ia/sis	condition of	15
-iatrics	medical specialty	17
iatr/o	physician	104
-iatry	medical specialty	17
-ic	pertaining to	19
-ical	pertaining to	19
-ics	medical specialty	17
idr/o	sweat, perspiration	613
-ile	pertaining to	19
ile/o	ileum	289
ili/o	ilium	518
im-	not	31
immun/o	immunity, immune system	222
in-	not	31
infra-	below	74
in/o	fiber, muscle fiber	589
insul/o	pancreatic islets	432
inter-	between	74
intra-	in, within	74
ir-, irit/o, irid/o	iris	516
-ism	condition of	15
iso-	equal, same	34
-ist	specialist	17
-itis	inflammation	100
jejun/o	jejunum	289
juxta-	near, beside	74
kali	potassium	224
kary/o	nucleus	50
kerat/o	cornea, keratin, horny layer of skin	515, 613
kine, kinesi/o, kinet/o	movement	589
labi/o	lip	288
labyrinth/o	labyrinth (inner ear)	505
lacrim/o	tear, lacrimal apparatus	514
lact/o	milk	393
-lalia	speech, babble	466
lapar/o	abdominal wall	72
laryng/o	larynx	255
lent/i	lens	515
-lepsy	seizure	466
leuk/o-	white, colorless, white blood cell	31, 322
leukocyt/o	white blood cell	222
-lexia	reading	466

WORD PART	MEANING	REFERENCE PAGE
lingu/o	tongue	288
lip/o	fat, lipid	54
lith	calculus, stone	98
-logy	study of	17
lumb/o	lumbar region, lower back	72
lymphaden/o	lymph node	180
lymphangi/o	lymphatic vessel	180
lymph/o	lymph, lymphatic system, lymphocyte	180, 222
lymphocyt/o	lymphocyte	222
lysis	separation, loosening, dissolving, destruction	101
-lytic	dissolving, reducing, loosening	143
macro-	large, abnormally large	34
mal-	bad, poor	99
malacia	softening	101
mamm/o	breast, mammary gland	392
mania	excited state, obsession	466
mast/o	breast, mammary gland	392
medull/o	inner part, medulla oblongata, spinal cord	464
mega-, megalo-	large, abnormally large	35
-megaly	enlargement	100
melan/o-	black, dark, melanin	31, 613
mening/o, meninge/o	meninges	463
men/o, mens	month, menstruation	390
mes/o	middle	37
-meter	instrument for measuring	125
metr/o	measure	518
metr/o, metr/i	uterus	391
-metry	measurement of	125
micro-	small, one millionth	35
-mimetic	mimicking, simulating	143
mon/o	one	29
morph/o	form, structure	50
muc/o	mucus, mucous membrane	51
multi-	many	29
muscul/o	muscle	589
myc/o	fungus, mold	103
myel/o	bone marrow, spinal cord	222, 463, 547
my/o	muscle	589
myring/o	tympanic membrane	505
myx/o	mucus	51
narc/o	stupor, unconsciousness	144, 464
nas/o	nose	255
nat/i	birth	393
natri	sodium	224
necrosis	death of tissue	102

WORD PART	MEANING	REFERENCE PAGE
neo-	new	35
nephr/o	kidney	327
neur/o, neur/i	nervous system, nerve	463
noct/i	night	338
non-	not	31
normo-	normal	35
nucle/o	nucleus	50
nyct/o	night, darkness	128
ocul/o	eye	515
odont/o	tooth, teeth	288
-odynia	pain	100
-oid	like, resembling	19
olig/o-	few, scanty, deficiency of	34
-oma	tumor	100
onc/o	tumor	98
onych/o	nail	613
oo	ovum	390
oophor/o	ovary	390
ophthalm/o	eye	515
-opia	eye, vision	517
-opsia	vision	517
opt/o	eye, vision	515
orchid/o, orchi/o	testis	360
or/o	mouth	288
ortho-	straight, correct, upright	35
-ory	pertaining to	19
osche/o	scrotum	360
-ose	sugar	54
-o/sis	condition of	16
-osmia	sense of smell	502
oste/o	bone	547
ot/o	ear	505
-ous	pertaining to	19
ovari/o	ovary	390
ov/o	ovum	390
-oxia	oxygen (level of)	254
ox/y	oxygen, sharp, acute	224, 416
pachy-	thick	99
palat/o	palate	288
palpebr/o	eyelid	514
pan-	all	34
pancreat/o	pancreas	291
papill/o	nipple	50
para-	near, beside	74
para	woman who has given birth	393
parathyr/o, parathyroid/o	parathyroid	432

WORD PART	MEANING	REFERENCE PAGE
paresis	partial paralysis	466
path/o, -pathy	disease, any disease of	98, 100
ped/o	foot, child	73, 557
pelvi/o	pelvis	548
-penia	decrease in, deficiency of	221
per-	through	33
peri-	around	74
perine/o	perineum	392
periton, peritone/o	peritoneum	72
-pexy	surgical fixation	126
phac/o, phak/o	lens	515
phag/o	eat, ingest	53
pharmac/o	drug	144
pharyng/o	pharynx	255
-phasia	speech	466
phil, -philic	attracting, absorbing	53
phleb/o	vein	179
phobia	fear	466
phon/o	sound, voice	124
-phonia	voice	254
phot/o	light	124
phren/o	diaphragm	256
phrenic/o	phrenic nerve	256
pituitar	pituitary hypophysis	432
plas, -plasia	formation, molding, development	53
-plasty	plastic repair, plastic surgery, reconstruction	126
-plegia	paralysis	466
pleur/o	pleura	256
-pnea	breathing	254
pneum/o, pneumat/o	air, gas, lung respiration	256
pneumon/o	lung	256
pod/o	foot	73
-poiesis	formation, production	221
poikilo-	varied, irregular	35
poly-	many, much	29
post-	after, behind	36
pre-	before, in front of	36
presby-	old	515, 518
prim/i-	first	29
pro-	before, in front of	36
proct/o	rectum	290
prostat/o	prostate	360
prote/o	protein	54
pseudo-	false	35
psych/o	mind	464
ptosis	dropping, downward displacement, prolapse	102
ptysis	spitting	263
pulm/o, pulmon/o	lung	256

WORD PART	MEANING	REFERENCE PAGE
pupill/o	pupil	516
pyel/o	renal pelvis	327
pylor/o	pylorus	289
py/o	pus	98
pyr/o, pyret/o	fever, fire	98, 144
quadr/i-	four	29
rachi/o	spine	548
radicul/o	root of spinal nerve	463
radi/o	radiation, x-ray	124
re-	again, back	35
rect/o	rectum	290
ren/o	kidney	327
reticul/o	network	51
retin/o	retina	516
retro-	behind, backward	74
-rhage, -rhagia	bursting forth, profuse flow, hemorrhage	100
-rhaphy	surgical repair, suture	126
-rhea	flow, discharge	100
-rhexis	rupture	100
rhin/o	nose	255
sacchar/o	sugar	54
sacr/o	sacrum	548
salping/o	tube, oviduct, eustachian (auditory) tube	391, 505
-schisis	fissure, splitting	100
scler/o	hard, sclera (of eye)	98, 515
sclerosis	hardening	98, 101
-scope	instrument for viewing or examining	125
-scopy	examination of	125
seb/o	sebum, sebaceous gland	613
semi-	half, partial	29
semin	semen	360
sial/o	saliva, salivary gland, salivary duct	288
sider/o	iron	224
sigmoid/o	sigmoid colon	289
sinistr/o	left	37
-sis	condition of	15
somat/o	body	51
-some	body	51
somn/i, somn/o	sleep	464
son/o	sound, ultrasound	124
spasm	sudden contraction, cramp	102
sperm/i	semen	360
spermat/o	spermatozoa	360
spir/o	breathing	256
splen/o	spleen	180
spondyl/o	vertebra	548

WORD PART	MEANING	REFERENCE PAGE
staped/o, stapedi/o	stapes	505
staphyl/o	grapelike cluster, staphylococcus	103
stasis	suppression, stoppage	102
steat/o	fatty	54
stenosis	narrowing, constriction	102
steth/o	chest	72
stoma, stomat/o	mouth	288
-stomy	surgical creation of an opening	126
strept/o-	twisted chain, streptococcus	103
sub-	below, under	74
super-	above, excess	34
supra-	above	74
syn-, sym-	together	37
synov/i	synovial joint, synovial membrane	547
tachy-	rapid	99
tel/e-, tel/o-	end	37
ten/o, tendin/o	tendon	589
terat/o	malformed fetus	403
test/o	testis	360
tetra-	four	29
thalam/o	thalamus	464
therm/o	heat, temperature	124
thorac/o	chest, thorax	72
thromb/o	blood clot	222
thrombocyt/o	platelet, thrombocyte	222
thym/o	thymus gland	180
thyr/o, thyroid/o	thyroid	432
toc/o	labor	393
-tome	instrument for incising (cutting)	126
-tomy	incision, cutting	126
ton/o	tone	589
tonsill/o	tonsil	180
tox/o, toxic/o	poison, toxin	98, 144
trache/o	trachea	255
trans-	through	33
tri-	three	29
trich/o	hair	613
-tripsy	crushing	126
trop,- tropic	act(ing) on, affect(ing)	143
troph/o, -trophy, -trophia	feeding, growth, nourishment	53
tympan/o	tympanic cavity (middle ear), tympanic membrane	505
un-	not	31
uni-	one	29
ureter/o	ureter	328
urethr/o	urethra	328
-uria	urine, urination	328

WORD PART	MEANING	REFERENCE PAGE
ur/o	urine, urinary tract	328
urin/o	urine	328
uter/o	uterus	391
uve/o	uvea (of eye)	515
vagin/o	sheath, vagina	391
valv/o, valvul/o	valve	178
varic/o	twisted and swollen vein	191
vascul/o	vessel	179
vas/o	vessel, duct, vas deferens	144, 179, 360
ven/o, ven/i	vein	179
ventricul/o	cavity, ventricle	178, 464
vertebr/o	vertebra, spinal column	548
vesic/o	urinary bladder	328
vesicul/o	seminal vesicle	360
vestibul/o	vestibule, vestibular apparatus (of ear)	505
vir/o	virus	103
vulv/o	vulva	392
xanth/o-	yellow	31
xero-	dry	99
-y	condition of	15

Meanings and Their Corresponding Word Parts

MEANING	WORD PART(S)	REFERENCE PAGE
abdomen	abdomin/o, celi/o	72
abdominal wall	lapar/o	72
abnormal	dys-	99
abnormally high	hyper-	34
abnormally large	macro-, mega-, megalo-	34, 35
abnormally low	hypo-	34
above	super-, supra-	34, 74
absence	a-, an-, dis-	31
absorb(ing)	phil, -philic	53
accumulation of fluid	edema	101
act of recording data	-graphy	125
act(ing) on	trop, -tropic	53, 143
acute	ox/y	416
adrenal gland	adren/o, adrenal/o	432
adrenaline	adren/o	432
adrenal	adren/o	432
adrenal cortex	adrenocortic/o	432
affect(ing)	trop, -tropic	53
after	post-	36
again	re-	35
against	anti-, contra-	31, 143, 144
air	aer/o, pneumat/o	124, 256
all	pan-	34
amnion	amnio	393
anus	an/o	290
any disease of	-pathy	100
aorta	aort/o	179
arm	brachi/o	73
around	circum-, peri-	74
arteriole	arteriol/o	179
artery	arter/o, arteri/o	179
atrium	atri/o	178
attract(ing)	phil, -philic	53
away from	ab-, ex/o-	33, 37
babble	-lalia	466
bacillus	bacill/i, bacill/o	103

MEANING	WORD PART(S)	REFERENCE PAGE
back	re-	35
backward	retro-	74
bacterium	bacteri/o	103
bad	mal-	99
before	ante-, pre-, pro-	36
behind	post-, retro-	36, 74
below	hypo-, infra-, sub-	34, 74
beside	para-, juxta-	74
between	inter-	74
bile	bili, chol/e, chol/o	291
bile duct	cholangi/o	291
binding	-desis	126
birth	nat/i	393
black	melan/o-	31, 163
bladder	cyst/o, cyst/i	98, 328
bladder (urinary)	cyst/o, vesic/o	98
blood	hem/o, hemat/o	222
blood (condition of)	-emia, -hemia	221
blood clot	thromb/o	222
blue	cyan/o-	30
body	somat/o, -some	51
bone	oste/o	547
bone marrow	myel/o	222, 463, 547
brain	encephal/o	464
breaking	clasis, clasia	100
breast	mamm/o, mast/o	392
breathing	-pnea, spir/o	254, 256
bronchiole	bronchiol	255
bronchus	bronch/i, bronch/o	255
bursa	burs/o	547
bursting forth	-rhage, -rhagia	100
calcium	calc/i	224
calculus	lith	98
calyx	cali, calic	327
cancer	carcin/o	98
carbon dioxide	-capnia	254
carcinoma	carcin/o	98
cartilage	chondr/o	547
cavity	ventricul/o	178, 464
cecum	cec/o	289
cell	-cyte, cyt/o	50
cerebellum	cerebell/o	464
cerebral cortex	cortic/o	464
cerebrum	cerebr/o	464

MEANING	WORD PART(S)	REFERENCE PAGE
cervix	cervic/o	391
chain (twisted)	strept/o	103
cheek	bucc/o	288
chemical	chem/o	144
chest	thorac/o, steth/o	72
child	ped/o	557
choroid	chori/o, choroid/o	516
ciliary body	cycl/o	516
ciliary muscle	cycl/o	516
clitoris	clitor/o, clitorid/o	352
clot	thromb/o	222
coccyx	coccy, coccyg/o	548
cochlea	cochle/o	505
cold	cry/o	124
colon	col/o, colon/o	289
color	chrom/o, chromat/o	124
colorless	leuk/o-	31
common bile duct	choledoch/o	291
condition of	-ia, -ia/sis, -ism, -o/sis, -sis, -y	5
condition of blood	-emia, -hemia	222
constriction	stenosis	102
contraction (sudden)	spasm	102
cornea	corne/o, kerat/o	515
correct	ortho-	35
cramp	spasm	102
cranium	crani/o	548
crushing	-tripsy	126
cutting	-tomy	126
cutting instrument	-tome	126
cyst	cyst/o, cyst/i	98
dark	melan/o-	31, 613
darkness	nyct/o	128
data	-gram	125
death of tissue	necrosis	102
decreased, decrease in	hypo-, -penia	34, 221
deficiency of	oligo-, -penia	221
destruction	lysis	101
development	plas, -plasia	53
diaphragm	phren/o	256
different	hetero-	34
difficult	dys-	99
dilatation, dilation	ectasia, ectasis	101
dim	ambly-	522
discharge	-rhea	100
disease	path/o, -pathy	98

MEANING	WORD PART(S)	REFERENCE PAGE
dissolving	lysis, -lytic	143
double	dipl/o-	29
down	de-	31
dropping, downward displacement	ptosis	102
drug	pharmac/o	144
dry	xero-	99
duct	vas/o	179
duodenum	duoden/o	289
ear	ot/o	505
easy	eu-	34
eat	phag/o	53
egg	oo, ov/o	390
electricity	electr/o	124
embryo	embry/o	393
embryonic cell	-blast, blast/o	53
end	tel/e, tel/o, acro	37, 73
endocrine	endocrin/o	432
enlargement	-megaly	100
enzyme	-ase	54
epididymis	epididym/o	360
epinephrine	adren/o	432
equal	iso-, equi-	34
esophagus	esophag/o	289
eustachian (auditory) tube	salping/o	505
examination of	-scopy	125
excess	hyper-, super-	34
excision	-ectomy	126
excited state	mania	466
expansion	dilation, dilatation, ectasia, ectasis	101
extremity	acro	73
eye	ocul/o, ophthalm/o, opt/o, -opia	515, 517
eyelid	blephar/o, palpebr/o	514
false	pseudo-	35
fascia	fasci/o	589
fat	adip/o, lip/o	54
fatty	steat/o	54
fear	phobia	466
feeding	troph/o, -trophy, -trophia	53
fetus	fet/o	393
fetus (malformed)	terat/o	403
fever	pyr/o, pyret/o	98, 144
few	oligo-	34
fiber	fibr/o, in/o	50, 589
filled sac or pouch	cyst/o, cyst/i	98
finger	dactyl/o	73

MEANING	WORD PART(S)	REFERENCE PAGE
fire	pyr/o, pyret/o	98
first	prim/i-	29
fissure	-schisis	100
fixation (surgical)	-pexy	126
flow	-rhea	100
fluid	hydr/o	54
foot	ped/o, pod/o	73
form	morph/o	50
formation	gen, genesis, plas, -plasia, -poiesis	53, 221
four	quadr/i, tetra-	29
fungus	myc/o	103
fusion	-desis	126
gall	chol/e, chol/o	291
gallbladder	cholecyst/o	291
ganglion	gangli/o, ganglion/o	463
gas	aer/o, pneum/o, pneumon/o, pneumat/o	124, 256
gland	aden/o	51
glomerulus	glomerul/o	327
glucose	gluc/o, glyc/o	54
good	eu-	34
grapelike cluster	staphyl/o	103
growth	troph/o, -trophy, -trophia	53
gum	gingiv/o	288
hair	trich/o	613
half	hemi-, semi-	29
hard	scler/o	98
hardening	sclerosis	98, 101
head	cephal/o	72
hearing	acous, acus, audi/o, cus	505
heart	cardi/o	178
heat	therm/o	124
hemorrhage	-rhage, -rhagia	100
hernia	-cele	100
hidden	crypt/o	364
horny layer of skin	kerat/o	613
hypophysis	hypophys, pituitar	432
islets (pancreatic)	insul/o	432
ileum	ile/o	289
ilium	ili/o	548
immature cell	blast/o, -blast	53
immune system	immun/o	222
immunity	immun/o	222
in	end/o-, intra-	37, 74
in front of	pre-, pro-	36
incision of	-tomy	126

MEANING	WORD PART(S)	REFERENCE PAGE
incomplete	atel/o-	263
increased	hyper-	34
inflammation	-itis	100
ingest	phag/o	53
instrument for incising (cutting)	-tome	126
instrument for measuring	-meter	125
instrument for recording data	-graph	125
instrument for viewing or examining	-scope	125
intestine	enter/o	289
iris	ir, irid/o, irit/o	516
iron	ferr/i, ferr/o, sider/o	224
irregular	poikilo-	35
jaw	gnath/o	288
jejunum	jejun/o	289
joint	arthr/o	547
keratin	kerat/o	613
kidney	nephr/o, ren/o	327
labor	toc/o	393
labyrinth	labyrinth/o	505
lack of	a-, an-	31
lacrimal apparatus	dacry/o, lacrim/o	514
lacrimal sac	dacryocyst/o	514
large	macro-, mega-, megalo-	34, 35
larynx	laryng/o	255
left	sinistr/o-	37
lens	lent/i, phac/o, phak/o	515
leukocyte	leuk/o, leukocyt/o	222
level of carbon dioxide	-capnia	254
level of oxygen	-oxia	254
light	phot/o	124
like	-form, -oid	19
lip	labi/o	288
lipid	lip/o	54
liver	hepat/o	291
localized dilation	-cele	100
loosening	lysis, -lytic	101, 143
loss	de-	31
lumbar region, lower back	lumb/o	72
lung, lungs	pneum/o, pneumat/o, pneumon/o, pulm/o, pulmon/o	256
lymph, lymphatic system	lymph/o	180
lymph node	lymphaden/o	180

MEANING	WORD PART(S)	REFERENCE
lymphatic vessel	lymphangi/o	180
lymphocyte	lympho, lymphocyt/o	222
male	andr/o	358
malformed fetus	terat/o	403
mammary gland	mamm/o, mast/o	392
many	multi-, poly-	29
marrow	myel/o	222
measure	metr/o	518
measuring instrument	-meter	125
measurement of	-metry	125
medical specialty	-ics, -iatrics, iatry	17
medulla oblongata	medull/o	464
melanin	melan/o	613
meninges	mening/o, meninge/o	463
menstruation	men/o, mens	390
middle	meso-	37
milk	galact/o, lact/o	393
mimicking	-mimetic	143
mind	psych/o	464
mold	myc/o	103
molding	plas, -plasia	53
month	men/o, mens	390
mouth	or/o, stoma, stomat/o	288
movement	kine, kinesi/o, kinet/o	589
much	poly-	29
mucus	muc/o, myx/o	51
mucous membrane	muc/o	51
muscle	my/o, muscul/o	589
muscle fiber	in/o	589
nail	onych/o	613
narrowing	stenosis	102
near	ad-, juxta-, para-	33, 74
neck	cervic/o	72, 391
nerve, nervous system, nervous tissue	neur/o, neur/i	463
network	reticul/o	51
neuroglia	gli/o	463
new	neo-	35
night	noct/i, nyct/o	338
nipple	papill/o	51
nitrogen compounds	azot/o	224
normal	eu-, normo-	34, 35
nose	nas/o, rhin/o	255
not	a-, an-, in-, im-, non-, un-	31
nourishment	troph/o, -trophy, -trophia	53
nucleus	kary/o, nucle/o	50

MEANING	WORD PART(S)	REFERENCE PAGE
obsession	mania	466
old	presby-	515, 518
old age	ger/e, ger/o	32
one	mon/o-, uni-	29
one side	hemi-	29
opening (created surgically)	-stomy	126
opposite	contra-	31, 144
origin	gen, genesis	53
other	hetero-	34
out, outside	ec-, ecto-, ex/o, extra-	37, 74
outer portion	cortic/o	464
ovary	ovari/o, oophor/o	390
over	hyper-, epi-	34, 74
oviduct	salping/o	391
ovum	oo, ov/o	390
oxygen	ox/y, -oxia	224, 254
pain	-algia, -odynia	98, 100
pain	-algesia, alg/o, algi/o, algesi/o	98, 100, 144, 502
painful	dys-	99
palate	palat/o	288
pancreas	pancreat/o	291
pancreatic islets	insul/o	432
paralysis	-plegia	466
paralysis (partial)	paresis	466
parathyroid	parathyr/o, parathyroid/o	432
partial	semi-	29
partial paralysis	paresis	466
pelvis	pelvi/o	548
perineum	perine/o	352
peritoneum	periton, peritone/o	72
perspiration	hidr/o, idr/o	613
pertaining to	-ac, -al, -ar, -ary, -ial, -ic, -ical, -ile,	
	-ory, -ous	19
pharynx	pharyng/o	255
phrenic nerve	phrenic/o	256
physician	iatr/o	104
pituitary	pituitar, hypophys	432
plastic repair, plastic surgery	-plasty	126
platelet	thrombocyt/o	222
pleura	pleur/o	256
poison	tox/o, toxic/o	98, 144
poor	mal-	99
potassium	kali	224
pouch (filled)	cyst/o, cyst/i	98
pregnant woman	gravida	393
pressure	bar/o	124
production	-poiesis	221

MEANING	WORD PART(S)	REFERENCE PAGE
productive cell	blast/o, -blast	53
profuse flow	-rhage, -rhagia	100
prolapse	ptosis	102
prostate	prostat/o	360
protein	prote/o	54
puncture	centesis	126
pupil	pupill/o	516
pus	py/o	98
pylorus	pylor/o	289
radiation	radi/o	124
rapid	tachy-	99
reading	-lexia	466
reconstruction	-plasty	126
record of data	-gram	125
recording data (act of)	-graphy	125
rectum	rect/o, proct/o	290
red	erythr/o-	30
red blood cell	erythr/o, erythrocyt/o	222
reducing	-lytic	143
removal	de-, dis-	31
removal (surgical)	-ectomy	126
renal pelvis	pyel/o	327
repair (plastic)	-plasty	126
repair (surgical)	-rhaphy	126
respiration	pneum/o, pneumon/o, pneumat/o	256
resembling	-form, -oid	19
retina	retin/o	516
rib	cost/o	548
right	dextr/o-	37
root of spinal nerve	radicul/o	463
rupture	-rhexis	100
sac (filled)	cyst/o, cyst/i	98
sacrum	sacr/o	548
saliva, salivary gland, salivary duct	sial/o	288
same	equi-, homo-, homeo-, iso-	34
sclera (of eye)	scler/o	515
scanty	oligo-	34
scrotum	osche/o	360
sebum, sebaceous gland	seb/o	613
seizure	-lepsy	466
self	auto-	229
semen	semin, sperm/i, spermat/o	360
seminal vesicle	vesicul/o	360
sensation	-esthesia, esthesi/o	502, 593
sense of smell	-osmia	502

MEANING	WORD PART(S)	REFERENCE PAGE
sense of taste	-geusia	502
separation	dis-, -lysis	31, 101
sharp	ox/y	416
sheath	vagin/o	391
sigmoid colon	sigmoid/o	289
simulating	-mimetic	143
skin	derm/o, dermat/o	613
skull	crani/o	548
sleep	somn/o, somn/i, hypn/o	144, 464
slow	brady-	99
small	micro-	35
smell (sense of)	-osmia	502
sodium	natri	224
softening	malacia	101
sound	phon/o, son/o, acous, acus, cus	124, 505
specialist	-ian, -ist, -logist	17
specialty	-ics, -iatrics, -iatry	17
speech	-phasia, -lalia	466
sperm, spermatozoa	sperm/i, spermat/o	360
spinal column	vertebr/o	548
spinal cord	myel/o, medulla	463
spine	rachi/o	548
spitting	ptysis	263
spleen	splen/o	180
splitting	-schisis	100
stain	chrom/o, chromat/o	124
stapes	staped/o, stapedi/o	505
staphylococcus	staphyl/o	103
starch	amyl/o	54
stomach	gastr/o	289
stone	lith	98
stoppage	stasis	102
straight	ortho-	35
streptococcus	strept/o	103
structure	morph/o	50
study of	-logy	17
stupor	narc/o	144, 464
sugar	glyc/o, sacchar/o, -ose	54
sudden contraction	spasm	102
suppression	stasis	102
surgery (plastic)	-plasty	126
surgical creation of an opening	-stomy	126
surgical fixation	-pexy	126
surgical removal	-ectomy	126
surgical repair	-rhaphy	126
suture	-rhaphy	126

MEANING	WORD PART(S)	REFERENCE PAGE
sweat	hidr/o, idr/o	613
swelling	edema	101
synovial fluid, joint, membrane	synov/i	547
tap	centesis	126
taste (sense of)	-geusia	502
tear	dacry/o, lacrim/o	514
teeth	dent/o, denti, odont/o	288
temperature	therm/o	124
tendon	ten/o, tendin/o	589
testis	test/o, orchid/o, orchi/o	360
thalamus	thalam/o	464
thick	pachy-	99
thorax	thorac/o	72
three	tri-	29
thrombocyte	thrombocyt/o	222
through	dia-, per-, trans-	33
thymus gland	thym/o	180
thyroid	thyr/o, thyroid/o	432
time	chron/o	124
tissue	hist/o, histi/o	50
tissue death	necrosis	102
toe	dactyl/o	73
together	syn-, sym-	37
tone	ton/o	589
tongue	gloss/o, lingu/o	288
tonsil	tonsill/o	180
tooth	-dent/o, dent/i, odont/o	288
toward	ad-	33
toxin	tox/o, toxic/o	144
trachea	trache/o	255
true	eu-	34
tube	salping/o	391, 505
tumor	onc/o, -oma	98, 100
twice	bi-, di-	29
twisted chain	strept/o	103
twisted and swollen vein	varic/o	191
two	bi-, di-, dipl/o-	29
tympanic cavity	tympan/o	505
tympanic membrane	myring/o, tympan/o	505
ultrasound	son/o	124
unchanging	homo-, homeo-	34
unconsciousness	narc/o	464
under	hypo-, sub-	34, 74
unequal	hetero-	34
upright	ortho-	35

MEANING	WORD PART(S)	REFERENCE PAGE
ureter	ureter/o	328
urethra	urethr/o	328
urinary bladder	cyst/o, vesic/o	328
urine, urinary tract, urination	ur/o, -uria	328
uterus	hyster/o, metr/o, metr/i, uter/o	391
uvea	uve/o	515
vagina	colp/o, vagin/o	391
valve	valv/o, valvul/o	178
varied	poikilo-	35
vas deferens	vas/o	360
vein	ven/o, ven/i, phleb/o	179
vein (twisted, swollen)	varic/o	191
ventricle	ventricul/o	178, 464
vertebra	spondyl/o, vertebr/o	548
vessel	angi/o, vas/o, vascul/o	144, 179, 360
vestibular apparatus, vestibule	vestibul/o	505
virus	vir/o	103
vision	opt/o, -opia, -opsia	515, 517
voice	phon/o, -phonia	124, 254
vomiting	emesis	298
vulva	episi/o, vulv/o	352
water	hydr/o	54
white	leuk/o-	31
white blood cell	leuk/o, leukocyt/o	222
widening	ectasia, ectasis, dilation, dilatation	101
within	end/o-, intra-	37, 74
without	a-, an-, de-	31
woman	gyn/o, gynec/o	390
woman who has given birth	para	393
work	erg/o	124
x-ray	radi/o	124
yellow	xanth/o-	31

Metric Measurements

UNIT	ABBREVIATION	METRIC EQUIVALENT	U.S. EQUIVALENT
UNITS OF LENGTH			
kilometer	km	1,000 meters	0.62 miles; 1.6 km/mile
meter*	m	100 cm; 1,000 mm	39.4 inches; 1.1 yards
centimeter	cm	1/100 m; 0.01 m	0.39 inches; 2.5 cm/inch
millimeter	mm	1/1,000 m; 0.001 m	0.039 inches; 25 mm/inch
micrometer	µm	1/1,000 mm; 0.001 mm	
UNITS OF WEIGHT			
kilogram	kg	1,000 g	2.2 lb
gram*	g	1,000 mg	0.035 oz; 28.5 g/oz
milligram	mg	1/1,000 g; 0.001 g	
microgram	µg, mcg	1/1,000 mg; 0.001 mg	
UNITS OF VOLUME			
liter*	L	1,000 mL	1.06 qt
deciliter	dL	1/10 L; 0.1 L	
milliliter	mL	1/1,000 L; 0.001 L	0.034 oz; 29.4 mL/oz
microliter	µL	1/1,000 mL; 0.001 mL	

*Basic unit.

Suggested Readings

Anderson DM, Keith J, Novak PD. Dorland's Illustrated Medical Dictionary. 29th Ed. Philadelphia: Saunders, 2000.

Aschenbrenner DS, Cleveland LW, Venable SJ. Drug Therapy in Nursing. Baltimore: Lippincott, Williams and Wilkins, 2002.

Bellington DA, Laughlin MM. Pharmacology for Technicians. St. Paul: Paradigm Publications, 1999.

Bickley LS, Hoekelman RA. Bates' Guide to Physical Examination. 7th Ed. Baltimore: Lippincott, Williams & Wilkins, 1999.

Black JG. Microbiology. 5th Ed. New York: John Wiley, 2002.

Burton GG, Hodgkin JE, Ward JJ, Hess D, Pilbeam SP, Tietsort J. Respiratory Care: A Guide to Clinical Practice. 4th Ed. Philadelphia: Lippincott-Raven, 1997.

Burton GR, Engelkirk PG. Microbiology for the Health Sciences. 6th Ed. Philadelphia: Lippincott-Raven, 2000.

Clayton BD, Stock YN. Basic Pharmacology for Nurses. 12th Ed. St. Louis: Mosby, 2001.

Cohen BJ, Wood DL. Memmler's The Human Body in Health and Disease. 9th Ed. Philadelphia: Lippincott-Raven, 2000.

Cormack DH. Essential Histology. 2nd Ed. Philadelphia: Lippincott-Raven, 2001.

DerMarderosian A. The Review of Natural Products. St. Louis: Facts and Comparisons, 2001.

Erkonen WE, Smith WL. Radiology 101. Baltimore: Lippincott, Williams & Wilkins, 1998.

Fetrow CW, Avila JR. Complementary & Alternative Medicines. 2nd Ed. Springhouse, PA: Springhouse Corporation, 2001.

Fischbach F. A Manual of Laboratory and Diagnostic Tests. 6th Ed. Philadelphia: Lippincott-Raven, 2000.

Fogel BS, Schifter RB, Rao SM. Synopsis of Neuropsychiatry. Baltimore: Lippincott, Williams & Wilkins, 2000.

Fontaine KL. Healing Practices. Upper Saddle River, NJ: Prentice Hall, 2000.

Groer M. Advanced Pathophysiology. Baltimore: Lippincott, Williams & Wilkins, 2001.

Jablonski S. Dictionary of Medical Acronyms & Abbreviations. 4th Ed. Philadelphia: Hanley and Belfus, 2001.

Martini F. Fundamentals of Anatomy and Physiology. 5th Ed. Englewood Cliffs, NJ: Prentice-Hall, 2000.

McCann JAS. Diseases. 3rd Ed. Springhouse, PA: Springhouse Corporation, 2000.

Physicians' Desk Reference. Oradell, NJ: Medical Economics Books, published yearly.

Pillitteri A. Maternal and Child Health Nursing. 4th Ed. Baltimore: Lippincott, Williams & Wilkins, 2002.

Porth CM. Pathophysiology. 6th Ed. Baltimore: Lippincott, Williams & Wilkins, 2002.

Rosdahl CB. Textbook of Basic Nursing. 7th Ed. Baltimore: Lippincott, Williams & Wilkins, 1999.

Rubin E. Essential Pathology. 3rd Ed. Baltimore: Lippincott, Williams & Wilkins, 2001.

Smeltzer SC, Bare BG. Brunner & Suddarth's Textbook of Medical-Surgical Nursing. 9th Ed. Baltimore: Lippincott, Williams & Wilkins, 2000.

Stedman's Medical Dictionary. 27th Ed. Baltimore: Lippincott, Williams & Wilkins, 2000.

Taber's Cyclopedic Medical Dictionar. 19th Ed. Philadelphia: F.A. Davis, 2001.

Taylor C, Lillis C, LeMone C. Fundamentals of Nursing. 4th Ed. Philadelphia: Lippincott-Raven, 2001.

Tortora GJ, Grabowski SR. Principles of Anatomy and Physiology. 10th Ed. New York: John Wiley, 2002.

Index

Page numbers in *italics* denote figures; those followed by a t denote tables.

Notes

Notes

Notes

Flashcards

An excellent way to learn this new vocabulary is by using flashcards. These have proved so successful that a section of flashcards has been included. They are presented in chapter order so that they can be removed in sequence as you progress through the book. Of course, these cards represent only a portion of the necessary vocabulary, and you should add to the collection with cards of your own. Blank cards are included for this purpose. Note also that the flashcards are the size of one half of a 3" x 5" index card. You can make additional cards by cutting index cards in half.

13. continuous ambulatory peritoneal dialysis
14. blood urea nitrogen
15. end-stage renal disease
16. human immunodeficiency virus

17. cystometrogram
18. physiologic saline solution
19. extracorporeal shock wave lithotripsy

ANSWERS TO CROSSWORD PUZZLE

Urinary System